Medical Radiology

Diagnostic Imaging

Series Editors

Hans-Ulrich Kauczor
Paul M. Parizel
Wilfred C. G. Peh

The book series *Medical Radiology – Diagnostic Imaging* provides accurate and up-to-date overviews about the latest advances in the rapidly evolving field of diagnostic imaging and interventional radiology. Each volume is conceived as a practical and clinically useful reference book and is developed under the direction of experienced editors, who are world-renowned specialists in the field. Book chapters are written by expert authors in the field and are richly illustrated with high quality figures, tables and graphs. Editors and authors are committed to provide detailed and coherent information in a readily accessible and easy-to-understand format, directly applicable to daily practice.

Medical Radiology – Diagnostic Imaging covers all organ systems and addresses all modern imaging techniques and image-guided treatment modalities, as well as hot topics in management, workflow, and quality and safety issues in radiology and imaging. The judicious choice of relevant topics, the careful selection of expert editors and authors, and the emphasis on providing practically useful information, contribute to the wide appeal and ongoing success of the series. The series is indexed in Scopus.

Marc Mespreuve • Karl Waked

MRI of the Wrist

A Practical Case-Based Approach

Springer

Marc Mespreuve
Faculty of Medicine and Health Sciences
University of Ghent
Ghent, Belgium

Karl Waked
Plastic and Reconstructive Surgery
Free University of Brussels
Jette, Belgium

ISSN 0942-5373 ISSN 2197-4187 (electronic)
Medical Radiology
ISSN 2731-4677 ISSN 2731-4685 (electronic)
Diagnostic Imaging
ISBN 978-3-031-63972-2 ISBN 978-3-031-63973-9 (eBook)
https://doi.org/10.1007/978-3-031-63973-9

This Springer imprint is published by the registered company Springer Nature Switzerland AG
The registered company address is: Gewerbestrasse 11, 6330 Cham, Switzerland

Preface

The idea for this project was initiated during the teaching courses as professor at the postgraduate medical education of the Department of Medical Imaging at the University of Ghent, Belgium (scientific chair Prof. Dr. K. Verstraete).

The need for a "pictorial essay of MRI of the wrist" in addition to the, albeit rare, up-to-date general textbooks seemed relevant. Not only colleagues who were less familiar with this specific topic showed interest but also residents in training and other interested radiologists and clinicians were fond of the proposed project.

The theoretical part of this book is limited to the essentials as are the references to additional literature. Therefore, the basic understanding and knowledge of osteoarticular MRI is needed to fully comprehend the illustrated pathologies.

The two major parts—traumatic pathology and non-traumatic pathology–are only based on the clinical presentation of the patients. There is, however, an overflow between both entities (e.g., repetitive microtrauma, acute trauma with non-traumatic underlying pathology, etc.).

The aim of this book is to provide an extra tool to the reader to take up the challenge of analysing in depth a wrist MRI by illustrating extensively not only the typical textbook pathology but also the less obvious and combined pathologies, which are displayed in different sequences.

Mostly, standard PA and lateral radiography views are added to allow a detailed comparison with the MRI images but also in the conviction that a wrist MRI exam should always be reported in conjunction with the available and less than 2-week-old standard views (at least four views: PA, lateral, clenched fist, and semi-pronated in ulnar deviation).

Sometimes, a case may be open for discussion…but that is also part of the goal of this book.

As "you only see what you know", it is important to realize that several anomalies may frequently be revealed, if searched for. One should certainly not be satisfied with finding the most obvious pathology. There may also be a disagreement between the MRI results and the initial clinical information. Therefore, a second consult with the clinician is part of the standard procedure in (complex) wrist pathology.

All the images in this book are real patient cases and were analysed and discussed in close collaboration with hand surgeons, orthopaedic surgeons, and clinicians. Therefore, the description and diagnosis and the clinician's point of view are integrated throughout the selected images in this book.

Ghent, Belgium Marc Mespreuve
Jette, Belgium Karl Waked

Contents

Abbreviations

AP	AnteroPosterior
apl	abductor pollicis longus
AS	Abutment syndrome
ASC	ArthroSynovial cyst
AVN	Avascular necrosis
Ax	Axial
BMO	Bone marrow oedema
C	Capitate bone
cart	cartilage
CE	Contrast enhancement
CMC	CarpoMetaCarpal
Cor	Coronal
CPPD	Calcium pyrophosphate deposition disease
CT	Carpal tunnel
CTS	Carpal tunnel syndrome
DISI	Dorsal intercalated segment instability
dist	distal
dors	dorsal
DRUJ	Distal RadioUlnar joint
ecb	extensor carpi radialis brevis
ecl	extensor carpi radialis longus
ecu	extensor carpi ulnaris
ed	extensor digitorum
edm	extensor digiti minimi
epb	extensor pollicis brevis
epl	extensor pollicis longus
fcr	flexor carpi radialis
fcu	flexor carpi ulnaris
fd	flexor digitorum
fdp	flexor digitorum profundus
fds	flexor digitorum superficialis
FlR	flexor retinaculum
fpl	flexor pollicis longus
Gc	Guyon canal
H	Hamate bone
h	hamulus
I (-VI)	extensor compartment 1 (to VI)

IA	IntraArticular
L	Lunate bone
LT	LunoTriquetral
LTL	LunoTriquetral ligament
MC	MetaCarpal
MC-A	MidCarpal arthrography
MC-J	MetaCarpal joint
MedC-J	MedioCarpal joint
MH	Meniscus homologue
mn	median nerve
OA	OsteoArthritis
P	Pisiform bone
palm	palmar
(pl)	palmaris longus
pl	pollicis longus
PQ	Pronator Quadratus
PR	Prestyloid Recessus
prox	proximal
PsA	Psoriatic Arthritis
R Triq	Radiotriquetral ligament
R	Radius
ra	radial artery
RA	Rheumatoid arthritis
rad	radial
RCJ	Radiocarpal joint
RD	Radial deviation
rlt	radiolunotriquetral ligament
rsc	radioscaphocapitatum ligament
rul	radio-ulnar ligament
S Triq	Scaphotriquetral ligament
S	Scaphoid bone
Sag	Sagittal
SI	Signal intensity
SL	ScaphoLunate
SLL	ScaphoLunate ligament
(S)(O)CM	(Synovial) (Osteo)Chondromatosis
St	Styloid process
sup	superficial
T(ra)	Trapezium bone
t(ra)	trapezoid bone
T1WI	T1-Weighted Image
T1WI-FS	T1-Weighted Image Fat-Suppressed
T2WI	T2-Weighted Image
T2WI-FS	T2-Weighted Image Fat-Suppressed
TFC	Triangular FibroCartilago
TFCC	Triangular FibroCartilaginous Complex
TLis	Tuberculum of lister
Tra Triq	Trapeziotriquetral ligament

Tri	Triquetral bone
TriP	TriquetroPisiform
tub	tuberculum
U	Ulna
UA	Ulnar abutment
ua	ulnar artery
UCL	Ulnar collateral ligament
UD	Ulnar deviation
UL	Ulnolunate ligament
un	ulnar nerve
Utriq	Ulnotriquetral ligament

Part I

Section on Anatomy and Technique

Anatomy

Contents

The wrist is considered as the most complex anatomical and biomechanical structure in the human body (Loredo et al. 2005; MacLean et al. 2021). Hence, a thorough knowledge is essential.

The anatomy on MRI is usually easier to analyse in the axial plane on T1-weighted images fat-suppressed (T1WI-FS). The longitudinal continuity of a lot of structures helps their identification in the consecutive axial planes. Correlation with the coronal and sagittal plane can easily be achieved by positioning the 3D MRI cursor in the axial image(s).

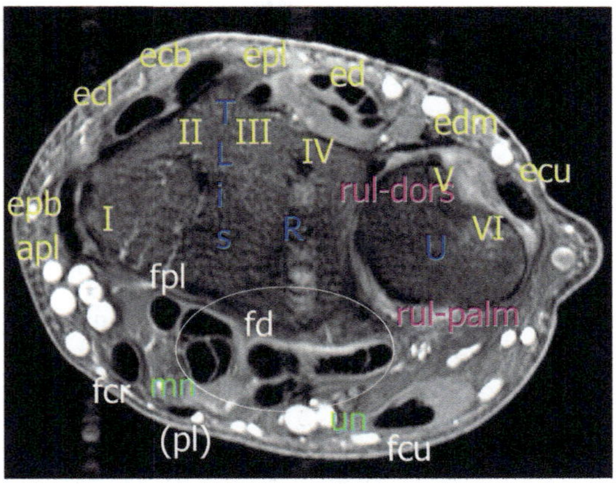

Fig. 1 Proximal cross-sectional view (Ax. T1-WI FS) at the level of the distal radius and ulna. Six dorsal extensor compartments numbered I to VI from radial to ulnar. The flexor tendons and median and ulnar nerves are illustrated at the palmar side of the wrist

1 Axial General MRI Anatomy

Starting proximally (Figs. 1 and 2) at the distal radius (R) and ulna (U), from radial to ulnar six extensor compartments—numbered I to VI—are delineated (Table 1).

M. Mespreuve, K. Waked, *MRI of the Wrist*, Medical Radiology,
https://doi.org/10.1007/978-3-031-63973-9_1

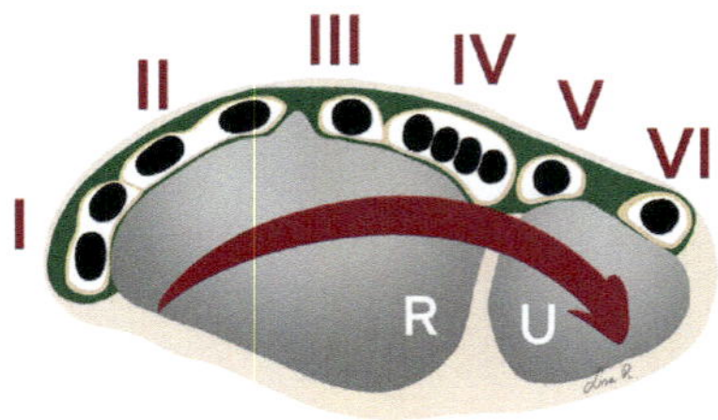

Fig. 2 The extensor retinaculum (green). The retinaculum subdivides the extensor region in six compartments (I-VI) and holds the tendons on-site. (Illustrated by Lisa Ramaut, MD)

Table 1 Extensor compartments of the wrist

Compartment	Tendon(s)	Abbreviation
I	Abductor pollicis longus Extensor pollicis brevis	apl epb
II	Extensor carpi radialis longus Extensor carpi radialis brevis	ecl ecb
III	Extensor pollicis longus (variable position II-IV)	epl
IV	Extensor digitorum	ed
V	Extensor digiti minimi	edm
VI	Extensor carpi ulnaris	ecu

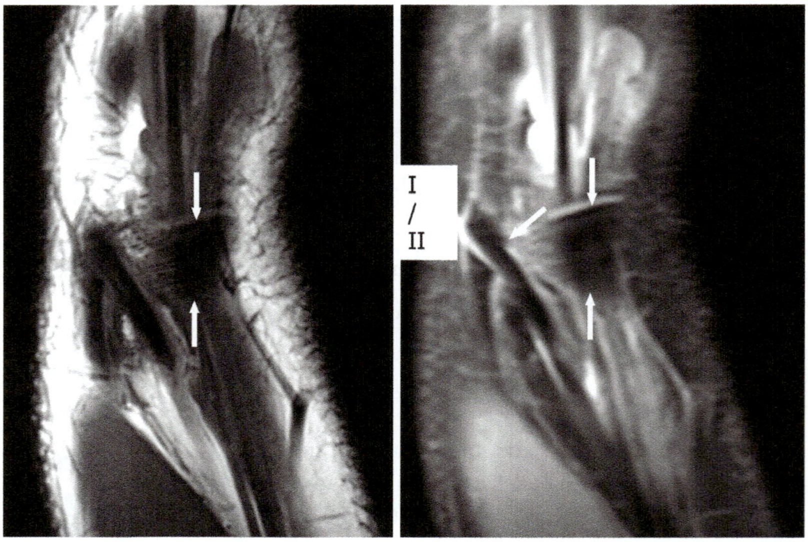

Fig. 3 The extensor retinaculum (Cor T1-WI and T2 WI-FS). The low signal band of the extensor retinaculum at the level of the (proximal) crossover of the tendons of compartment I over II (radially)

The extensor tendons are held in place by the extensor retinaculum, surrounding the tendons and subdividing the extensor region (Fig. 2). On the coronal images, the extensor retinaculum may be seen as a low signal band at the (proximal) crossover of the tendons of compartment I over II (Fig. 3).

An important dorsal landmark is the tuberculum of Lister (TLis) (Bhat et al. 2011)

The palmar tendinous structures from radial to ulnar are the flexor carpi radialis (fcr), the flexor pollicis longus (fpl), the flexor digitorum (fd), and the flexor carpi ulnaris (fcu).

The palmaris longus (pl) is inconsistently present centrally and most superficial (running over the flexor retinaculum).

Two important nerves must be delineated as well: the median nerve (mn) runs at the radial side between the fcr (superficial) and the fpl and fd (deep); the ulnar nerve (un) runs medially between the fd (deep) and fcu (superficial).

At the distal radio-ulnar joint (Ekenstam and Hagert 1985; Nakamura 2012; Schmitt et al. 2003), the dorsal and palmar radio-ulnar ligaments (rul) are noted.

More distally (Fig. 4), the triangular fibrocartilage (TFC) appears between the radial notch and the ulnar styloid process (St). The radial (ra) and ulnar (ua) arteries may be delineated between multiple venous structures at the radial side of respectively the median (mn) and ulnar (un) nerve.

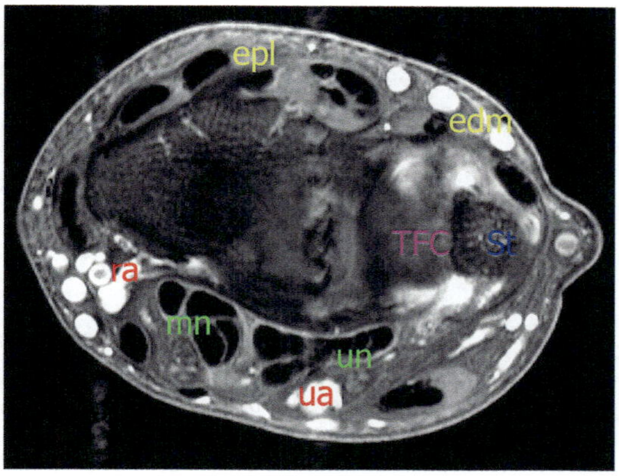

Fig. 4 The triangular fibrocartilage (Ax. T1-WI FS). The TFC appears between the radial notch and the ulnar styloid process (St). The radial and ulnar arteries are located at the radial side of respectively the median (mn) and ulnar (un) nerve

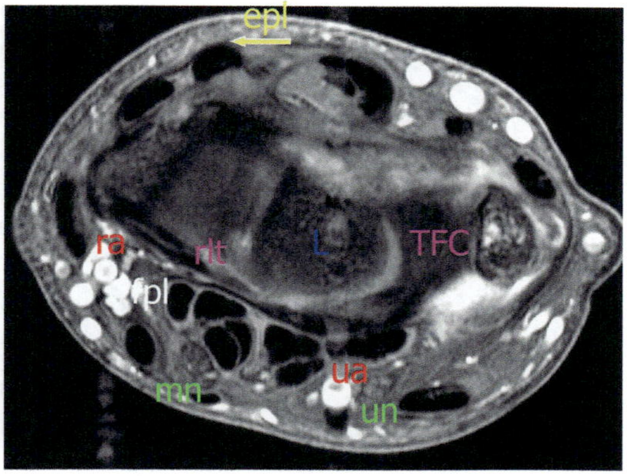

Fig. 5 The level of the proximal pole of the lunate bone (Ax. T1-WI FS). Dorsally, the distal crossover of the epl and at the palmar side the radial part of the palmar extrinsic radiolunate ligament appears at the level of the proximal pole of the lunate bone

The proximal pole of the lunate carpal bone (L) appears (Fig. 5) centrally, as does the radial part of the palmar extrinsic radiolunate ligament (rlt). At the dorsal side, the extensor pollicis longus tendon (epl; III) starts crossing over the tendons of compartment II (distal crossover).

The bones of the proximal carpal row (scaphoid (S), lunate (L), and triquetral (Tri) bone) are delineable, with the intrinsic ligaments (scapholunate (sl), lunotriquetral (lt)) running between them, as well as the palmar extrinsic radiolunate ligament (rlt) (Figs. 6 and 7). The ulnar snuff box is an anatomical landmark at the ulnar side between the ulnar flexor and extensor tendons.

At the level of the triquetropisiform joint (Fig. 8), which is located at the entrance of the carpal tunnel, the lunate bone is positioned between a part of the palmar radio-scapho-capitate (rsc) and the radiolunate (rlt) ligament. The median nerve is situated very superficially, under the proximal part of the flexor retinaculum (Fl R). The triangular Gyon canal (Gc) has its base against the pisiform bone and the flexor retinaculum at its bottom. Consequently, the ulnar artery and nerve are isolated from the carpal tunnel at this level. The flexor carpi ulnaris (fcu) tendon inserts on the pisiform bone. Dorsally, an ulnar part of the extrinsic radio-triquetral ligament (rtriq) appears.

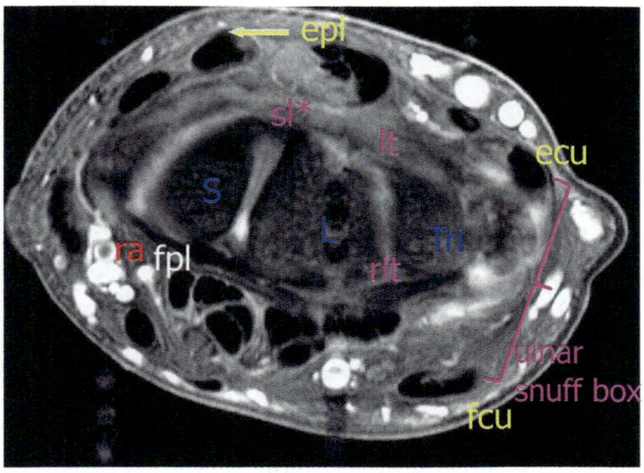

Fig. 6 The proximal carpal row (Ax. T1-WI FS). The bones of the proximal carpal row composed of the scaphoid (S), lunate (L), and triquetral (Tri) bone. The intrinsic ligaments (scapholunate (sl), lunotriquetral (lt)) are running between them. The ulnar part of the palmar extrinsic radiolunate ligament (rlt) is noted as is the ulnar snuff box

The proximal pole of capitate bone (C) is now centrally located (Fig. 9) and the carpal tunnel fully extended. The radial artery (ra) moves radio-dorsally.

Moving further on (Figs. 10 and 11) to the proximal part of the distal carpal row (Bonnel and Allieu 1984) (formed by the trapezoid (tra) and hamate (H) bone), the median nerve (mn) continues its superficial trajectory under the distal part of the flexor retinaculum. At the radial side, the radial snuff box—another important

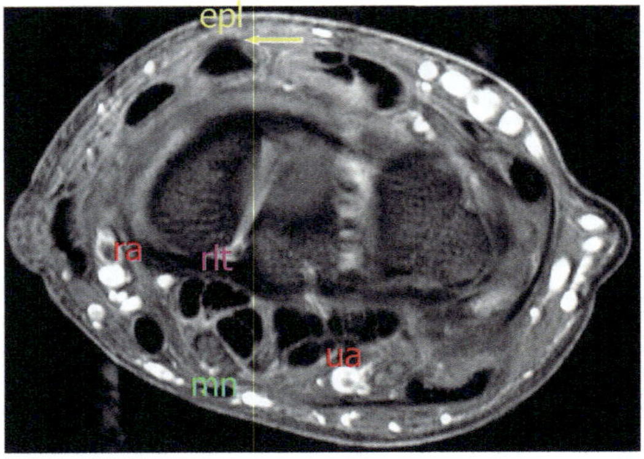

Fig. 7 The proximal carpal row (more distally) (Ax. T1-WI FS). The radial part of the palmar extrinsic radiolunate ligament (rlt)

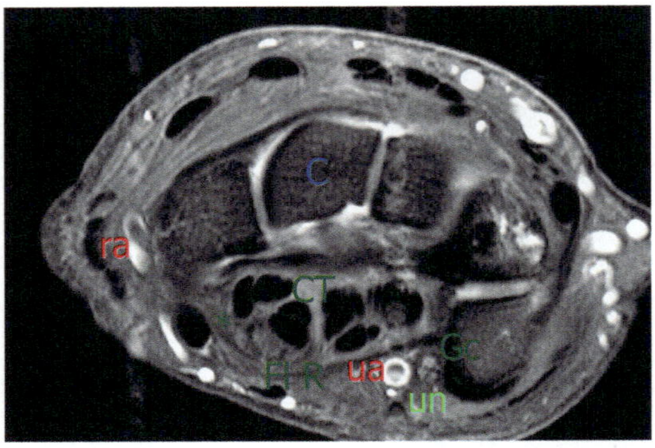

Fig. 9 The carpal tunnel (Ax. T1-WI FS). The proximal pole of capitate bone (C) is centrally located. The radial artery (ra) moves radio-dorsally

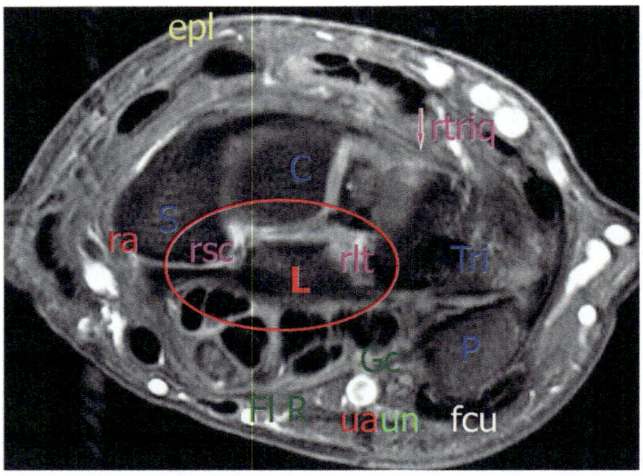

Fig. 8 Entrance of the carpal tunnel (Ax. T1-WI FS). At the level of the triquetropisiform joint (Tri-P), the L is positioned between a part of the palmar radioscaphocapitate (rsc) and the radiolunate (rlt) ligament. The median nerve is situated superficially, under the flexor retinaculum (Fl R). The triangular Gyon canal (Gc) has its base against the pisiform bone with the flexor retinaculum at its bottom and contains the ulnar artery and nerve. Dorsally, an ulnar part of the extrinsic radio-triquetral ligament (rtriq) appears

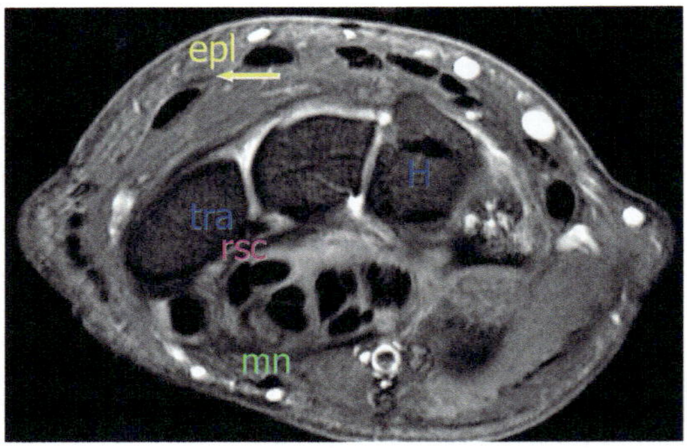

Fig. 10 Proximal part of the distal carpal row (Ax. T1-WI FS). The proximal part of the distal carpal row formed by trapezoid (tra) and hamate (H) bone). The median nerve (mn) continues its superficial trajectory

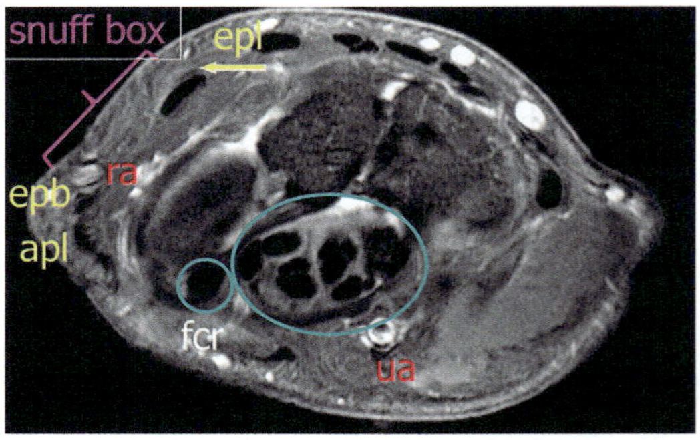

Fig. 11 The distal carpal row (Ax. T1-WI FS). The radial snuff box is bordered by the epl (medially) and the epb and apl (laterally). The radial artery is situated dorsally and runs along the floor of the snuff-box

anatomical landmark—is noted, bordered by the epl (medially) and the epb and apl (laterally). Meanwhile, the radial artery is situated dorsally and runs along the floor of the snuff box. The flexor carpi radialis (fcr) is separated from the other flexor tendons and runs closely to the tuberculum of the trapezium bone (Tra) (Fig. 12). The deep flexor tendons are more separated from the superficial tendons and located at the bottom of the carpal tunnel. The carpal tunnel thus contains all four superficial and deep flexor digitorum tendons, as well as the flexor pollicis longus, located most laterally and superficial to the scaphoid bone (S). The ulnar nerve passes superficial from

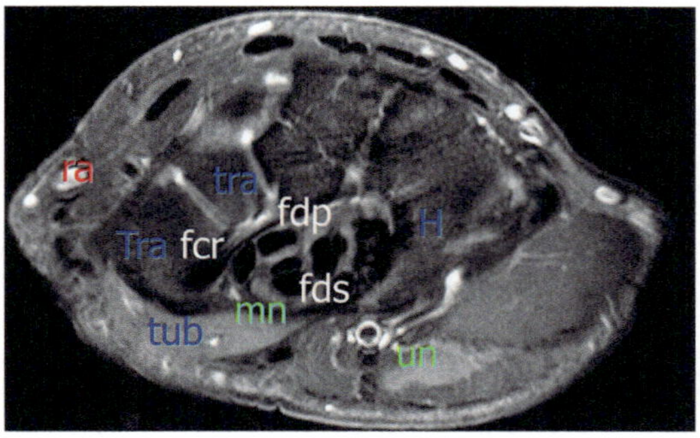

Fig. 12 The distal carpal row at the level of the tuberculum (tub) (Ax. T21-WI FS). The flexor carpi radialis (fcr) is separated from the other flexor tendons and runs closely to the tuberculum of the trapezium bone (Tra). The deep flexor tendons are more separated from the superficial tendons and located at the bottom of the carpal tunnel

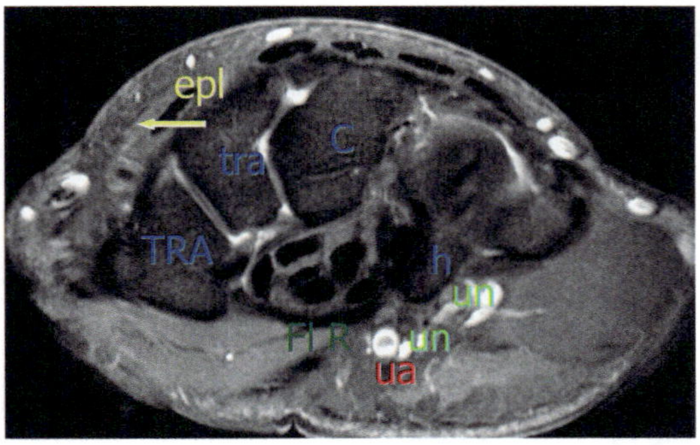

Fig. 13 The distal carpal row at the level of the hamulus (h) (Ax. T21-WI FS). The ulnar nerve passed between the pisiform bone (lateral) and the hamulus (medial) and splits in a superficial and deep branch. The deep branch of the ulnar nerve accompanies the deep branch of the ulnar artery

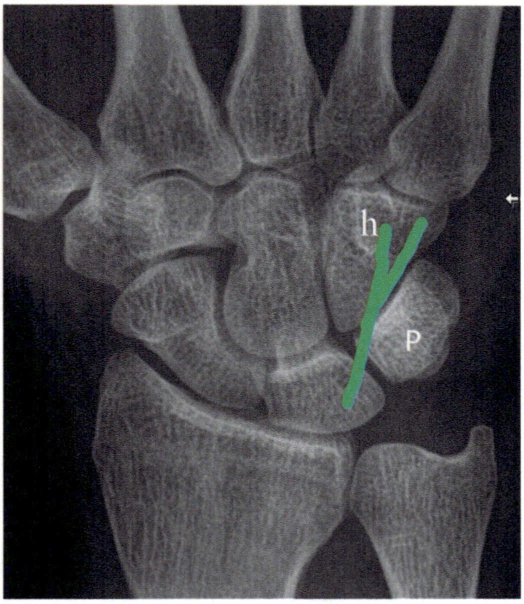

Fig. 14 Schematic drawing of the ulnar nerve trajectory. The ulnar nerve passes between the pisiform bone (laterally) and the hamulus (medially) and splits in a superficial and deep branch

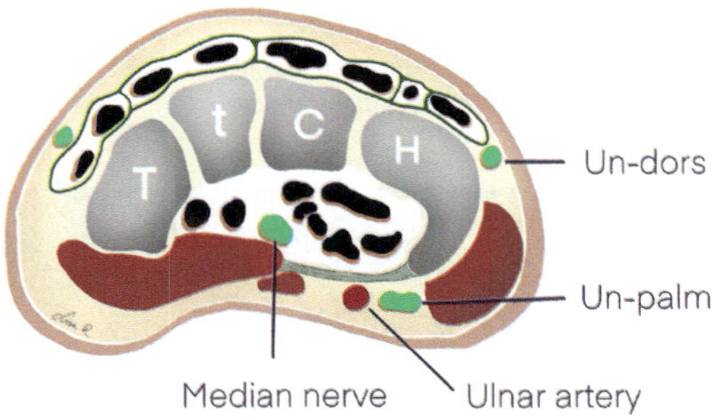

Fig. 15 Schematic drawing of the nerves at the level of the hamulus. The deep dorsal (un-dors) and superficial palmar branch (un-palm) of the ulnar nerve. (Illustrated by Lisa Ramaut, MD)

the flexor retinaculum, between the pisiform bone (lateral) and the hamulus (medial) and splits in a superficial and deep branch (Figs. 13 and 14). Interestingly, the deep branch of the ulnar nerve accompanies the deep branch of the ulnar artery.

The four distal carpal row bones (trapezium (TRA), trapezoid (tra), capitate (C), and hamate with the hamulus (h)) form the distal part of the bony carpal tunnel (Fig. 13), limited at the palmar side by the flexor retinaculum (Fl R). The two branches of the ulnar nerve (un) are situated superficially and at the ulnar side of the hamulus (Figs. 13 and 14) and give rise to a deep dorsal (un-dors) and superficial palmar branch (un-palm) (Fig. 15).

The bases of the metacarpals (Gunther 1984; Nakamura et al. 2001a; Theumann et al. 2002; Zancolli et al. 1987) appear (Figs. 16, 17, and 18), while the epl continues its crossing course. The median nerve is splitting into 5–6 components, while a superficial palmar branch runs superficially from the flexor retinaculum as does

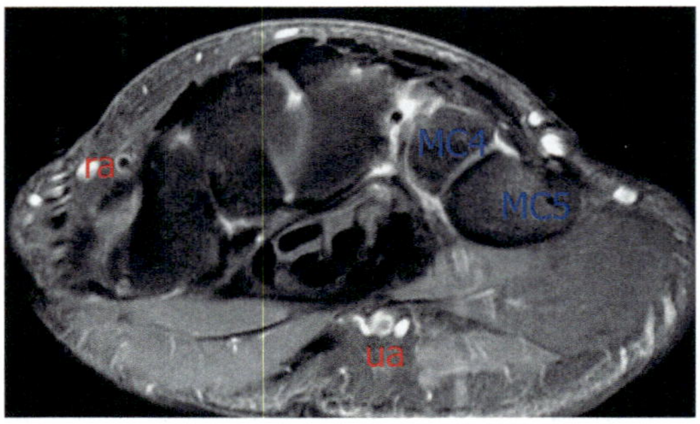

Fig. 16 The bases of the ulnar metacarpals (Ax. T1-WI FS). The bases of the metacarpals appear

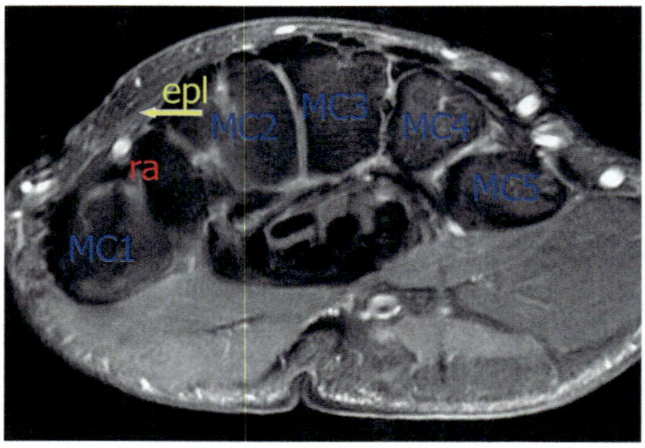

Fig. 17 The bases of the metacarpals (Ax. T1-WI FS). The epl continues its crossing course

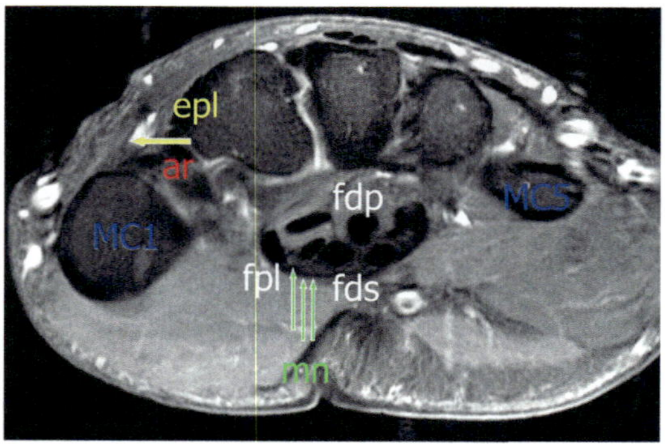

Fig. 18 The proximal metacarpals (Ax. T1-WI FS). The median nerve is splitting into 5–6 components

a recurrent superficial branch (Fig. 19), which in normal conditions are difficult to distinguish.

T2-weighted images fat-suppressed (T2WI-FS) may be useful in identifying specific structures due to the internal fascicular signal of the small ulnar nerve and the flow void of the ulnar artery (Figs. 20, 21, 22, 23, and 24). The virtual Parona space (Fig. 25) (a "highway" between the forearm and the hand, located between the Pronator Quadratus muscle (deep) and fdp (superficial), and just proximal to the carpal tunnel) and the potential presence of liquid (pathognomonic for a horse shoe abscess), the separation between the fcr (Fig. 26) and the rest of the flexor tendons of the carpal tunnel and the patency of vascular structures (Fig. 27) is better illustrated.

For the exact delineation of the joint capsule (containing the extrinsic ligaments) versus the overlying tendons, an arthrography technique is needed (Fig. 28).

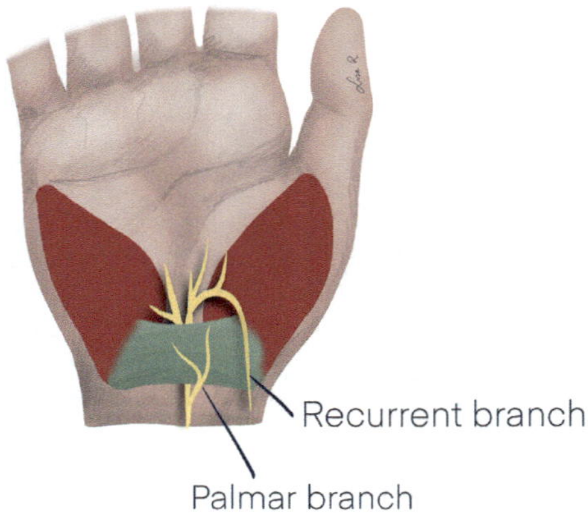

Fig. 19 Schematic drawing of the two important branches of the median nerve. The superficial palmar branch runs superficially from the flexor retinaculum as does a recurrent superficial branch. (Illustrated by Lisa Ramaut, MD)

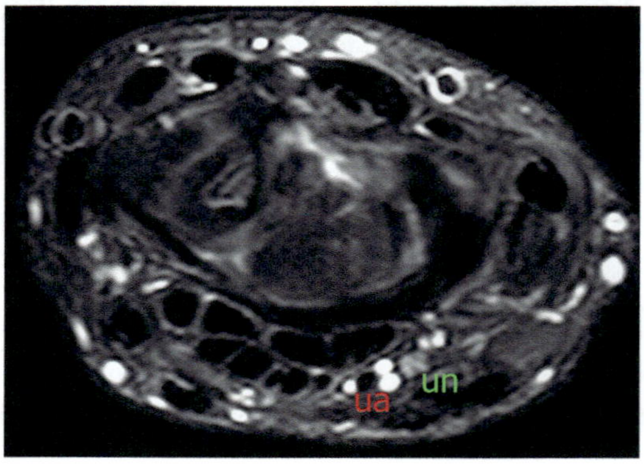

Fig. 20 The ulnar nerve (Ax. T2-WI FS). The internal fascicular signal of the small ulnar nerve

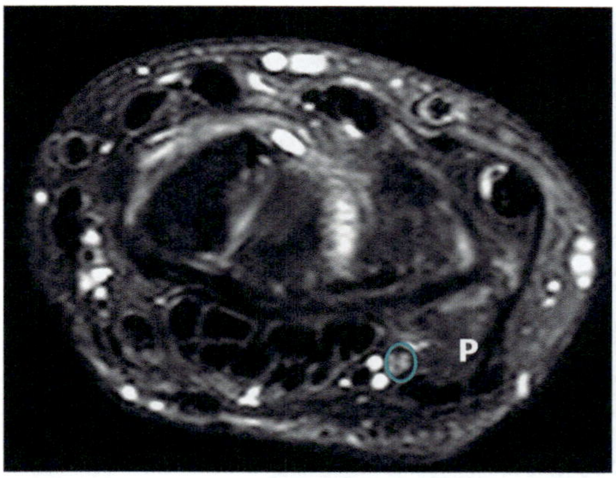

Fig. 21 The ulnar nerve continued (Ax. T2-WI FS). The higher signal of the small ulnar nerve at the level of the P

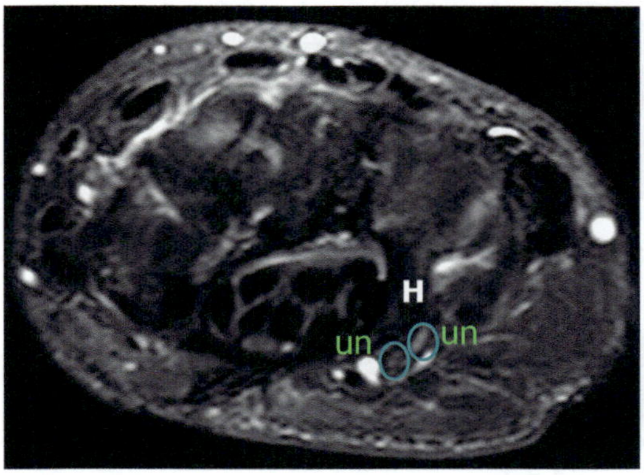

Fig. 22 The ulnar nerve continued (Ax. T2-WI FS). The higher signal of the small ulnar nerve branches at the level of the hamulus

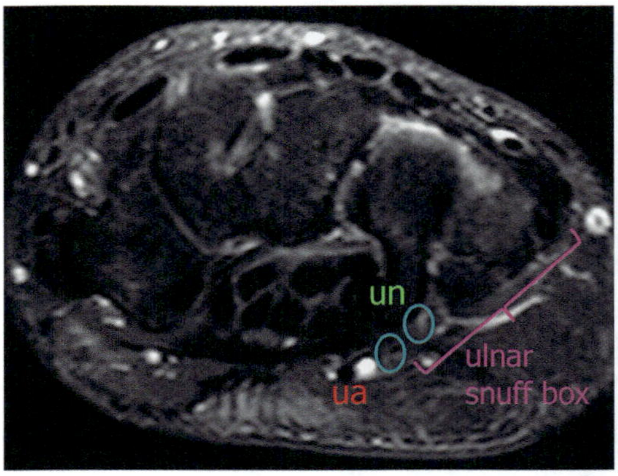

Fig. 23 The ulnar artery (Ax. T2-WI FS). Flow void of the ulnar artery

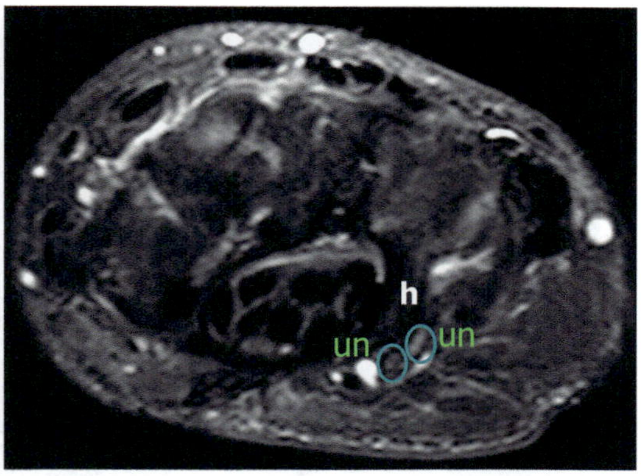

Fig. 24 The ulnar nerve continued (Ax. T2-WI FS). Splitting of the ulnar nerve, higher signal with fascicules

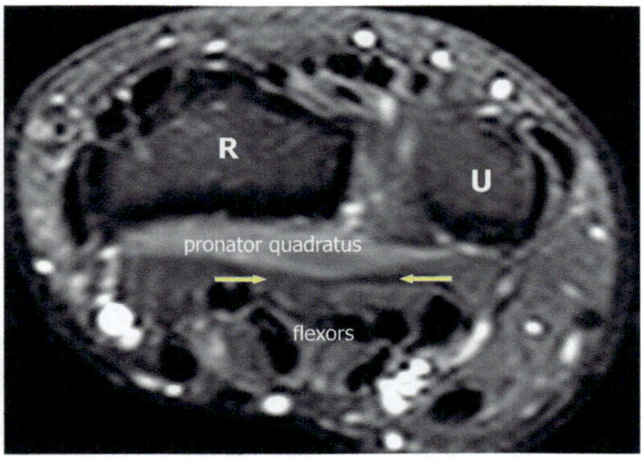

Fig. 25 The virtual space of Parona (Ax. T2-WI FS)

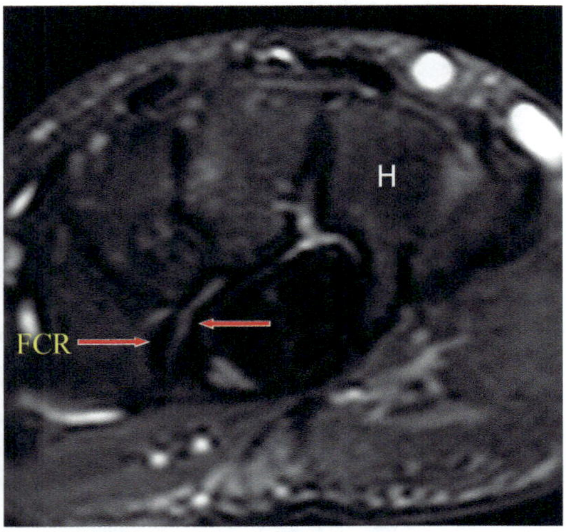

Fig. 26 (Ax. T2-WI FS). There is a clear separation between the fcr and the rest of the flexor tendons

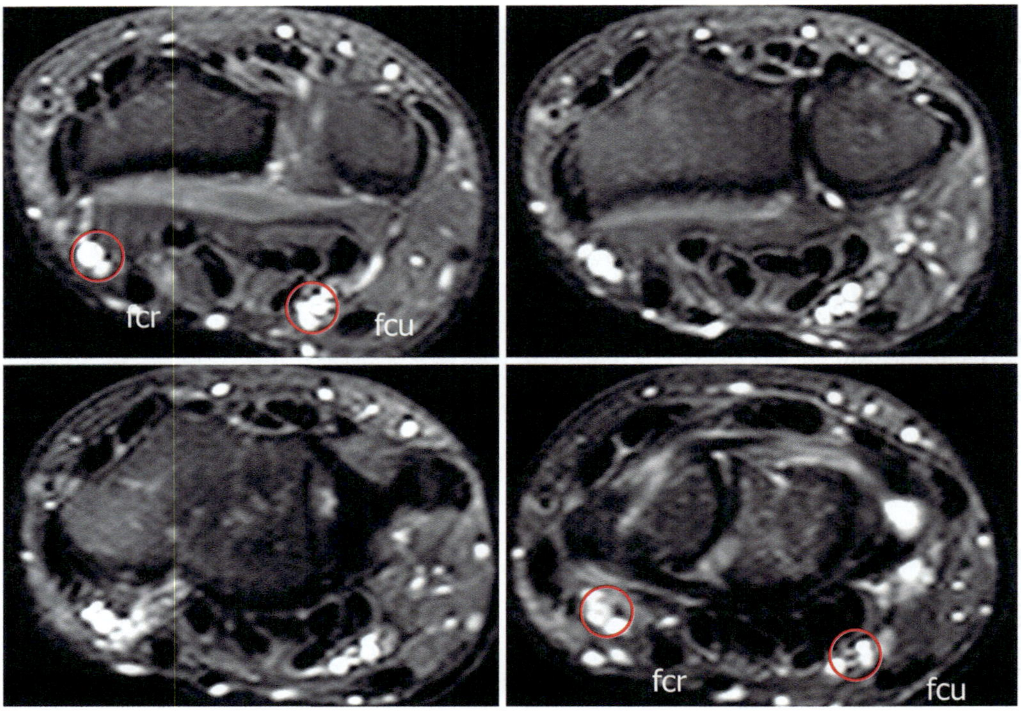

Fig. 27 Ax. T2-WI FS at several locations. Homogenous high signal on the trajectory of the arteries

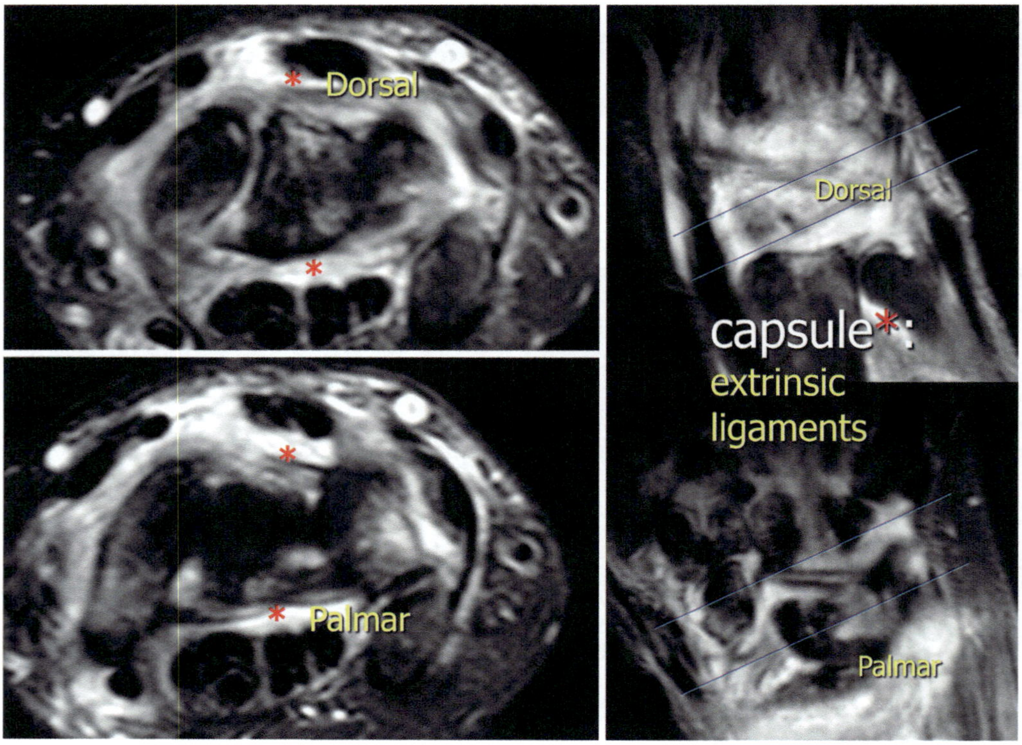

Fig. 28 MR arthrography (Ax. and Cor T2-WI FS). Visualization of the joint capsule (Ax) containing the extrinsic ligaments (Cor)

2 Ligaments

A lot of ligamentous structures (MacLean et al. 2021; Boutry et al. 2005; Davis and Blankenbaker 2010; Gitto and Draghi 2016; Gitto et al. 2017; Pulos and Bozentka 2015; Ringler 2013; Ringler and Murthy 2015; Scheck et al. 1999; Zlatkin and Rosner 2006) form connections between the carpal bones (intrinsic ligaments) as well as connections between the carpal and adjacent bones (extrinsic ligaments). Optimally, axial images are combined with coronal and/or sagittal images to visualise the complex trajectory of these ligaments.

2.1 Intrinsic Ligaments

The bones of the distal carpal row are connected by firm intrinsic (Lee et al. 2017; Manley et al. 2013; Schmid et al. 2005; Sennwald et al. 1994; Zdravkovic et al. 1994) interosseous ligaments (trapeziotrapezoid, capitotrapezoid, and capitohamate ligament) (Fig. 29). These limit the midcarpal joint distally, although there is a connection with the carpo-metacarpal joint (M-joint) through the central interruption of the trapeziotrapezoid ligament (Figs. 30 and 31). The distal extensions of the M-joint between the metacarpal bases II–V are limited by the intermetacarpal ligaments

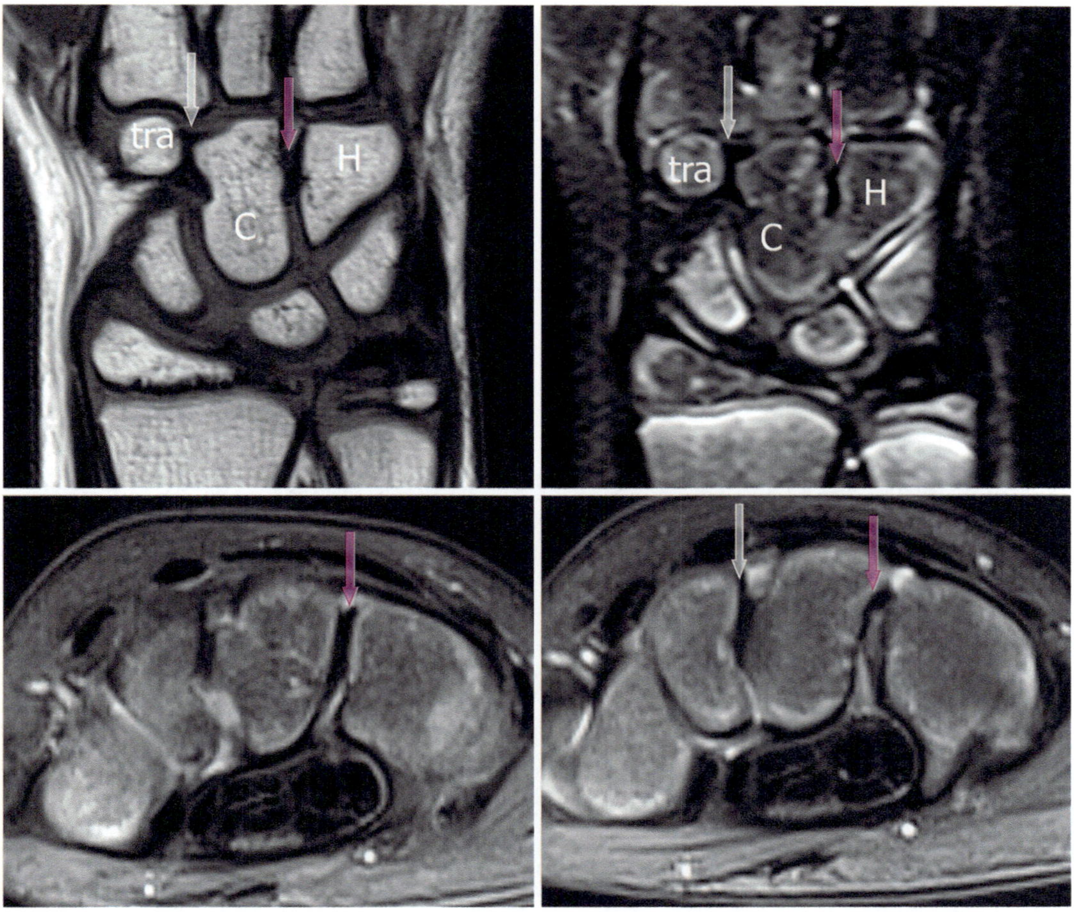

Fig. 29 The capitotrapezoid (white) and capitohamate (pink) ligament of distal carpal row (Cor T1-WI, T2-WI FS, and Ax T1-WI FS)

(Fig. 31). Special attention must be given to the variable configuration of the quadrangular joint (Figs. 32 and 33).

The capsular borders of the dorsal side of the CMC-joint are in close contact with the tendon insertions of the extensor carpi radialis longus and brevis, respectively, at the dorsal side of the base of MC II and III (Fig. 34).

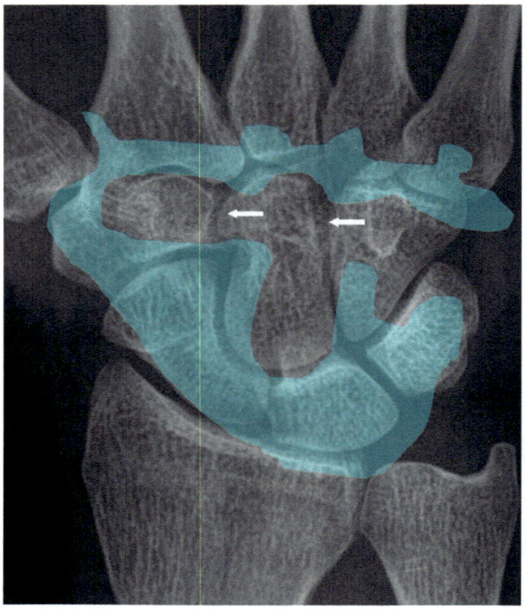

Fig. 30 Schematic drawing of the midcarpal arthrogram. No contrast passing (arrows) through the capitotrapezoid and capitohamate ligament of distal carpal row

The scapholunate (SL) and lunotriquetral (LT) intrinsic ligaments of the proximal carpal row are essential structures for the wrist motion. The scapholunate ligament (Shahabpour et al. 2015) mostly presents centrally as a triangular structure situated proximally between the scaphoid and lunate bone (Fig. 35). However, its form changes as the ligament has a horseshoe or C-shaped aspect in the sagittal plane. The ligamentous attachment to the adjacent bones varies. The central part attaches to the cartilage, whereas the dorsal and ventral parts attach to the cortex of the scaphoid bone and by Sharpey fibres to the lunate bone (Fig. 36). The most important dorsal part (Fig. 37), due to its C-shaped configuration, seems to extend between the carpal bones (Figs. 36 and 37). In children, the ligament is situated more eccentric in the SL bony space due to the remaining presence of a large cartilaginous part at the proximal pole of the scaphoid bone (Fig. 38). Midcarpal arthrography (Fig. 39) shows the exact location and continuity of the SL. The lunotriquetral ligament (Ritt et al. 1998) is smaller and mostly bandlike or triangular (Figs. 40, 41, and 42). The form also changes as the ligament has a similar horseshoe shape in the sagittal plane.

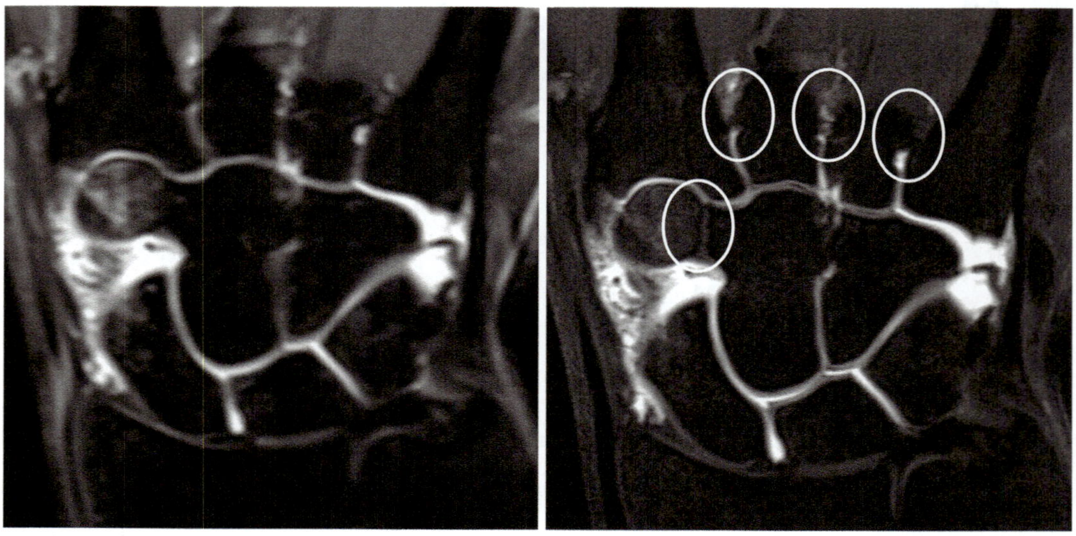

Fig. 31 Midcarpal Cor T1-WI FS arthrography. The midcarpal joint is in normal communication with the M-joint through the Tra-tra space. The intermetacarpal spaces are distally limited by small ligaments

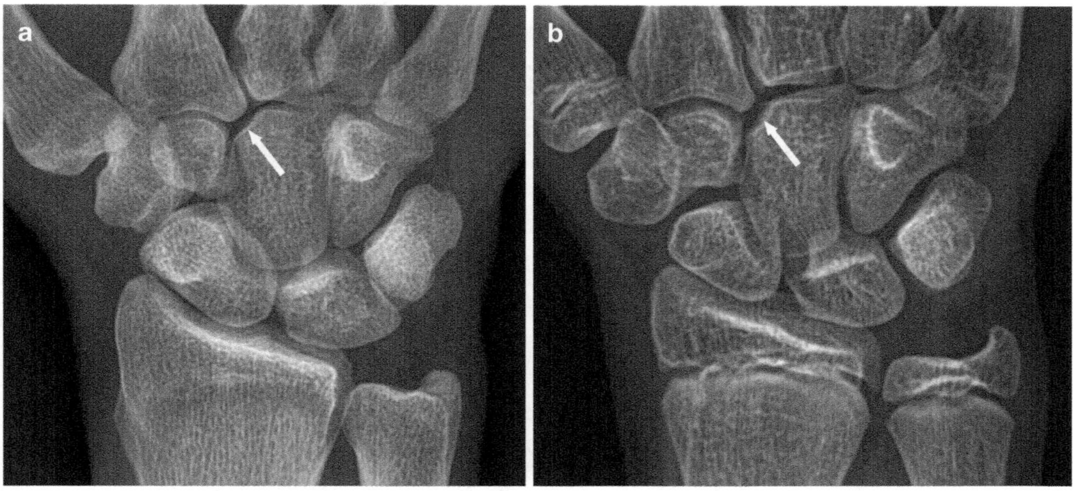

Fig. 32 Standard PA view. The quadrangular space in adult (**a**) and child (**b**)

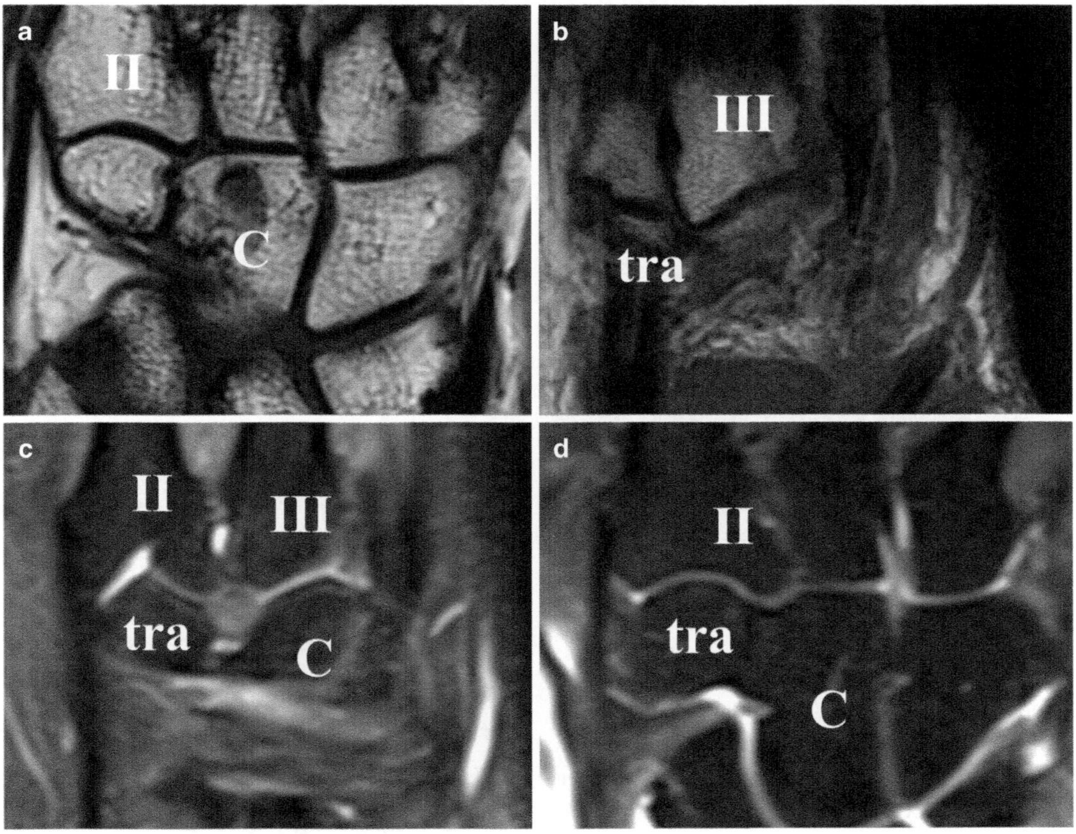

Fig. 33 Cor T1-WI (**a**, **b**) and Cor T2-WI FS (**c**, **d**). Variable configurations of the quadrangular joint: MC II—C contact (**a**); MC III—tra contact (**b**); interposition of styloid bone between MC II, III, tra and C (**c**) and coalition tra-C in contact with MC II (**d**)

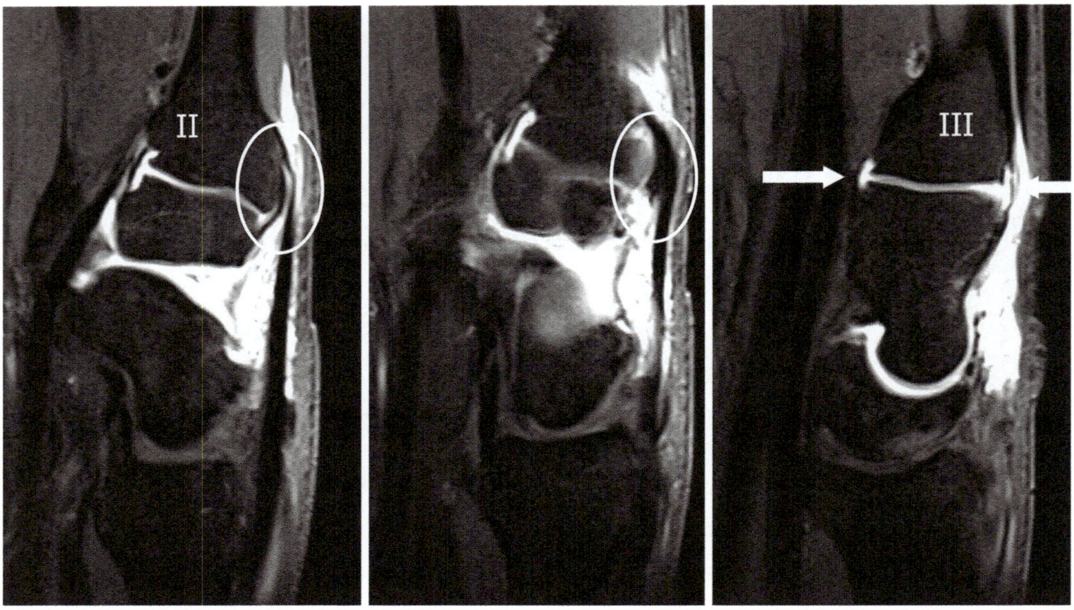

Fig. 34 MR GRE arthrography. Close contact between the insertion tendons of the ecl and ecb and, respectively, the dorsal capsule of the MC II and MC III joint (ovals). Contrast in the MC joints limited by the ventral and dorsal part of the capsule (arrows)

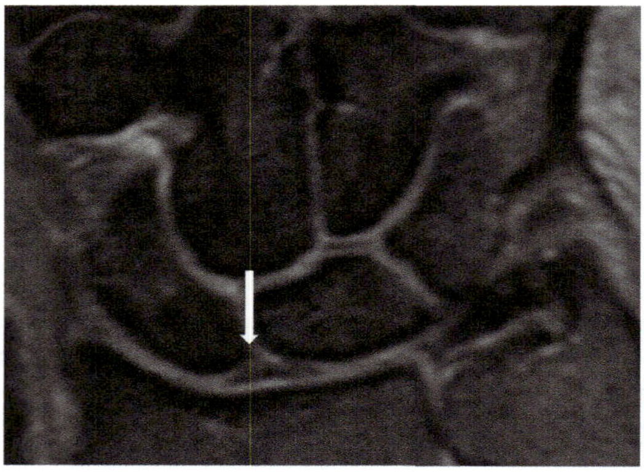

Fig. 35 Cor T2-WI FS. A triangular homogenous low signal SL is proximally positioned between the S and L

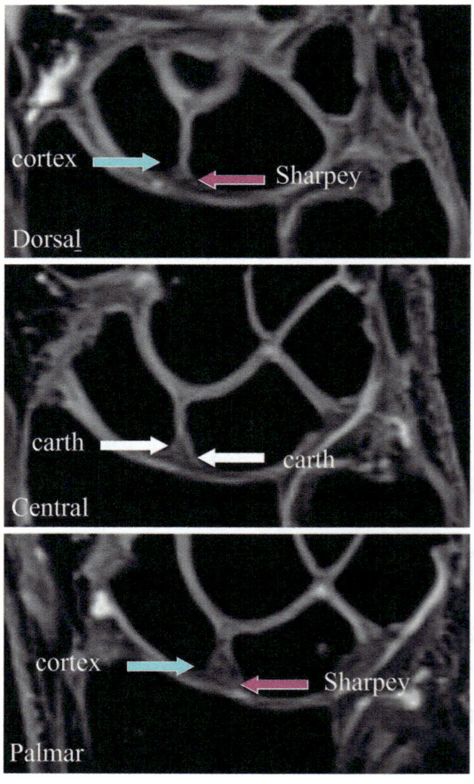

Fig. 36 Cor GRE. The ligament is attached to the ventral and dorsal cortex on the S side and by Sharpey fibers on the L side. Centrally it is fixated on the cartilage

The ligamentous attachment to the adjacent bones varies (Fig. 41). The most important part is the palmar component (Fig. 41).

Although the triangular fibrocartilaginous complex (TFCC) (Nakamura et al. 2001b; Zhan et al. 2020) (Fig. 43) is not an intrinsic ligament, it is often mentioned together with the SL and LT. This complex structure contains seven components, which are summarised in Table 2. A small cartilage band is interposed (Fig. 44) between the radial notch and the triangular

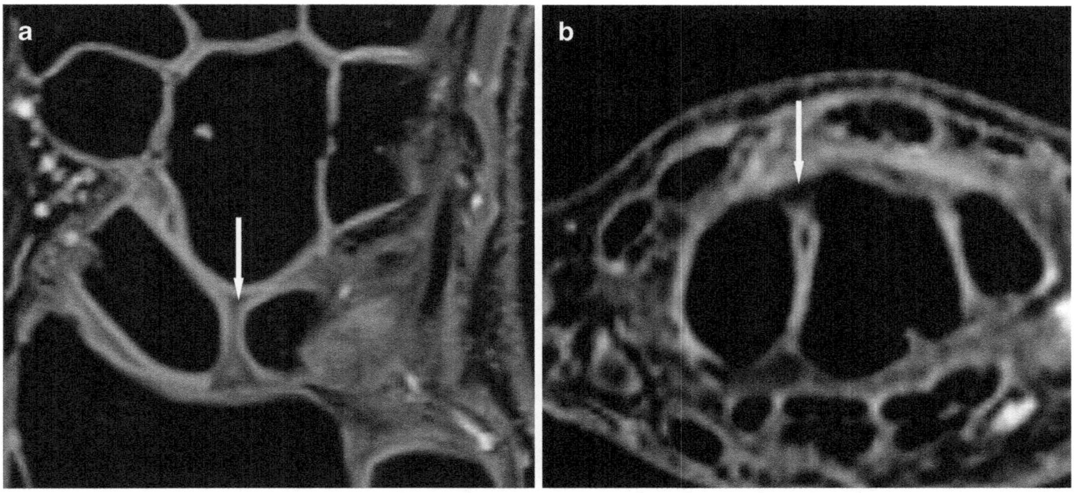

Fig. 37 Cor (**a**) and Ax (**b**) GRE. The dorsal part of the SL (arrows) is the most important part

Fig. 38 Cor GRE (**a**), proton density (**b**), T1-WI (**c**) imaging and standard PA view (**d**). Pseudo-widening of the SL joint space and eccentric position of the low signal ligament (arrows) in the SL bony space due to a large still cartilaginous part of the proximal pole of the scaphoid bone in a child

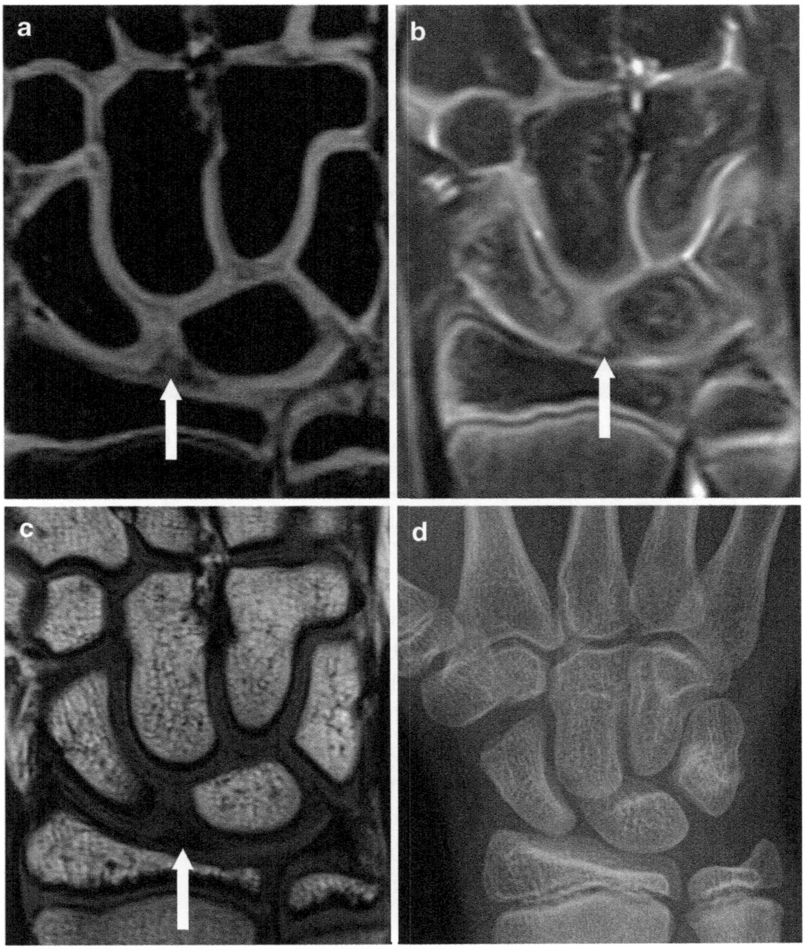

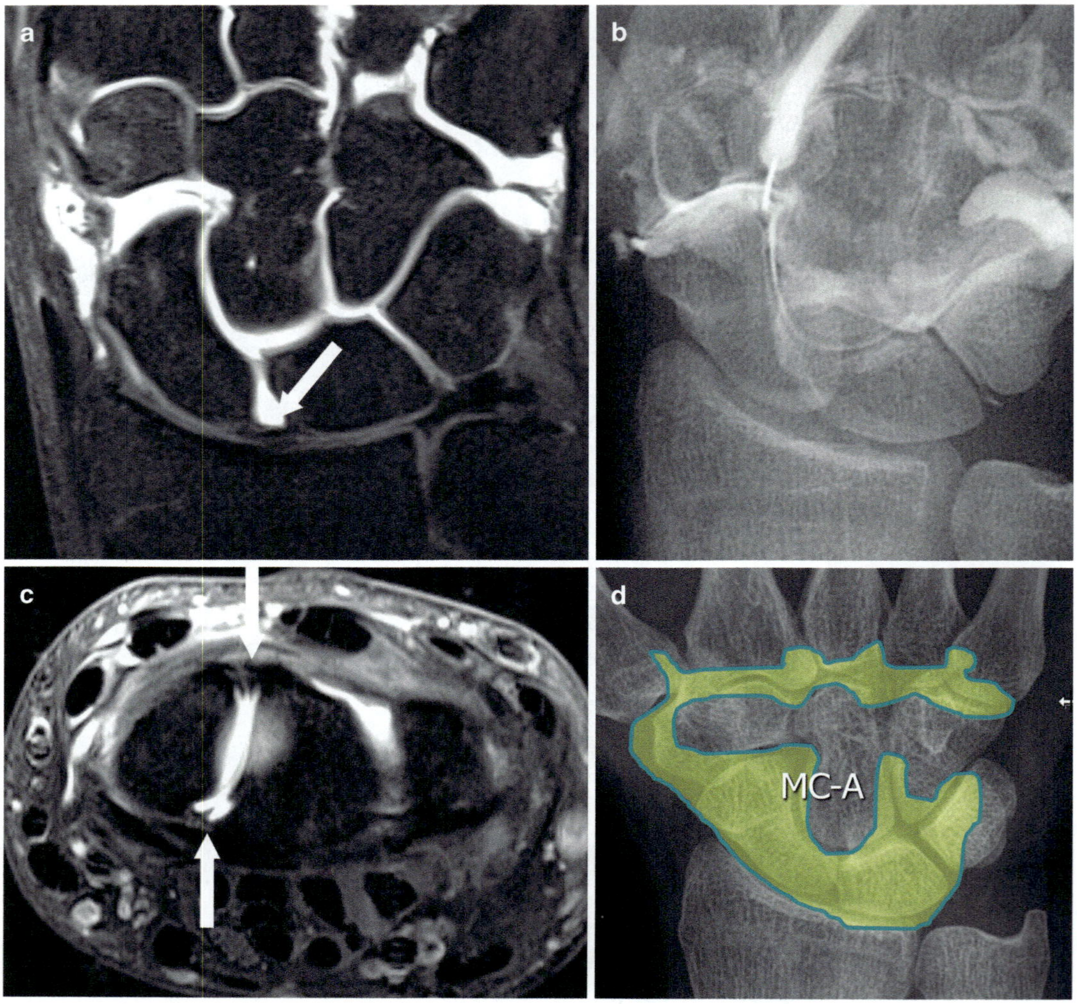

Fig. 39 Midcarpal arthrography Cor and Ax T1-WI FS (**a**, **b**), standard PA arthrography view (**c**) with schematic drawing of MCA (**d**). The space between the S and L is opacified by contrast and delineates the distal border of the SL. The interpretation of the continuity needs at least coronal (**a**) and axial (**b**) images. The observation during the injection and the arthrography views (**c**, **d**) are an integral part of the examination

structure. The poorly vascularised central disc has a well vascularised double insertion on the ulnar styloid process near the base (ulnar notch) and near the tip (Figs. 43a, 44a, and 45a). The TFCC separates the radiocarpal joint (RCJ) from the distal radio-ulnar joint (DRUJ) (Fig. 43b) and provides stability to the latter joint. The base of the meniscus homologue (Figs. 43b and 45b) rests on the ulnar collateral ligament and delineates the entrance to the prestyloid capsule recessus of the radiocarpal joint (Fig. 45c, d). At the palmar and dorsal side, the radio-ulnar ligament maintains the position of the ulnar head in the radial notch (Fig. 46a). Two small palmar ligaments connect the TFCC and the palmar radio-ulnar ligament to the lunate (ulnolunar) and triquetral (ulnotriquetral) bones (Fig. 46b, c).

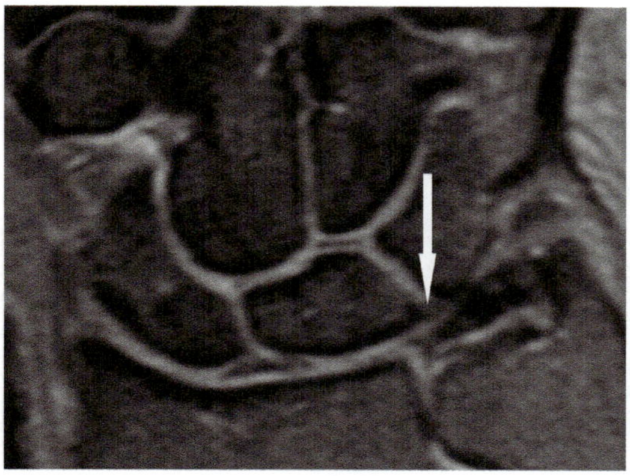

Fig. 40 Cor T2-WI FS. A bandlike homogenous low signal LT is proximally positioned between the L and Tri

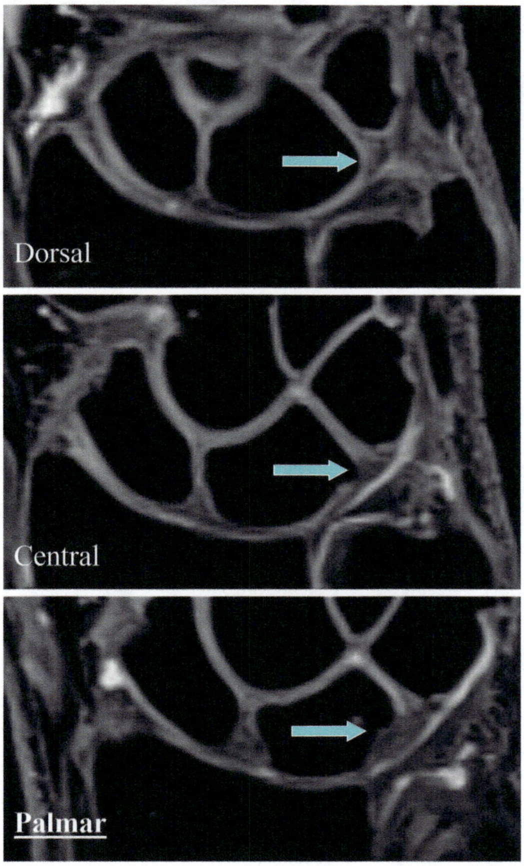

Fig. 41 Cor GRE. The form of the LT changes and the palmar component is the strongest of the three parts

Rarely mentioned ligaments are the intrinsic ligament between the trapezium and scaphoid bone (Fig. 47) as well as those between the hamate and triquetrum proximally and the base of the fifth metacarpal distally (Fig. 48).

2.2 Extrinsic Ligaments

To achieve a clear and structured approach, the extrinsic ligament (Shahabpour et al. 2011) nomenclature is derived from their bony insertion points. Most of them run in an oblique 3D-direction and thus need to be evaluated on successive images.

2.2.1 Palmar Side

On MRI images, two V-shaped structures are considered (Figs. 49, 50, 51, 52, 53, 54, and 55). Distally, the V located on the radial side is formed by the radioscaphocapitate ligament (1), continuing on the ulnar side as a proximal (5a) and distal (5b) part of the scaphocapitate-triquetral ligament (5; Prendergast ligament). Proximally, the radial component of the V is formed by the radiolunotriquetral ligament (2). The ulnar component consists of the small ulnolunar (3) and ulnotriquetral (4) ligaments.

The sometimes-mentioned deltoid ligament refers to the radioscaphocapitate ligament continued by the scaphocapitate-triquetral ligament (Fig. 54).

At the radial side, the space of Poirier is situated between the radioscaphocapitate (1) and radiolunotriquetral (2) ligament (Fig. 50).

The classical "palmar V" is composed of (1), (2), and (5) (Fig. 49).

Obermann (1991) first introduced the term "proximal palmar V" ((2), (3) and (4)) (Fig. 49).

A fairly large number of the ligaments form a central fixed column (T-form, formed by the distal carpal row and the L) (Fig. 54b). The radial (S) and ulnar columns (Tri) allow for the carpal mobility.

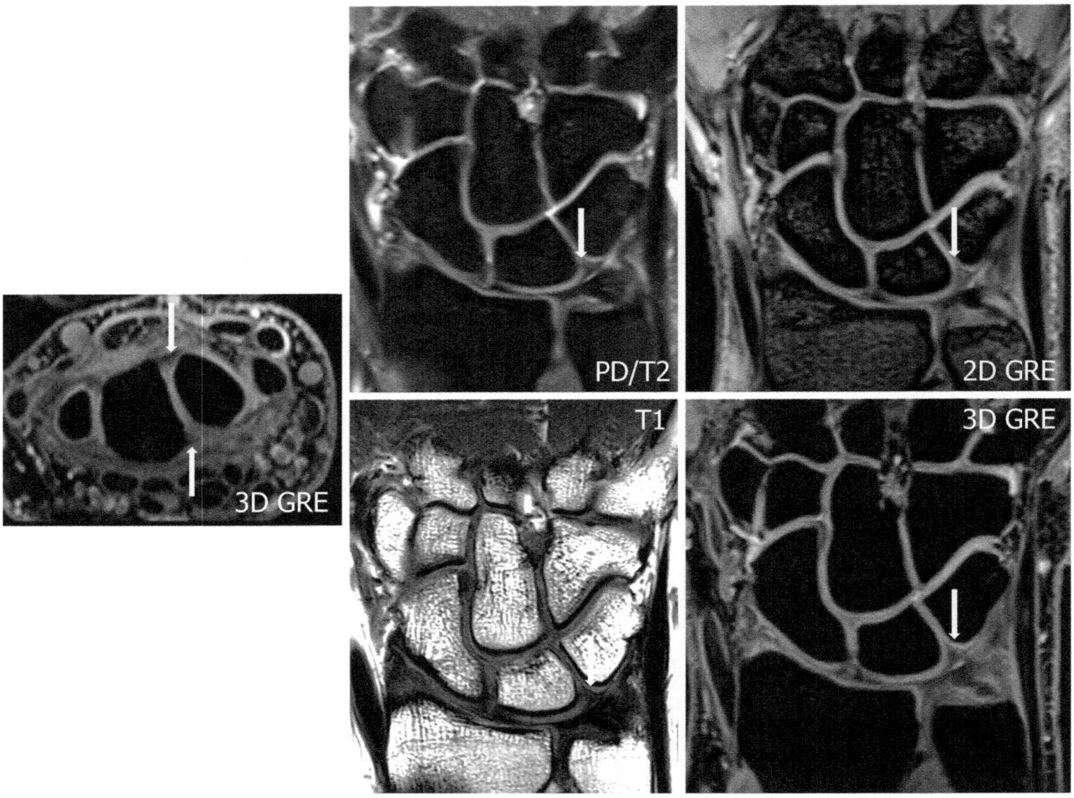

Fig. 42 Different imaging sequences of the LT. The form, signal, and continuity should be evaluated in two orthogonal dimensions

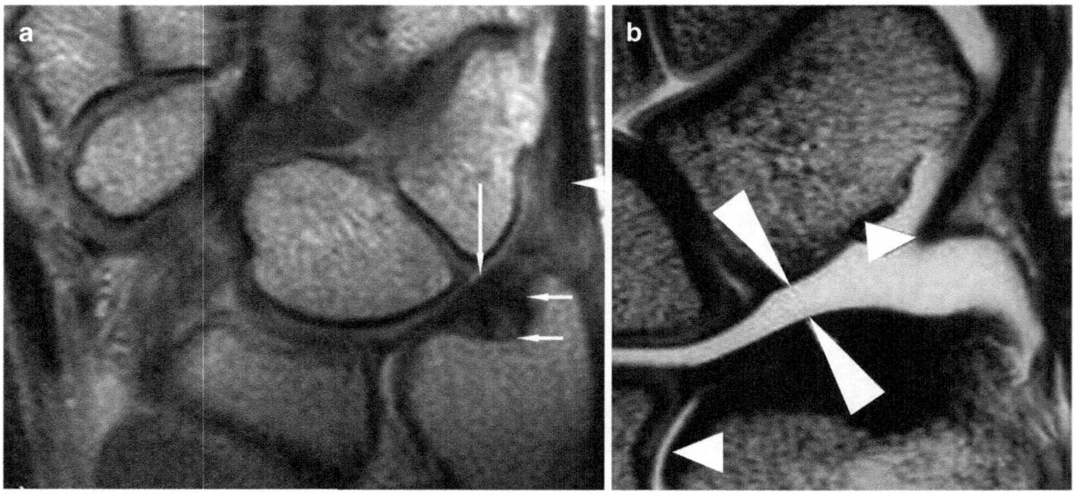

Fig. 43 T1-WI (**a**) and MR-arthrography (**b**). The TFCC (A-Ad) has a double insertion on the ulnar styloid (A-double Alr). It separates the RCJ (B-double AH) from the DRUJ (B-Ahr). The meniscus homologue (B-Ahl) rests on the ulnar collateral ligament (A-Ahr)

Table 2 Components of the TFCC-complex

Components		Abbreviation
Triangular fibrocartilage	Central articular disc	TFC-AD
Double ulnar attachment	Tip of the styloid ulnar notch	
Palmar and dorsal radio-ulnar ligament		rul (palm/ dors)
Meniscus homologue		MH
Ulnar collateral ligament		UCL
Ulnocarpal ligaments	Ulnolunate and ulnotriquetral	UL and Utriq
Tendon sheath of extensor carpi ulnaris		ecu

2.2.2 Dorsal Side

The main ligaments converge to the dorsum of the triquetral bone (Figs. 56 and 57). Their origin is located, respectively, on the radius (1), the scaphoid (2), and the trapezium (3) bone. The often-used term "dorsal intercarpal ligament" refers to (1) and (2).

The ulnotriquetral (4) and the radial collateral ligaments (5) can also be visualised. Note that (2) and (3) are connecting carpal bones and should theoretically be considered as "intrinsic".

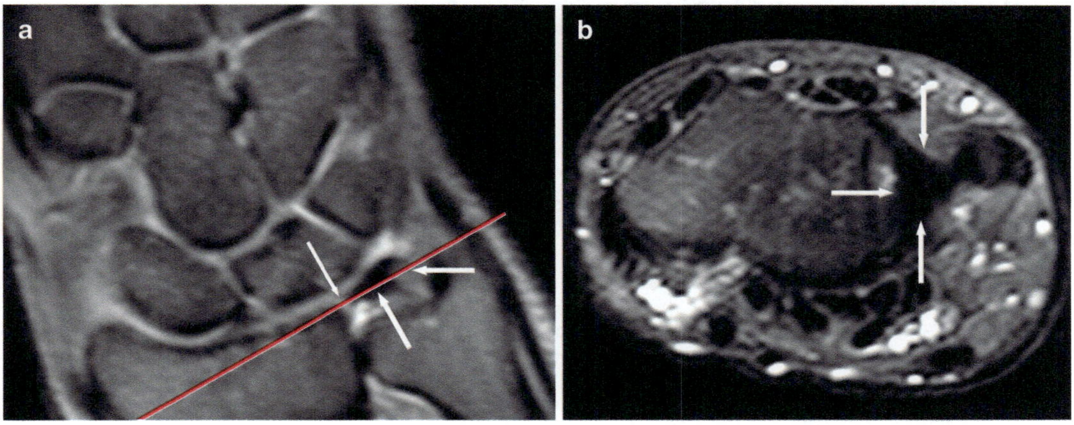

Fig. 44 Cor proton density (**a**) and Ax T2-WI FS (**b**) (at the level of the red line in **a**). There is a small band at the radial sigmoid notch (A-AOdl) between the central disc (A-AOar, B-arrows) and the highly vascularized ulnar insertion (A-Alr)

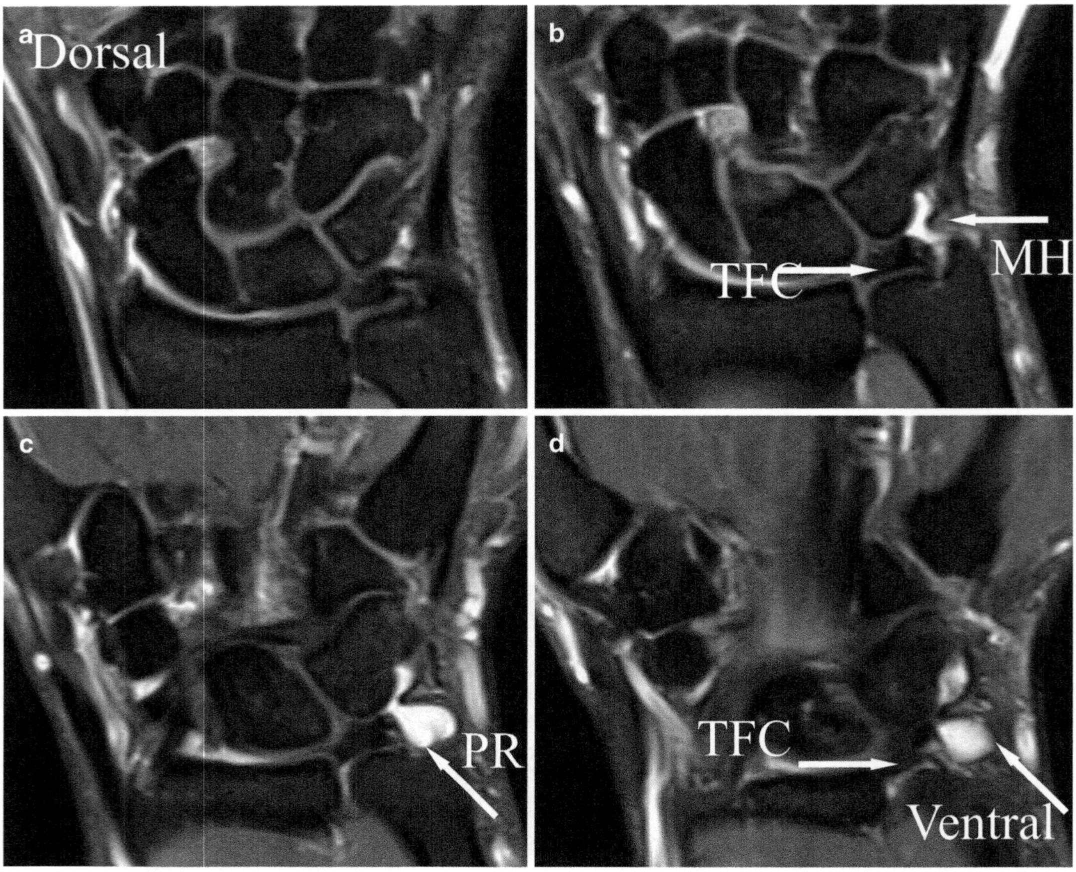

Fig. 45 Ax T2-WI FS (**a**–**d**; from dorsal to ventral). Ventrally, there is a small connection of the RCJ to the prestyloid recess (PR). The meniscus homologue (MH) margins it distally

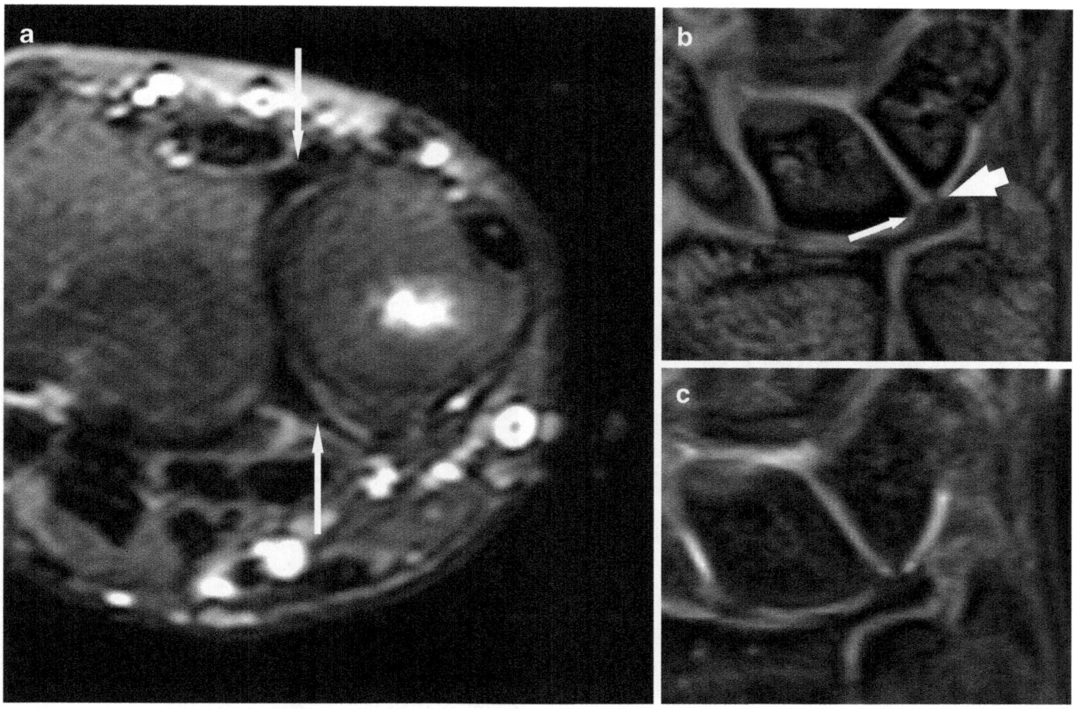

Fig. 46 Ax T2-WI FS (**a**), Cor 2D-GRE (**b**) and 3D-GRE (**c**). The palmar (A-Ad) and dorsal (A-Aa) radio-ulnar ligaments assist in fixing the moving ulnar head in the sigmoid notch. Two small ligaments (**b**, **c**), the ulnolunar (B-AOar) and ulnotriquetral (B-AOdr), may be delineated between the TFCC and, respectively, the L and Tri

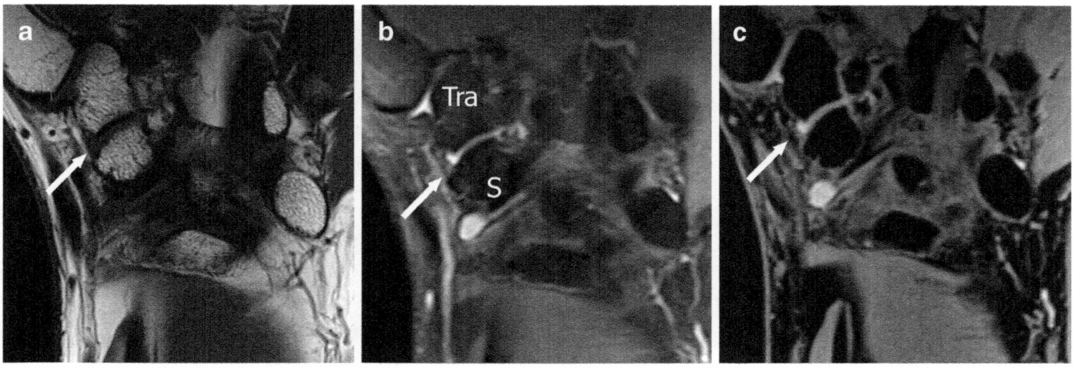

Fig. 47 Cor T1-WI (**a**), Cor T2-WI FS (**b**), and 3D-GRE (**c**). The scaphotrapezial ligament limits the mediocarpal joint radially

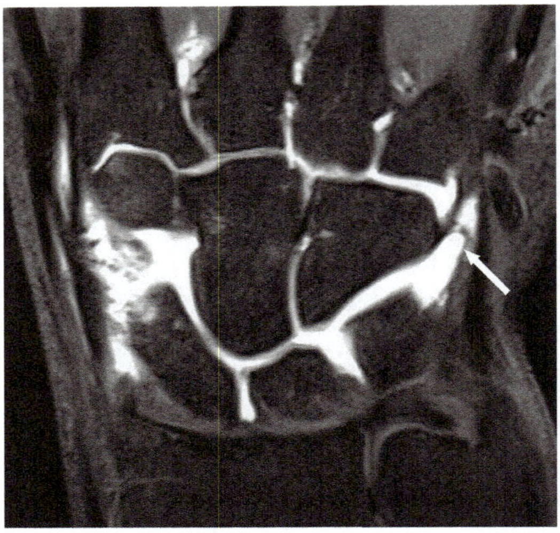

Fig. 48 Cor T1-WI FS arthrography. The triquetrohamate ligament limits the mediocarpal joint ulnarly

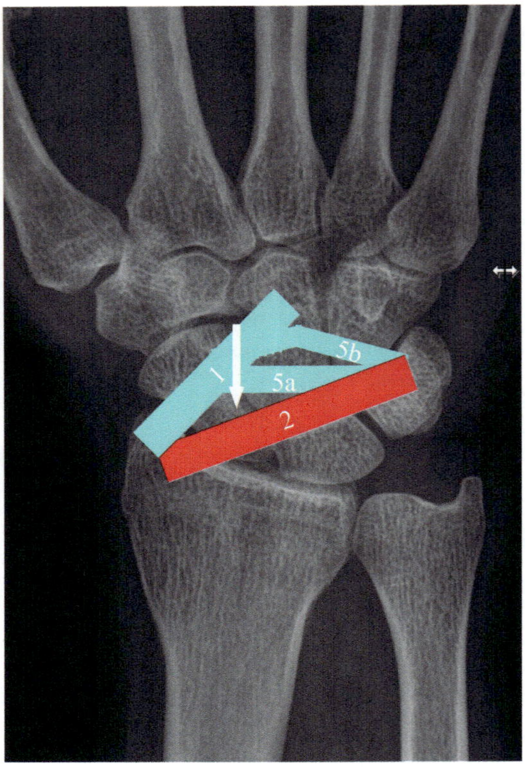

Fig. 50 Schematic representation of the space of Poirier (arrow)

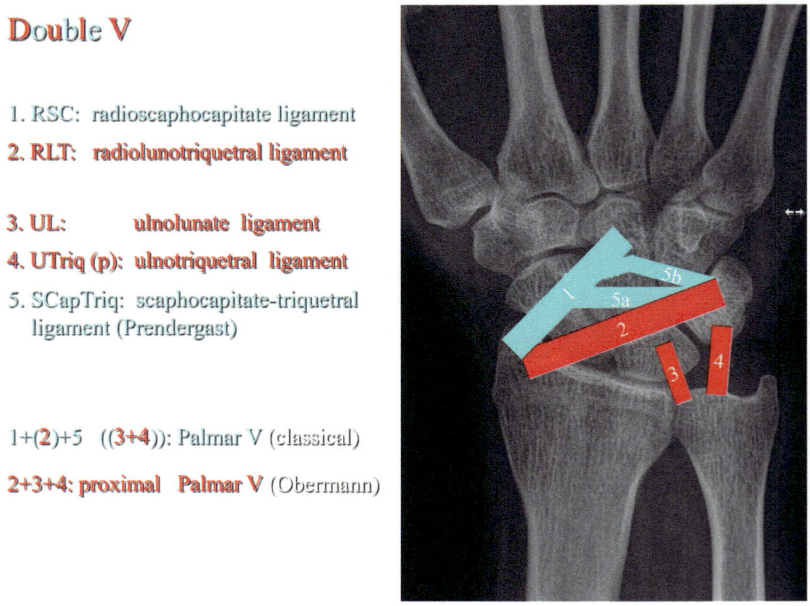

Fig. 49 Schematic representation of the carpal extrinsic ligaments at the palmar side illustrating the proximal (red) and distal (green) V-pattern

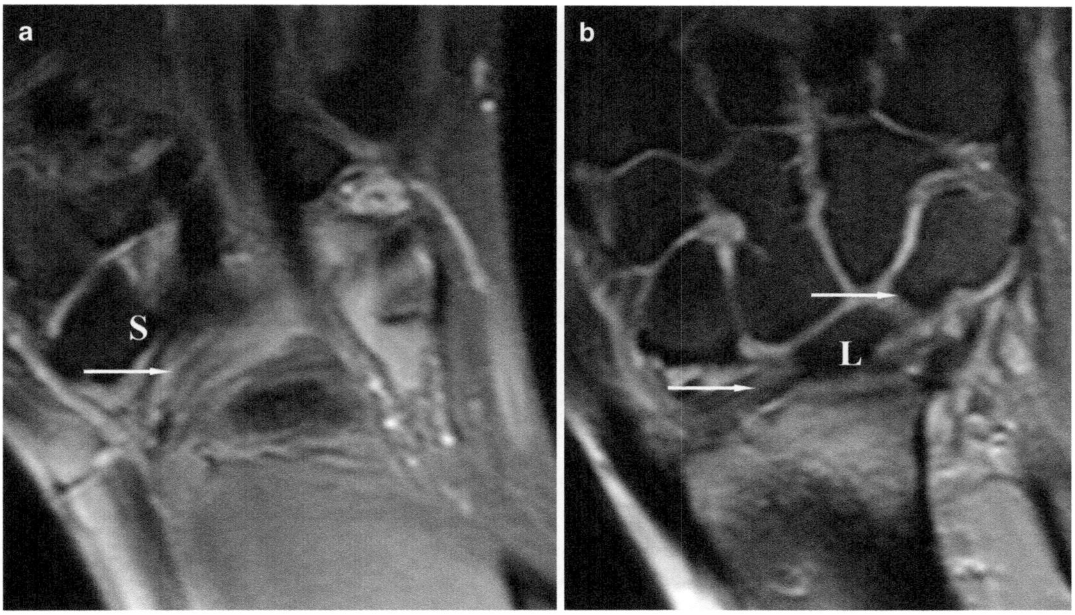

Fig. 51 Cor proton density images. The RSC (**a**) and RLT (**b**) ligaments show linear small low signal bands in alternation with higher signal bands

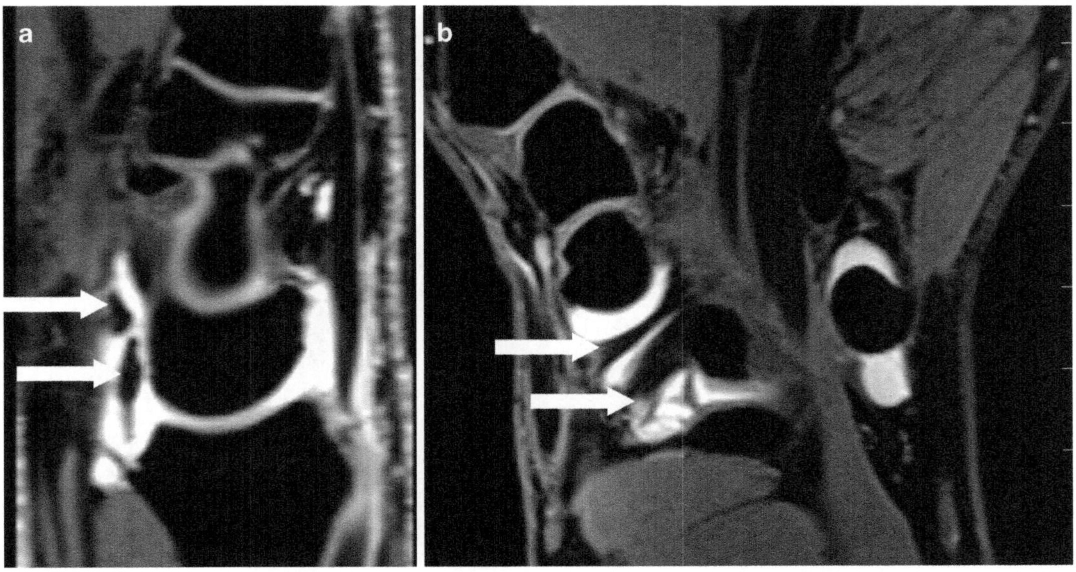

Fig. 52 Sag (**a**) and Cor 3D-GRE (**b**) arthrography. The RSC (upper arrows) and the RLT (lower arrows) are continuously delineated by the contrast at the palmar side

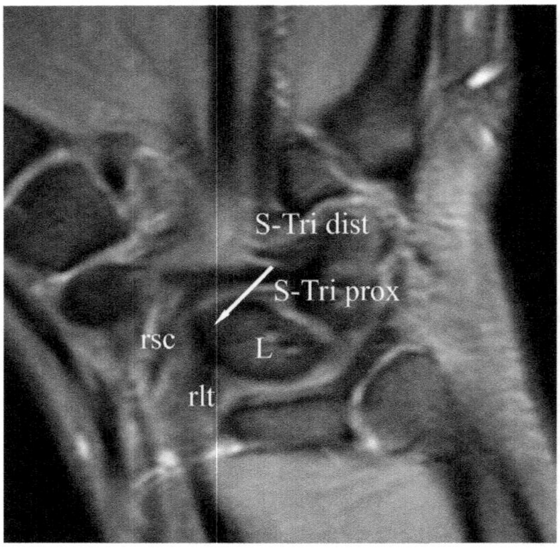

Fig. 53 Cor proton density images. The distal V starts radially as RSC and continues at the ulnar side as scapho(capitate)triquetral ligament. The space of Poirier (arrow) is situated between the RSC and RLT

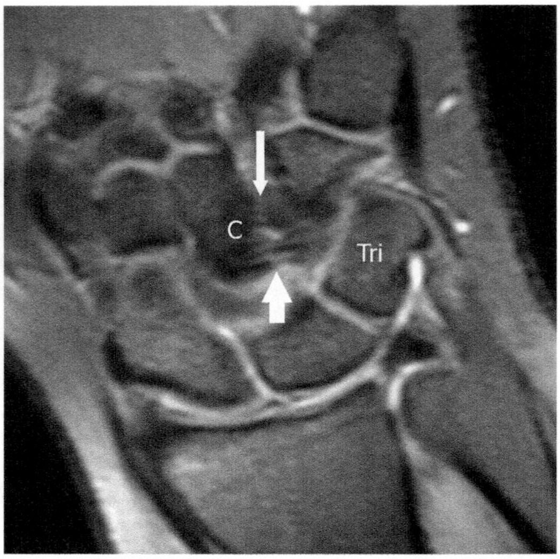

Fig. 55 Cor proton density images. The proximal (Aa) and distal (Ad) component of the (S)-C-Tri ligament

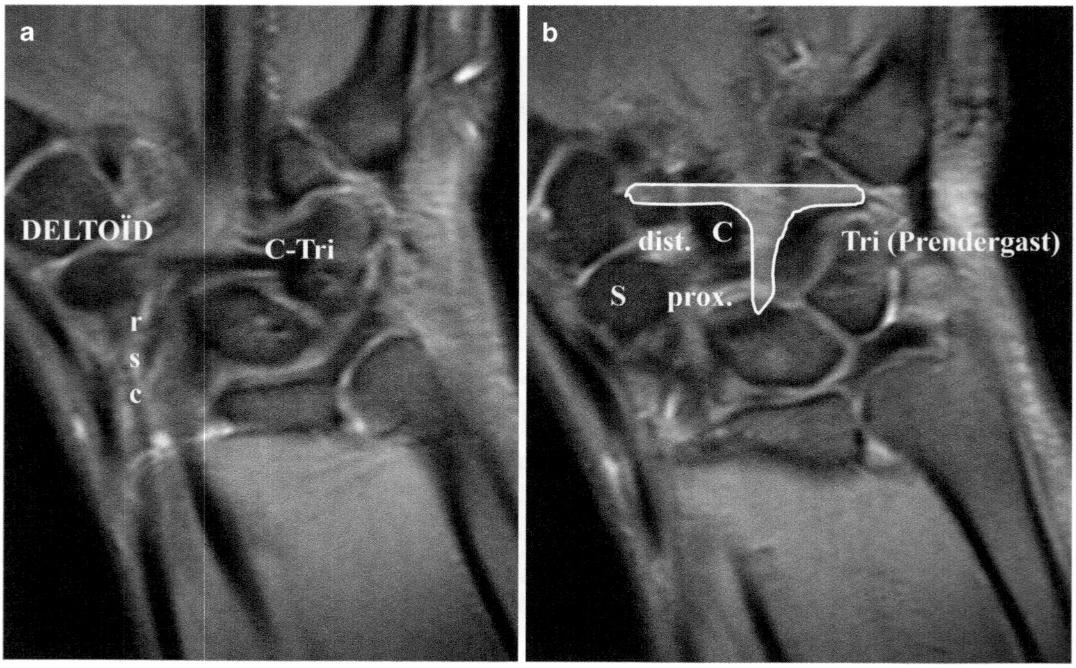

Fig. 54 Cor proton density images. The radial rsc continues in the ulnar C-Triq component to form the deltoid ligament (**a**). Due to the ligaments, a three-column carpal complex is formed (**b**)

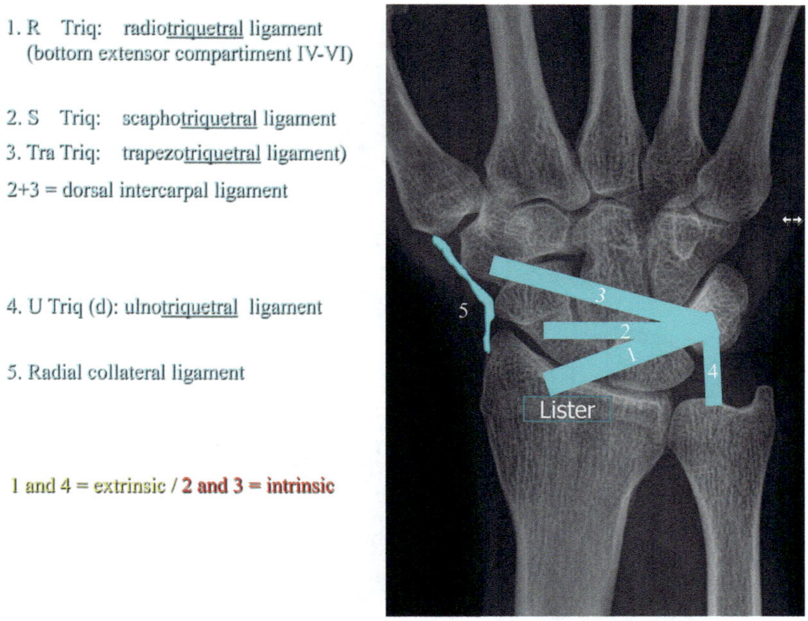

Fig. 56 Schematic representation of the carpal extrinsic ligaments at the dorsal side, mainly converging to the Tri

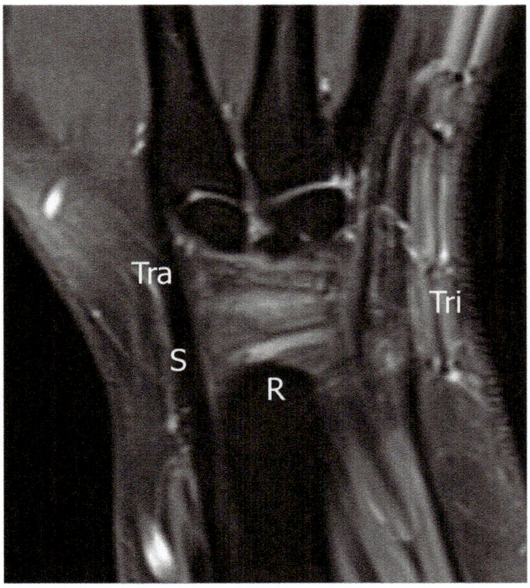

Fig. 57 Cor proton density image. The main carpal extrinsic ligaments at the dorsal side, mainly converging to the Tri

3 Cartilage

The so-called cartilaginous component (Zheng et al. 2010) (Figs. 58 and 59) is well seen on different MRI sequences, in contrast to the radiological transparency of the growth cartilage and the bony precursors. T1-WI shows an intermediate signal of the cartilage (A). The signal is well delineated and homogenously high, mainly on T2-WI (B), Flash-2D (C), and less explicit on DESS-3D (D). The fibrocartilage of the TFCC is of intermediate (B-D) to low (A) signal. Special attention should be given to the pseudo-widening of the scapholunate joint, due to the eccentric development of the scaphoid bone (Fig. 60). After bony differentiation, the signal is altered in a low signal at the cortex, a high fat signal at the medullar parts on T1-WI (Fig. 59i–l), and a low signal on PD-T2-WI (Fig. 59a, b, e–h).

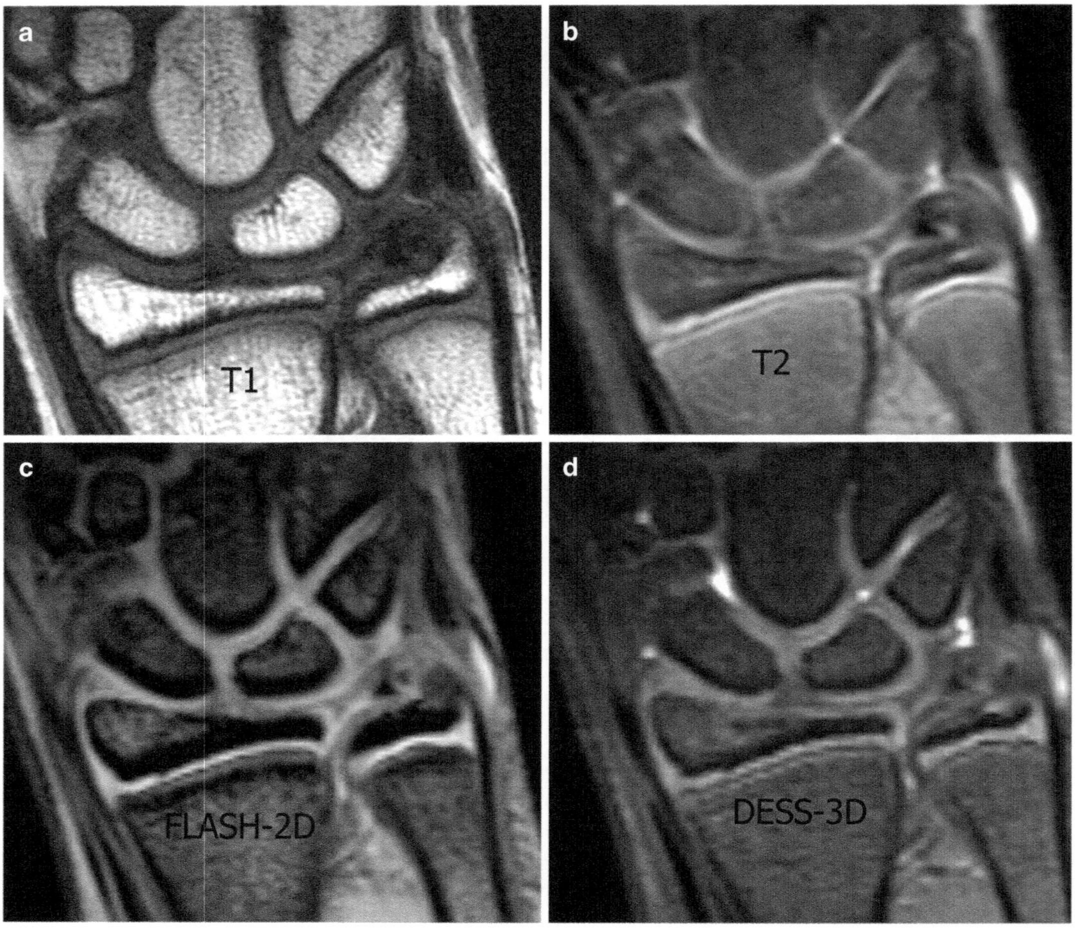

Fig. 58 Cor T1-WI (**a**), T2-WI (**b**), Flash-2D (**c**) and DESS-3D (**d**). The signal of the (fibro)cartilage depends on the sequence, but the cartilage is well delineated and homogenous in all

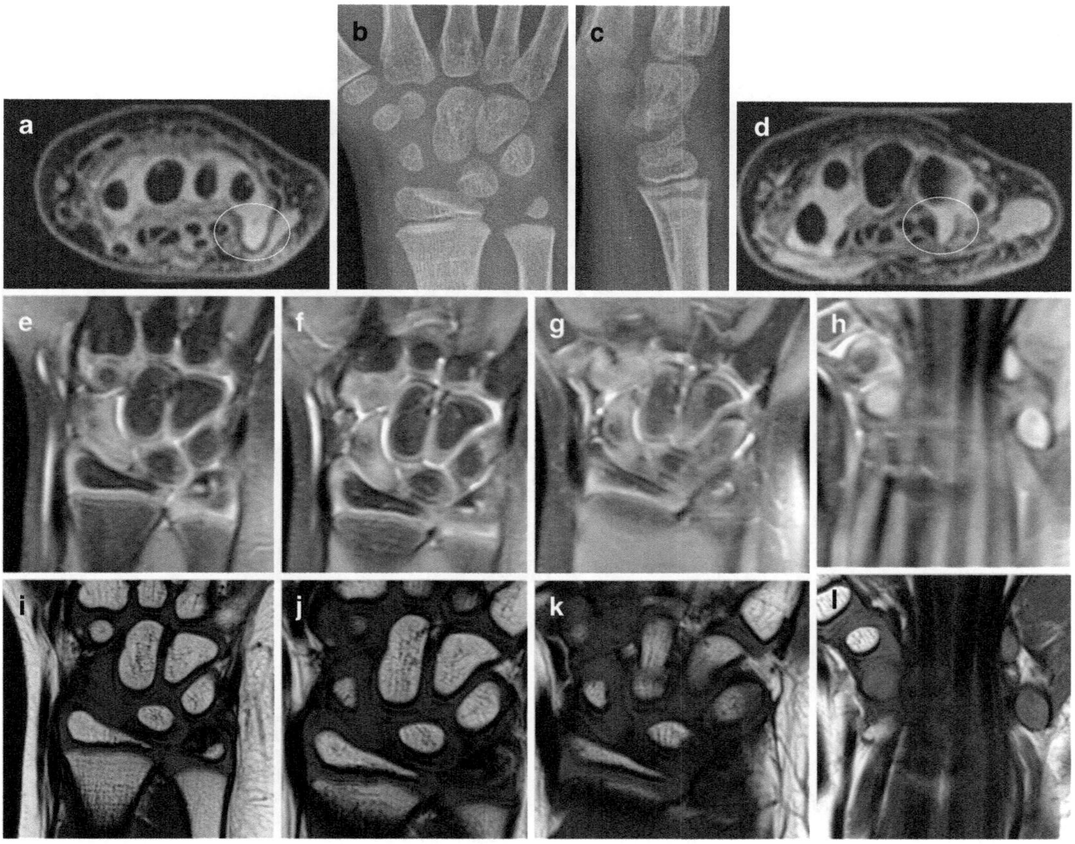

Fig. 59 Ax and Cor proton-density (**a**, **d**, **e**–**h**), standard PA and lateral view (**b**, **c**), Cor T1-WI (I-L). The cartilaginous parts are well displayed, in contrast to standard views

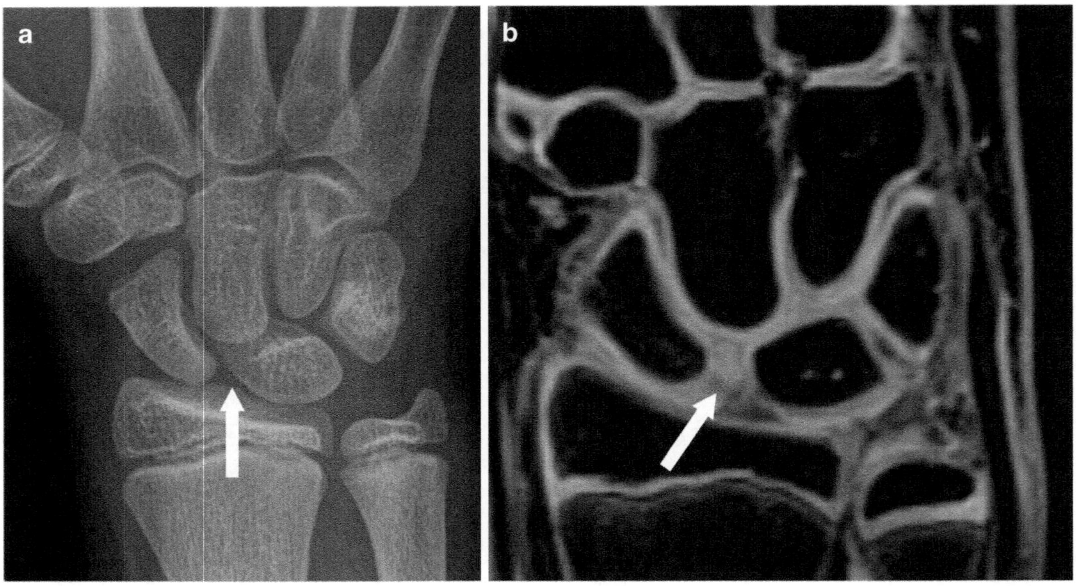

Fig. 60 Standard PA view (**a**) and Cor T2-WI FS (**b**). Pseudo-widening of the scapholunate joint (**a**) due to the eccentric osteogenic differentiation of the scaphoid bone (b)

4 Median and Ulnar Nerve

At the entrance of the carpal tunnel, at the level of the pisiform bone (Fig. 61a), the median nerve runs as an oval structure close to the flexor retinaculum. At the exit, at the level of the hamulus, the nerve has a rather flat configuration (Fig. 61b). However, the rotational position of the median nerve may vary, from vertical between the flexor pollicis longus and the superficial flexor digitorum tendons (Fig. 62a) to horizontal, superficially of the flexor digitorum tendons (Fig. 62b).

The ulnar nerve is at the level of the pisiform bone separated from the carpal canal and runs through the Guyon canal (Figs. 9 and 21), together with the ulnar artery. It leaves the canal laterally, between the pisiform bone and the hamulus, and splits into a superficial and deep branch lateral from the hamulus (Figs. 12 and 24).

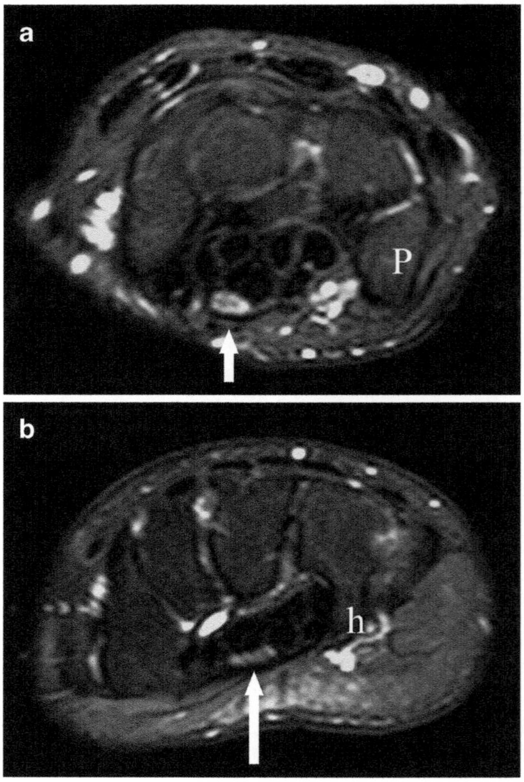

Fig. 61 Ax T2-WI FS. At the level of the pisiform bone (**a**), the median nerve runs as an oval structure close to the flexor retinaculum. At the level of the hamulus, the nerve has a flat configuration (**b**)

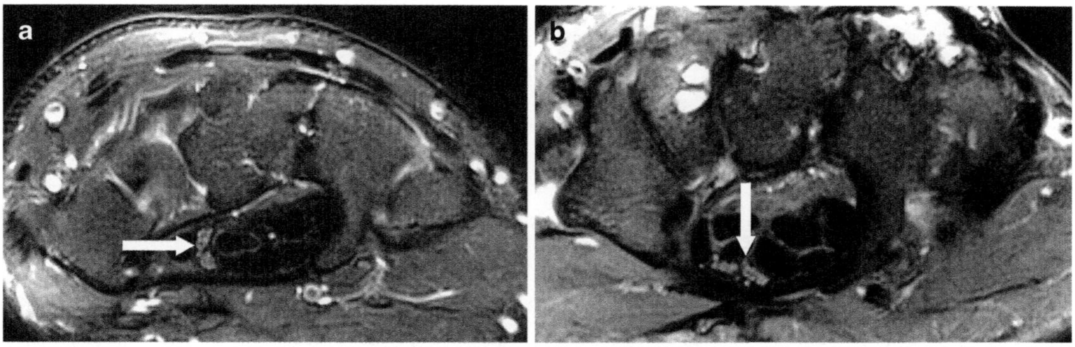

Fig. 62 Ax T2-WI FS. Varying rotational position of the median nerve, from deeper vertical between the fpl and fds (**a**) to horizontal superficially from the fds (**b**)

5 Variants and Congenital Anomalies

Numerous tendinous and osseous variants and anomalies exist (Freyschmidt et al. 2003; Keats 1981; Köhler and Zimmer 1989; Lawson 1985, 1994; Nayak et al. 2008; Oberg et al. 2010; Philip-Sarles 2008; Poznanski and Holt 1971; Stein et al. 2011; Timins 1999).

The number of tendons may vary (Albright and Linburg 1978; Chang et al. 2017; Elias and Schulter-Ellis 1985; Gümüşalan et al. 1997; Harvie et al. 2004; Jones et al. 1997; Martinoli et al. 2010; Meraj et al. 2017; Rixey et al. 2021; Rodríguez-Niedenführ et al. 2002; Schön et al. 1992; Sookur et al. 2008; Zeiss and Guilliam-Haidet 1996) from the absence of a tendon (Fig. 63; extensor pollicis brevis in compartment I) to a supernumerary tendon (Fig. 64; extensor carpi radialis accessories in compartment II).

Bones of the carpus may form a fibrous or bony coalition (Alemohammad et al. 2009; Burnett 2011; Cockshott 1963; Defazio et al. 2013; Devilliers Minnaar 1952; Ganos and Imbriglia 1991; Garn et al. 1971; Henry 1945; Mertens et al. 2023; Metz et al. 1993; Stäbler et al. 1999; Wharton and Ahearne 2021) (Fig. 65) and accessory carpal bones may be present as well (Berko et al. 2015; Greenspan and Gerscovich 1993; Hulten 1928; Kalantari et al. 2007) (Fig. 66).

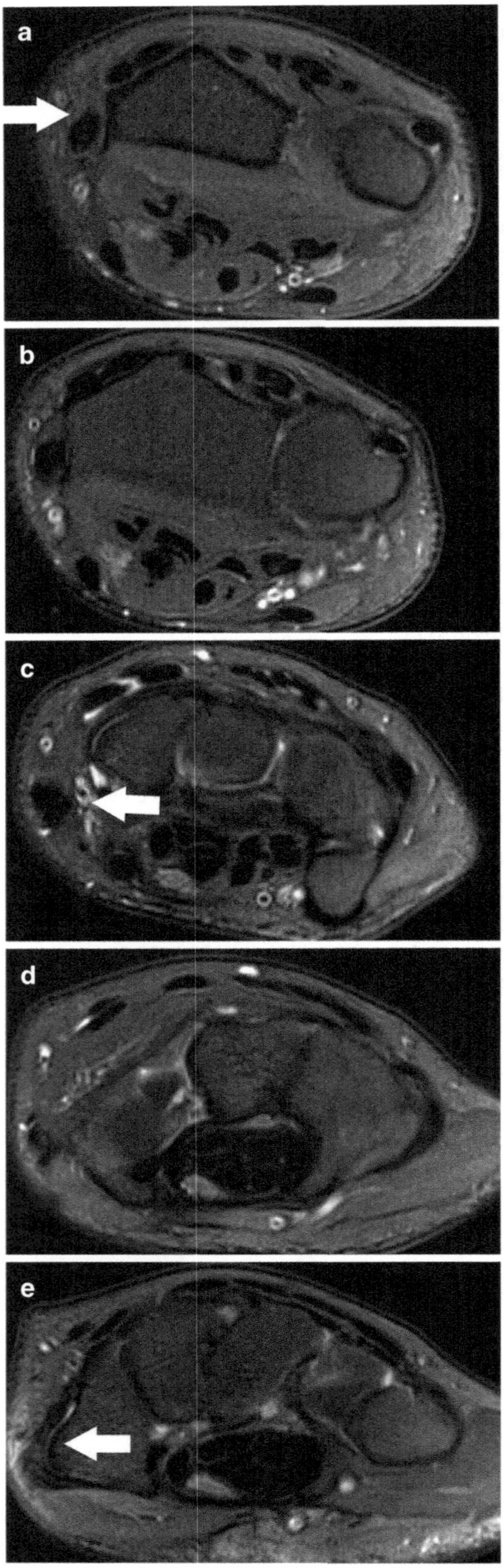

Fig. 63 Ax T2-WI FS. Absence of the extensor pollicis brevis tendon in compartment I (**a**–**e**)

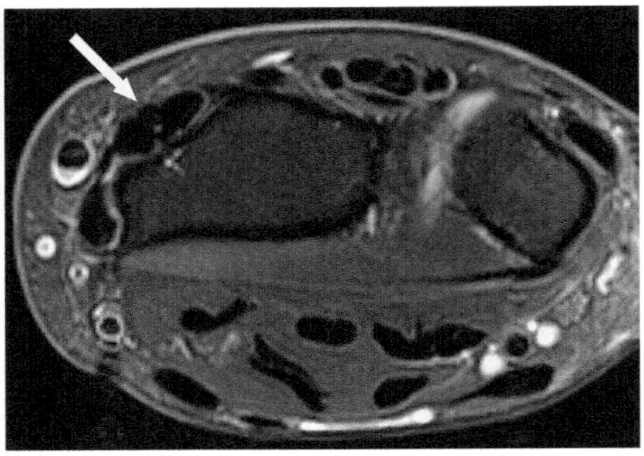

Fig. 64 Ax T2-WI FS. Supernumerary extensor carpi radialis accessories tendon in compartment II

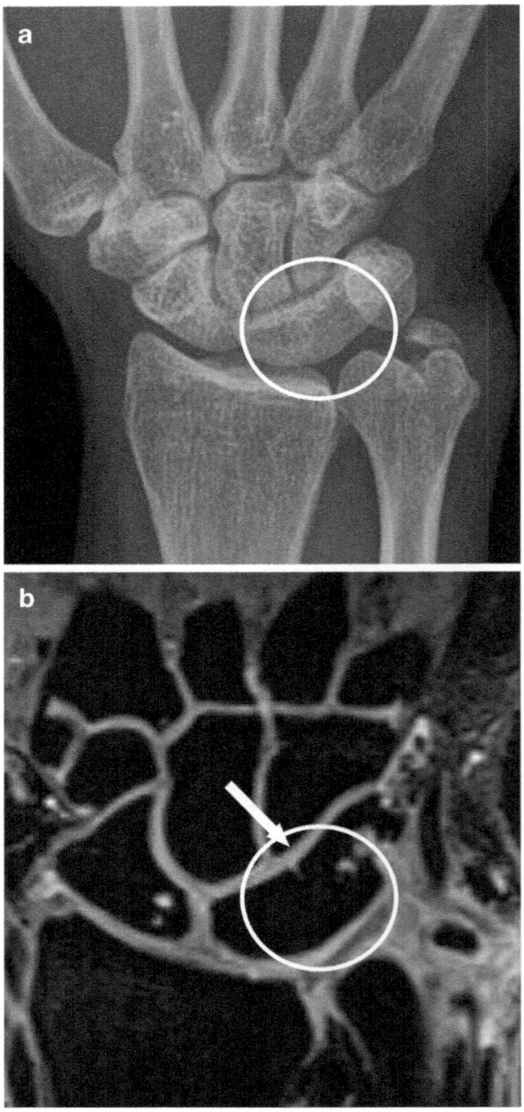

Fig. 65 Standard PA view (**a**) and Cor 3D-GRE (**b**). Bony L-T coalition

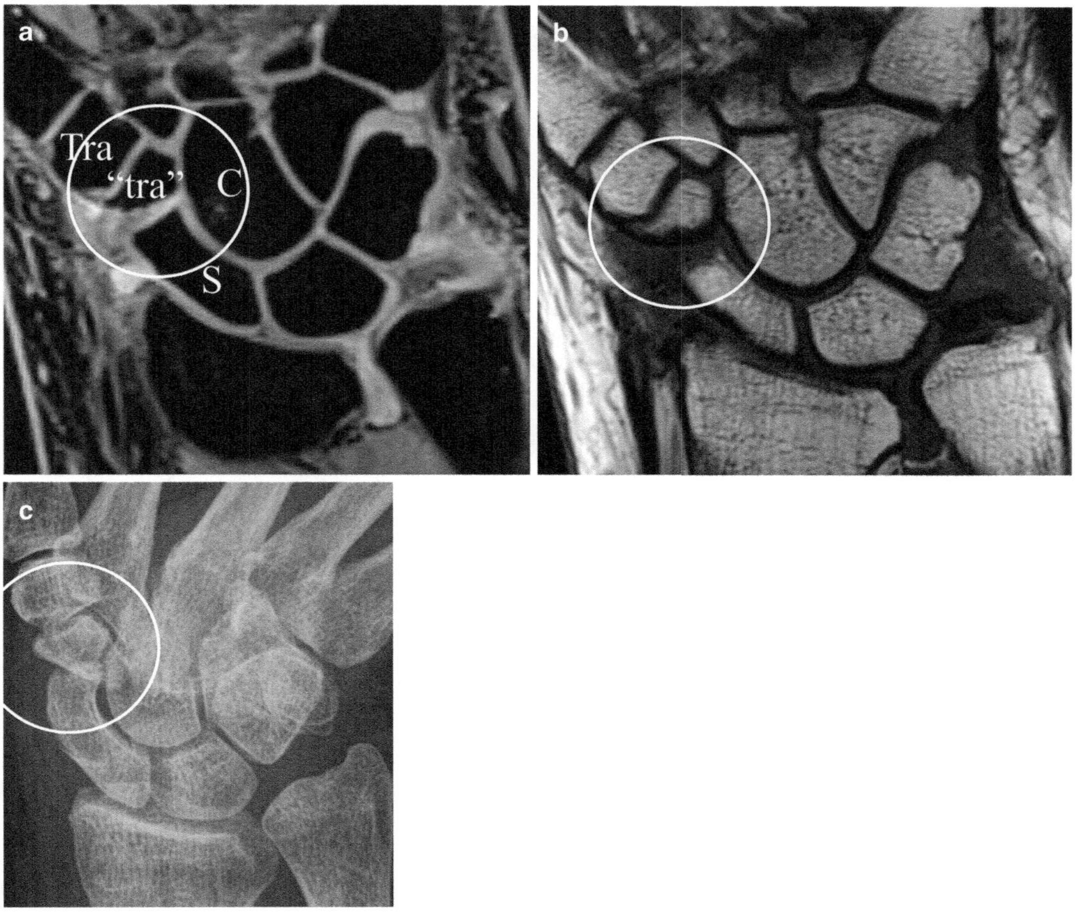

Fig. 66 Cor 3D-GRE (**a**), Cor T1-WI (**b**), and standard PA view (**c**). Accessory carpal bone between the Tra ans S

References

Albright JA, Linburg RM (1978) Common variations of the radial wrist extensors. J Hand Surg Am 3(2):134–138. https://doi.org/10.1016/s0363-5023(78)80060-4. PMID: 632542

Alemohammad AM, Nakamura K, El-Sheneway M, Viegas SF (2009) Incidence of carpal boss and osseous coalition: an anatomic study. J Hand Surg Am 34(1):1–6. https://doi.org/10.1016/j.jhsa.2008.08.025. Epub 2008 Dec 10. PMID: 19081681

Berko NS, Kurian J, Taragin BH, Thornhill BA (2015) Imaging appearances of musculoskeletal developmental variants in the pediatric population. Curr Probl Diagn Radiol 44(1):88–104. https://doi.org/10.1067/j.cpradiol.2014.06.002. Epub 2014 Nov 10. PMID: 25512169

Bhat AK, Kumar B, Acharya A (2011) Radiographic imaging of the wrist. Indian J Plast Surg 44(2):186–196. https://doi.org/10.4103/0970-0358.85339. PMID: 22022028; PMCID: PMC3193630

Bonnel F, Allieu Y (1984) Les articulations radio-cubito-carpienne et médio-carpienne. Organisation anatomique et bases biomécaniques [Radioulnocarpal and mediocarpal articulations. Anatomic organization and biomechanical bases]. Ann Chir Main 3(4):287–296. https://doi.org/10.1016/s0753-9053(84)80002-2. French. PMID: 6397151

Boutry N, Lapegue F, Masi L, Claret A, Demondion X, Cotten A (2005) Ultrasonographic evaluation of normal extrinsic and intrinsic carpal ligaments: preliminary experience. Skeletal Radiol 34(9):513–521. https://doi.org/10.1007/s00256-005-0929-4. Epub 2005 Jul 12. PMID: 16010593

Burnett SE (2011) Hamate-pisiform coalition: morphology, clinical significance, and a simplified classification scheme for carpal coalition. Clin Anat 24(2):188–196. https://doi.org/10.1002/ca.21086. Epub 2010 Nov 10. PMID: 21322040

Chang CY, Kheterpal AB, Vicentini JRT, Huang AJ (2017) Variations of anatomy on MRI of the first extensor compartment of the wrist and association with DeQuervain tenosynovitis. Skeletal Radiol

46(8):1047–1056. https://doi.org/10.1007/s00256-017-2639-0. Epub 2017 Apr 7. PMID: 28389821
Cockshott WP (1963) Carpal fusions. Am J Roentgenol Radium Therapy, Nucl Med 89:1260–1271. PMID: 14021907
Davis KW, Blankenbaker DG (2010) Imaging the ligaments and tendons of the wrist. Semin Roentgenol 45(3):194–217. https://doi.org/10.1053/j.ro.2009.12.005. PMID: 20483115
Defazio MV, Cousins BJ, Miversuski RA Jr, Cardoso R (2013) Carpal coalition: a review of current knowledge and report of a single institution's experience with asymptomatic intercarpal fusion. Hand (N Y) 8(2):157–163. https://doi.org/10.1007/s11552-013-9498-5. Erratum in: Hand (N Y). 2013 Jun;8(2):245. PMID: 24426912; PMCID: PMC3653005
Devilliers Minnaar AB (1952) Congenital fusion of the lunate and triquetral bones in the South African Bantu. J Bone Joint Surg Br 34-B(1):45–48. https://doi.org/10.1302/0301-620X.34B1.45. PMID: 12999869
Ekenstam F, Hagert CG (1985) Anatomical studies on the geometry and stability of the distal radio ulnar joint. Scand J Plast Reconstr Surg 19(1):17–25. https://doi.org/10.3109/02844318509052861. PMID: 4023639
Elias LS, Schulter-Ellis FP (1985) Anomalous flexor superficialis indicis: two case reports and literature review. J Hand Surg Am 10(2):296–299. https://doi.org/10.1016/s0363-5023(85)80128-3. PMID: 3980950
Freyschmidt J, Brossmann J, Wiens J, Sternberg A (2003) Freyschmidt. "Koehler/Zimmer" Borderlands of normal and early pathologic findings in skeletal radiography, 5th revised edn. Thieme Medical Publishers, New York. https://doi.org/10.1055/b-002-85526
Ganos DL, Imbriglia JE (1991) Symptomatic congenital coalition of the pisiform and hamate. J Hand Surg Am 16(4):646–650. https://doi.org/10.1016/0363-5023(91)90188-h. PMID: 1880361
Garn SM, Frisancho AR, Poznanski AK, Schweitzer J, McCann MB (1971) Analysis of triquetral-lunate fusion. Am J Phys Anthropol 34(3):431–433. https://doi.org/10.1002/ajpa.1330340313. PMID: 5120558
Gitto S, Draghi F (2016) Normal sonographic anatomy of the wrist with emphasis on assessment of tendons, nerves, and ligaments. J Ultrasound Med 35(5):1081–1094. https://doi.org/10.7863/ultra.15.06105. Epub 2016 Apr 1. PMID: 27036166
Gitto S, Messina C, Mauri G, Aliprandi A, Sardanelli F, Sconfienza LM (2017) Dynamic high-resolution ultrasound of intrinsic and extrinsic ligaments of the wrist: how to make it simple. Eur J Radiol 87:20–35. https://doi.org/10.1016/j.ejrad.2016.12.002. Epub 2016 Dec 5. PMID: 28065372
Greenspan A, Gerscovich EO (1993) Bilateral os centrale carpi: a rare congenital variant. J Hand Surg Am 18(4):586–587. https://doi.org/10.1016/0363-5023(93)90294-D. PMID: 8349961
Gümüşalan Y, Kalaycioğlu A, Yazar F, Arifoğlu Y, Sinav A (1997) Accessory extensor carpi radialis muscle and interconnecting muscular bundle. Acta Anat (Basel) 159(1):57–60. PMID: 9522898
Gunther SF (1984) The carpometacarpal joints. Orthop Clin North Am 15(2):259–277. PMID: 6728445
Harvie P, Patel N, Ostlere SJ (2004) Prevalence and epidemiological variation of anomalous muscles at guyon's canal. J Hand Surg Br 29(1):26–29. https://doi.org/10.1016/j.jhsb.2003.08.004. PMID: 14734065
Henry MG (1945) Anomalous fusion of the scaphoid and the greater multangular bone. Arch Surg 50(5):240–241. https://doi.org/10.1001/archsurg.1945.01230030249004
Hulten O (1928) Uber Anatomische Variationen der Handgelenkknochen. Acta Radiol 9(2):155–168. https://doi.org/10.3109/00016922809176658
Jones M, Abrahams PH, Sañudo JR, Campillo M (1997) Incidence and morphology of accessory heads of flexor pollicis longus and flexor digitorum profundus (Gantzer's muscles). J Anat 191(Pt 3):451–455. https://doi.org/10.1046/j.1469-7580.1997.19130451.x. PMID: 9419002; PMCID: PMC1467702
Kalantari BN, Seeger L, Motamedi K et al (2007) Accessory ossicles and sesamoid bones: spectrum of pathology and imaging evaluation. Appl Radiol 10:28–37
Keats TE (1981) Some new normal roentgen variants that may simulate disease. Curr Probl Diagn Radiol 10(3):1–52. https://doi.org/10.1016/0363-0188(81)90006-2. PMID: 6791877
Köhler A, Zimmer EA (1989) Grenzen des normalen und anfänge des pathologischen im röntgenbild des skeletts. George Thieme Verlag, Stutgart, pp 80–103
Lawson JP (1985) Symptomatic radiographic variants in extremities. Radiology 157(3):625–631. https://doi.org/10.1148/radiology.157.3.4059550. PMID: 4059550
Lawson JP (1994) International skeletal society lecture in honor of Howard D. Dorfman. Clinically significant radiologic anatomic variants of the skeleton. AJR Am J Roentgenol 163(2):249–255. https://doi.org/10.2214/ajr.163.2.8037009. PMID: 8037009
Lee RK, Griffith JF, Ng AW, Law EK, Tse WL, Wong CW, Ho PC (2017) Intrinsic carpal ligaments on MR and multidetector CT arthrography: comparison of axial and axial oblique planes. Eur Radiol 27(3):1277–1285. https://doi.org/10.1007/s00330-016-4436-x. Epub 2016 Jun 10. PMID: 27287482
Loredo RA, Sorge DG, Garcia G (2005) Radiographic evaluation of the wrist: a vanishing art. Semin Roentgenol 40(3):248–289. https://doi.org/10.1053/j.ro.2005.01.014. PMID: 16060116
MacLean S, Amarasooriya M, Bain GI (2021) Functional anatomy of the wrist. In: Arthroscopy and endoscopy of the elbow, wrist and hand. Springer, Cham, pp 553–561. https://doi.org/10.1007/978-3-030-79423-1_67
Manley M, Boardman M, Goitz RJ (2013) The carpal insertions of the transverse carpal ligament. J Hand Surg Am 38(4):729–732. https://doi.org/10.1016/j.jhsa.2013.01.015. PMID: 23537443

Martinoli C, Perez MM, Padua L, Valle M, Capaccio E, Altafini L, Michaud J, Tagliafico A (2010) Muscle variants of the upper and lower limb (with anatomical correlation). Semin Musculoskelet Radiol 14(2):106–121. https://doi.org/10.1055/s-0030-1253155. Epub 2010 May 18. PMID: 20486022

Meraj S, Gyftopoulos S, Nellans K, Walz D, Brown MS (2017) MRI of the extensor tendons of the wrist. AJR Am J Roentgenol 209(5):1093–1102. https://doi.org/10.2214/AJR.17.17791. Epub 2017 Aug 31. PMID: 28858545

Mertens K, Mespreuve M, Vanhoenacker FM (2023) Lunotriquetral coalition. Semin Musculoskelet Radiol 27(3):378–380. https://doi.org/10.1055/s--0043-1766108. Epub 2023 May 25. PMID: 37230136

Metz VM, Schimmerl SM, Gilula LA, Viegas SF, Saffar P (1993) Wide scapholunate joint space in lunotriquetral coalition: a normal variant? Radiology 188(2):557–559. https://doi.org/10.1148/radiology.188.2.8327715. PMID: 8327715

Nakamura T (2012) Anatomy and biomechanics of the distal radioulnar joint (DRUJ). In: Arthroscopic management of ulnar pain. Springer, Berlin/Heidelberg, pp 15–23. https://doi.org/10.1007/978-3-642-30544-3_2

Nakamura K, Patterson RM, Viegas SF (2001a) The ligament and skeletal anatomy of the second through fifth carpometacarpal joints and adjacent structures. J Hand Surg Am 26(6):1016–1029. https://doi.org/10.1053/jhsu.2001.26329. PMID: 11721245

Nakamura T, Takayama S, Horiuchi Y, Yabe Y (2001b) Origins and insertions of the triangular fibrocartilage complex: a histological study. J Hand Surg Br 26(5):446–454. https://doi.org/10.1054/jhsb.2001.0562. PMID: 11560427

Nayak SR, Krishnamurthy A, Prabhu LV, Rai R, Ranade AV, Madhyastha S (2008) Anatomical variation of radial wrist extensor muscles: a study in cadavers. Clinics (Sao Paulo) 63(1):85–90. https://doi.org/10.1590/s1807-59322008000100015. PMID: 18297212; PMCID: PMC2664178

Oberg KC, Feenstra JM, Manske PR, Tonkin MA (2010) Developmental biology and classification of congenital anomalies of the hand and upper extremity. J Hand Surg Am 35(12):2066–2076. https://doi.org/10.1016/j.jhsa.2010.09.031. PMID: 21134615

Philip-Sarles N (2008) Malformations congénitales de la main et génétique [Genetics of congenital hand malformations]. Chir Main 27(Suppl 1):S7–S20. https://doi.org/10.1016/j.main.2008.07.011. French. Epub 2008 Aug 20. PMID: 18838287

Poznanski AK, Holt JF (1971) The carpals in congenital malformation syndromes. Am J Roentgenol Radium Therapy, Nucl Med 112(3):443–459. https://doi.org/10.2214/ajr.112.3.443. PMID: 5570355

Pulos N, Bozentka DJ (2015) Carpal ligament anatomy and biomechanics. Hand Clin 31(3):381–387. https://doi.org/10.1016/j.hcl.2015.04.007. PMID: 26205699

Ringler MD (2013) MRI of wrist ligaments. J Hand Surg Am 38(10):2034–2046. https://doi.org/10.1016/j.jhsa.2013.02.042. Epub 2013 May 6. PMID: 23660198

Ringler MD, Murthy NS (2015) MR imaging of wrist ligaments. Magn Reson Imaging Clin N Am 23(3):367–391. https://doi.org/10.1016/j.mric.2015.04.007. PMID: 26216769

Ritt MJ, Bishop AT, Berger RA, Linscheid RL, Berglund LJ, An KN (1998) Lunotriquetral ligament properties: a comparison of three anatomic subregions. J Hand Surg Am 23(3):425–431. https://doi.org/10.1016/S0363-5023(05)80460-5. PMID: 9620183

Rixey A, Wenger D, Baffour F, Kakar S, McKenzie G (2021) Accessory abductor digiti minimi muscle, less muscular than thought: an update on prevalence, morphology, and review of the literature. Skeletal Radiol 50(8):1687–1695. https://doi.org/10.1007/s00256-021-03728-5. Epub 2021 Feb 3. PMID: 33533963

Rodríguez-Niedenführ M, Vázquez T, Golanó P, Parkin I, Sañudo JR (2002) Extensor digitorum brevis manus: anatomical, radiological and clinical relevance. A review. Clin Anat 15(4):286–292. https://doi.org/10.1002/ca.10027. PMID: 12112357

Scheck RJ, Romagnolo A, Hierner R, Pfluger T, Wilhelm K, Hahn K (1999) The carpal ligaments in MR arthrography of the wrist: correlation with standard MRI and wrist arthroscopy. J Magn Reson Imaging 9(3):468–474. https://doi.org/10.1002/(sici)1522-2586(199903)9:3<468::aid-jmri16>3.0.co;2-t. PMID: 10194719

Schmid MR, Schertler T, Pfirrmann CW, Saupe N, Manestar M, Wildermuth S, Weishaupt D (2005) Interosseous ligament tears of the wrist: comparison of multi-detector row CT arthrography and MR imaging. Radiology 237(3):1008–1013. https://doi.org/10.1148/radiol.2373041450. PMID: 16304116

Schmitt R, Christopoulos G, Meier R, Coblenz G, Fröhner S, Lanz U, Krimmer H (2003) Direkte MR-Arthrographie des Handgelenks im Vergleich zur Arthroskopie: Eine prospektive Studie an 125 Patienten [Direct MR arthrography of the wrist in comparison with arthroscopy: a prospective study on 125 patients]. Rofo 175(7):911–919. https://doi.org/10.1055/s-2003-40434. German. PMID: 12847645

Schön R, Kraus E, Boller O, Kampe A (1992) Anomalous muscle belly of the flexor digitorum superficialis associated with carpal tunnel syndrome: case report. Neurosurgery 31(5):969–970. https://doi.org/10.1227/00006123-199211000-00026; discussion 970–971. PMID: 1436428

Sennwald GR, Zdravkovic V, Oberlin C (1994) The anatomy of the palmar scaphotriquetral ligament. J Bone Joint Surg Br 76(1):147–149. PMID: 8300661

Shahabpour M, De Maeseneer M, Pouders C, Van Overstraeten L, Ceuterick P, Fierens Y, Goubau J, De Mey J (2011) MR imaging of normal extrinsic wrist ligaments using thin slices with clinical and surgical correlation. Eur J Radiol 77(2):196–201. https://doi.org/10.1016/j.ejrad.2010.05.043. PMID: 20599335

Shahabpour M, Staelens B, Van Overstraeten L, De Maeseneer M, Boulet C, De Mey J, Scheerlinck T (2015) Advanced imaging of the scapholunate ligamentous complex. Skeletal Radiol 44(12):1709–1725.

https://doi.org/10.1007/s00256-015-2182-9. Epub 2015 Jul 30. PMID: 26219592

Sookur PA, Naraghi AM, Bleakney RR, Jalan R, Chan O, White LM (2008) Accessory muscles: anatomy, symptoms, and radiologic evaluation. Radiographics 28(2):481–499. https://doi.org/10.1148/rg.282075064. PMID: 18349452

Stäbler A, Glaser C, Reiser M, Resnick D (1999) Symptomatic fibrous lunato-triquetral coalition. Eur Radiol 9(8):1643–1646. https://doi.org/10.1007/s003300050901. PMID: 10525882

Stein JM, Cook TS, Simonson S, Kim W (2011) Normal and variant anatomy of the wrist and hand on MR imaging. Magn Reson Imaging Clin N Am 19(3):595–608. https://doi.org/10.1016/j.mric.2011.05.007; ix. PMID: 21816333

Theumann NH, Pfirrmann CW, Chung CB, Antonio GE, Trudell DJ, Resnick D (2002) Ligamentous and tendinous anatomy of the intermetacarpal and common carpometacarpal joints: evaluation with MR imaging and MR arthrography. J Comput Assist Tomogr 26(1):145–152. https://doi.org/10.1097/00004728-200201000-00026. PMID: 11801922

Timins ME (1999) Osseous anatomic variants of the wrist: findings on MR imaging. AJR Am J Roentgenol 173(2):339–344. https://doi.org/10.2214/ajr.173.2.10430131. PMID: 10430131

Wharton RMH, Ahearne D (2021) Bilateral STT arthrodesis in a young patient with occult proximal row coalition. J Wrist Surg 11(6):546–549. https://doi.org/10.1055/s-0041-1740137. PMID: 36504535; PMCID: PMC9731740

Zancolli EA, Ziadenberg C, Zancolli E Jr (1987) Biomechanics of the trapeziometacarpal joint. Clin Orthop Relat Res 220:14–26. PMID: 3594983

Zdravkovic V, Sennwald GR, Fischer M, Jacob HA (1994) The palmar wrist ligaments revisited, clinical relevance. Ann Chir Main Memb Super 13(5):378–382. https://doi.org/10.1016/s0753-9053(05)80078-x. PMID: 7531477

Zeiss J, Guilliam-Haidet L (1996) MR demonstration of anomalous muscles about the volar aspect of the wrist and forearm. Clin Imaging 20(3):219–221. https://doi.org/10.1016/0899-7071(95)00013-5. PMID: 8877177

Zhan H, Bai R, Qian Z, Yang Y, Zhang H, Yin Y (2020) Traumatic injury of the triangular fibrocartilage complex (TFCC)-a refinement to the Palmer classification by using high-resolution 3-T MRI. Skeletal Radiol 49(10):1567–1579. https://doi.org/10.1007/s00256-020-03438-4. Epub 2020 May 5. PMID: 32372253

Zheng ZZ, Shan H, Li X (2010) Fat-suppressed 3D T1-weighted gradient-echo imaging of the cartilage with a volumetric interpolated breath-hold examination. AJR Am J Roentgenol 194(5):W414–W419. https://doi.org/10.2214/AJR.09.2423. PMID: 20410387

Zlatkin MB, Rosner J (2006) MR imaging of ligaments and triangular fibrocartilage complex of the wrist. Radiol Clin North Am 44(4):595–623. https://doi.org/10.1016/j.rcl.2006.04.010; ix. PMID: 16829252

MRI Techniques

Contents

The most essential in MRI techniques (Davis and Blankenbaker 2010; Girgis and Epstein 2000; Lee et al. 2013a; Magee 2009; Ochman et al. 2017; Oneson et al. 1997; Quinn et al. 1989; Ringler and Murthy 2015; Shahabpour et al. 2011, 2015; Stecco et al. 2019; Zheng et al. 2010; Zlatkin and Rosner 2006) is the use of a dedicated wrist coil (Fig. 1) in order to realise an optimal image resolution. The wrist should be as much as possible in the centre of the gantry. Therefore, the patient is positioned in the "superman position" and immobilised with pillows in a 30° right or left oblique anterior position depending on the wrist to be examined.

The coronal slices are parallel to the dorsal side of the wrist. A first general approach needs coronal plain T1- and T2-weighted sequences. At least one sequence should be isotropic with a reconstruction of images in the three orthogonal dimensions (Fig. 2).

As 1.5 Tesla machines are still in a majority position, and in order to show the possibility of achieving a good resolution, an overview of a possible standard diagram of sequences is displayed (Table 1). In principle, these are always implemented as a basic study.

Supplementary mobility images (Boutin et al. 2013; Chaudhari et al. 2023; Li et al. 2022; MacLean et al. 2021; Rauch et al. 2018; Shaw et al. 2019; Sulkers et al. 2018) in pro- and supination (Fig. 3) may be added to evaluate the ulnar head position at the DRUJ. A series of short 2D GRE sequences without wrist coil in five different positions from radial to ulnar deviation (Fig. 4) may be added as well and/or eventually correlated with classical motion X-rays (Fig. 5).

Additional sequences after IV contrast enhancement (Sulkers et al. 2018; Barbieri et al. 2013; Bashir et al. 2014; Boeren et al. 2023; Dakkak et al. 2020; Fujimori et al. 2017; Mysling et al. 2013; Ruston et al. 2013) will depend on the pathology or specific clinical information.

MR arthrography (Cerezal et al. 2005; Lee et al. 2013b; Mutimer et al. 2008; Scheck et al. 1999; Schmid et al. 2005; Theumann et al. 2002) (Fig. 6) is always considered only in a second time for possible ligamentous lesions or after surgical repair, and after consulting the referring physician(s) concerning the result of the plain MRI. The midcarpal arthrography is preferred if only one compartment is injected, and Cor T1-WI with FS and 3D-GRE imaging are implemented.

M. Mespreuve, K. Waked, *MRI of the Wrist*, Medical Radiology,
https://doi.org/10.1007/978-3-031-63973-9_2

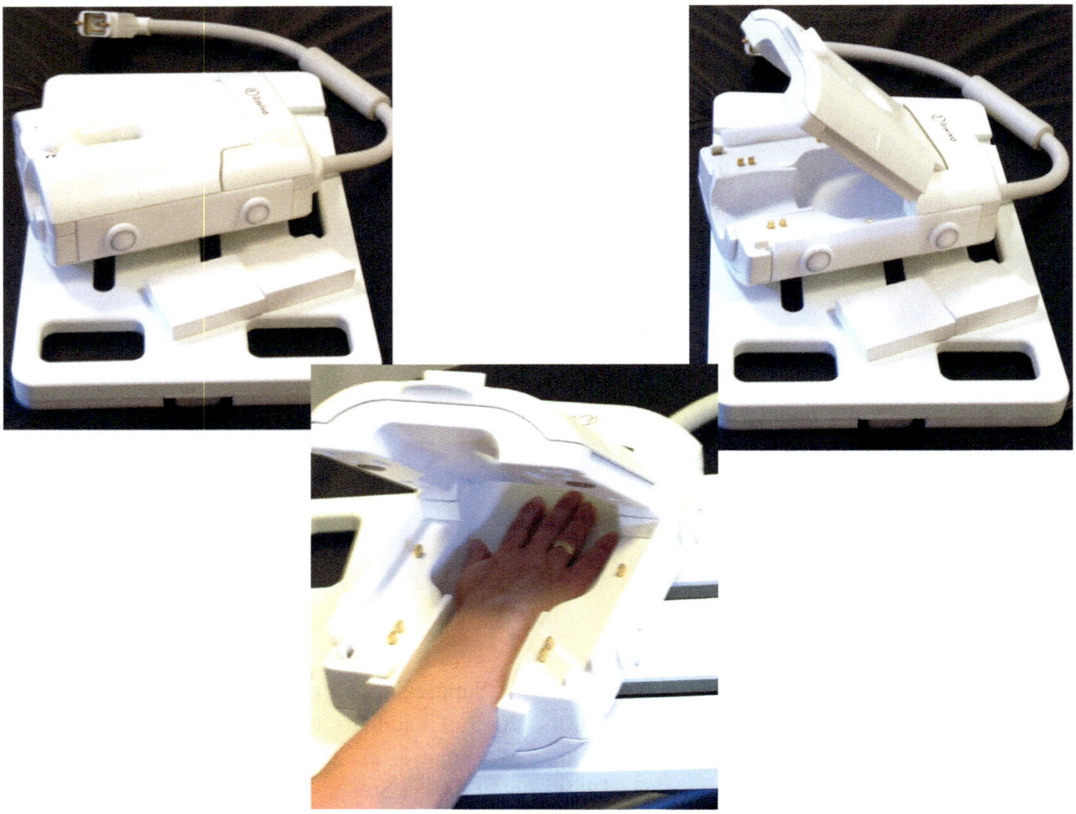

Fig. 1 Dedicated wrist coil. The use of a dedicated wrist coil is essential

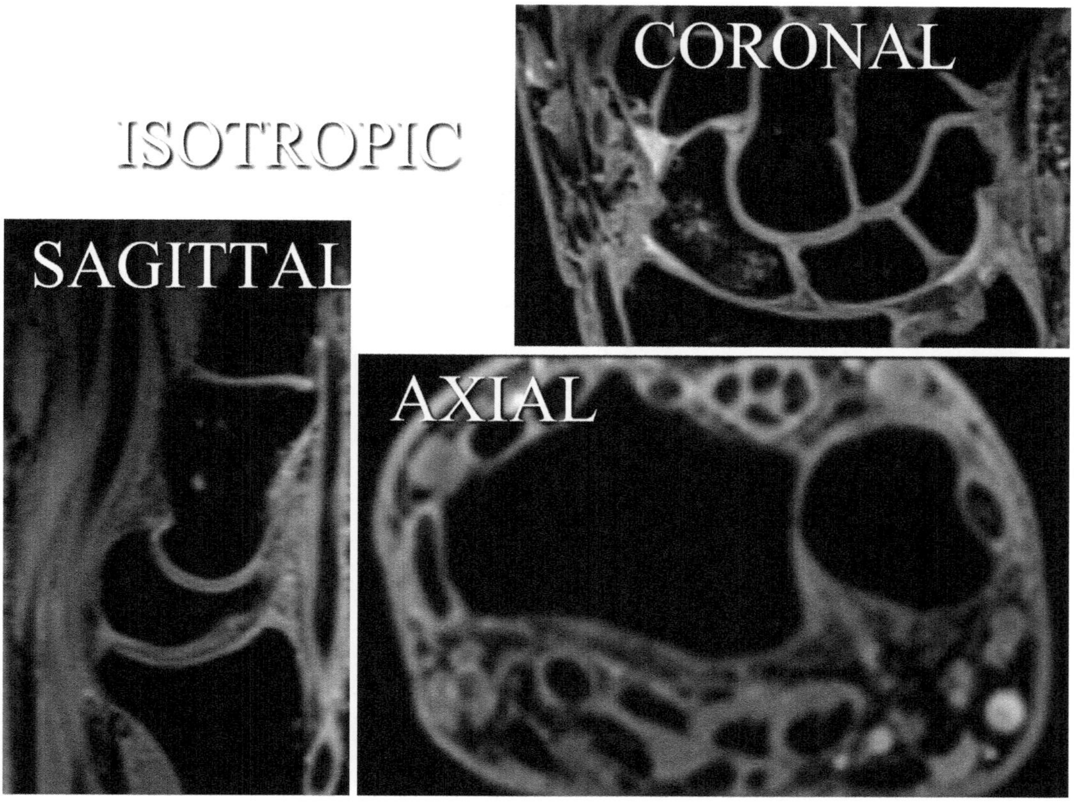

Fig. 2 Isotropic 3D-GRE with reconstructions in the three dimensions

Table 1 Standard diagram of sequences on 1.5 Tesla machines

		TR	TE	FOV (cm)	Slice (mm)	Gap (%)	matrix	NEX	kHz	ETL	Time (sec)	TOT
Pd/T2 FS	Cor	3500	26/91	120	2	20	256 (70%)	3	130	5	3′ 18″	
T1-SE	Cor	479	22	120	2	20	512 (75%)	1	65	/	3′ 36″	
2D T2*GE (FLASH)	Cor	369	15	120	2	20	256 (70%)	3	60	/	3′ 21″	
3D T2*GE (DESS) of True FISP	Cor Cor	23,59 10,54	8,31 4,75	120 120	0.5 0.5	20 20	256 (90%) 256 (100%)	1 1	150 235	/ /	5′ 00″ 4′ 24″	
PD-TSE FS	Ax	1950	27	100	3	10	320 (80%)	2	130	5	2′ 26″	**16′ 25″ 16′ 27″**

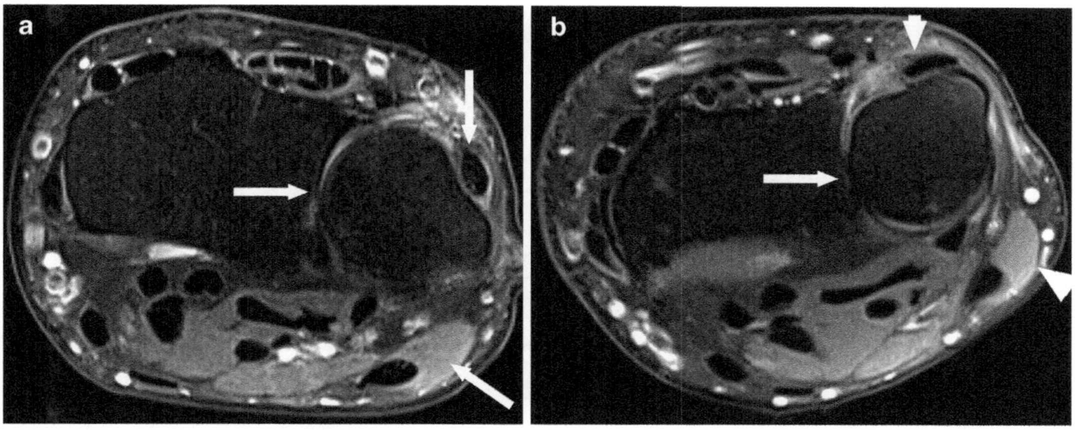

Fig. 3 Ax T2-WI FS. Mobility images in pro- and supination. The U remains centered, the ECU does not leave the sulcus, and the FCU moves laterodorsally

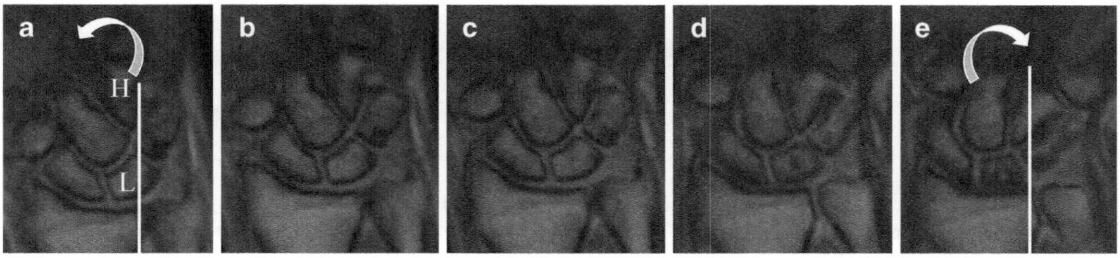

Fig. 4 Short Cor 2D-GRE (TR 7.7; TE 3.28; EC 1; khz 90; thk 6). Mobility of the carpal bones in maximal (**a**) and intermediate (**b**) radial deviation, over neutral position (**c**), to intermediate (**d**) and maximal (**e**) ulnar deviation

Fig. 5 Standard PA view in maximal radial and ulnar deviation. Mobility of the carpal bones at the radio- and mediocarpal joint

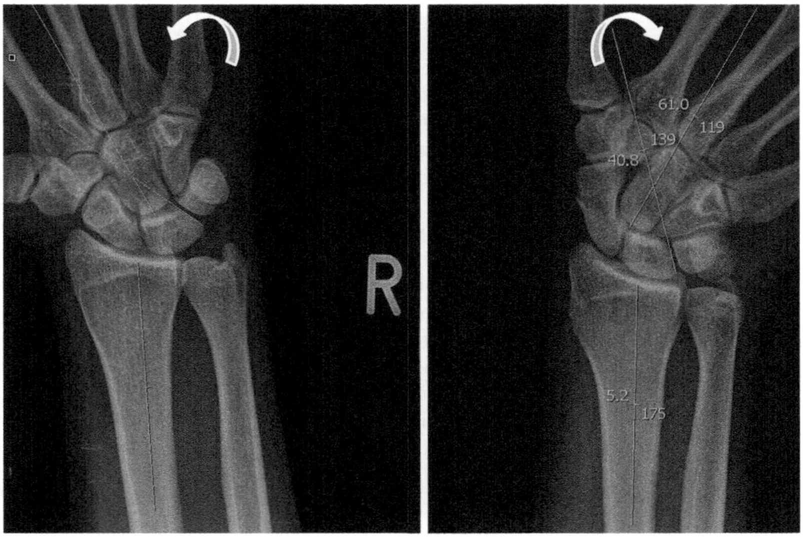

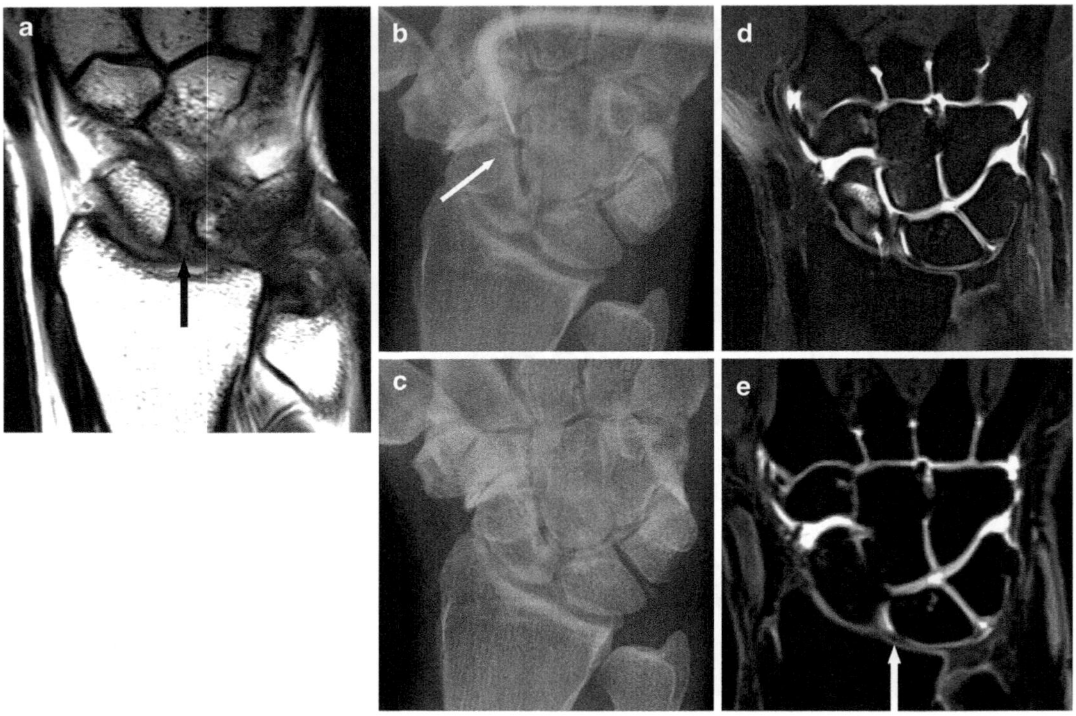

Fig. 6 Cor T1-WI (**a**); Standard PA view during midcarpal injection (**b**), and after mobilisation (**c**); Cor T1-WI FS (**d**), and 3D GRE (**e**). Plain MRI after surgery (**a**) shows a doubtful configuration of the SL ligament. After a midcarpal diluted gadolinium contrast injection (**b**) and mobilisation (**c**), a coronal T1-WI FS and a 3D GRE imaging show a continuously delineated SL ligament without contrast leakage to the radiocarpal joint

References

Barbieri F, Parascandolo P, Vosilla L, Cesario L, Viano G, Cimmino MA (2013) Assessing MRI erosions in the rheumatoid wrist: a comparison between RAMRIS and a semiautomated segmentation software. Ann Rheum Dis 71(Suppl 3):709–709. https://doi.org/10.1136/annrheumdis-2012-eular.1253

Bashir W, Aziz A, Jidaal I (2014) Imaging of skeletal extremity trauma: a review. Trauma 16:300–317. https://doi.org/10.1177/1460408614542920

Boeren AMP, Niemantsverdriet E, Verstappen M, Wouters F, Bloem JL, Reijnierse M, van der Helm-van Mil AHM (2023) Towards a simplified fluid-sensitive MRI protocol in small joints of the hand in early arthritis patients: reliability between modified Dixon and regular Gadolinium enhanced TSE fat saturated MRI-sequences. Skeletal Radiol 52(6):1193–1202. https://doi.org/10.1007/s00256-022-04238-8. Epub 2022 Nov 28. PMID: 36441238

Boutin RD, Buonocore MH, Immerman I, Ashwell Z, Sonico GJ, Szabo RM, Chaudhari AJ (2013) Real-time magnetic resonance imaging (MRI) during active wrist motion – initial observations. PLoS One 8(12):e84004. https://doi.org/10.1371/journal.pone.0084004. PMID: 24391865; PMCID: PMC3877133

Cerezal L, Abascal F, García-Valtuille R, Del Piñal F (2005) Wrist MR arthrography: how, why, when. Radiol Clin North Am 43(4):709–731. https://doi.org/10.1016/j.rcl.2005.02.004, viii. PMID: 15893533

Chaudhari AJ, Lim Y, Cui SX, Bayne CO, Szabo RM, Boutin RD, Nayak KS (2023) Real-time MRI of the moving wrist at 0.55 tesla. Br J Radiol 96(1151):20230298. https://doi.org/10.1259/bjr.20230298. Epub 2023 Oct 11. PMID: 37750944; PMCID: PMC10607422

Dakkak YJ, Matthijssen XME, van der Heijde D, Reijnierse M, van der Helm-van Mil AHM (2020) Reliability of magnetic resonance imaging (MRI) scoring of the metatarsophalangeal joints of the foot according to the rheumatoid arthritis MRI score. J Rheumatol 47(8):1165–1173. https://doi.org/10.3899/jrheum.190258. Epub 2019 Sep 15. PMID: 31523041; PMCID: PMC7115895

Davis KW, Blankenbaker DG (2010) Imaging the ligaments and tendons of the wrist. Semin Roentgenol 45(3):194–217. https://doi.org/10.1053/j.ro.2009.12.005. PMID: 20483115

Fujimori M, Nakamura S, Hasegawa K, Ikeno K, Ichikawa S, Sutherland K, Kamishima T (2017) Cartilage quantification using contrast-enhanced MRI in the wrist of rheumatoid arthritis: cartilage loss is associated with bone marrow edema. Br J Radiol 90(1077):20170167. https://doi.org/10.1259/bjr.20170167. Epub 2017 Jul 14. PMID: 28707530; PMCID: PMC5858812

Girgis WS, Epstein RE (2000) Magnetic resonance imaging of the hand and wrist. Semin Roentgenol 35(3):286–296. https://doi.org/10.1053/sroe.2000.7339. PMID: 10939130

Lee YH, Choi YR, Kim S, Song HT, Suh JS (2013a) Intrinsic ligament and triangular fibrocartilage complex (TFCC) tears of the wrist: comparison of isovolumetric 3D-THRIVE sequence MR arthrography and conventional MR image at 3 T. Magn Reson Imaging 31(2):221–226. https://doi.org/10.1016/j.mri.2012.06.024. Epub 2012 Sep 7. PMID: 22959873

Lee RK, Ng AW, Tong CS, Griffith JF, Tse WL, Wong C, Ho PC (2013b) Intrinsic ligament and triangular fibrocartilage complex tears of the wrist: comparison of MDCT arthrography, conventional 3-T MRI, and MR arthrography. Skeletal Radiol 42(9):1277–1285. https://doi.org/10.1007/s00256-013-1666-8. Epub 2013 Jun 28. PMID: 23812413

Li J, Rath B, Hildebrand F, Eschweiler J (2022) Wrist bone motion during flexion-extension and radial-ulnar deviation: an MRI study. Life (Basel) 12(10):1458. https://doi.org/10.3390/life12101458. PMID: 36294894; PMCID: PMC9605103

MacLean S, Amarasooriya M, Bain GI (2021) Functional anatomy of the wrist. In: Arthroscopy and endoscopy of the elbow, wrist and hand. Springer, Cham, pp 553–561. https://doi.org/10.1007/978-3-030-79423-1_67

Magee T (2009) Comparison of 3-T MRI and arthroscopy of intrinsic wrist ligament and TFCC tears. AJR Am J Roentgenol 192(1):80–85. https://doi.org/10.2214/AJR.08.1089. PMID: 19098183

Mutimer J, Green J, Field J (2008) Comparison of MRI and wrist arthroscopy for assessment of wrist cartilage. J Hand Surg Eur 33(3):380–382. https://doi.org/10.1177/1753193408090395. PMID: 18562375

Mysling P, Dam E, Zaim S, Genant HK, Fuerst T, Lillholm M (2013) An evaluation of a novel technique for fully automatic synovitis quantification from pre- and post-contrast wrist MRI. Ann Rheum Dis 71(Suppl 3):303–304. https://doi.org/10.1136/annrheumdis-2012-eular.2404

Ochman S, Wieskötter B, Langer M, Vieth V, Raschke MJ, Stehling C (2017) High-resolution MRI (3T-MRI) in diagnosis of wrist pain: is diagnostic arthroscopy still necessary? Arch Orthop Trauma Surg 137(10):1443–1450. https://doi.org/10.1007/s00402-017-2747-2. Epub 2017 Aug 14. PMID: 28808768

Oneson SR, Timins ME, Scales LM, Erickson SJ, Chamoy L (1997) MR imaging diagnosis of triangular fibrocartilage pathology with arthroscopic correlation. AJR Am J Roentgenol 168(6):1513–1518. https://doi.org/10.2214/ajr.168.6.9168716. PMID: 9168716

Quinn SF, Belsole RJ, Greene TL, Rayhack JM (1989) Advanced imaging of the wrist. Radiographics 9(2):229–246. https://doi.org/10.1148/radiographics.9.2.2928572. PMID: 2928572

Rauch A, Arab WA, Dap F, Dautel G, Blum A, Gondim Teixeira PA (2018) Four-dimensional CT analysis of wrist kinematics during radioulnar deviation. Radiology 289(3):750–758. https://doi.org/10.1148/radiol.2018180640. Epub 2018 Sep 25. PMID: 30251928

Ringler MD, Murthy NS (2015) MR imaging of wrist ligaments. Magn Reson Imaging Clin N Am 23(3):367–391. https://doi.org/10.1016/j.mric.2015.04.007. PMID: 26216769

Ruston J, Konan S, Rubinraut E, Sorene E (2013) Diagnostic accuracy of clinical examination and magnetic resonance imaging for common articular wrist pathology. Acta Orthop Belg 79(4):375–380. PMID: 24205765

Scheck RJ, Romagnolo A, Hierner R, Pfluger T, Wilhelm K, Hahn K (1999) The carpal ligaments in MR arthrography of the wrist: correlation with standard MRI and wrist arthroscopy. J Magn Reson Imaging 9(3):468–474. https://doi.org/10.1002/(sici)1522-2586(199903)9:3<468::aid-jmri16>3.0.co;2-t. PMID: 10194719

Schmid MR, Schertler T, Pfirrmann CW, Saupe N, Manestar M, Wildermuth S, Weishaupt D (2005) Interosseous ligament tears of the wrist: comparison of multi-detector row CT arthrography and MR imaging. Radiology 237(3):1008–1013. https://doi.org/10.1148/radiol.2373041450. PMID: 16304116

Shahabpour M, De Maeseneer M, Pouders C, Van Overstraeten L, Ceuterick P, Fierens Y, Goubau J, De Mey J (2011) MR imaging of normal extrinsic wrist ligaments using thin slices with clinical and surgical correlation. Eur J Radiol 77(2):196–201. https://doi.org/10.1016/j.ejrad.2010.05.043. PMID: 20599335

Shahabpour M, Staelens B, Van Overstraeten L, De Maeseneer M, Boulet C, De Mey J, Scheerlinck T (2015) Advanced imaging of the scapholunate ligamentous complex. Skeletal Radiol 44(12):1709–1725. https://doi.org/10.1007/s00256-015-2182-9. Epub 2015 Jul 30. PMID: 26219592

Shaw CB, Foster BH, Borgese M, Boutin RD, Bateni C, Boonsri P, Bayne CO, Szabo RM, Nayak KS, Chaudhari AJ (2019) Real-time three-dimensional MRI for the assessment of dynamic carpal instability. PLoS One 14(9):e0222704. https://doi.org/10.1371/journal.pone.0222704. PMID: 31536561; PMCID: PMC6752861

Stecco A, Arioli R, Buemi F, Parziale G, Trisoglio A, Soligo E, Cerini P, Leigheb M, Brambilla M, Di Nardo G, Guzzardi G, Carriero A (2019) Overcoming metallic artefacts from orthopaedic wrist volar plating on a low-field MRI scanner. Radiol Med

124(5):392–399. https://doi.org/10.1007/s11547-018-0973-5. Epub 2018 Dec 17. PMID: 30560500

Sulkers GSI, Strackee SD, Schep NWL, Maas M (2018) Wrist cineradiography: a protocol for diagnosing carpal instability. J Hand Surg Eur 43(2):174–178. https://doi.org/10.1177/1753193417694820. Epub 2017 Mar 1. PMID: 28488457; PMCID: PMC5791518

Theumann NH, Pfirrmann CW, Chung CB, Antonio GE, Trudell DJ, Resnick D (2002) Ligamentous and tendinous anatomy of the intermetacarpal and common carpometacarpal joints: evaluation with MR imaging and MR arthrography. J Comput Assist Tomogr 26(1):145–152. https://doi.org/10.1097/00004728-200201000-00026. PMID: 11801922

Zheng ZZ, Shan H, Li X (2010) Fat-suppressed 3D T1-weighted gradient-echo imaging of the cartilage with a volumetric interpolated breath-hold examination. AJR Am J Roentgenol 194(5):W414–W419. https://doi.org/10.2214/AJR.09.2423. PMID: 20410387

Zlatkin MB, Rosner J (2006) MR imaging of ligaments and triangular fibrocartilage complex of the wrist. Radiol Clin North Am 44(4):595–623. https://doi.org/10.1016/j.rcl.2006.04.010, ix. PMID: 16829252

Part II

Section on Traumatic Pathology

Fractures of the Carpal Bones

Contents

1 General

Fractures may occur in all the eight of the carpal bones (Balci et al. 2015; Bashir et al. 2014; Bencardino and Rosenberg 2006; Bhat et al. 2011; Bruno et al. 2019; Gilula 1979; Jørgsholm et al. 2016; Lee et al. 2021; Lok et al. 2014; Loredo et al. 2005; Matthews et al. 2019; Meyer 1991; Nance et al. 2017; Rettig 2003; Welling et al. 2008; Yaghoubian et al. 2001) (Fig. 1). Although the pisiform bone is by some authors considered as a sesamoid bone and "not a real carpal bone", we will include it in this discussion.

The radial column is mostly affected, especially the scaphoid bone (Fig. 1; Table 1). Standard X-ray views are still the first technique to evaluate the status of the carpal bones. However, it is fairly known that about 33% of all carpal bone fracture are missed and the distribution changes a lot when cross-sectional imaging is used (Welling et al. 2008; Borgeskov et al. 1966) (Table 1: CT versus plain film). Moreover, MRI has a very high sensitivity for detecting fractures in general thanks to its additional sensitivity for signal changes. For scaphoid fractures, MRI is even considered as the golden standard (Couzens et al. 2014; Eriksen and Ringe 2012;

M. Mespreuve, K. Waked, *MRI of the Wrist*, Medical Radiology,
https://doi.org/10.1007/978-3-031-63973-9_3

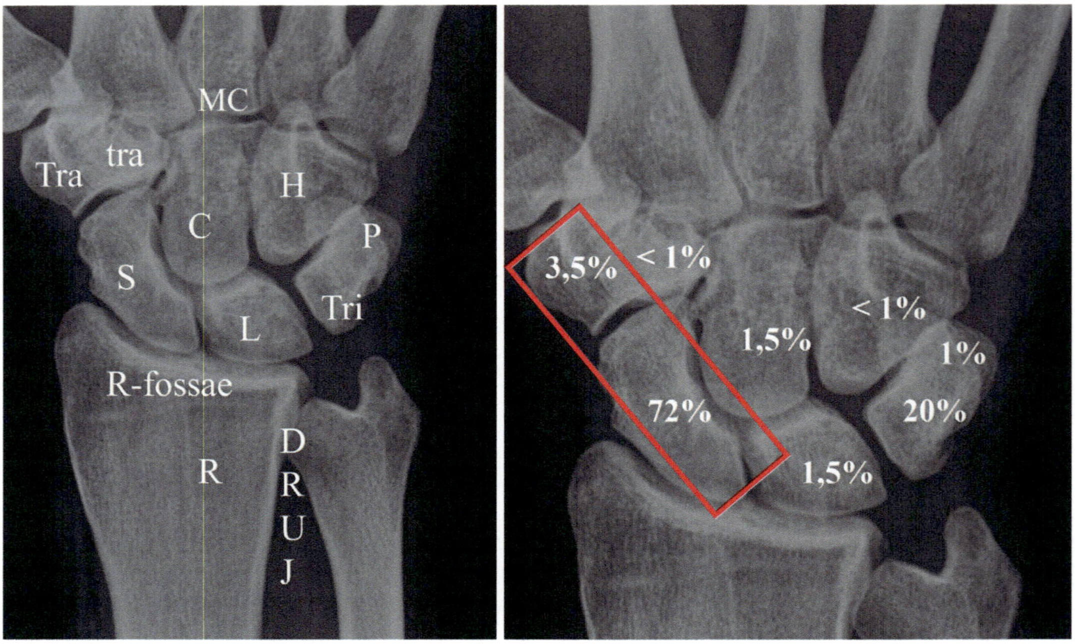

Fig. 1 Distribution (%) of fractures over the carpus on standard views (Borgeskov et al. 1966)

Table 1 Distribution of fractures on plain film and CT

Bone	X-rays (% of distribution) (Borgeskov et al. 1966)	CT (% of distribution) (Welling et al. 2008)	≠
Scaphoid	**72**	42	
Lunate	1.5	**8**	**
Triquetral	**20**	13	
Pisiform	1	**3**	*
Trapezium	3.5	**8**	*
Trapezoïd	< 1	**8**	**
Capitate	1.5	**5**	*
Hamate	< 1	**13**	***

Faccioli et al. 2010; Gornitzky and Carrigan 2016; Khalid et al. 2006; Mack et al. 2003; Ochman et al. 2017; Quinn et al. 1989; Ruston et al. 2013) (Figs. 2 and 3), mainly to evaluate avascular necrosis of the proximal pole. CT cross-sectional imaging will also reveal most fractures (Fig. 4), but MRI has the added advantage of avoiding radiation. Both CT and MRI are not hindered by a cast (Fig. 5). However, in the acute phase, access to the CT is easier and may frequently reveal (an) unexpected fracture(s) and dislocation(s) (Fig. 6).

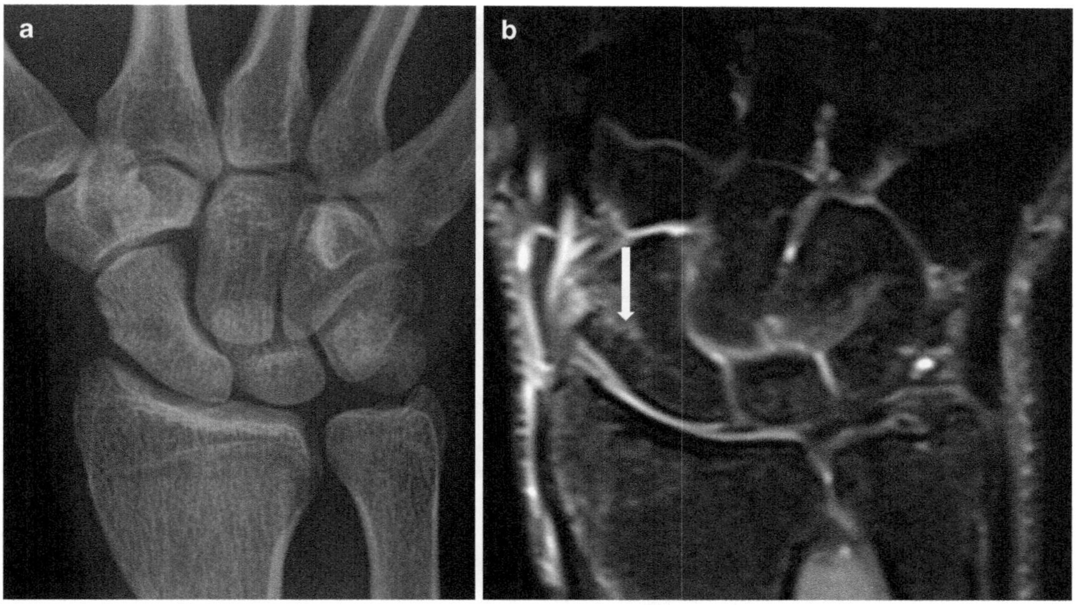

Fig. 2 Standard PA view (**a**) and Cor T2-WI FS (**b**). The standard PA view does not reveal a fracture of the S (**a**). On MRI, a high signal longitudinal fracture line is clearly seen in the acute phase

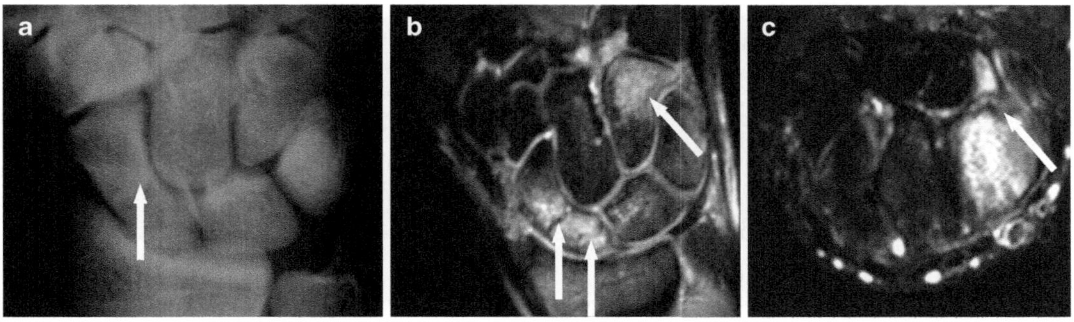

Fig. 3 Standard PA view (**a**) and Cor T2-WI FS (**b**, **c**). The standard PA view did reveal a transverse fracture of the S waist (**a**) in the acute phase. After the cast immobilization period, a control MRI showed a second proximal oblique low signal fracture line in the residual extended S oedema. Moreover, a second fracture can be noticed clearly at the base of the hamulus (**b**, **c**) also with extended BMO of the H

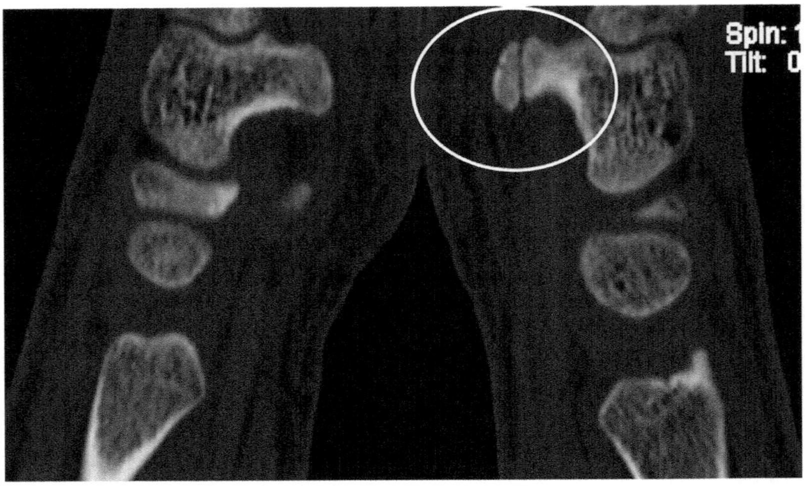

Fig. 4 Sagittal reconstruction of a bilateral CT. Cross-sectional imaging will reveal most carpal fractures

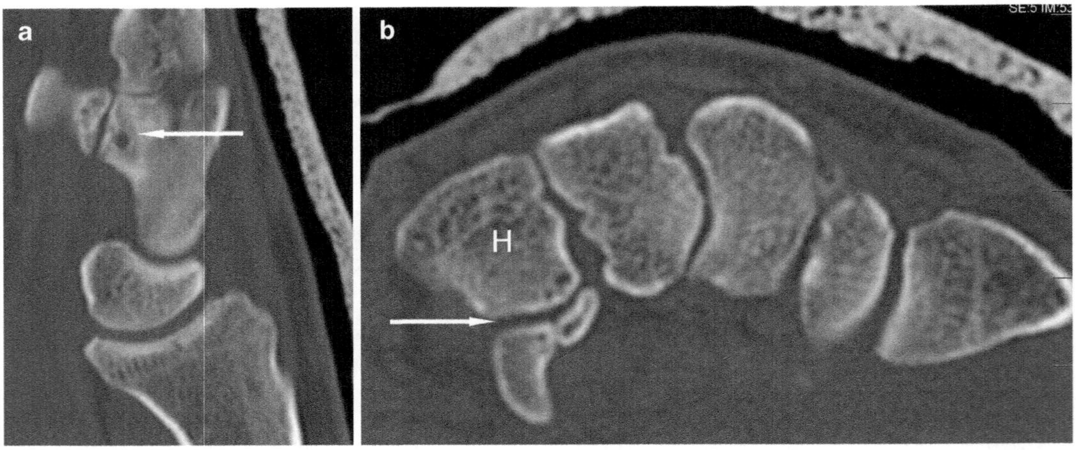

Fig. 5 Sagittal (**a**) and transverse (**b**) reconstructions of CT with the wrist in a cast. Old fracture at the base of the hamulus with cortical lining and secondary degenerative alterations

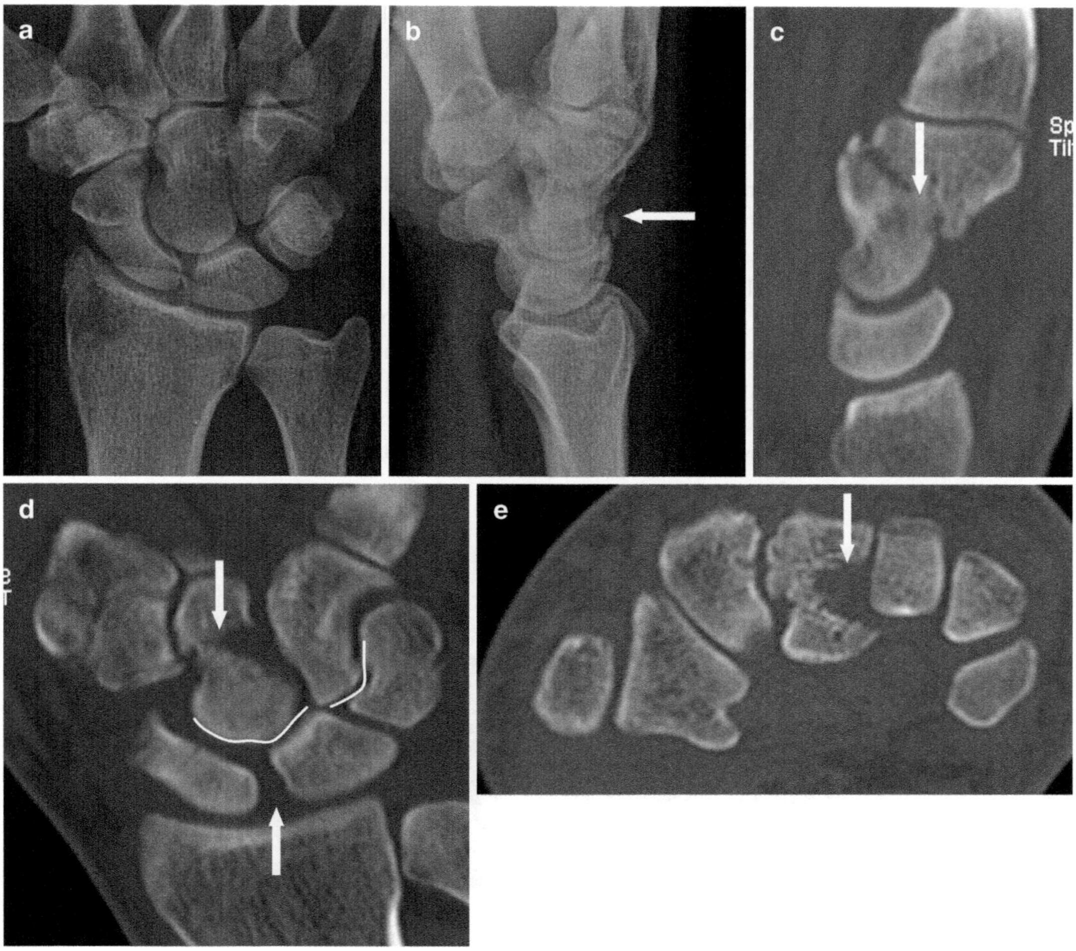

Fig. 6 Standard PA (**a**) and lateral (**b**) view; sagittal (**c**), coronal (**d**), and transverse (**e**) reconstructions of CT. Acute trauma with only a small midcarpal fragment posteriorly (**a**, **b**), an oblique capitate fracture (**c**–**e**) (Ad), clear widening of the SL joint (**d**) (Aa), and an interrupted arc shape with step off sign at the second and third line of Gilula (**d**)

2 Scaphoid Bone Fractures

The S fracture (Bergh et al. 2014; Dean et al. 2021; Johnson et al. 2013; Margo and Seely 1963; Rajayogeswaran et al. 2013; Rowan and Downing 2017; Rua et al. 2019; Vilke 1999) is the most common fracture of the carpal bones (Fig. 1; Table 1). 70% of all carpal bone fractures are located at the waist of the S in adults. Standard views may not reveal a fracture of the S in the acute phase, while on MRI, a high signal at the fine fracture line (Fig. 2) can clearly be seen on T2-WI FS images. Control MRI after the cast immobilisation period may also show additional fractures of the (carpal) bones (Fig. 3b, c; Aa), diagnosed as a low signal fracture line in the residual extended bone marrow oedema.

Of all complete fractures, 50% are unstable. Moreover, 30% of the waist fractures may cause avascular necrosis. So early and correct diagnosis is important not only to treat the fracture but also to prevent complications.

3 Triquetral Bone Fractures

The triquetral bone is the second most affected carpal bone in case of trauma (Welling et al. 2008; Borgeskov et al. 1966; Garcia-Elias 1987). Mostly, a small bone fragment (Figs. 7a, b and 8a) is noticed posteriorly of the proximal carpal row. A low signal of the Tri is found on T1-WI (Fig. 7c) and a high signal on T2-WI FS (Fig. 7d) due to the (residual) bone marrow oedema. Frequently, the complete posterior part of the triquetral bone is broken off and relocated (Figs. 7e and 8c). This includes a detachment of the triquetral insertion of the most important dorsal extrinsic ligaments between the Tra, S, R, and the Tri. Additional laceration of the palmar ligament should also be looked for (Fig. 9). As a result of these ligamentous lesions, the carpus may slide as a whole to the ulnar side (see also: ulnar translation type 1). Large fragments or new bone formation in smaller fragments may eventually lead to a neo-articulation with the original fracture location (Fig. 10). Secondary degeneration may appear at the site with subcortical cysts (Fig. 10d) and BMO (Fig. 10e).

The Tri is the main insertion point of the dorsal stabilisers of the wrist. Early diagnosis and treatment is therefore a must.

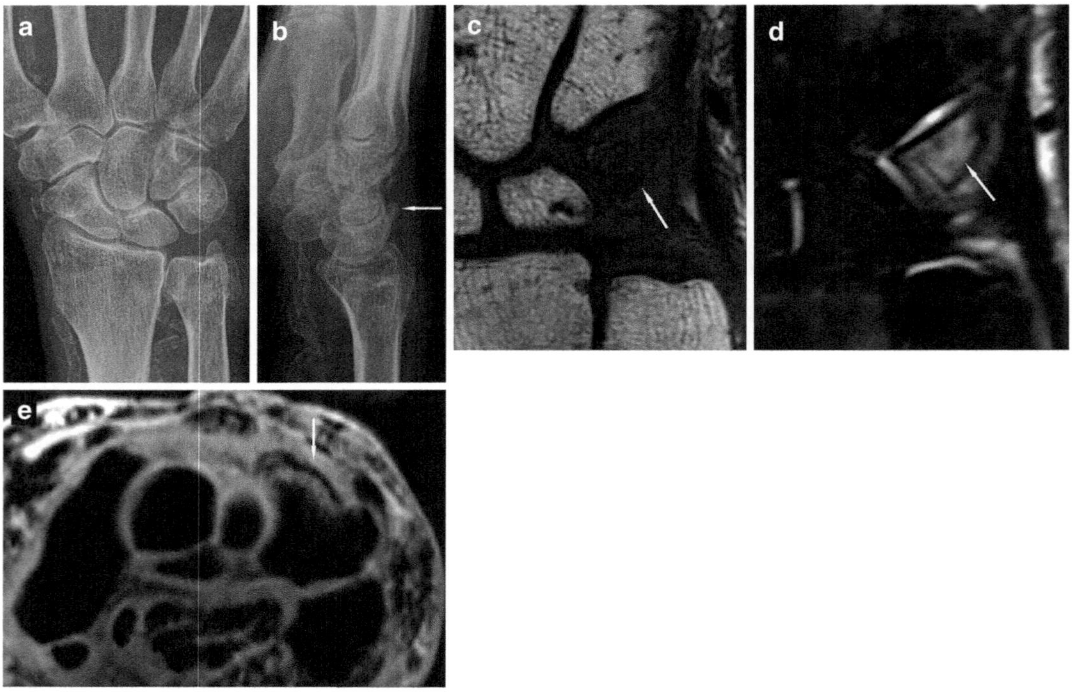

Fig. 7 Standard PA (**a**) and lateral (**b**) view; Cor T1-WI (**c**), T2-WI FS (**d**), and Ax 3D GRE (**e**). Only a small bone fragment (**a**, **b**) is noticed posteriorly of the proximal carpal row. A low signal of the Tri is found on T1-WI (**c**) and a high signal on T2-WI FS (**d**) due to the (residual) BMO. The complete posterior part of the triquetral bone is broken off and slightly relocated (**e**)

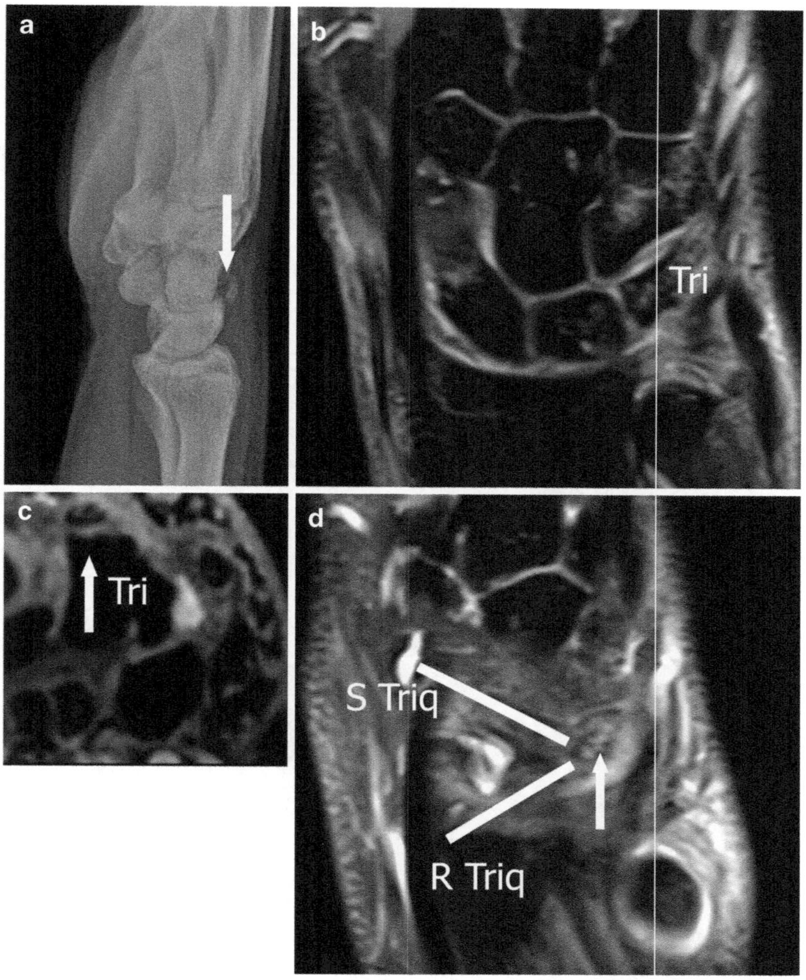

Fig. 8 Standard lateral view (**a**); Cor T2-WI FS (**b**, **d**), and Ax 3D GRE (**c**). The small fragment posteriorly of the proximal carpal row (**a**) corresponds with a part of the fracture (**b**) of the complete dorsal side of the triquetral bone (**c**). The fragment and the depicted attached ligaments (S triq and R Triq) are displaced radially versus the white line through the normal position (**b**, **d**) on the more dorsal image (**d**)

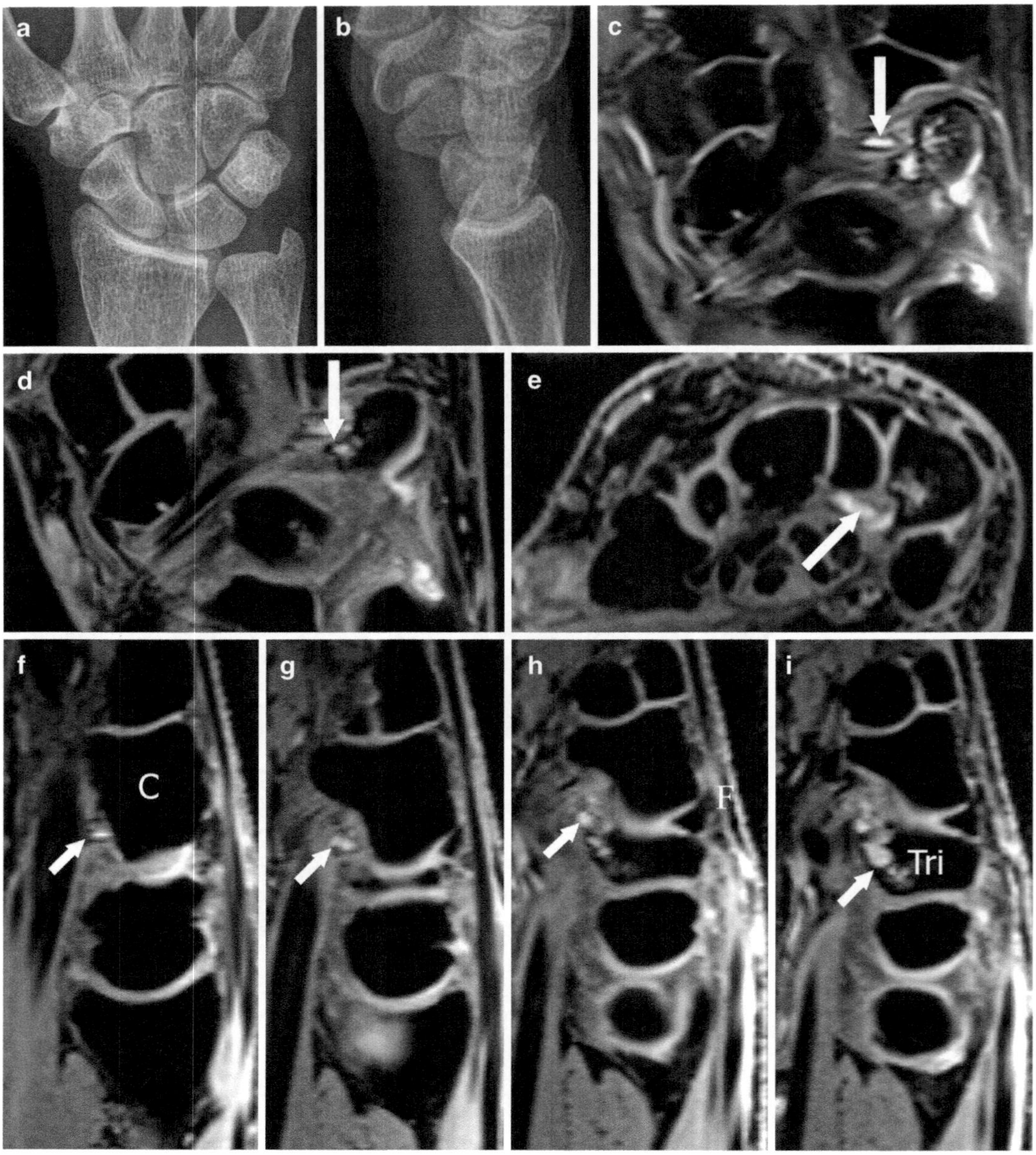

Fig. 9 Standard PA (**a**) and lateral view (**b**); Cor T2-WI FS (**c**) and 3D GRE (**d**); Ax 3D GRE (**e**); and Sag 3D GRE (**f**–**i**). No bony abnormalities on the palmar side on the standard views (**a**, **b**). Part of the ulnar component of the palmar-V (C-Tri) (**c**–**i**) is lacerated

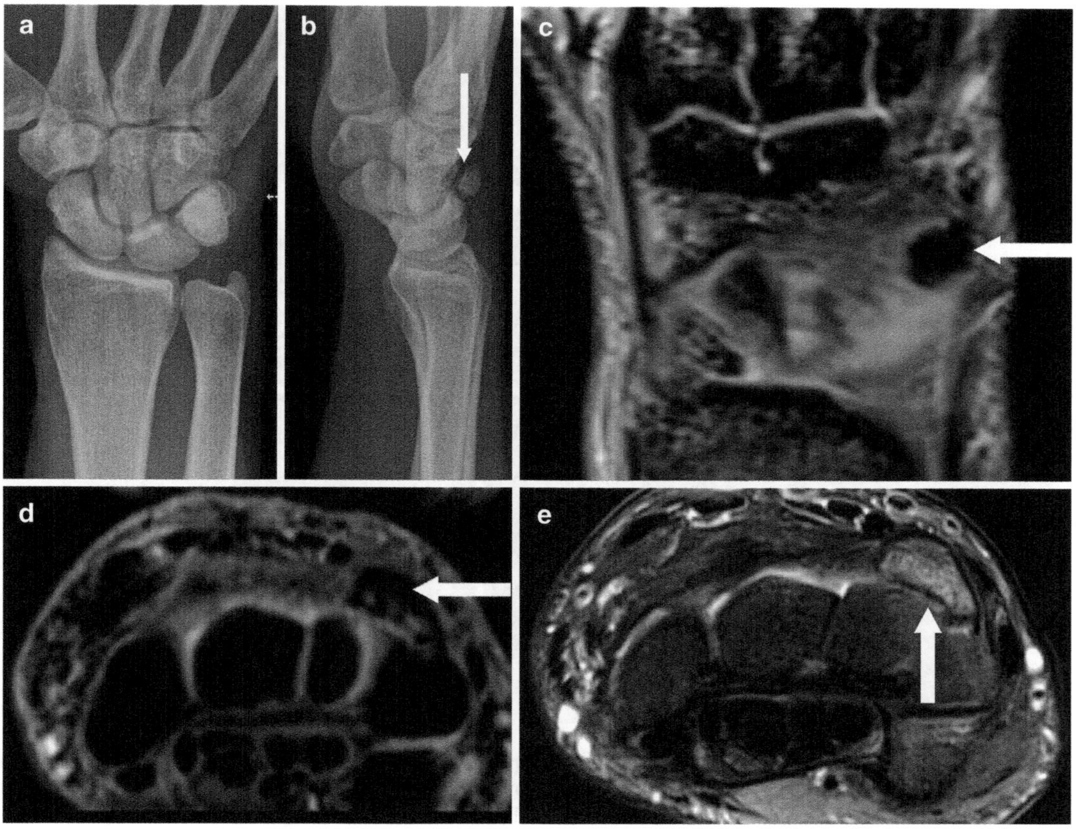

Fig. 10 Standard PA (**a**) and lateral view (**b**); Cor 2D GRE (**c**); Ax 3D GRE (**d**); and T2-WI FS (**e**). The large fragment posteriorly of the carpal region (**b**, **c**) neo-articulates with the Tri (**d**, **e**), and shows subcortical cysts (**d**) and BMO (**e**)

4 Lunate Bone Fractures

The dorsal side of the lunate bone is mostly affected (Rowan and Downing 2017; Goodman et al. 2019; Muppavarapu and Capo 2015; Patel and Quiz. 2010) (Fig. 11) and is hardly visible on standard views (Fig. 11a, b). The cross-sectional and signal sensitive MRI images on the other hand clearly show the classical signs of a fracture (Fig. 11c–e). But also fractures of the palmar horn are possible. Often neglected and barely (Fig. 12a–c) or not visible on standard views, palmar horn fractures can be clearly illustrated by cross-sectional imaging (by MRI (Figs. 12d–f and 13a–d) without radiation or by CT (Fig. 13e, f)).

MRI may also help in the differential diagnosis between fractures of the posterior horn of the Tri (Fig. 14a, c) and the L (Fig. 14b, d). Although the former is by far the most frequent, a rare fracture of the L or a combined fracture of Tri and L should always be excluded (Fig. 15). It should also be noted that the X-ray ratio of 93% Tri versus 7% L fractures changes to 62% Tri versus 38% L fractures when applying MRI, illustrating the importance of cross-sectional imaging (Fig. 2). Likewise, a fracture of the proximal dorsal border of the H should be excluded (Fig. 16). On standard (lateral) views, the dorsal fragment may be caused by a variety of fractures (Tri, L, H or C fracture; Fig. 17).

As the L is prone to avascular necrosis, an early diagnosis and treatment is preferrable.

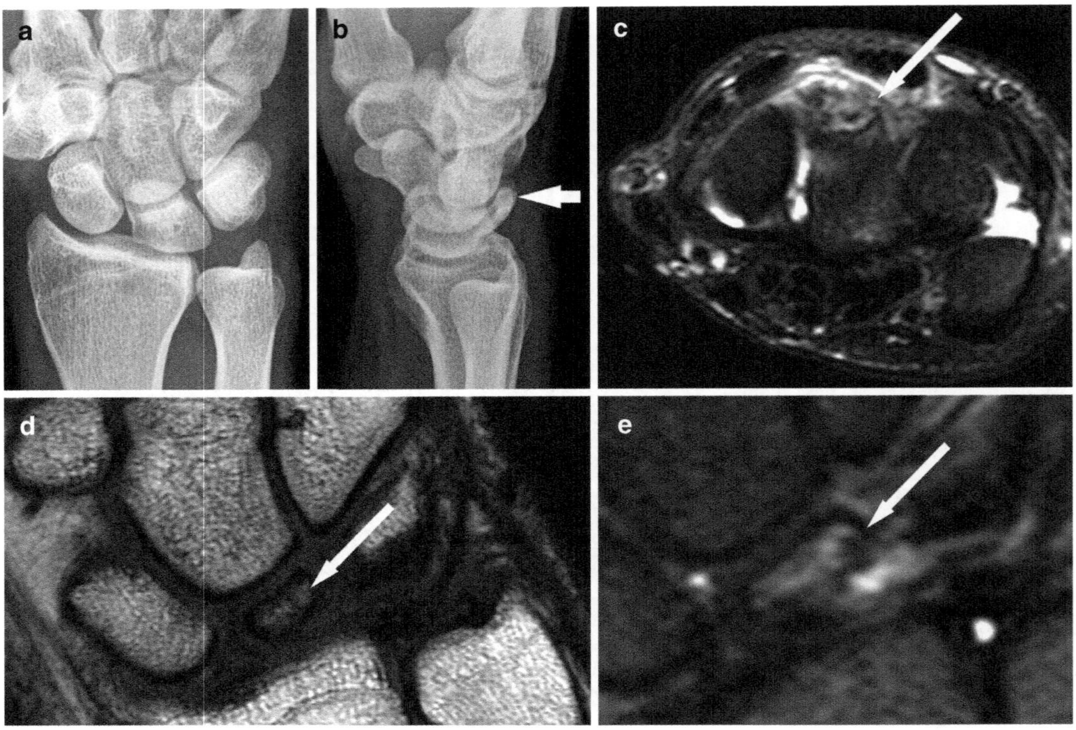

Fig. 11 Standard PA (**a**) and lateral view (**b**); Ax T2-WI FS (**c**); Cor T1-WI (**d**); and T2-WI FS (**e**). The lateral view shows a small density projected almost entirely on the posterior pole region of the lunate (**b**). MRI shows a multi-fragmentary fracture of the dorsal pole (**c**) with BMO in a larger bone fragment (**d, e**)

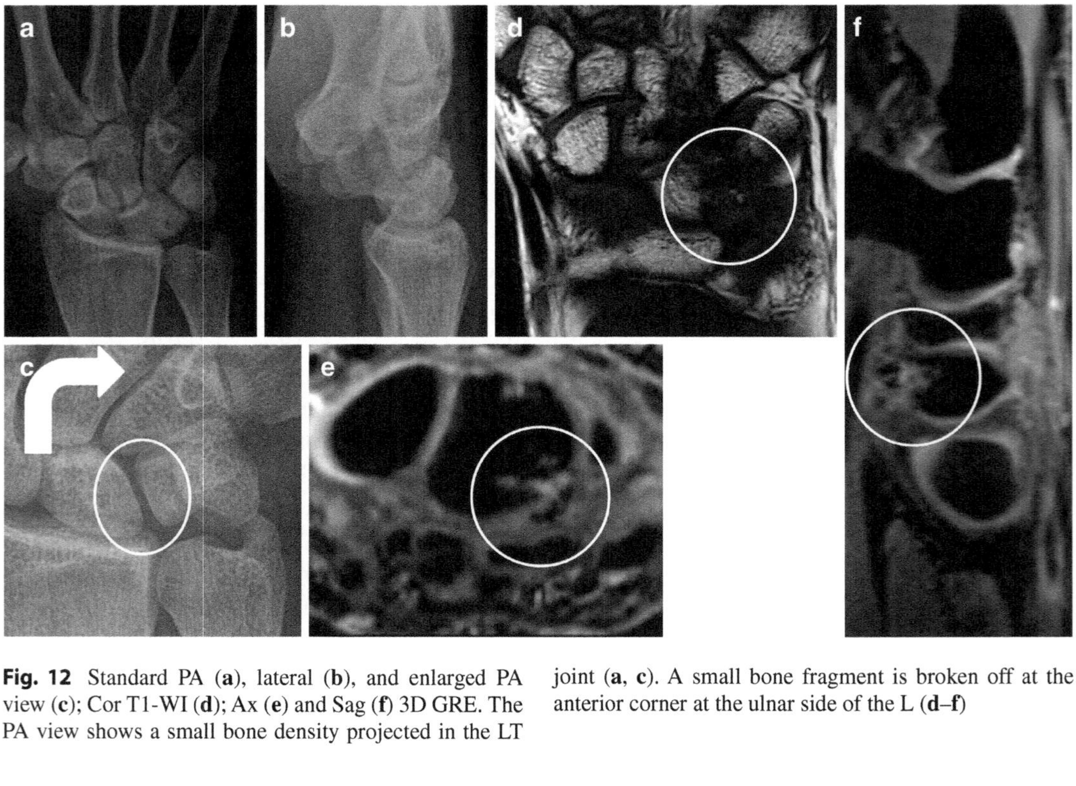

Fig. 12 Standard PA (**a**), lateral (**b**), and enlarged PA view (**c**); Cor T1-WI (**d**); Ax (**e**) and Sag (**f**) 3D GRE. The PA view shows a small bone density projected in the LT joint (**a, c**). A small bone fragment is broken off at the anterior corner at the ulnar side of the L (**d–f**)

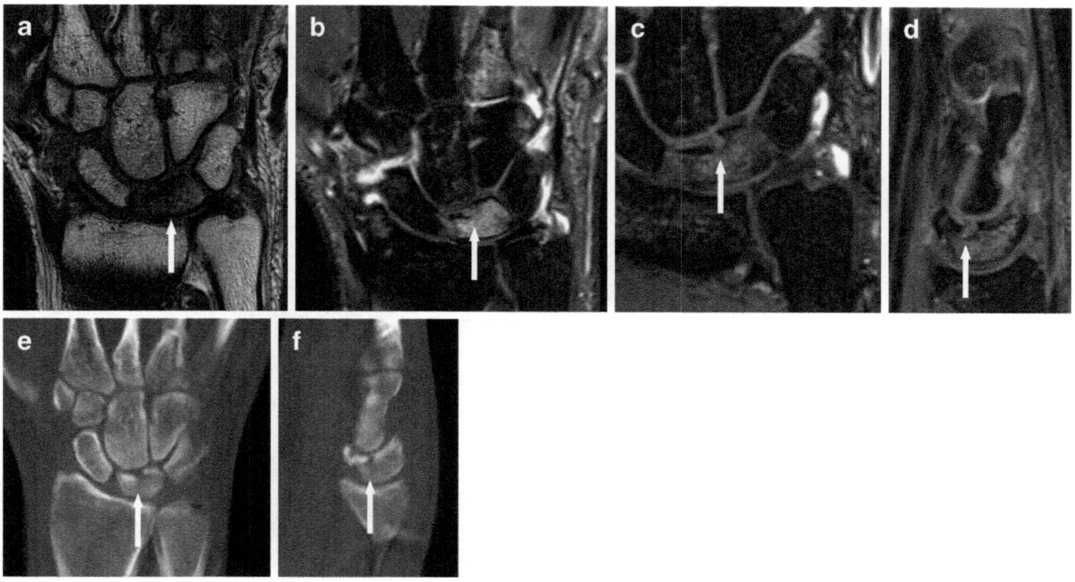

Fig. 13 Cor T1-WI (**a**) and T2WI FS (**b**); Cor (**c**) and Sag 3D GRE (**d**); Cor (**e**) and Sag (**f**) CT images. The extensive BMO of the L (**a**, **b**) is due to a fracture of the anterior horn (**c**, **d**). The 3D GRE correlates perfectly with the available CT images (**e**, **f**)

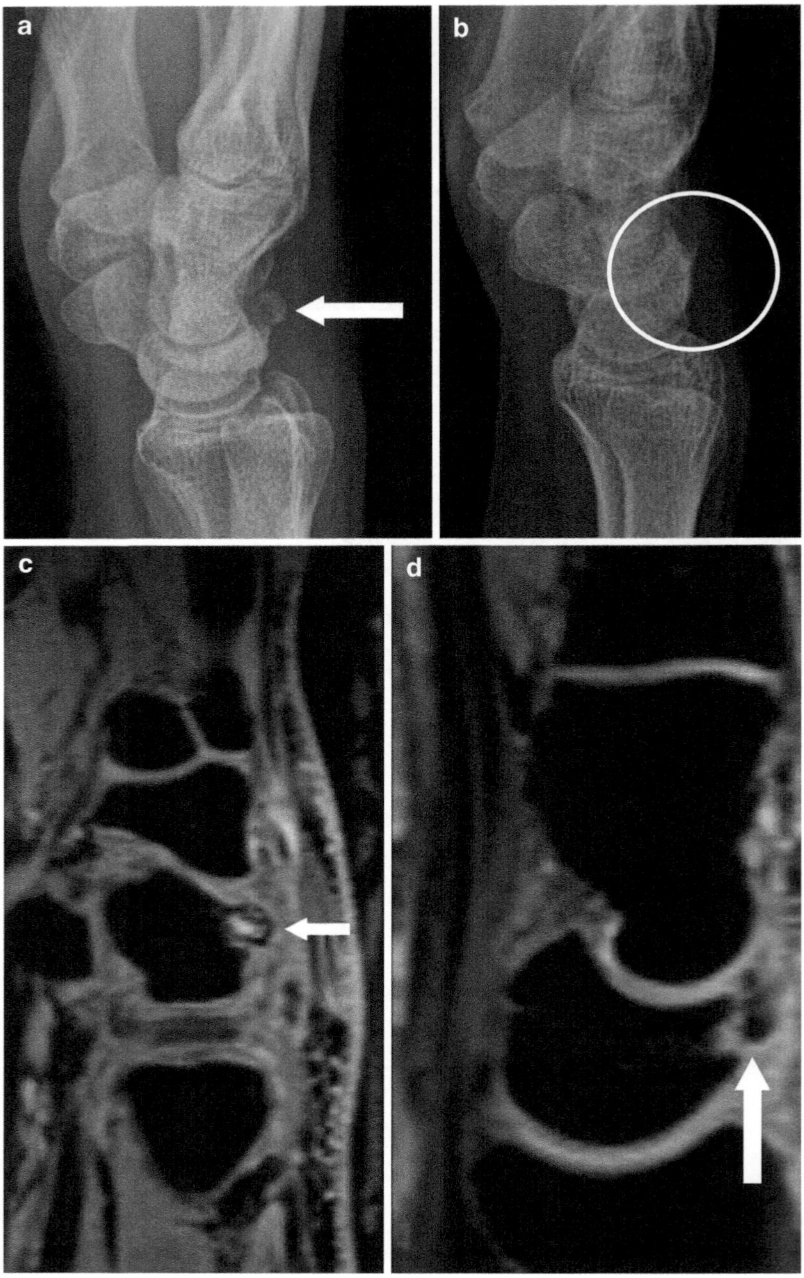

Fig. 14 Standard Lateral (**a**, **b**) and Sag 3D GRE (**c**, **d**). The small fragment posteriorly of the proximal carpal row (**a**, **b**) corresponds with the fracture of the dorsal side of the triquetral bone (**c**) or lunate bone (**d**)

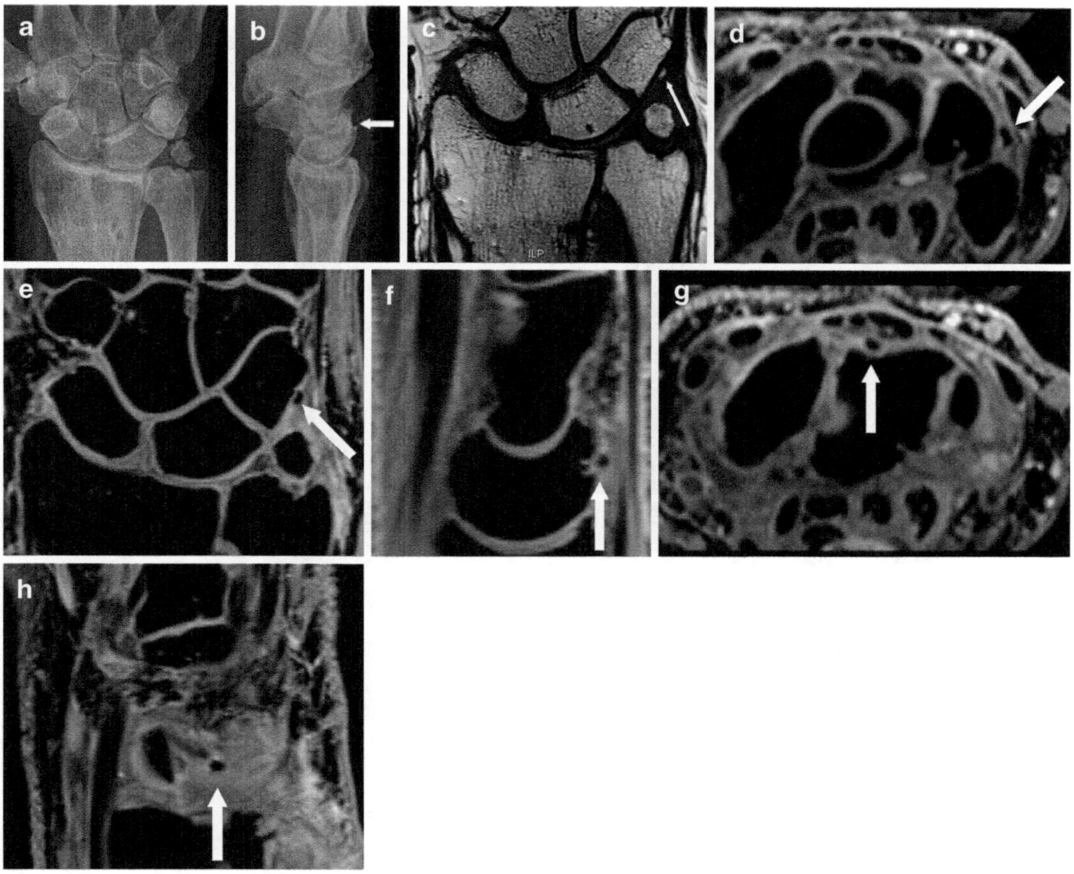

Fig. 15 Standard PA (**a**) and lateral (**b**) view; Cor T1-WE (**c**); Ax (**d**, **g**), Cor (**e**, **h**), and Sag (**f**) 3D GRE. A small fragment posteriorly of the proximal carpal row is present (B), but there is not only a fracture of the posterior border of the Tri (**c**–**e**), but also of the L (**f**–**h**)

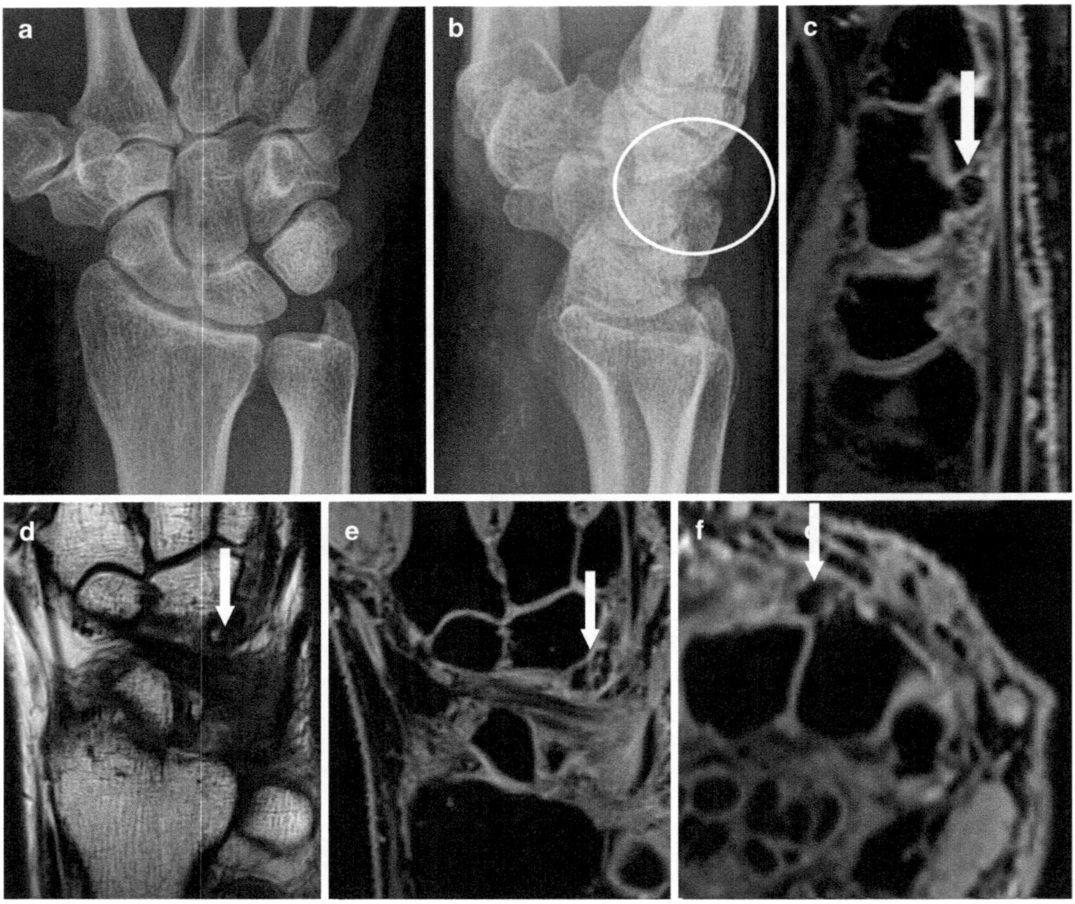

Fig. 16 Standard PA (**a**) and lateral (**b**) view; Sag 3D GRE (**c**); Cor T1-WE (**d**); Cor (**e**) and Sag (**f**) 3D GRE. A small more distal fragment posteriorly of the carpal row is present (**b**), due to a posterior border fracture of the H (**c–f**)

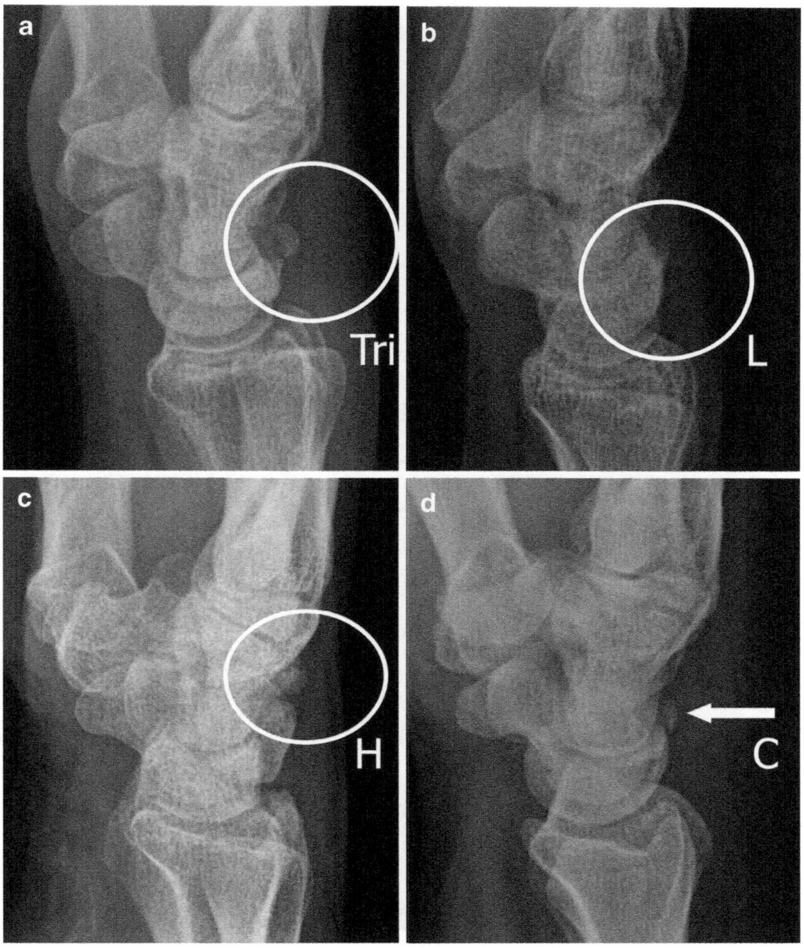

Fig. 17 Standard Lateral views. Various illustrated carpal fractures, Tri (**a**; 14 C), L (**b**; 14 D), H (**c**; 16 E) or C (**d**; 6 C), may cause a dorsal fragment approximately at the same place

5 Trapezium Bone Fractures

This rare fracture (Balci et al. 2015; Bencardino and Rosenberg 2006; Bhat et al. 2011; Bruno et al. 2019; Borgeskov et al. 1966; Couzens et al. 2014; Gornitzky and Carrigan 2016; Khalid et al. 2006) (Figs. 18, 19, and 20) may, especially if the tuberculum is broken (Figs. 19 and 20), have secondary implications (tendinitis, fissuration, and rupture) towards the adjacent flexor carpi radialis tendon (Fig. 20).

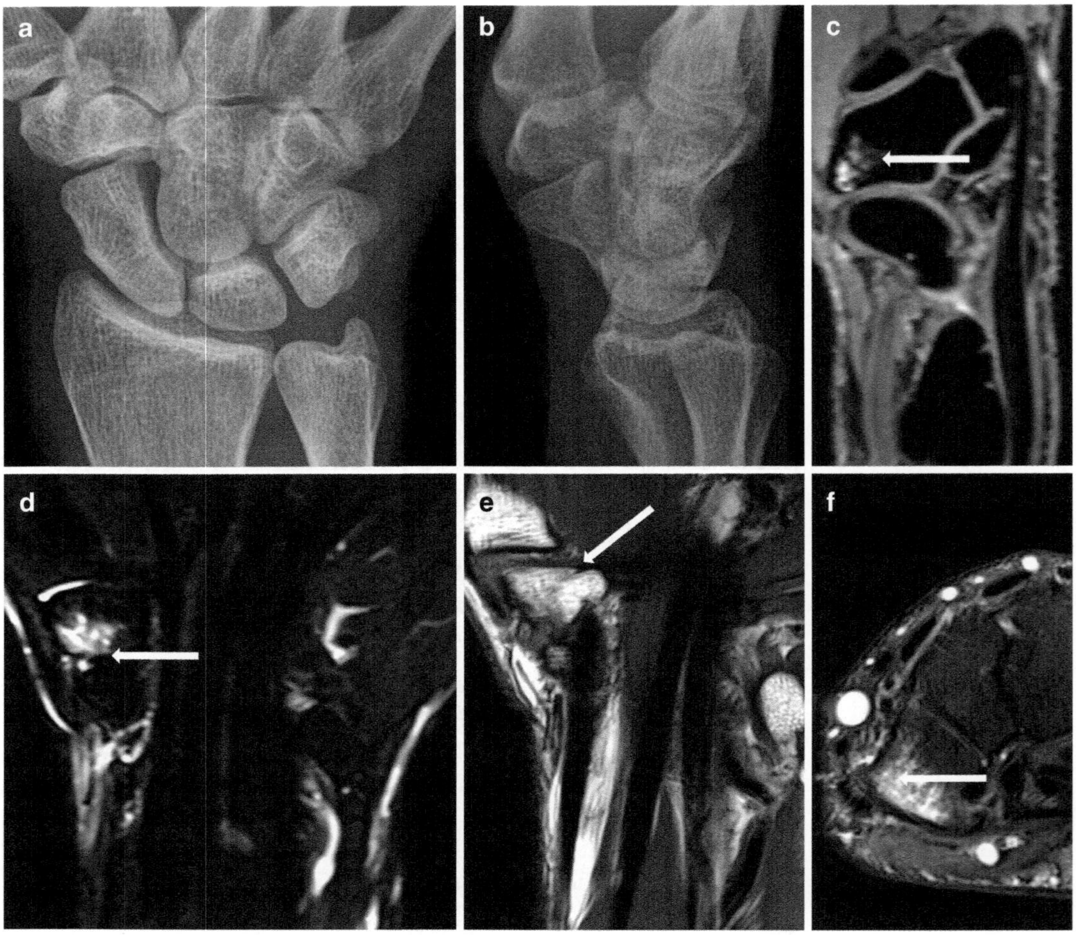

Fig. 18 Standard PA (**a**) and lateral (**b**) view; Sag 3D GRE (**c**); Cor T2-WE FS (**d**); Cor T1-WI (**e**); and Ax T2-WI FS (**f**). No abnormalities were observed on standard views (**a**, **b**). A low signal fracture line was discovered in the zone of BMO (**c**–**f**)

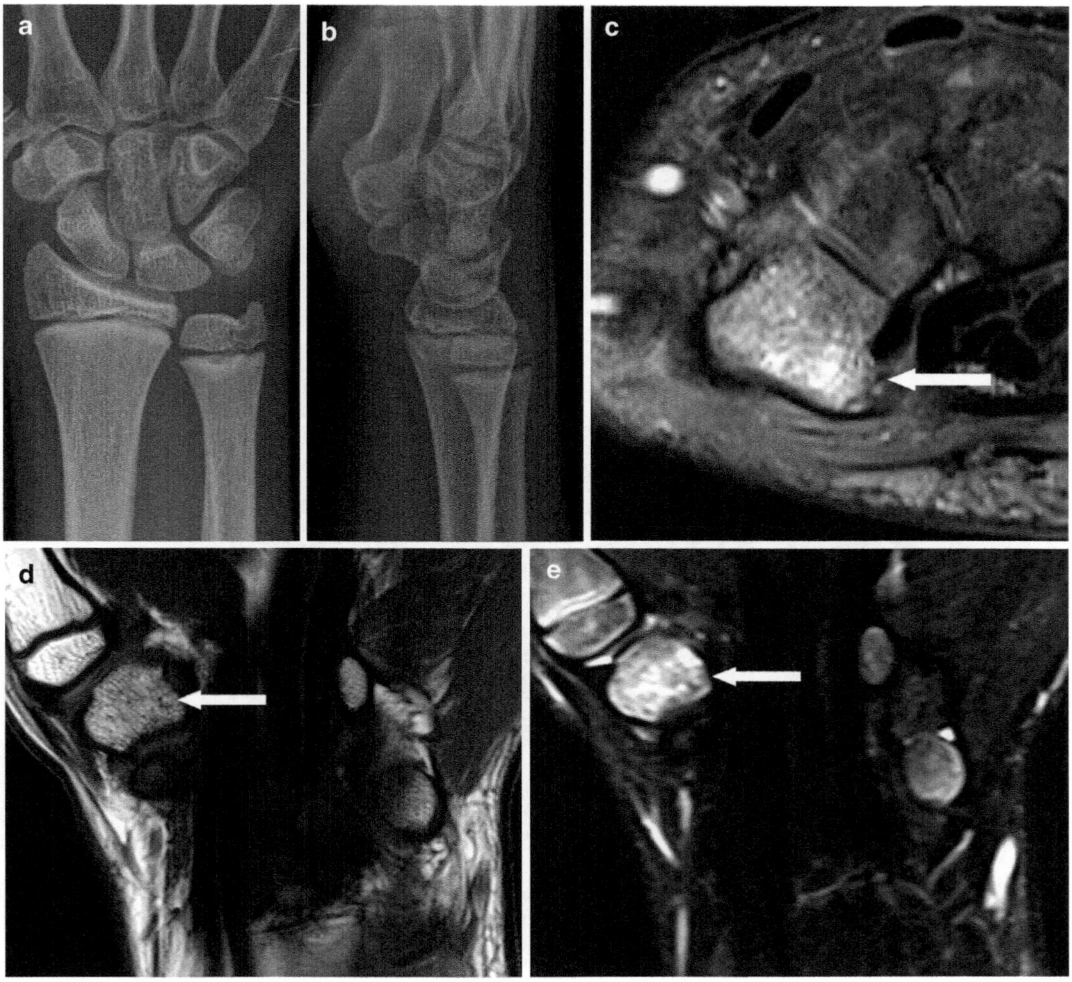

Fig. 19 Standard PA (**a**) and lateral (**b**) view; Ax T2-WE FS (**c**); Cor T1-WI (**e**); and T2-WI FS (**e**). No abnormalities were observed on the standard views (**a**, **b**) in a child. A low signal fracture line was seen in this child at the base of the tubercle (**c**) with extensive bone marrow oedema of the Tra (**c–e**)

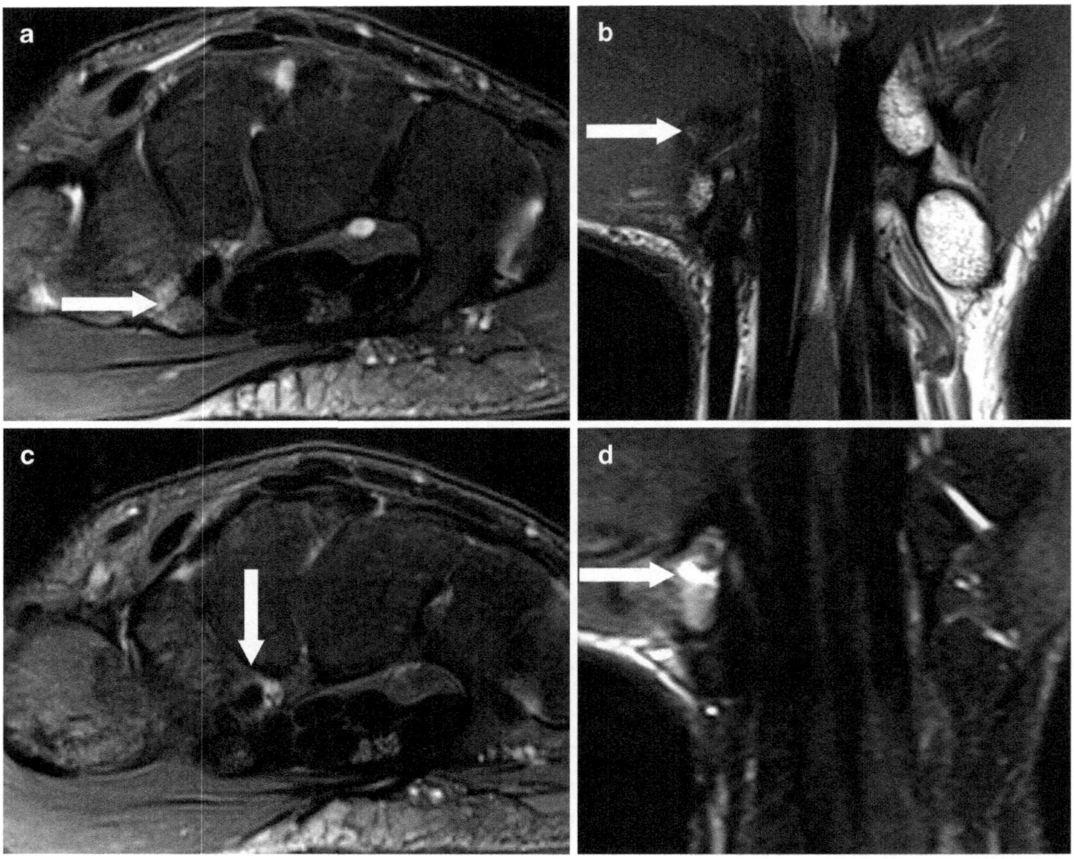

Fig. 20 Ax T2-WE FS (**a**, **c**); Cor T1-WI (**b**); and T2-WI FS (**d**). A low signal fracture line was seen at the tubercle (**a**) with limited BMO of the tubercle (**a**, **b**, and **d**) and tenosynovitis of the fcr tendon (**c**)

6 Trapezoid Bone Fractures

Isolated fractures of the tra (Balci et al. 2015; Borgeskov et al. 1966; Couzens et al. 2014; Gornitzky and Carrigan 2016) (Fig. 21) are extremely rare due to the protected position of the tra in the carpus. Diagnosis needs almost always cross-sectional imaging.

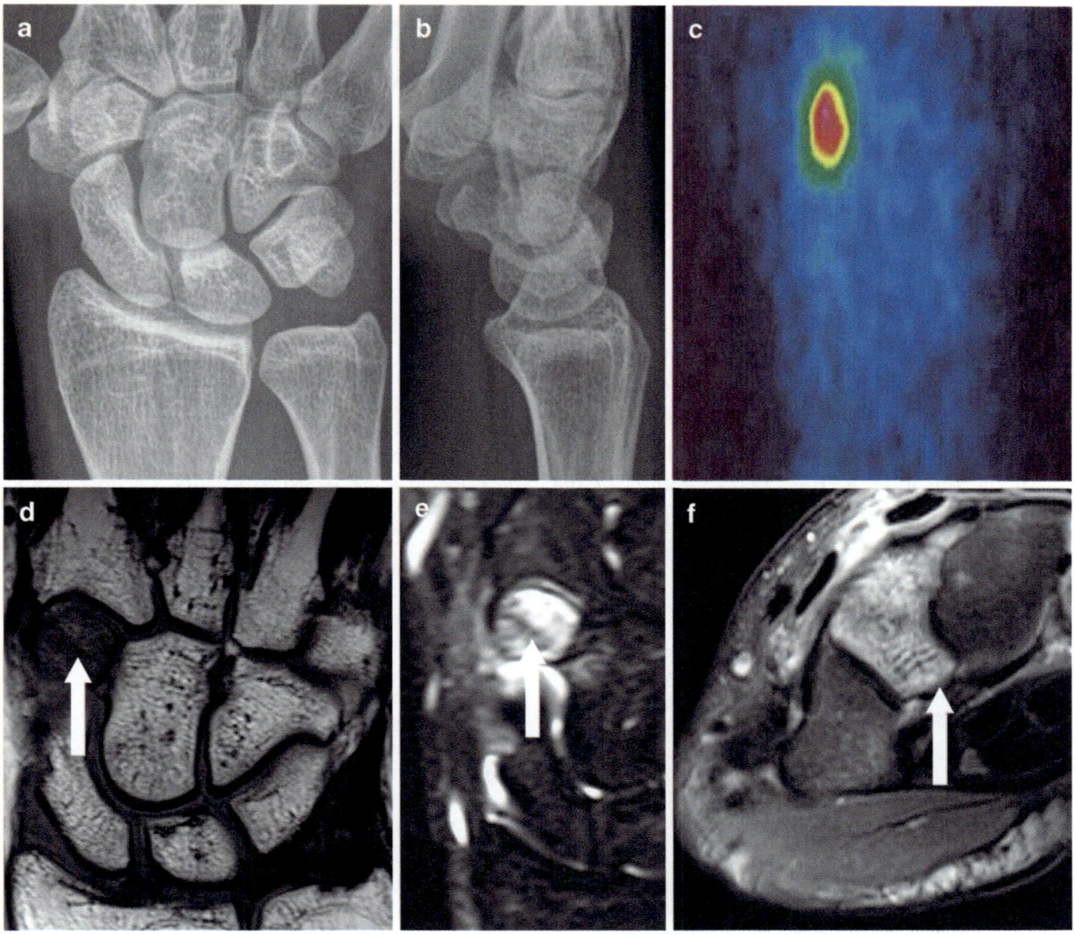

Fig. 21 Standard PA (**a**) and lateral (**b**) view; bone scintigraphy (**c**); Cor T1-WI (**d**) and Cor (**e**); and Ax (**f**) T2-WI FS. The standard view revealed no fracture (**a**, **b**) in contrast with the obvious elective high signal in the tra on bone scintigraphy (**c**). A low signal fracture line (**d**, **e**) was visible in the BMO of the tra (**d–f**)

7 Capitate Bone Fractures

The central position and the size of the capitate bone imply that the presence of a fracture (Welling et al. 2008; Borgeskov et al. 1966; Eriksen and Ringe 2012) (Fig. 6c–e) indicates that the trauma was severe. A thorough evaluation by cross-sectional imaging should always exclude associated trans-carpal fracture-luxation(s) and ligamentous lesions (Fig. 6d).

8 Hamate Bone Fractures

The base of the hamulus is prone to fractures (Gilula 1979; Welling et al. 2008; Borgeskov et al. 1966; Gornitzky and Carrigan 2016), but these fractures are often missed on standard views, certainly in emergency circumstances. Here as well, cross-sectional imaging as MRI (Fig. 3) or CT (Figs. 4 and 5) are essential. The fracture line at the base of the hamulus and extended BMO of the H (Fig. 3b, c) are obvious.

Laceration with palsy of the ulnar nerve which runs close to the hamulus may be an alarming symptom.

9 Pisiform Bone Fractures

In the event of an isolated fracture of this carpal or sesamoid bone (Gilula 1979; Loredo et al. 2005; Welling et al. 2008; Borgeskov et al. 1966; Mack et al. 2003) (Fig. 22), special attention should be given to the insertion and the continuity of the fcu tendon (Fig. 22). Fractures of the distal pole may have an impact on the ulnar nerve passing between the hamulus and the pisiform bone.

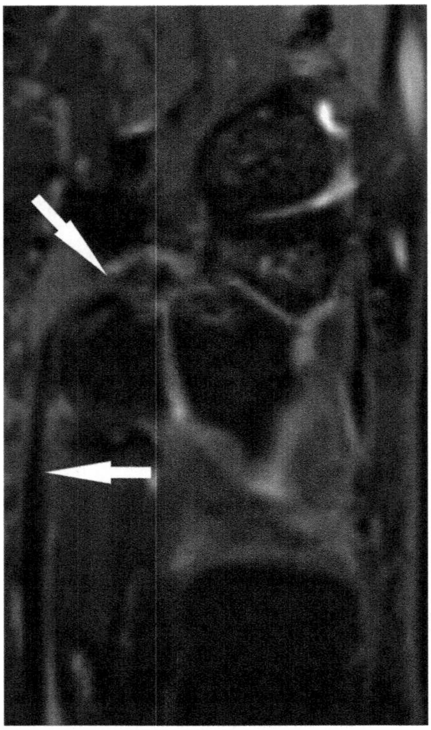

Fig. 22 Sag 3D GRE. The distal pole of the pisiform bone is fractured. The fcu tendon and its insertion on the P are intact

References

Balci A, Basara I, Çekdemir EY, Tetik F, Aktaş G, Acarer A, Özaksoy D (2015) Wrist fractures: sensitivity of radiography, prevalence, and patterns in MDCT. Emerg Radiol 22(3):251–256. https://doi.org/10.1007/s10140-014-1278-1. Epub 2014 Oct 18. PMID: 25325932

Bashir W, Aziz A, Jidaal I (2014) Imaging of skeletal extremity trauma: a review. Trauma 16:300–317. https://doi.org/10.1177/1460408614542920

Bencardino JT, Rosenberg ZS (2006) Sports-related injuries of the wrist: an approach to MRI interpretation. Clin Sports Med 25(3):409–432. https://doi.org/10.1016/j.csm.2006.02.007, vi. PMID: 16798135

Bergh TH, Lindau T, Soldal LA, Bernardshaw SV, Behzadi M, Steen K, Brudvik C (2014) Clinical scaphoid score (CSS) to identify scaphoid fracture with MRI in patients with normal x-ray after a wrist trauma. Emerg Med J 31(8):659–664. https://doi.org/10.1136/emermed-2012-202219. Epub 2013 May 31. PMID: 23727599

Bhat AK, Kumar B, Acharya A (2011) Radiographic imaging of the wrist. Indian J Plast Surg 44(2):186–196. https://doi.org/10.4103/0970-0358.85339. PMID: 22022028; PMCID: PMC3193630

Borgeskov S, Christiansen B, Kjaer A, Balslev I (1966) Fractures of the carpal bones. Acta Orthop Scand 37(3):276–287. https://doi.org/10.3109/17453676608989415

Bruno F, Arrigoni F, Palumbo P, Natella R, Maggialetti N, Reginelli A, Splendiani A, Di Cesare E, Bazzocchi A, Guglielmi G, Masciocchi C, Barile A (2019) The acutely injured wrist. Radiol Clin North Am 57(5):943–955. https://doi.org/10.1016/j.rcl.2019.05.003. Epub 2019 Jun 26. PMID: 31351543

Couzens G, Daunt N, Crawford R, Ross M (2014) Positive magnetic resonance imaging findings in the asymptomatic wrist. ANZ J Surg 84(7–8):528–532. https://doi.org/10.1111/ans.12552. Epub 2014 Feb 26. PMID: 24612468

Dean BJF, Little C, Riley ND, Sellon E, Sheehan W, Burford J, Hormbrey P, Costa ML (2021) Suspected scaphoid injuries managed by MRI direct from the emergency department: a single-centre prospective cohort study. Bone Jt Open 2(6):447–453. https://doi.org/10.1302/2633-1462.26.BJO-2021-0054.R1. PMID: 34182789; PMCID: PMC8244792

Eriksen EF, Ringe JD (2012) Bone marrow lesions: a universal bone response to injury? Rheumatol Int 32(3):575–584. https://doi.org/10.1007/s00296-011-2141-2. Epub 2011 Sep 8. PMID: 21901347

Faccioli N, Foti G, Barillari M, Atzei A, Mucelli RP (2010) Finger fractures imaging: accuracy of cone-beam computed tomography and multislice computed tomography. Skeletal Radiol 39(11):1087–1095. https://doi.org/10.1007/s00256-010-0911-7. Epub 2010 Mar 12. PMID: 20224906

Garcia-Elias M (1987) Dorsal fractures of the triquetrum-avulsion or compression fractures? J Hand Surg Am 12(2):266–268. https://doi.org/10.1016/s0363-5023(87)80285-x. PMID: 3559084

Gilula LA (1979) Carpal injuries: analytic approach and case exercises. AJR Am J Roentgenol 133(3):503–517. https://doi.org/10.2214/ajr.133.3.503. PMID: 111512

Goodman AD, Harris AP, Gil JA, Park J, Raducha J, Got CJ (2019) Evaluation, management, and outcomes of lunate and perilunate dislocations. Orthopedics 42(1):e1–e6. https://doi.org/10.3928/01477447-20181102-05. Epub 2018 Nov 7. PMID: 30403823

Gornitzky AL, Carrigan RB (2016) The diagnostic utility of MRI in the painful wrist: when to reconsider advanced imaging in the pediatric patient. Pediatrics (Evanston) 137(Suppl 3):596–596A. https://doi.org/10.1542/peds.137.Supplement_3.596A

Johnson MR, Fogarty BT, Alitz C, Gerber JP (2013) Non-FOOSH scaphoid fractures in young athletes: a case series and short clinical review. Sports Health 5(2):183–185. https://doi.org/10.1177/1941738112464762. PMID: 24427388; PMCID: PMC3658385

Jørgsholm P, Thomsen N, Besjakov J, Abrahamsson S, Björkman A (2016) MRI shows a high incidence of carpal fractures in children with posttraumatic radial-sided wrist tenderness. Acta Orthop 87(5):533–537. https://doi.org/10.1080/17453674.2016.1210940. Epub 2016 Jul 20. PMID: 27436058; PMCID: PMC5016915

Khalid M, Jummani Z, Kanagaraj K, Robinson D, Reed H (2006) Role of MRI in the diagnosis of occult wrist injury following foosh. J Hand Surg Br Vol 31:42–42. https://doi.org/10.1016/j.jhsb.2006.03.149

Lee GE, Forster GL, Freilich AM, DeGeorge BR Jr (2021) Magnetic resonance arthrography of the wrist: the impact on operative management of wrist injuries. J Wrist Surg 11(2):120–126. https://doi.org/10.1055/s-0041-1735305. PMID: 35478944; PMCID: PMC9038300

Lok RL, Griffith JF, Ng AW, Wong CW (2014) Imaging of radial wrist pain. Part II: pathology. Skeletal Radiol 43(6):725–743. https://doi.org/10.1007/s00256-014-1826-5. Epub 2014 Feb 14. PMID: 24522772

Loredo RA, Sorge DG, Garcia G (2005) Radiographic evaluation of the wrist: a vanishing art. Semin Roentgenol 40(3):248–289. https://doi.org/10.1053/j.ro.2005.01.014. PMID: 16060116

Mack MG, Keim S, Balzer JO, Schwarz W, Hochmuth K, Windolf J, Vogl TJ (2003) Clinical impact of MRI in acute wrist fractures. Eur Radiol 13(3):612–617. https://doi.org/10.1007/s00330-002-1600-2. Epub 2002 Sep 11. PMID: 12594566

Margo MK, Seely JA (1963) A statistical review of 100 cases of fracture of the carpal navicular bone. Clin Orthop Relat Res 31:102–105. PMID: 5888847

Matthews GS, Kiani B, Wuertzer SD, Powell JA, Roller BL, Lenchik L, Torabi M (2019) MRI of the wrist: algorithmic approach for evaluating wrist pain. Radiographics 39(2):447–448. https://doi.org/10.1148/rg.2019180157. PMID: 30844354

Meyer S (1991) Radiographic evaluation of wrist trauma. Semin Roentgenol 26(4):300–317. https://doi.org/10.1016/0037-198x(91)90028-m. PMID: 1745909

Muppavarapu RC, Capo JT (2015) Perilunate dislocations and fracture dislocations. Hand Clin 31(3):399–408. https://doi.org/10.1016/j.hcl.2015.04.002. PMID: 26205701

Nance EM, Byun DJ, Endo Y, Wolfe SW, Lee SK (2017) Dorsal wrist pain in the extended wrist-loading position: an MRI study. J Wrist Surg 6(4):276–279. https://doi.org/10.1055/s-0037-1599829. Epub 2017 Mar 8. PMID: 29085728; PMCID: PMC5658215

Ochman S, Wieskötter B, Langer M, Vieth V, Raschke MJ, Stehling C (2017) High-resolution MRI (3T-MRI) in diagnosis of wrist pain: is diagnostic arthroscopy still necessary? Arch Orthop Trauma Surg 137(10):1443–1450. https://doi.org/10.1007/s00402-017-2747-2. Epub 2017 Aug 14. PMID: 28808768

Patel AS, Macleod A (2010) Picture quiz. The perils of a "FOOSH". BMJ 340:b5438. https://doi.org/10.1136/bmj.b5438. PMID: 20053826

Quinn SF, Belsole RJ, Greene TL, Rayhack JM (1989) Advanced imaging of the wrist. Radiographics 9(2):229–246. https://doi.org/10.1148/radiographics.9.2.2928572. PMID: 2928572

Rajayogeswaran B, Daneshi M, Elias D, Mutiso L (2013) FOOSH – audit of the clinical scaphoid fracture pathway. Clin Radiol 68:S11. https://doi.org/10.1016/j.crad.2013.05.062

Rettig AC (2003) Athletic injuries of the wrist and hand. Part I: traumatic injuries of the wrist. Am J Sports Med 31(6):1038–1048. https://doi.org/10.1177/03635465030310060801. PMID: 14623677

Rowan CH, Downing ND (2017) Trans-scaphoid perilunate fracture dislocation: 'notjust a scaphoid fracture'. BMJ Case Rep 2017:bcr2017221041. https://doi.org/10.1136/bcr-2017-221041. PMID: 28739625; PMCID: PMC5624016

Rua T, Malhotra B, Vijayanathan S, Hunter L, Peacock J, Shearer J, Goh V, McCrone P, Gidwani S (2019) Clinical and cost implications of using immediate MRI in the management of patients with a suspected scaphoid fracture and negative radiographs results from the SMaRT trial. Bone Joint J 101-B(8):984–994. https://doi.org/10.1302/0301-620X.101B8.BJJ-2018-1590.R1. PMID: 31362557; PMCID: PMC6681676

Ruston J, Konan S, Rubinraut E, Sorene E (2013) Diagnostic accuracy of clinical examination and magnetic resonance imaging for common articular wrist pathology. Acta Orthop Belg 79(4):375–380. PMID: 24205765

Vilke GM (1999) FOOSH injury with snuff box tenderness. J Emerg Med 17(5):899–900. https://doi.org/10.1016/s0736-4679(99)00102-x. PMID: 10499710

Welling R, Jacobson J, Jamadar D, Chong S, Caoili E, Jebson P (2008) MDCT and radiography of wrist fractures: radiographic sensitivity and fracture patterns. Am Roentgen Ray Soc 190(1):10–16

Yaghoubian R, Goebel F, Musgrave DS, Sotereanos DG (2001) Diagnosis and management of acute fracture-dislocation of the carpus. Orthop Clin North Am 32(2):295–305. https://doi.org/10.1016/s0030-5898(05)70250-9, viii. PMID: 11331542

Complications of Fractures

Contents

1 General

Bone fractures may be "invisible" on standard views in an early stage (Fig. 1a, b). Discrete or indirect signs, as well as a clinical correlation, may indicate the need for further investigation (Fig. 1b). MRI is much more sensitive for fractures (Balci et al. 2015; Bashir et al. 2014; Bencardino and Rosenberg 2006; Girgis and Epstein 2000; Gornitzky and Carrigan 2016; Khalid et al. 2006; Mack et al. 2003) due to the cross-sectional imaging combined with signal alterations (Fig. 1c). Follow-up standard views (usually 1–2 weeks after the trauma) may

M. Mespreuve, K. Waked, *MRI of the Wrist*, Medical Radiology,
https://doi.org/10.1007/978-3-031-63973-9_4

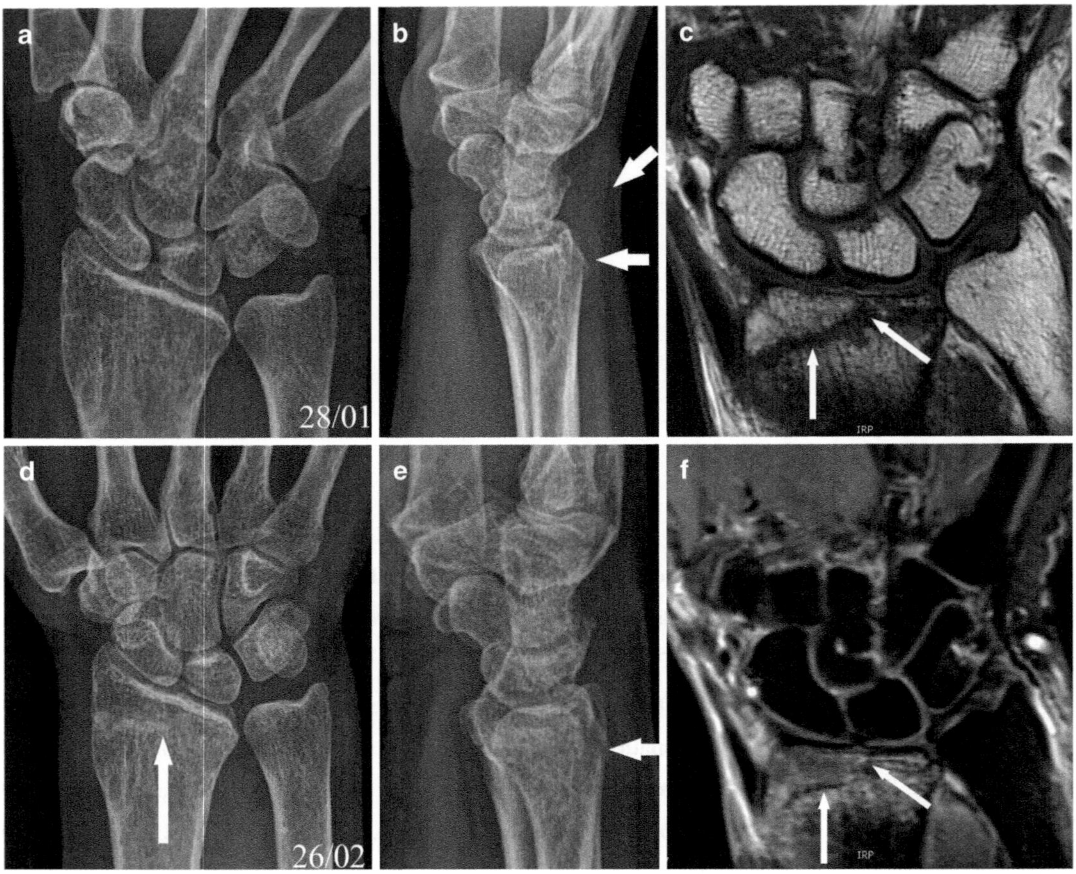

Fig. 1 Standard PA (**a**, **d**) and lateral (**b**, **e**) views; Cor T1-WI (**c**) and T2-WI FS (**f**). Standard views do not reveal a fracture (**a**, **b**). However, remark the small cortical irregularity dorsal of the R and mainly the soft tissue density posteriorly of the carpus and the obliteration of the adjacent subcutaneous fat plane. MRI clearly shows an intra-articular oblique fracture of the radial epiphysis (**c**). Periosteal bone reaction is obvious on control standard views 1 month later (**d**, **e**), as is the fracture line with surrounding BMO (**f**)

ultimately also clearly reveal the fracture (Fig. 1d, e). As the BMO may remain for up to 6 months (Fig. 1f), "missed" fractures can also be detected by follow-up MRI over a longer period. The evaluations of sequels of a trauma by standard views (Fig. 2a, b), especially in expert cases, frequently do not expose the complete status and additional fracture sequels are also highlighted by MRI (Avenarius et al. 2012) (Fig. 2c–f). In particular, fractures of the ulnar styloid (Fig. 2c), the sigmoid notch of the DRUJ (Fig. 2d), and the anterior (Fig. 2e) and posterior (Fig. 2f) border of the radial epiphysis (Arora et al. 2010) are frequently masked on standard views.

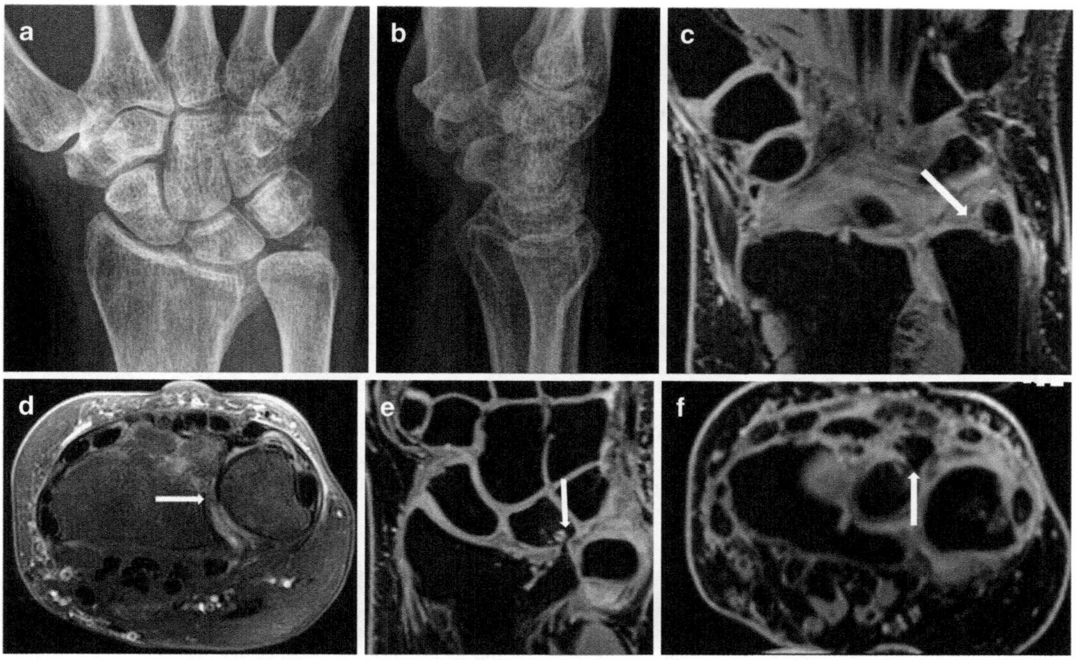

Fig. 2 Standard PA (**a**) and lateral (**b**) views; Cor 3D GRE (**c**); Ax T2-WI FS (**d**); and Cor (**e**) and Ax (**f**) 3D GRE. The sequels of a Pouteau fracture on standard views are obvious (**a**, **b**). However, there are also post-traumatic lesions with a fracture at the base of the ulnar styloid (**c**), the radial sigmoid notch (**d**) and at the palmar (**e**) and dorsal (**f**) border with displaced fragments of the radial epiphysis

2 Ulnar Styloid Fractures and Peri-Ulnar Lacerations

Standard views may show a number of non-healing ulnar styloid fractures (Hauck et al. 1996) (Fig. 3a). MRI additionally shows the surrounding BMO and subcortical cysts of the pseudarthrosis (Fig. 3b, c). The relation between the ulnar double insertion of the TFCC and the fragments may also clearly be delineated (Fig. 3b) and the stability evaluated (Fig. 4). The Gaulke classification defines a type I (Fig. 4d) ulnar styloid fracture at the tip, which correlates with a much more stable TFCC, than a larger broken fragment at the base of the styloid, labelled as a type II (Fig. 4e). Subtypes a (Fig. 4d, e) show a horizontal fracture line, subtypes b a fracture line running oblique towards the distal ulnar side, and in subtypes c, the fracture line runs oblique towards the proximal ulnar side.

Important deformations with sharp edges (Fig. 5a, b) may impact the ecu tendon as well. Repetitive strain causes inflammation (Fig. 5c–g) and fissuring (Fig. 5d–g), which may ultimately lead to tendon rupture and soft tissue oedema with swelling (Fig. 5a, g). A post-traumatic bony extension (callus) may also reduce the mobility of the tendon in its gutter (Fig. 5f).

The TFCC (Iordache et al. 2012) and its ulnar insertions should also be evaluated in depth after trauma, as the size of the broken bony fragment and the location of the fracture alone do not exclude nor confirm a lesion of the adjacent TFCC, nor of the ulnar insertions (Fig. 6). An avulsion fracture of the distal ulnar TFCC insertion may render the whole TFCC unstable (Fig. 6a, b, d). An avulsion fracture of the proximal ulnar insertion may be associated with a broken bony fragment or a fracture of the base of the styloid process (Fig. 6c).

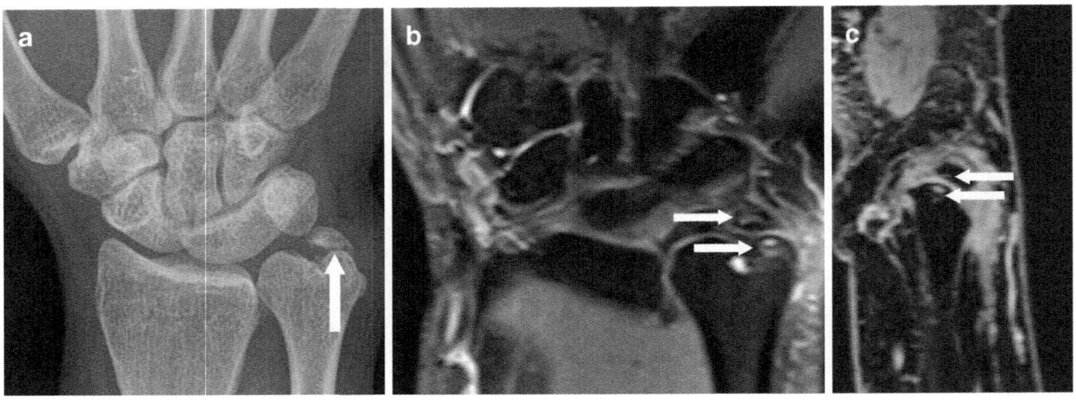

Fig. 3 Standard PA view (**a**); Cor T2-WI FS (**b**); and Sag 3D GRE (**c**). There is a sequel of a fracture at the ulnar styloid with sclerotic borders and a loose fragment (**a–c**). The neo-articulation between the remnant of the ulnar styloid and the loose fragment is surrounded by BMO and subcortical cysts (**b**, **c**)

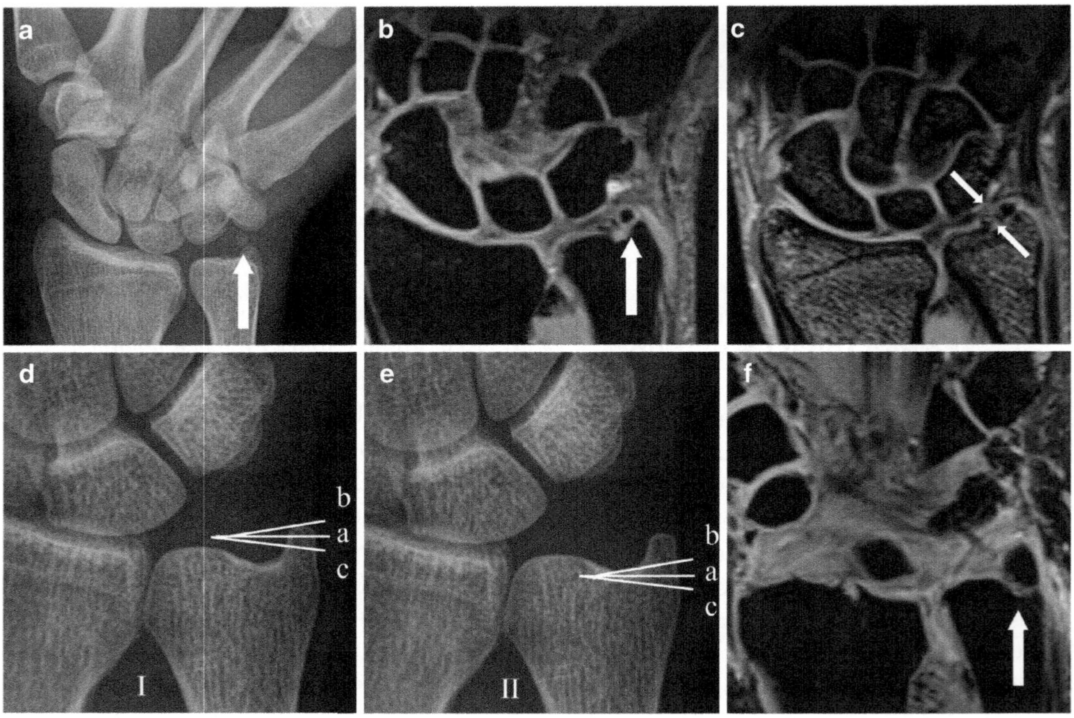

Fig. 4 Standard PA view (**a**); Cor 3D (**b**) and 2D (**c**) GRE; detail with marks on Standard PA views (**d**, **e**); Cor 3D GRE (**f**). A smaller fragment is broken at the tip in type I b (**a–d**), while a larger fragment is broken at the base in type II c (**e**, **f**). The location of the ulnar styloid fracture line at the tip (**d**; type I a-c) or at the base (**e**; type II a-c) is used to define the stability of the TFCC in the Gaulke classification

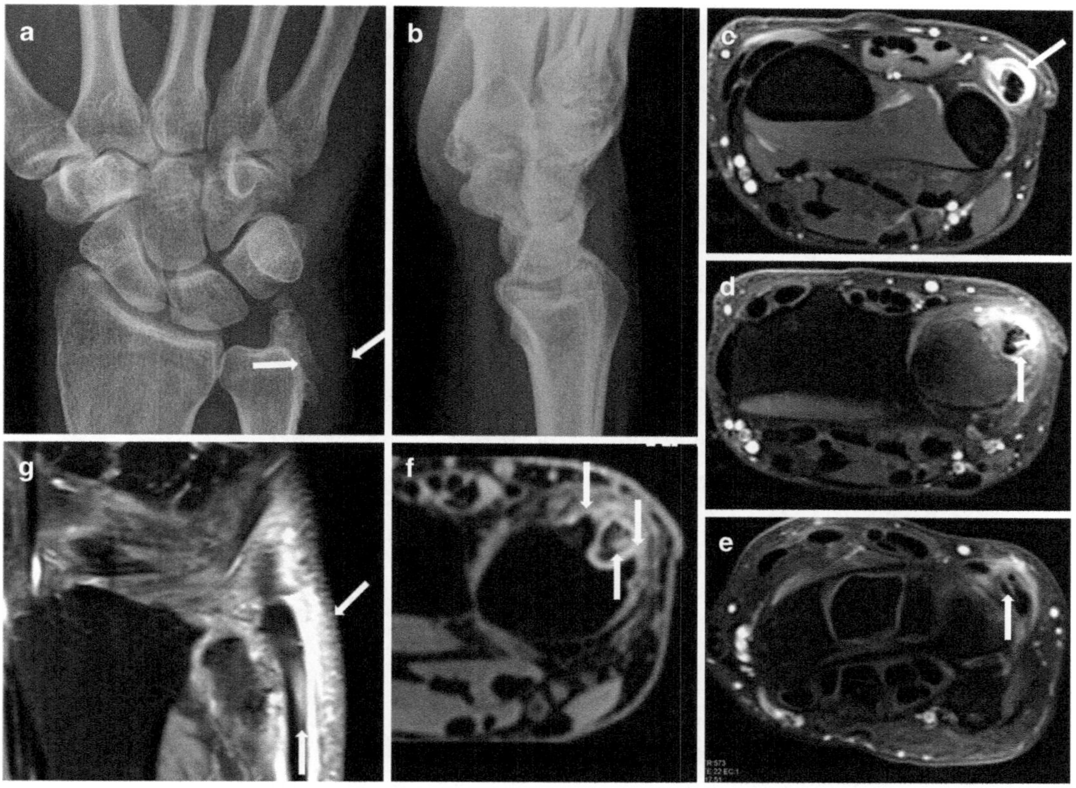

Fig. 5 Standard PA (**a**) and lateral views; Ax T2-WI FS (**c**–**e**); Ax 3D GRE (**f**); and Cor T2-WI FS. The ulnar styloid process is severely distorted with sharp edges and the adjacent soft tissues are swollen (Fig. 4a, b). Also, the tendon of the ecu is swollen (**c**–**e**), fissured (**d**–**g**), and surrounded by fluid in its sheath (Fig. 4c–g). A gutter-shaped bone extension partly surrounds the ecu at both sides (Fig. 4f)

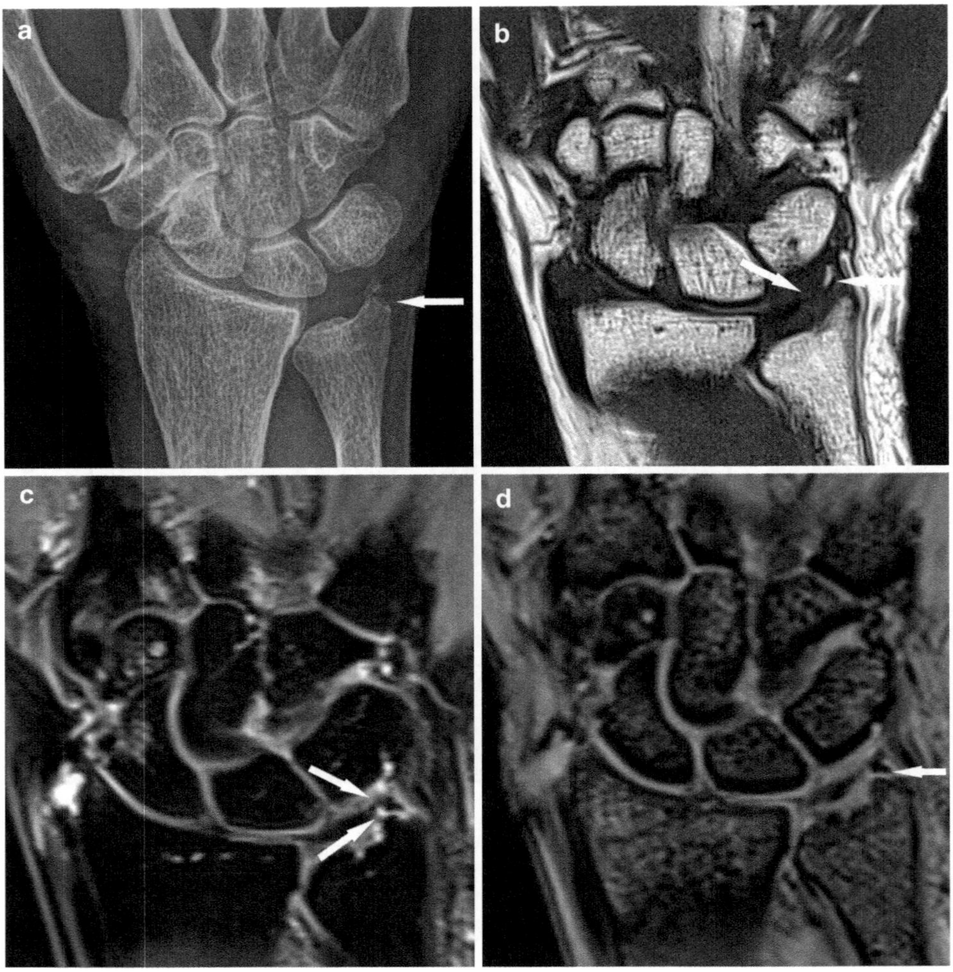

Fig. 6 Standard PA view (**a**); Cor T1-WI (**b**); Cor T2-WI FS (**c**); and 2D GRE (**d**). Only a small fragment of the tip is broken (**a**, **b**, **d**). The fibrocartilage of the TFCC seems intact (**b**, **c**) with its unstable distal ulnar insertion at the fragment (**a**, **b**, **d**), while the proximal insertion at the base of the styloid process is ruptured (**c**)

3 Distal Radioulnar Joint Fractures and Peri-Articular Lacerations

Due to its form and orientation, fractures of the DRUJ (Arora et al. 2010; Bouri et al. 2016; Carlsen et al. 2010; Ekenstam and Hagert 1985; Kwon et al. 2012; Lindau and Aspenberg 2002; Slattery et al. 2013; Stuart et al. 2000; Wechsler et al. 1987) are often disregarded. Even important and displaced fractures are often discovered (too) late (Fig. 7) and may lead to invalidating damage of the joint cartilage (Kim et al. 2012; Kohyama et al. 2015; Orbay et al. 2021) (Fig. 7c, d). Successful reduction of a DRUJ luxation does not, however, exclude bony sequels (second ulnar groove sign), tendinous (ecu), nor ligamentous lesions (rul) (Gillis et al. 2019) (Figs. 8c, d and 9c). The "successful" reduction of a luxation (Jenkins et al. 1987; Kim and Park 2008) needs a thorough evaluation with cross-sectional imaging, as residual subluxation (Lo et al. 2001; Malik et al. 2005; Mino et al. 1983; Morrissy and Nalebuff 1979) may remain undetected (Fig. 9). Prominent fractures in the acute phase may mislead the clinicians and radiologists and mask a (sub)luxation at the DRUJ (Fig. 10), especially in case of "normal" standard views (May et al. 2002; McMurray and Muralikuttan 2008; Mespreuve et al. 2015) (Fig. 11).

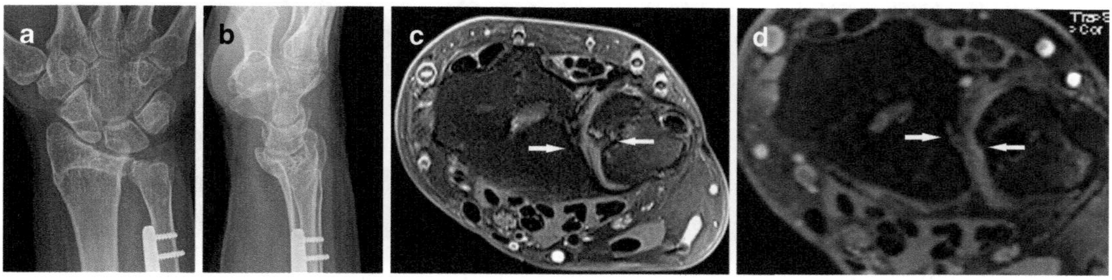

Fig. 7 Standard PA (**a**) and lateral (**b**) views; Ax T2-WI FS (**c**) and 3D GRE (**d**). After consolidation of an ulnar fracture, wrist rotation is partially hampered without major alterations at the DRUJ (**a**, **b**). A fracture sequel with step off is demonstrated at the radial sigmoid notch and at the ulnar head as well (**c**, **d**). The cartilage at the depressed sigmoid notch is irregular and focally reduced in thickness (**c**, **d**)

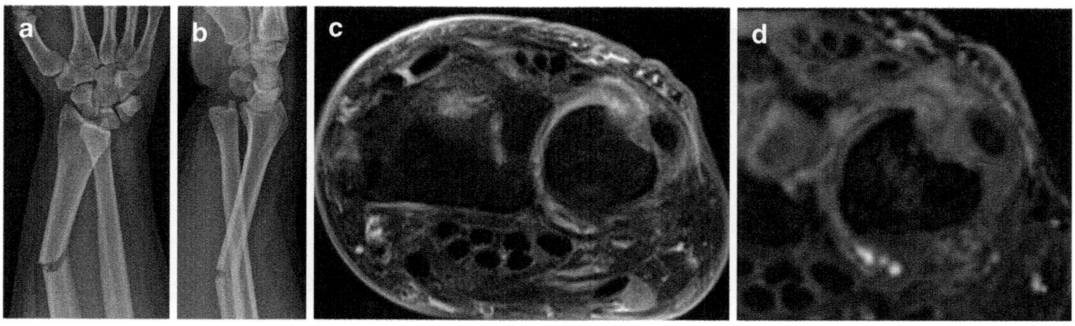

Fig. 8 Standard PA (**a**) and lateral (**b**) view; Ax T2-WI FS (**c**) and 3D GRE (**d**). After a rare anterior luxation of the ulna and a fracture of the radius (Galeazzi fracture-dislocation type I) with ulnodorsal angulation (**a**, **b**). The bony reduction is successful, but the distal radioulnar ligaments are destructed and barely visible (**c**, **d**). The gutter of the ecu is deformed and the tendon subluxated (**c**, **d**)

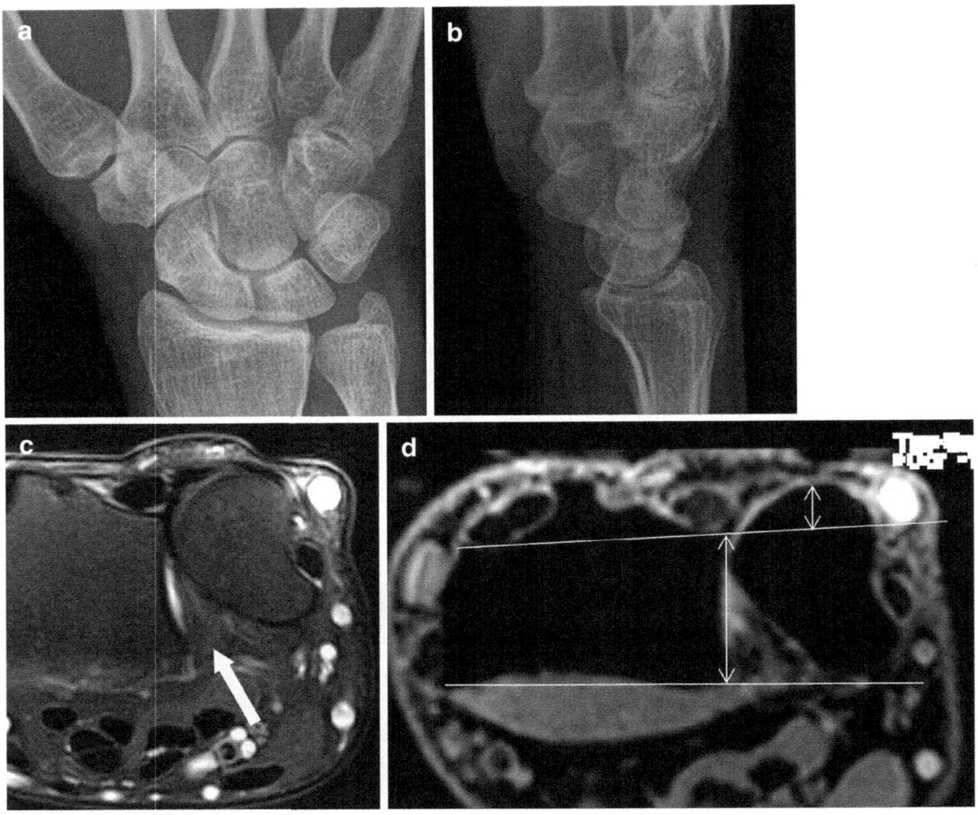

Fig. 9 Standard PA (**a**) and lateral (**b**) view; Ax T2-WI FS (**c**) and 3D GRE (**d**). After reduction of a dorsal ulna luxation, the standard views show no obvious pathology (**a**, **b**). However, the anterior rul is torn (**c**) and the ulna remains subluxated dorsally in pronation (**c**, **d**)

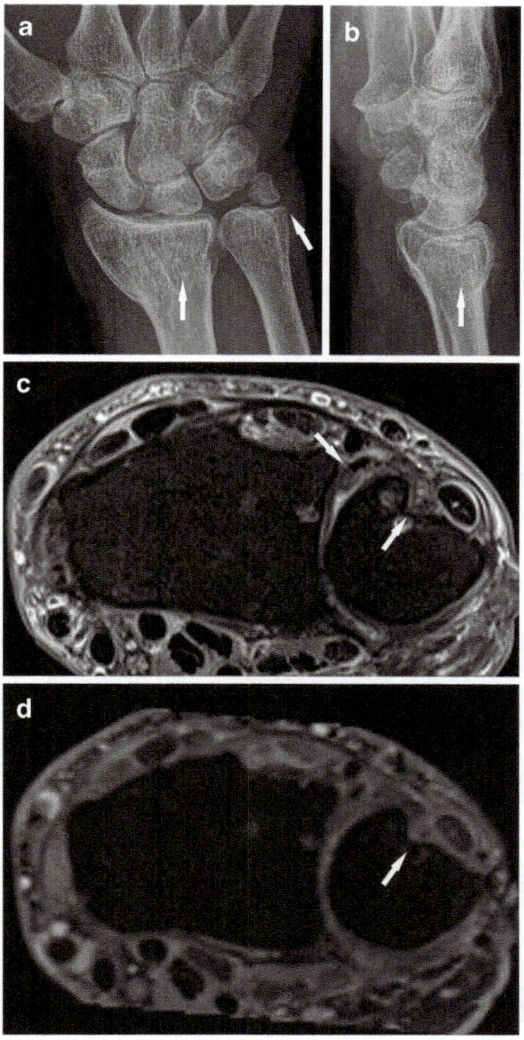

Fig. 10 Standard PA (**a**) and lateral (**b**) view; Ax T2-WI FS (**c**); and 3D GRE (**d**). There are prominent sequels of a Pouteau and ulnar styloid fracture (**a**, **b**). The second ulnar groove sign (**c**, **d**) and the laceration of the dorsal rul (**c**) are proof of an undiagnosed previous anterior luxation of the ulnar head

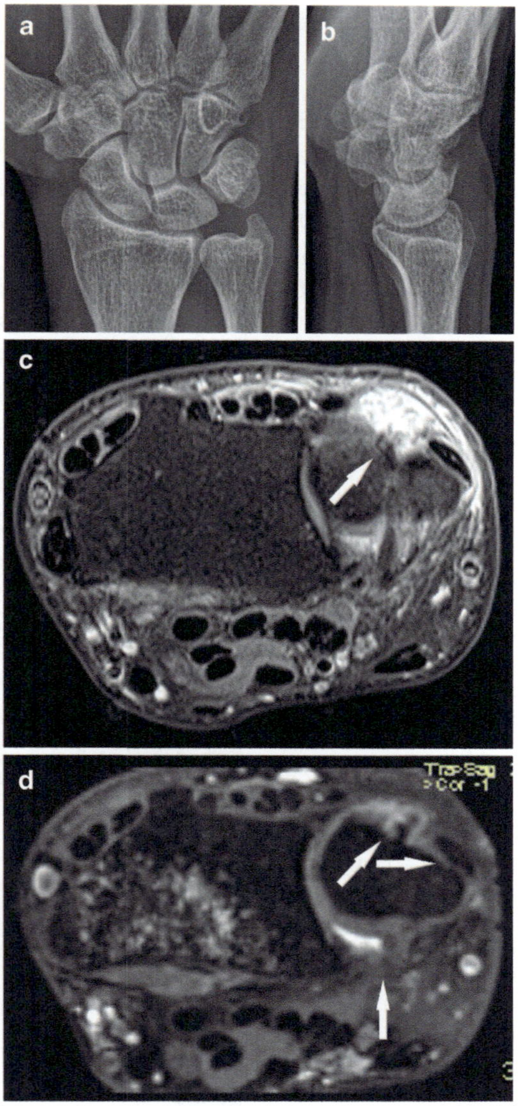

Fig. 11 Standard PA (**a**) and lateral (**b**) view; Ax T2-WI FS (**c**); and 3D GRE (**d**). Even without any sign of sequels of a fracture (**a**, **b**), the second ulnar groove sign (**c**, **d**) and the laceration of the palmar rul (**d**) are proof of a passed undiagnosed anterior luxation of the ulnar head. The ecu remains subluxated as well (**d**)

4 Scaphoid Pseudarthrosis

Pseudarthrosis after a scaphoid fracture is a serious mobility-restricting and osteoarthritis-inducing complication (Figs. 12 and 13). Early diagnosis of a delayed union (Perlik and Guilford 1991; Rowan and Downing 2017) is mandatory in order to prevent pseudarthrosis. MRI will provide early and spatial osseous and soft tissue information. The latter is important as well, as fractures/pseudarthrosis of the scaphoid do not exclude accompanying ligamentous injuries illustrated by MRI (Fig. 13c, d).

The space of Parona is a virtual tunnel, proximal to the carpal tunnel, which allows continuity from the distal forearm to the hand. A bone fragment may migrate through this space to the proximal carpal tunnel (Fig. 14) or even further. Interference with the adjacent soft tissue structures may cause long-term (nonspecific) symptoms.

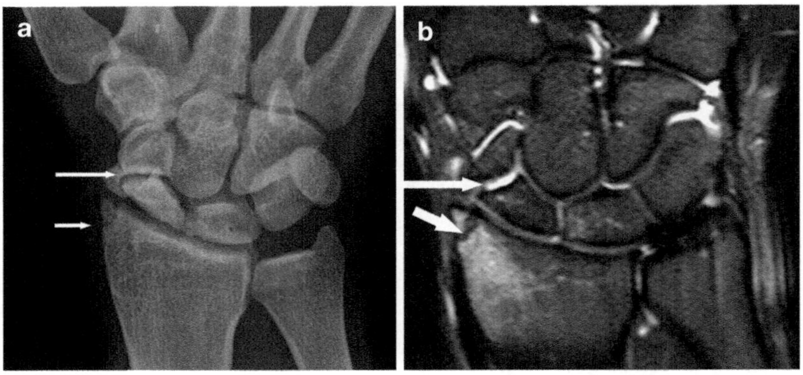

Fig. 12 Standard PA view (**a**); Cor T2-WI FS (**b**). Pseudarthrosis is present at the S waist (**a**, **b**) with fluid in the neo-joint space which has sclerotic borders with callus formation (**a**). A less obvious pseudarthrosis (**a**) with surrounding BMO (**b**) at the tip of the radial styloid process may be visualized as well

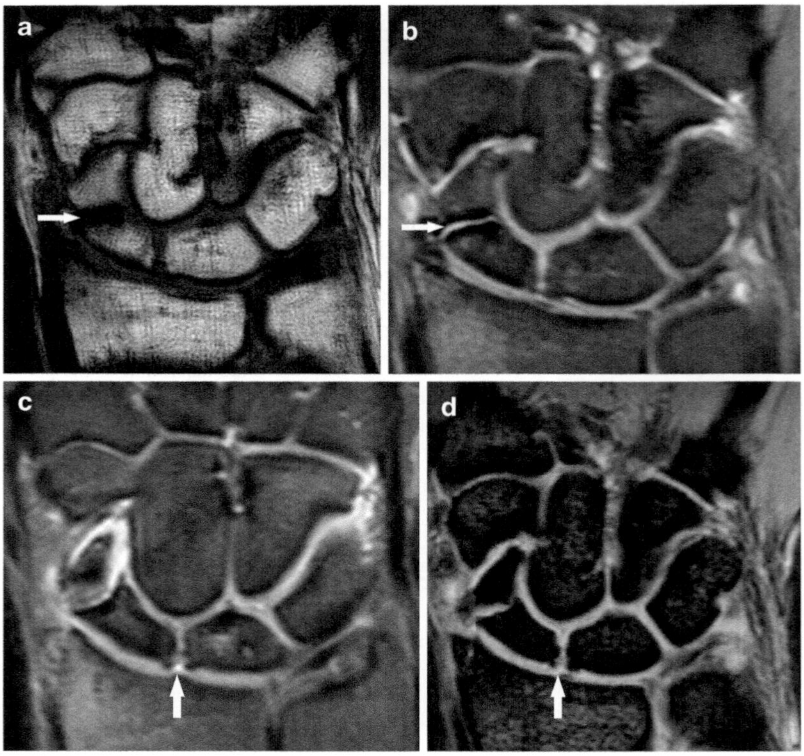

Fig. 13 Cor T1-WI (**a**), Cor PD WI (**b**, **c**), and 2D GRE (**d**). Pseudarthrosis at the S waist (**a**, **b**) is present, combined with a SL rupture (**c**, **d**)

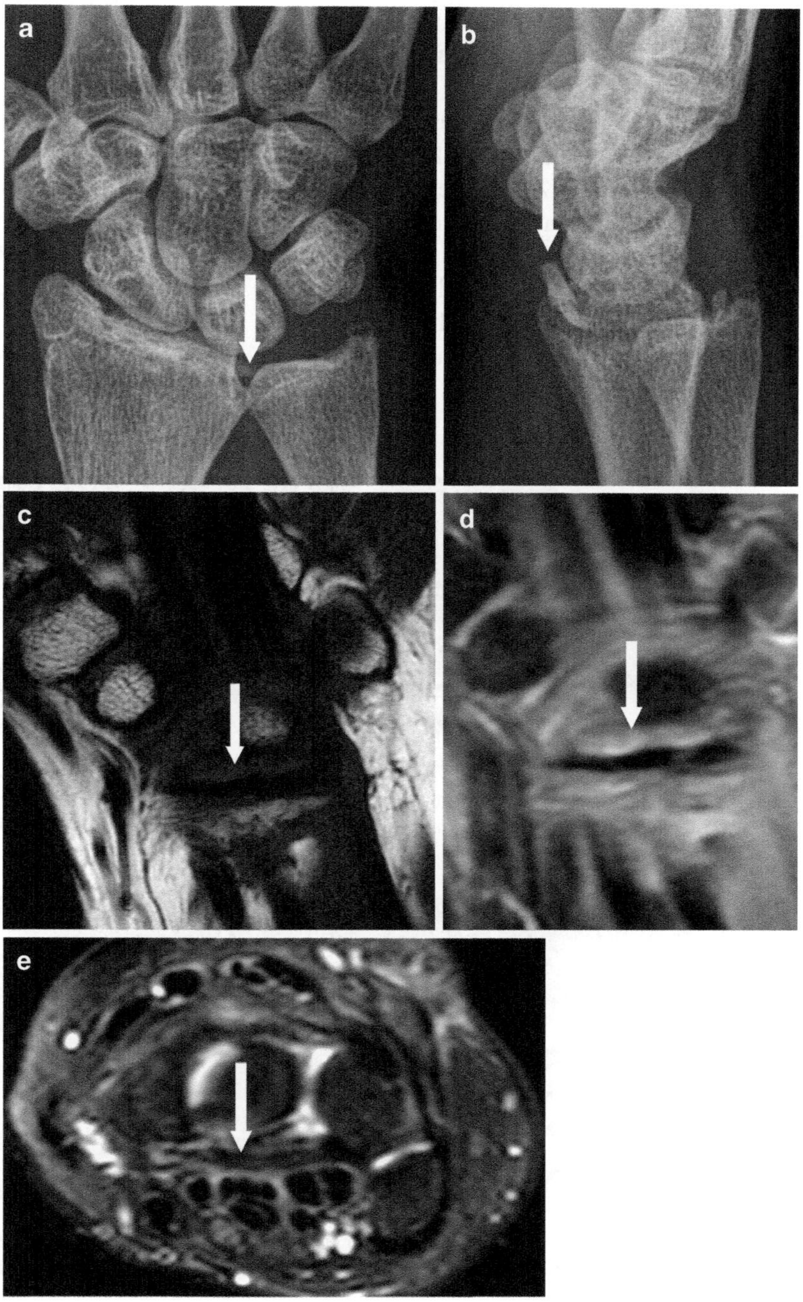

Fig. 14 Standard PA (**a**) and lateral (**b**) view; Cor T1-WI (**c**); Cor PD WI (**d**); and Ax T2-WI FS (**d**). Late control standard views show carpal migration towards the ulnar side (type 1) with a large bone fragment ventrally of the radiocarpal joint (**a**, **b**). The fragment (**c**–**e**) has migrated to the proximal carpal tunnel through the space of Parona (**e**)

5 Fracture Diagnosis and Differential Diagnosis

MRI may not only diagnose fractures (Jørgsholm et al. 2016) (Figs. 1 and 2), but also differentiate (Eriksen and Ringe 2012) them from other pathologies, such as avascular necrosis of the lunate or scaphoid bone. The typical, rather sharply delineated, band-shaped BMO pattern from anterior to posterior in the lunate bone allows the confirmation of a fracture (Fig. 15) and excludes avascular necrosis.

6 Post-Traumatic Carpal Boss

The typically affected CMC-III joint space may be altered by trauma and cause a secondary carpal boss (Fig. 16). However, the CMC II joint may be affected as well (Fig. 17). Even a combination of (a) post-traumatic lesion(s) (Fig. 18a, b) and an os styloideum fracture (Fig. 18c, d) may accidentally be discovered.

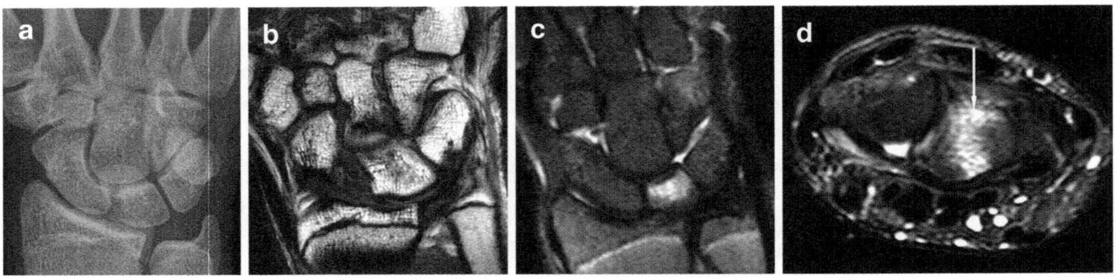

Fig. 15 Standard PA view (**a**); Cor T1-WI (**b**), Cor (**c**) and Ax T2-WI FS (**d**). Without an obvious trauma, but with persistent pain and despite of normal standard views (**a**), MRI shows BMO (**b**, **c**) with the typical band-shaped pattern from anterior to posterior in the L (**d**), which allows the radiologist to confirm a fracture

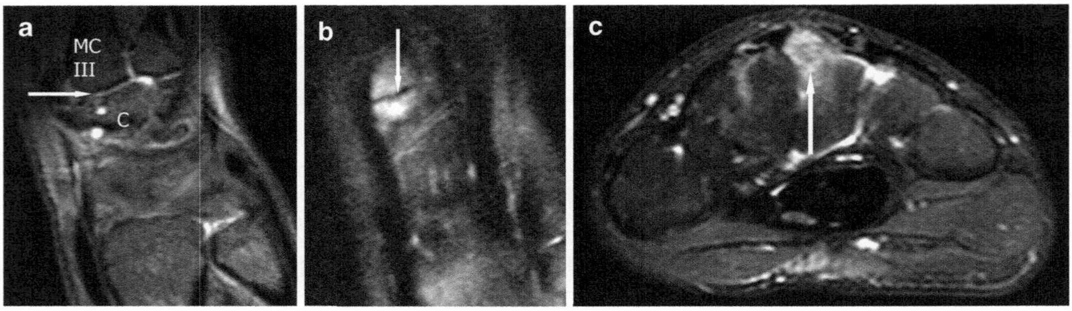

Fig. 16 Cor (**a**, **b**) and Ax T2-WI FS (**c**). After a previous trauma, the radial side of the CMC III joint is irregular and narrowed, with fluid in the joint space, surrounding bone marrow and soft tissue oedema

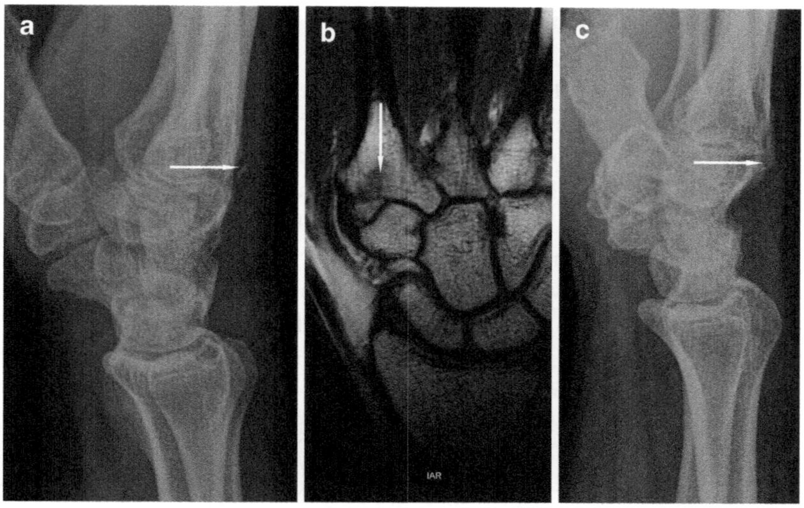

Fig. 17 Standard Lateral view (**a**, **c**); T1-WI FS (**b**). The standard lateral view reveals a broken fragment dorsally at the base of the MC region (**a**). MRI shows a fracture line and BMO at the base of the MC II (**b**). A follow-up standard lateral view shows a post-traumatic CB (**c**)

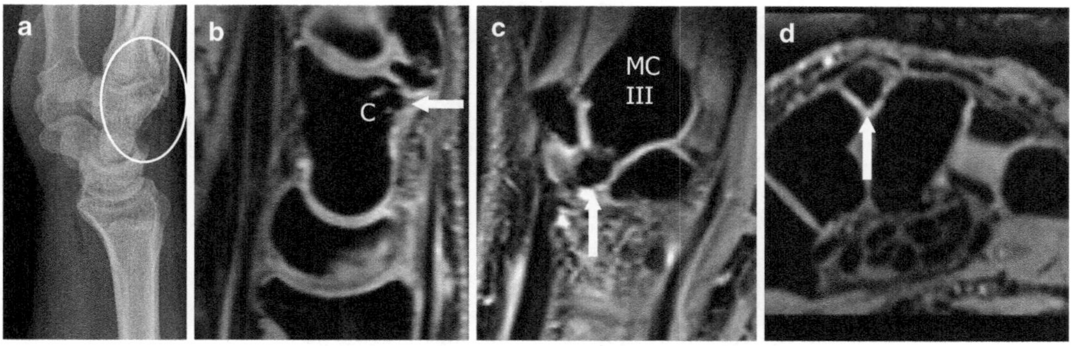

Fig. 18 Standard Lateral view (**a**); Sag (**b**), Cor (**c**), and Ax (**d**) 3D GRE. The standard lateral view shows some "irregularity" at the CMC joint (**a**). There is not only a post-traumatic sequel at the dorsal corner of the capitate bone (**b**), but also at the os styloideum at the quadrangular space (**c**, **d**), both predisposing to CB

7 Bone Deformation

The severe impaction of the radius may pass unnoticed on standard views (Knirk and Jupiter 1986), especially if the external margins of the bone remain intact (Fig. 19). Accidental associated findings, such as a dorsal U subluxation or a rupture of the palmar rul may indicate a severe trauma (Fig. 19).

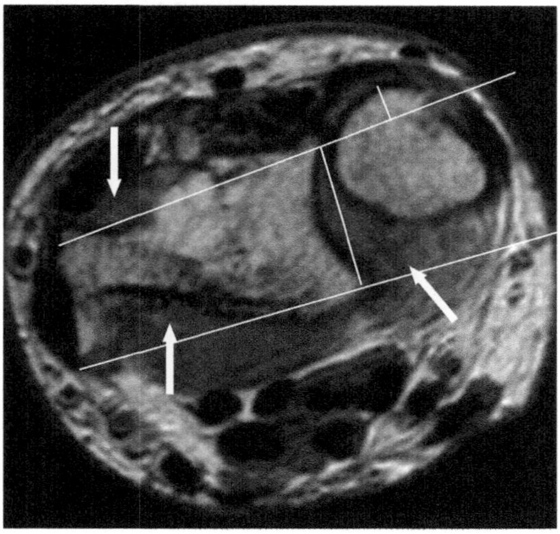

Fig. 19 Ax T1-WI. The radius is flattened in the AP direction ventrally and dorsally. The dorsal U subluxation and the rupture of the palmar rul are also accidental findings

8 Triquetropisiform Joint

This joint is frequently neglected in an urgent context due to the attention given to other (major) fractures and dislocations. A clear complete luxation (Fig. 20) is often discovered much later than at the time of trauma. The displacement may be less distinct (Fig. 21) in a subluxation.

Post-traumatic views may show calcification-like lesions at the T-P joint, which appear to be fragments broken off from the triquetral bone (Fig. 22). An old fracture of the P with a loose fragment and hydrops at the T-P joint are discovered rather frequently (Figs. 23 and 24) in symptomatic patients. The ligament between the pisiform bone and the hamulus may be torn as well (Figs. 24 and 25) whether (Fig. 25) or not in combination with a (sub)luxation at the T-P joint.

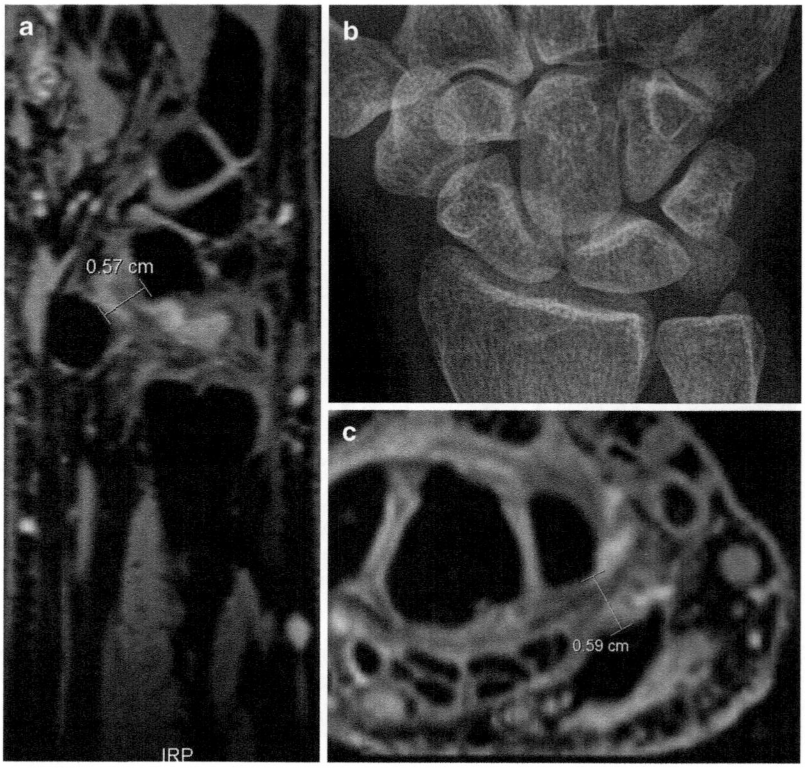

Fig. 20 Sag 3D GRE; Standard PA view (**b**); Ax 3D GRE. The pisiform bone is displaced and tilted (**a**). Retrospectively, the pisiform bone is projected to proximal and lateral on the standard view (**b**). There is no contact anymore with the triquetral bone due to this proximal and lateral luxation (**a**, **c**)

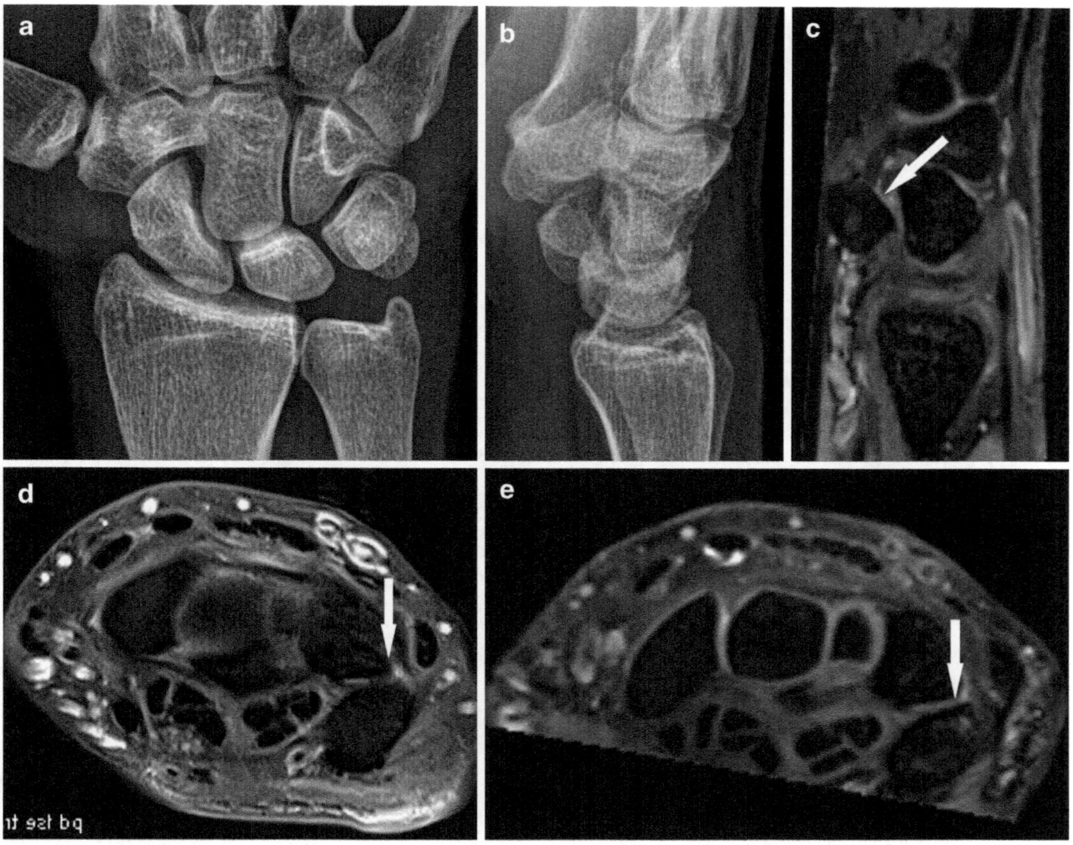

Fig. 21 Standard PA (**a**) and Lateral (**b**) views; Sag 3D GRE (**c**); Ax T2-WI FS (**d**); and Ax 3D GRE (**e**). Subluxation at the T-P joint without obvious alterations on standard views

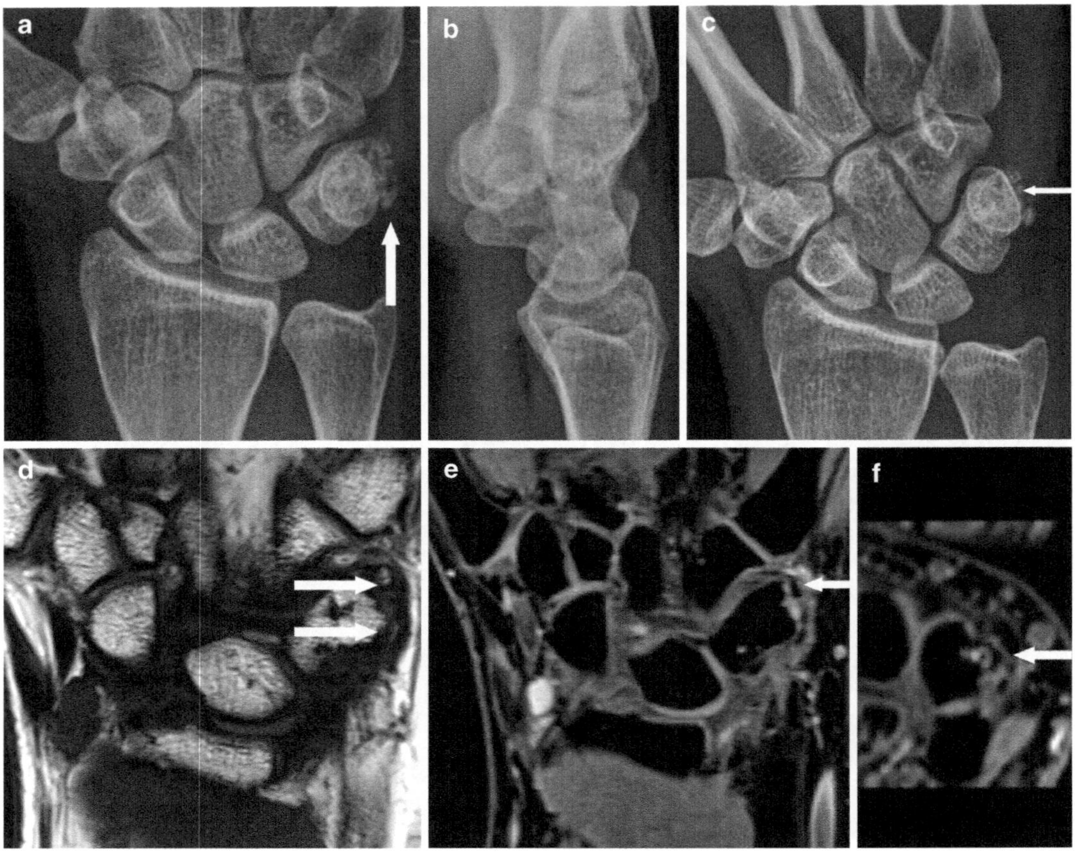

Fig. 22 Standard PA (**a**) and lateral (**b**) views; Standard PA view in radial deviation (**c**); Ax T1-WI (**d**); Cor (**e**) and Sag (**f**) 3D GRE. The calcification-like lesions at the T-P joint (**a**, **c**) appear to be fragments broken off from the triquetral bone (**d**–**f**)

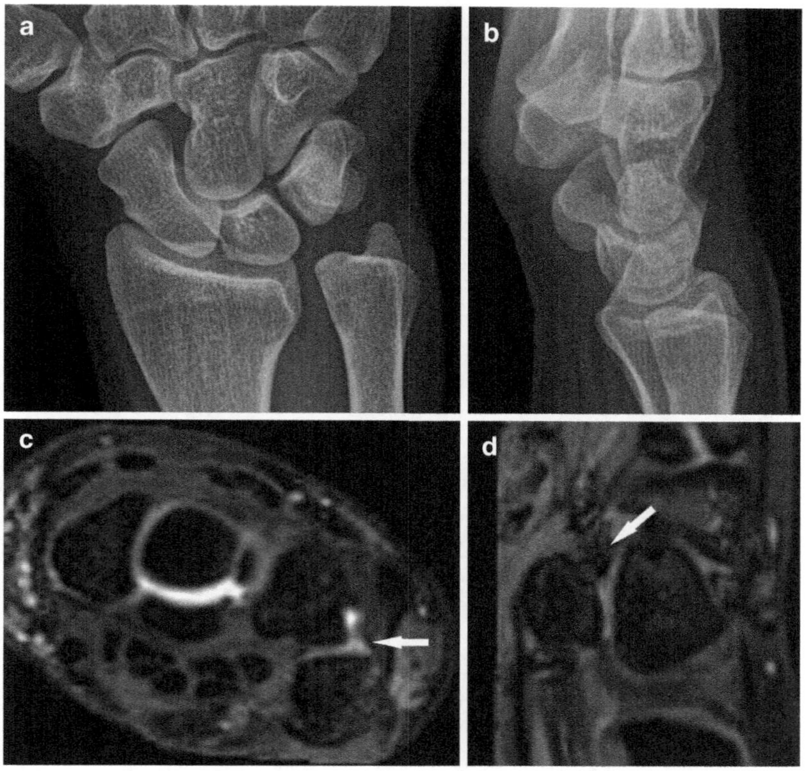

Fig. 23 Standard PA (**a**) and lateral (**b**) views; Ax (**c**) and Sag (**d**) 3D GRE. MRI shows an old distal fracture of the P with loose fragment and hydrops at the T-P joint

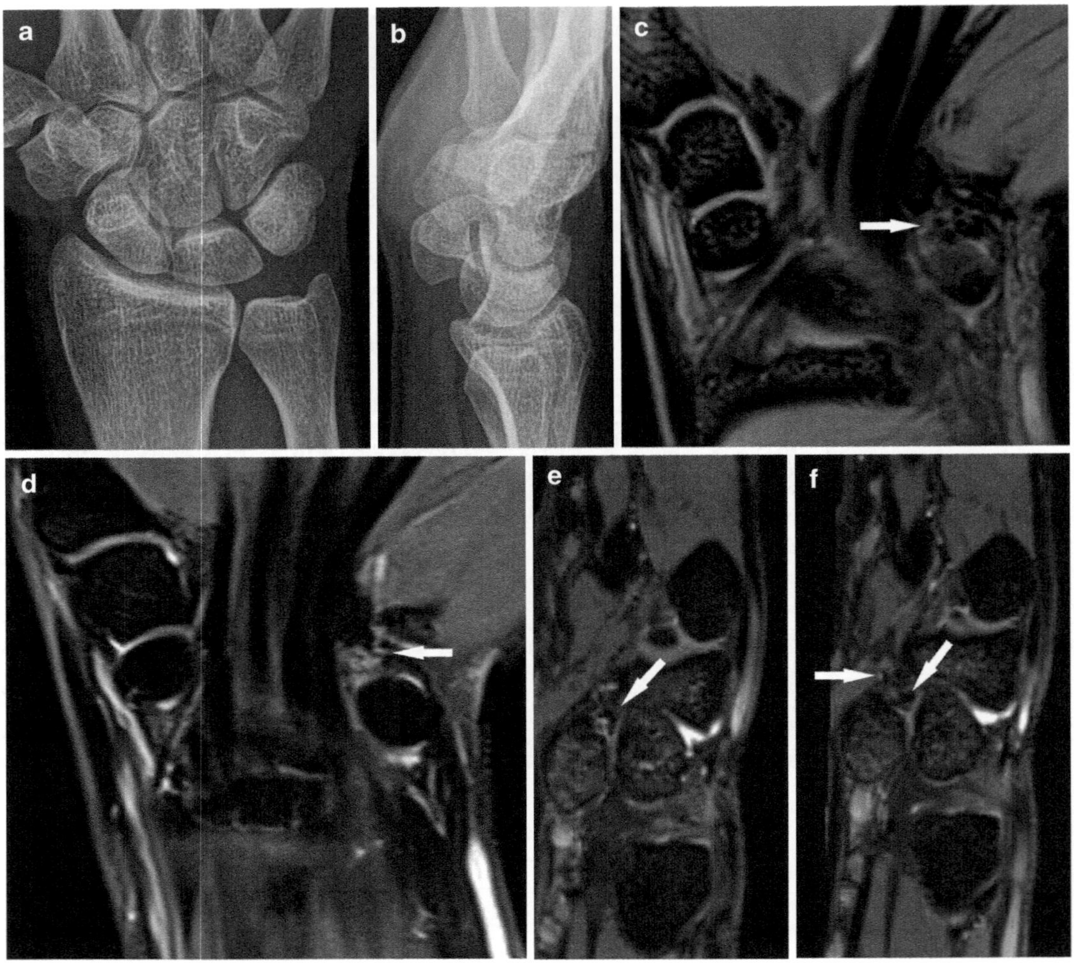

Fig. 24 Standard PA (**a**) and lateral (**b**) views; Cor 2D GRE (**c**) and T2-WI FS (**d**); Sag 3D GRE (**e**, **f**). Post-traumatic dotted low signals (**c**, **d**, **f**; horizontal arrows) at the location of an absent ligament between the pisiform bone and the hamulus and a distal P fracture (oblique arrows) (**e**, **f**)

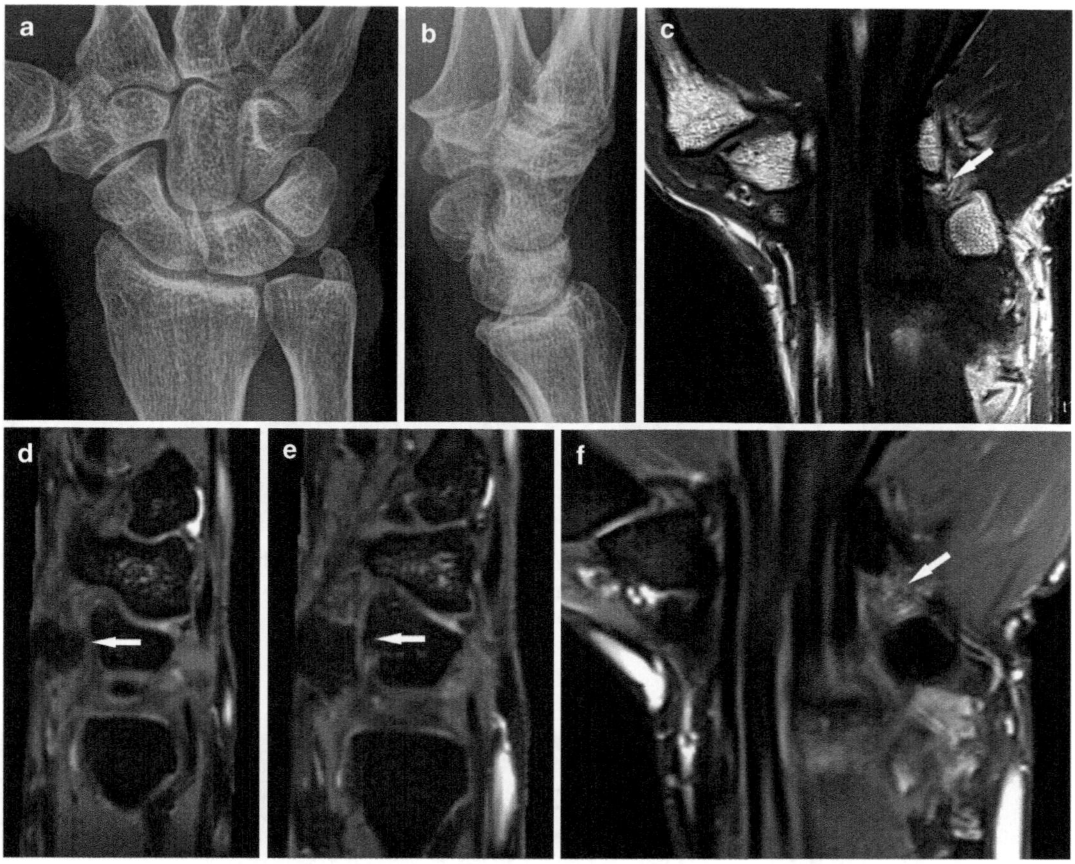

Fig. 25 Standard PA (**a**) and lateral (**b**) views; Cor T1-WI (**c**); Sag 3D GRE (**d**, **e**); and Cor T2-WI FS (**f**). A post-traumatic small bone fragment in the space of the absent T-P ligament (**c**–**f**) combined with a subluxation at the T-P joint (**e**)

9 Hamulus and Pisiform Bone Fractures

A fall on an outstretched hand (FOOSH-lesion) may also impact the prominent bony structures on the ulnar side of the wrist. As for the T-P joint, fractures of the P bone frequently pass unnoticed in the urgent phase of trauma (Figs. 22, 23, and 24). This also applies to the hamulus of the hamate bone (Zancolli 2001) (Fig. 26), which—in a traumatic setting—is often seen as a "spotlight" on T2-WI FS (Fig. 26h) due to the BMO.

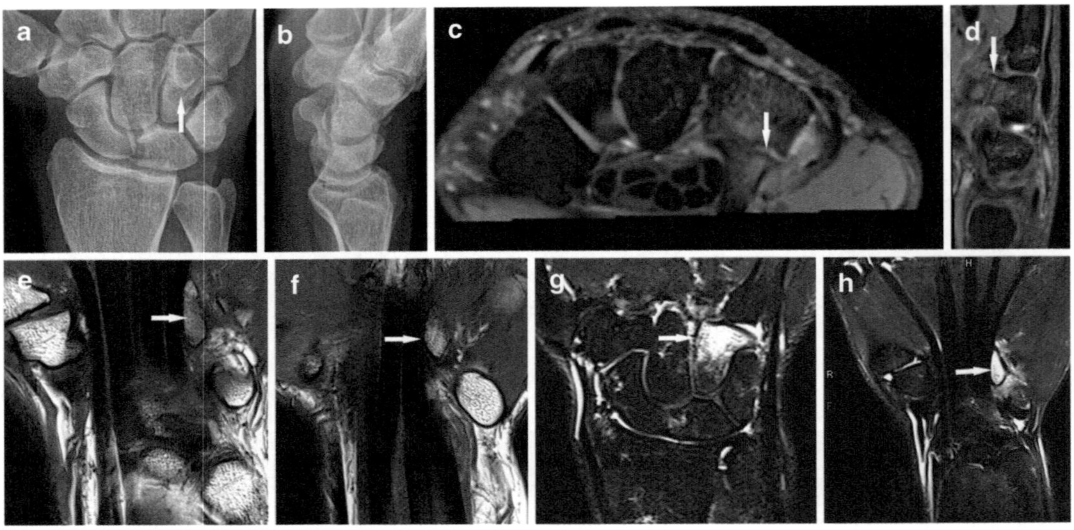

Fig. 26 Standard PA (**a**) and lateral (**b**) views; Ax (**c**) and Sag (**d**) 3D GRE; Cor T1-WI (**e**, **f**) and Cor T2-WI FS (**g**, **h**). Post-traumatic standard views show a normal aspect of the well delineated hamulus (**a**, **b**). Nevertheless, a fracture line is clearly seen at the base of the hamulus (**c**, **d**) with BMO at the distal part of the H and all over the hamulus (**e**, **f**)

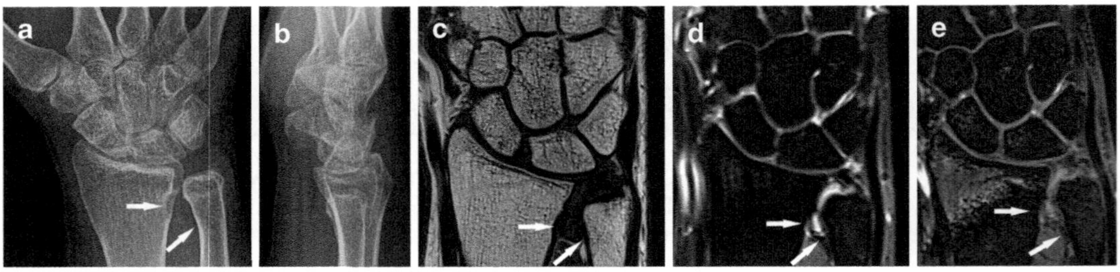

Fig. 27 Standard PA (**a**) and lateral (**b**) views; Cor T1-WI (**c**); Cor T2-WI FS (**d**); and 2D GRE (**e**). The post-traumatic bending of the distal U, the negative ulnar variance, and the shallow cortical indentation of the R on standard views (**a**, **b**) are also noticed on MRI (**c**–**e**). In addition, fluid in the DRUJ is demonstrated and—at the time of imaging—BMO around the indentation is excluded (**c**, **d**)

10 Negative Ulnar Variance and Impingement

The fracture and the post-traumatic bending of the distal U may result in a negative ulnar variance (Fig. 27a). Due to secondary impingement, a shallow cortical indentation of the R emerges (Fig. 27a, c–e). In addition, fluid in the DRUJ (Fig. 27d), and subsequently BMO around the indentation, are clinically significant.

11 Post-Traumatic Stylotriquetral Abutment

Post-traumatic deformation and/or enlargement of the ulnar styloid may lead to a secondary stylotriquetral abutment with kissing BMO and subcortical cysts (Fig. 28). Small displacements, due to an unconsolidated fracture, with pseudarthrosis at the base of a large styloid process may also initiate stylotriquetral abutment (Fig. 29).

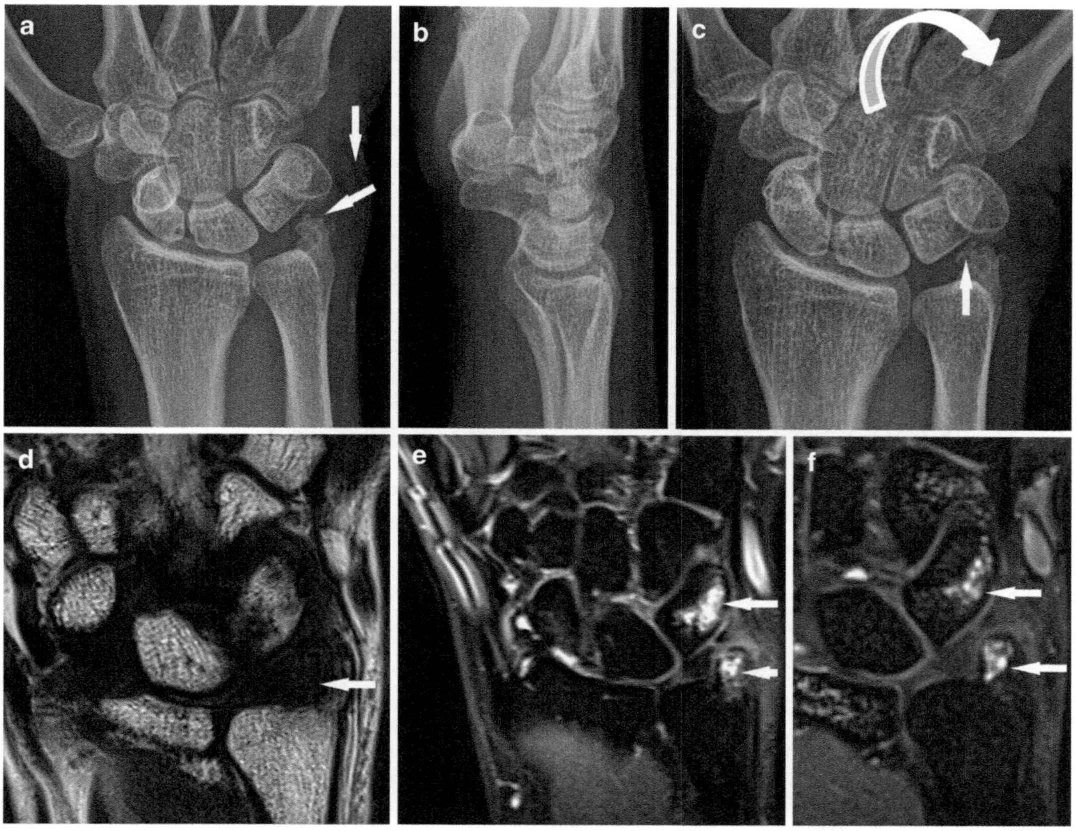

Fig. 28 Standard PA (**a**), lateral (**b**) and PA in ulnar deviation (**c**) views; Cor T1-WI (**d**); Cor T2-WI FS (**e**); and 3D GRE (**f**). The ulnar styloid process is deformed with adjacent soft tissue swelling after trauma (**a**–**c**). Ulnar deviation is almost completely lost (**c**). Kissing BMO and subcortical cysts at the Tri and ulnar styloid are prominent (**d**–**f**) indicating abutment

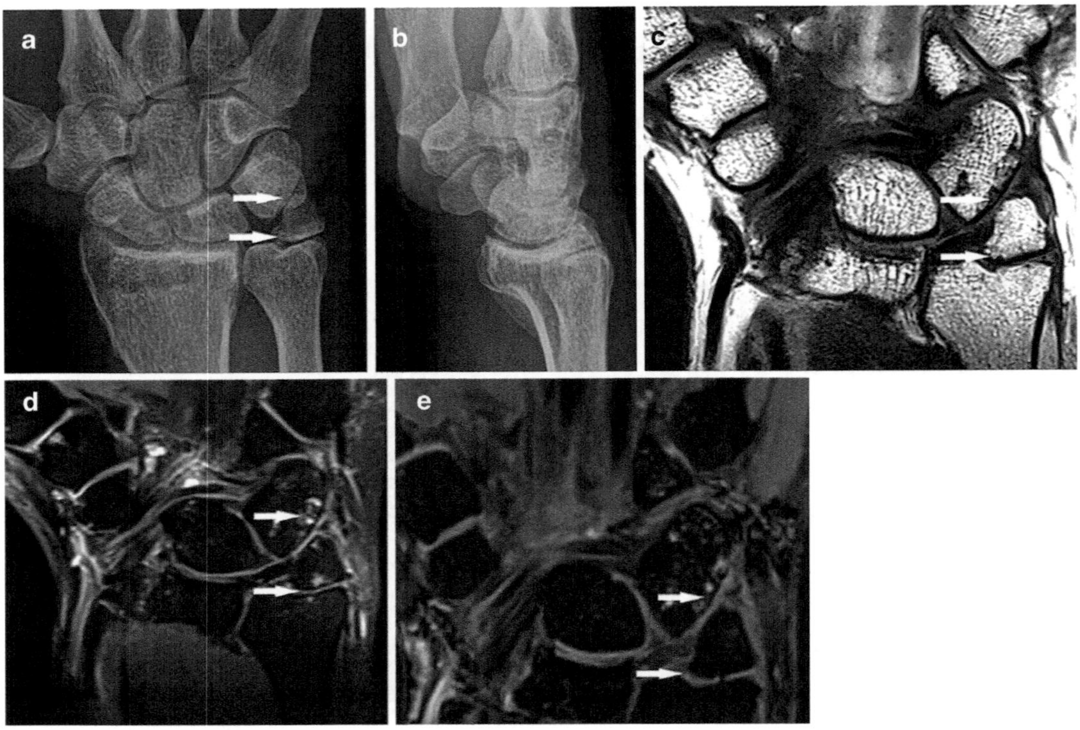

Fig. 29 Standard PA (**a**) and lateral (**b**) views; Cor T1-WI (**c**); Cor T2-WI FS (**d**); and 3D GRE (**e**). The ulnar styloid process is broken at the base with pseudarthrosis (**a**, **c**–**e**). The neo-articulation shows subcortical cysts (**d**, **e**) at the base of the styloid which is also slightly displaced distally resulting in a styloid triquetral abutment (**c**–**e**)

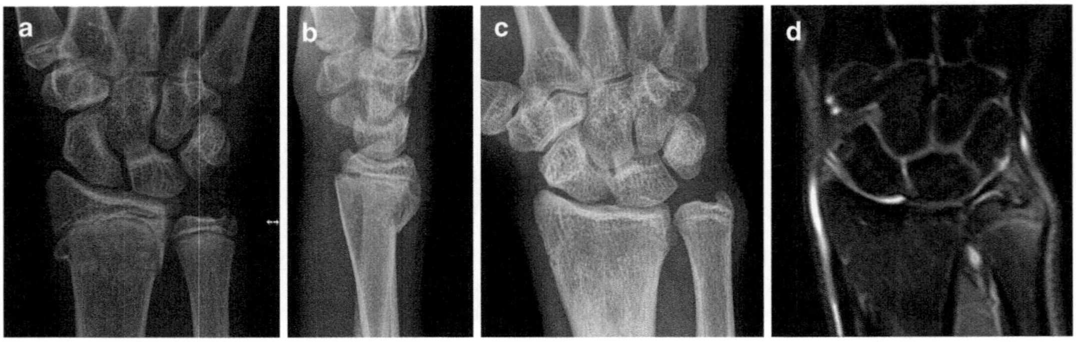

Fig. 30 Standard PA (**a**, **c**) and lateral (**b**) views; Cor T2-WI FS (**d**). Salter-Harris (type 2) fracture-epiphysiolysis of the distal R (and fracture of the tip of the ulnar styloid process) (**a**, **b**). After consolidation, there is a positive ulnar variance (**c**) due to a premature closure of the radial growth plate (**c**, **d**)

12 Post-Traumatic Positive Ulnar Variance

Salter-Harris fracture-epiphysiolysis of the distal R (Fig. 30a, b) may result in a premature closure of the radial growth plate in children (Fig. 30c, d). After consolidation, there is still growth at the (still faintly visible) ulnar growth plate, which ultimately results in a positive ulnar variance (Fig. 30c, d), a pre-determination for secondary ulnar abutment.

13 Gymnast Wrist

Due to the chronic microtraumas, small scattered ossification bridges cross the growth plates. This may ultimately lead to early closure of the growth plates. On standard views, the growth plate becomes irregular with an adjacent hazy and increasing bone density (Salter and Harris 1963) (Fig. 31a, b). In an earlier phase, the small bony bridges may already be observed on MRI (Fig. 31c–g).

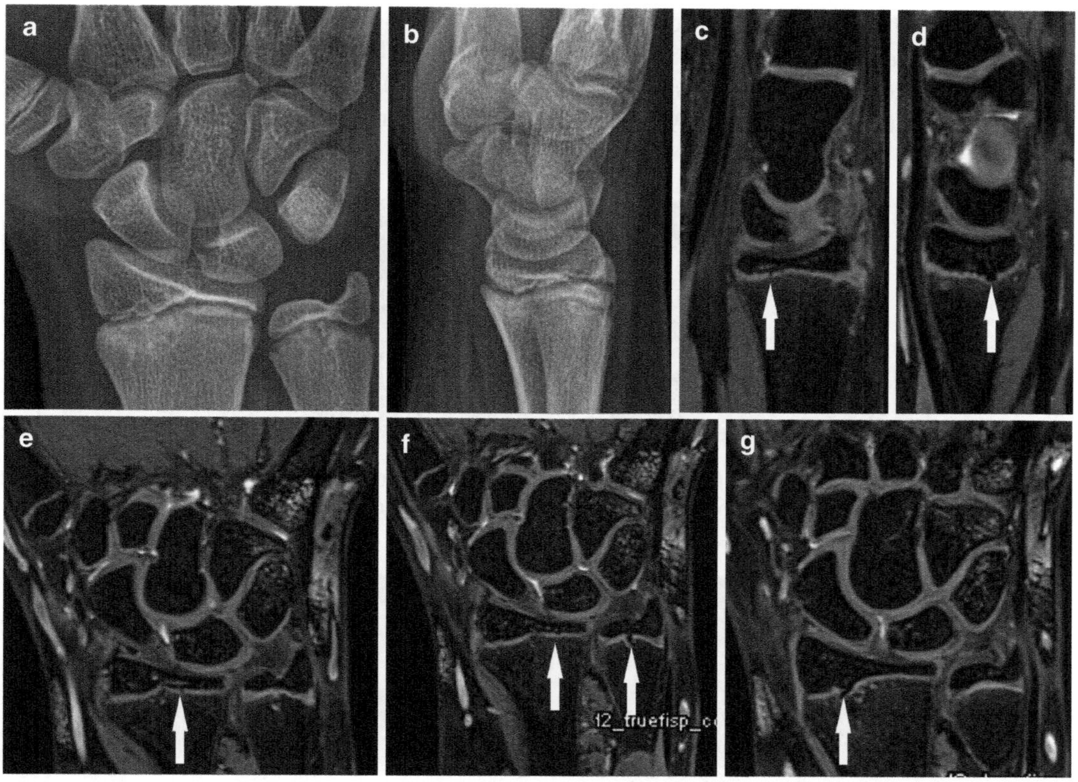

Fig. 31 Standard PA (**a**) and lateral (**b**) views; Sag (**c**, **d**); and Cor 3D GRE (**e**, **f**). Irregular delineation of and hazy increased bone density around the growth plates (**a**, **b**) appear on standard view. (Earlier) small-scattered ossification bridges may be demonstrated on MRI (**c**–**g**)

14 Post-Traumatic Soft Tissue Pathology

Good fracture consolidation in a correct position (Fig. 32a, b) may hide significant alterations of the tendons, such as a tendon luxation of the extensor compartment I (apl, epb) (Fig. 32c, d).

Another "hidden" post-traumatic soft tissue pathology may be a torn intrinsic scapholunate ligament (Gilula and Weeks 1978; Gondim Teixeira et al. 2016; Hafezi-Nejad et al. 2016; Langner et al. 2015; Metz et al. 1997; Ozçelik et al. 2005; Sulkers et al. 2018; Wolfe et al. 2012) with subsequent development of a pathognomonic radiopalmar arthrosynovial cyst (Fig. 33).

Lesions of the extrinsic ligaments (Gilula and Weeks 1978; Metz et al. 1997; Niacaris et al. 2015; Ramamurthy et al. 2016; Rubensson et al. 2018) (Fig. 34), even without apparent fracture sequels (Fig. 34a, b), should be searched for, especially in case of an ulnar carpal translation (Fig. 34a). The palmar (Fig. 34c–e, i) and dorsal (Fig. 34f–i) extrinsic ligaments should be screened thoroughly.

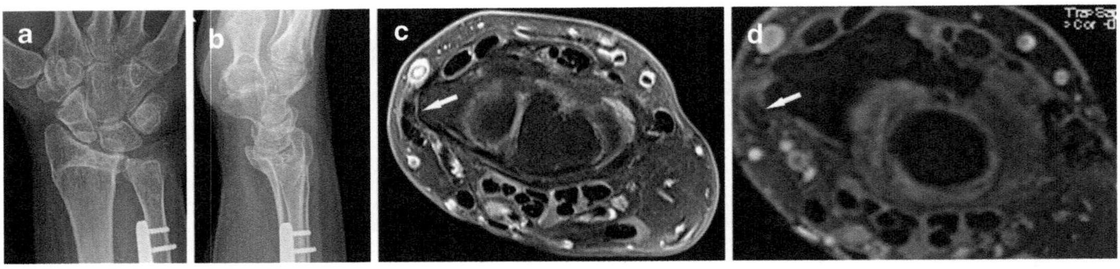

Fig. 32 Standard PA (**a**) and lateral (**b**) views; Ax T2-WI FS (**c**); and 3D GRE (**d**). Good consolidation of R, U and S-fracture (**a**, **b**). Luxation of the tendons of the extensor compartment I (**c**, **d**)

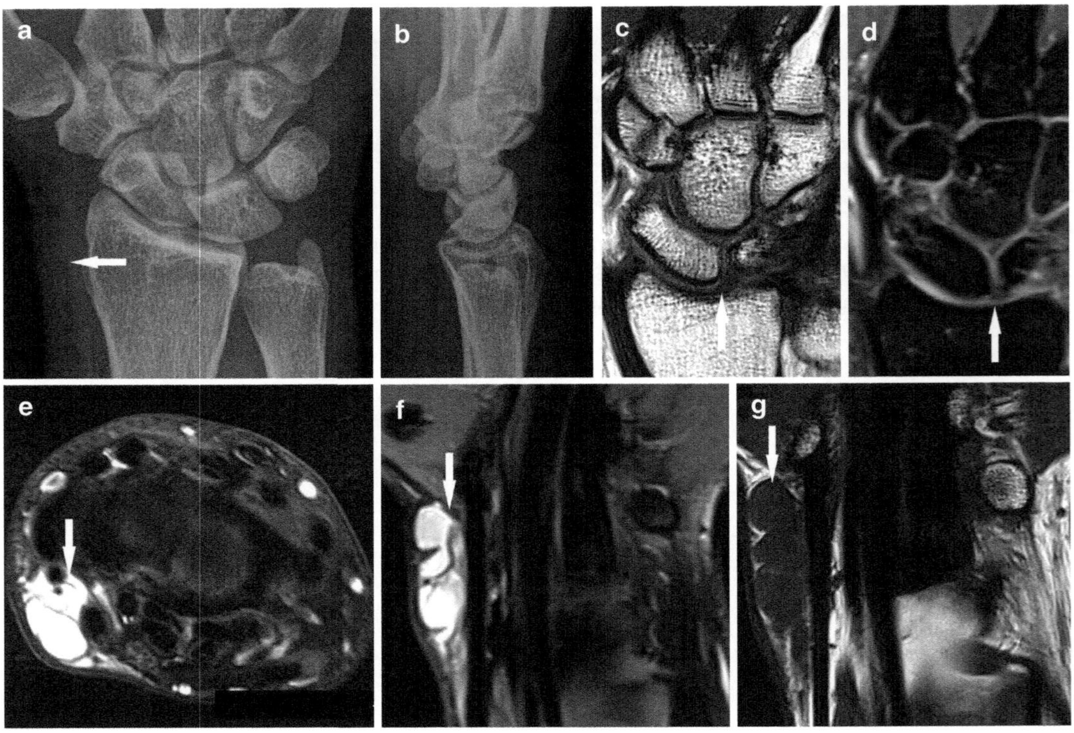

Fig. 33 Standard PA (**a**) and lateral (**b**) views; Cor T1-WI (**c**) and PD WI (**d**); Ax T2-WI FS (**e**); Cor T2-WI FS (**f**); and T1-WI (**g**). Soft tissue swelling adjacent to the R (**a**, **b**). A torn SL (**c**, **d**) is associated with a large arthrosynovial cyst (**e**–**g**)

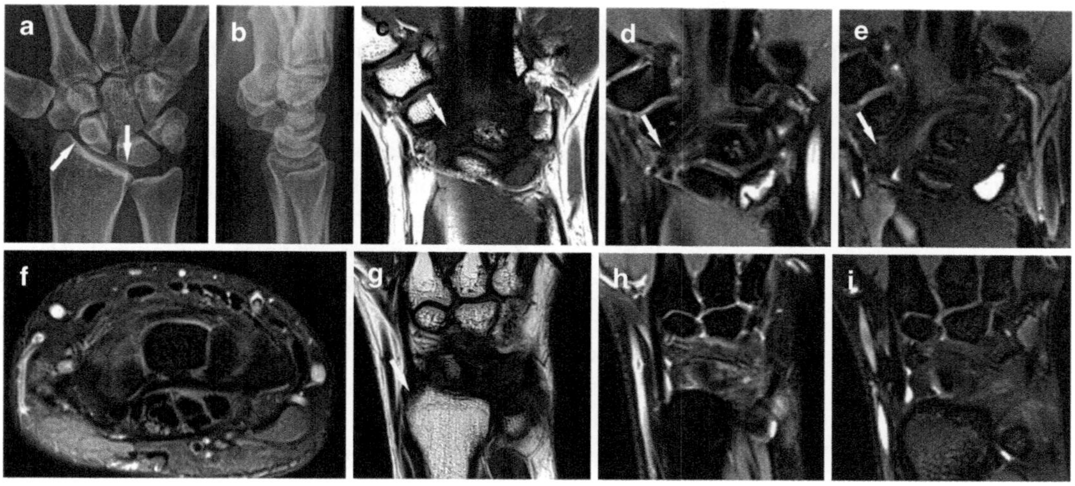

Fig. 34 Standard PA (**a**) and lateral (**b**) views; Cor T1-WI (**c**, **g**), T2-WI FS (**d**, **h**), and 2D GRE (**e**, **i**); Ax T2-WI FS (**f**). Ulnar translation of the carpus (type 1) with widening of the R-S space (**a**). The radial component of the palmar V is ruptured (**c**–**e**, **f**) and the dorsal main ligaments seem to be intact (**f**–**i**)

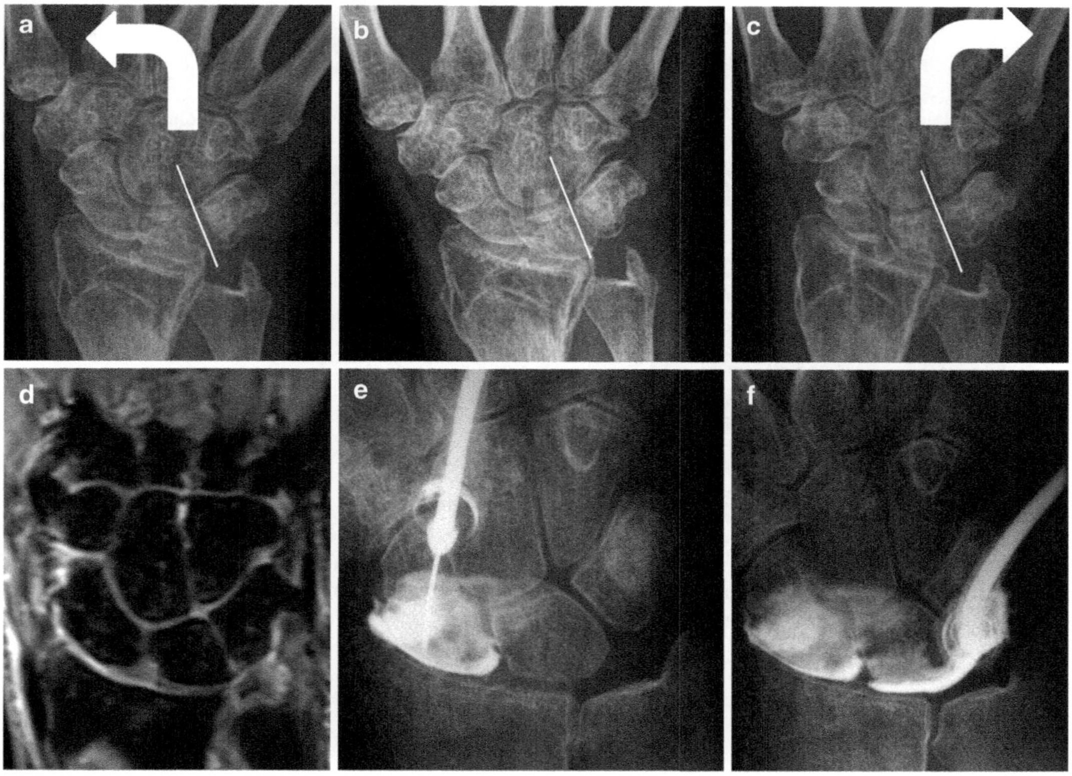

Fig. 35 Standard PA views in radial (**a**), neutral (**b**), and ulnar (**c**) deviation; Cor PD WI (**d**); wrist arthrography with double injection at the RC joint (**e**, **f**). Although the mobility of the carpus in radial and ulnar deviation is almost absent (**a**–**c**), no major pathology at MRI (**d**) could explain this restriction. A RC-arthrography showed an extreme capsule retraction of the RC joint with two compartments due to IA adhesions (**e**, **f**)

Motion standard views may in some (extreme) cases show a restricted mobility (Fig. 35a–c). The capsule is very difficult to evaluate on MRI (Fig. 35d). Arthrography of the wrist is still an indication to evaluate the shape and content of the capsule, especially if complemented by specific techniques such as double injection in the radial (Fig. 35e) and ulnar (Fig. 35f) part of the RC joint space. Not only an extremely restricted content and deformation of the RC joint capsule, but also an intra-articular adhesion, may sometimes be illustrated (Fig. 35e, f).

15 Cartilage

Obviously, the cartilage—in contrast with cortical deformation(s)—is only indirectly shown by standard views (Fig. 36a, b). The real condition of the cartilage needs a 3D evaluation (Avenarius et al. 2012; Hunt 2006; Tanabe et al. 2011), preferable initially by plain MRI (Mutimer et al. 2008) to determine the configuration and extent of the lesions. The extent of the cortical depression(s) (Fig. 36c–e) and the status of the (overlying) cartilage is evaluated (Fig. 36c–e). Certainly, in more complex post-traumatic deformations (Fig. 37), the 3D GRE techniques allow accurate analysis of the cortical depressions. In addition, loose bone fragments and/or calcifications may be found (Hunt 2006) (Fig. 37c–g).

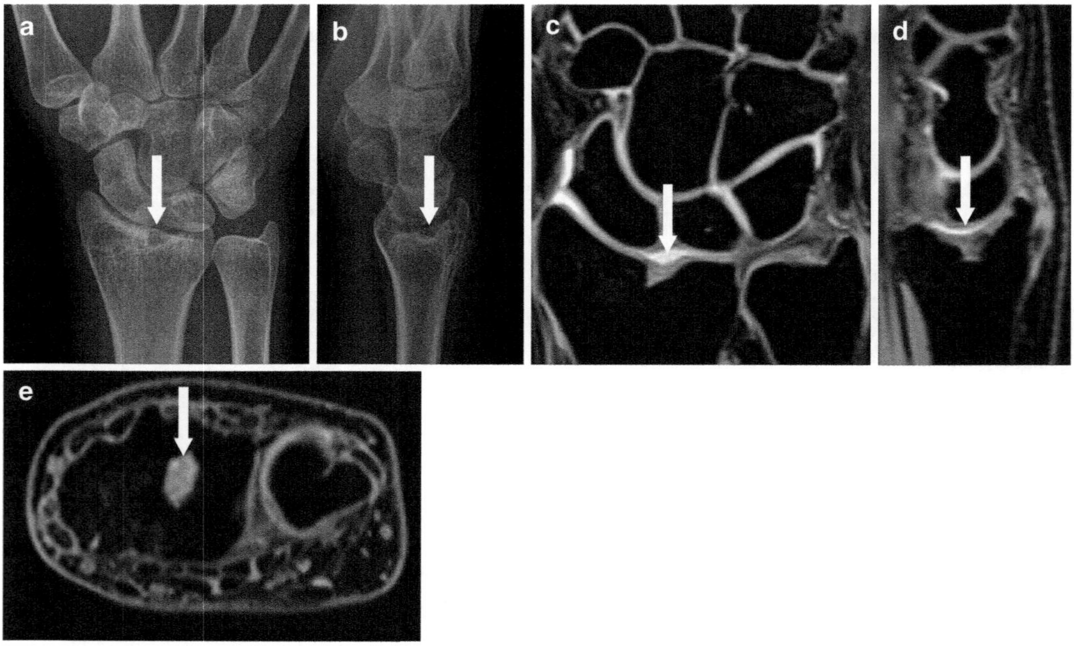

Fig. 36 Standard PA (**a**) and lateral views (**b**); Cor (**c**), Sag (**d**), and Ax (**e**) 3D GRE. The cortical depression at the distal radius epiphysis is clearly noticed on standard views (**a, b**). The real extent of the cortical depression and the step off at the surface of the cartilage is shown in MRI (**c–e**)

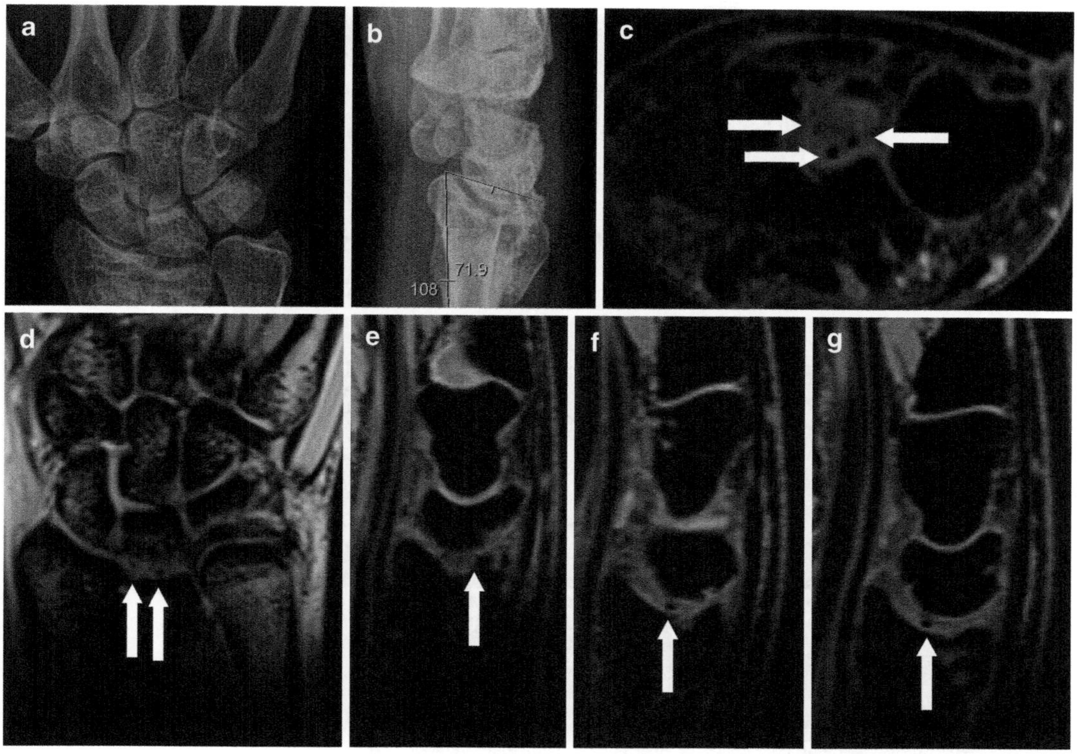

Fig. 37 Standard PA (**a**) and lateral (**b**) views; Ax (**c**), Cor (**d**), and Sag (**e**–**g**) 3D GRE. The irregular depression of the R (**a**, **b**) is better appreciated on a 3D MRI sequence (**c**–**g**). Small loose bone fragments at the depressed region are shown as are the small defects in the lunate bone (**c**–**g**)

16 Combined Pathology

The evaluation of trauma after surgery is challenging (Ochman et al. 2017) (Fig. 38). Metal artefacts may interfere. The comparison with previous MRI exams—if available—is a very valuable tool. Continuous bony fusions without BMO exclude new fractures. Post-traumatic (old) deformation of the (peri-)carpal bones and loose bone fragments should be looked for. Cartilage, ligaments, and nerves are frequently involved as well. Even after a common trauma, such as a Pouteau fracture, several other lesions (Fig. 39) may be present and interfere with the rehabilitation if not detected and/or treated properly.

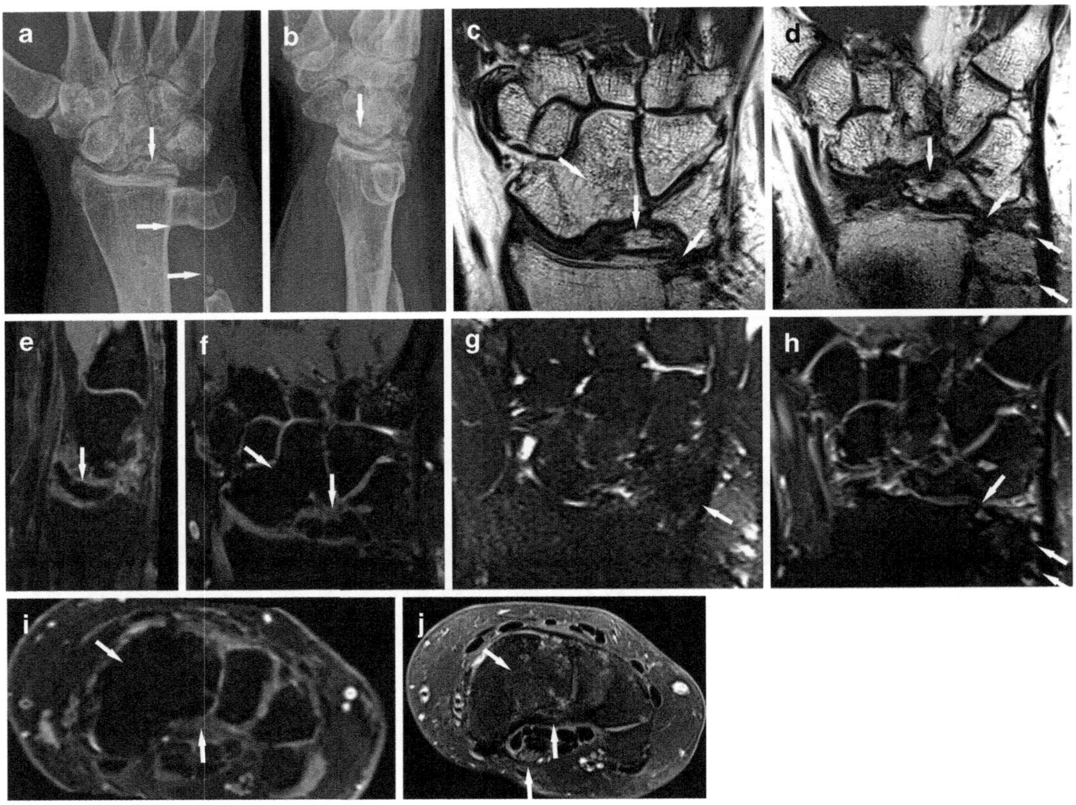

Fig. 38 Standard PA (**a**) and lateral (**b**) views; Cor T1-WI (**c**, **d**); Sag (**e**) and Cor (**f**) 3D GRE; Cor T2-WI (**g**, **h**); Ax 3D GRE (**i**); and T2-WI FS (**j**). Status after Suave-Kapandji surgery and bony fusion of S-C. The L is irregularly contoured and flattened without (new) traumatic lesion (**a**–**f**). The bony fusions are intact (**a**, **c**, **f**, **g**, **i**) without BMO after an additional trauma. There is a type IA tear of the TFCC (**h**). Fibrosis narrows the proximal carpal tunnel (**i**, **j**) and the median nerve shows signs of CTS (**j**)

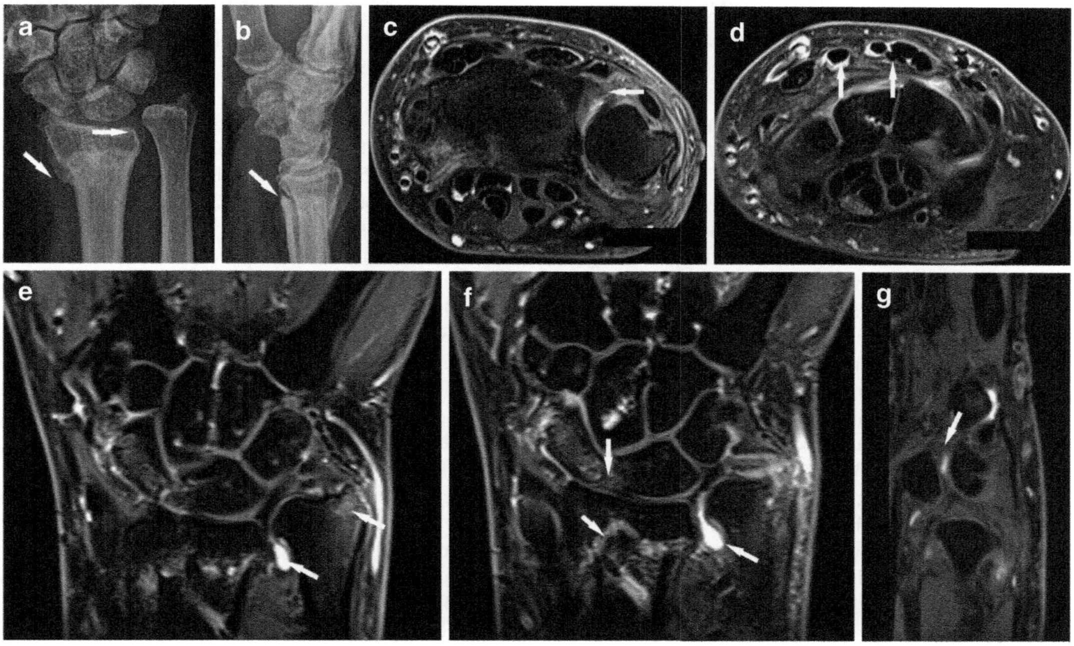

Fig. 39 Standard PA (**a**) and lateral (**b**) views; Ax (**c**, **d**) and Cor (**e**, **f**) T2-WI FS; Sag 3D GRE (**g**). Sequels of a Pouteau fracture with positive ulnar variance (**a**, **b**, **f**). Rupture of the dorsal rul (**c**); tenosynovitis of the extensor tendons (II, III and IV) (**d**); elongated but continuous TFCC and hydrops of the DRUJ (**e**, **f**); laceration of the SL (**f**) and subluxation at the TP joint (**g**)

References

Arora S, Grover SB, Batra S, Sharma VK (2010) Comparative evaluation of postreduction intra-articular distal radial fractures by radiographs and multidetector computed tomography. J Bone Joint Surg Am 92(15):2523–2532. https://doi.org/10.2106/JBJS.I.01617. PMID: 21048172

Avenarius DM, Ording Müller LS, Eldevik P, Owens CM, Rosendahl K (2012) The paediatric wrist revisited – findings of bony depressions in healthy children on radiographs compared to MRI. Pediatr Radiol 42(7):791–798. https://doi.org/10.1007/s00247-012-2354-x. Epub 2012 Mar 20. PMID: 22430482

Balci A, Basara I, Çekdemir EY, Tetik F, Aktaş G, Acarer A, Özaksoy D (2015) Wrist fractures: sensitivity of radiography, prevalence, and patterns in MDCT. Emerg Radiol 22(3):251–256. https://doi.org/10.1007/s10140-014-1278-1. Epub 2014 Oct 18. PMID: 25325932

Bashir W, Aziz A, Jidaal I (2014) Imaging of skeletal extremity trauma: a review. Trauma 16:300–317. https://doi.org/10.1177/1460408614542920

Bencardino JT, Rosenberg ZS (2006) Sports-related injuries of the wrist: an approach to MRI interpretation. Clin Sports Med 25(3):409–432. https://doi.org/10.1016/j.csm.2006.02.007, vi. PMID: 16798135

Bouri F, Fuad M, Elsayed Abdolenour A (2016) Locked volar distal radioulnar joint dislocation. Int J Surg Case Rep 22:12–14. https://doi.org/10.1016/j.ijscr.2016.03.012. Epub 2016 Mar 22. PMID: 27016647; PMCID: PMC4844664

Carlsen BT, Dennison DG, Moran SL (2010) Acute dislocations of the distal radioulnar joint and distal ulna fractures. Hand Clin 26(4):503–516. https://doi.org/10.1016/j.hcl.2010.05.009. PMID: 20951900

Ekenstam F, Hagert CG (1985) Anatomical studies on the geometry and stability of the distal radio ulnar joint. Scand J Plast Reconstr Surg 19(1):17–25. https://doi.org/10.3109/02844318509052861. PMID: 4023639

Eriksen EF, Ringe JD (2012) Bone marrow lesions: a universal bone response to injury? Rheumatol Int 32(3):575–584. https://doi.org/10.1007/s00296-011-2141-2. Epub 2011 Sep 8. PMID: 21901347

Gillis JA, Soreide E, Khouri JS, Kadar A, Berger RA, Moran SL (2019) Outcomes of the Adams-Berger ligament reconstruction for the distal radioulnar joint instability in 95 consecutive cases. J Wrist Surg 8(4):268–275. https://doi.org/10.1055/s--0039-1685235. Epub 2019 Apr 22. PMID: 31404256; PMCID: PMC6685731

Gilula LA, Weeks PM (1978) Post-traumatic ligamentous instabilities of the wrist. Radiology 129(3):641–651. https://doi.org/10.1148/129.3.641. PMID: 725039

Girgis WS, Epstein RE (2000) Magnetic resonance imaging of the hand and wrist. Semin Roentgenol 35(3):286–296. https://doi.org/10.1053/sroe.2000.7339. PMID: 10939130

Gondim Teixeira PA, De Verbizier J, Aptel S, Wack M, Dap F, Dautel G, Blum A (2016) Posterior radioscaphoid angle as a predictor of wrist degenerative joint disease in patients with scapholunate ligament tears. AJR Am J Roentgenol 206(1):144–150. https://doi.org/10.2214/AJR.15.14606. PMID: 26700346

Gornitzky AL, Carrigan RB (2016) The diagnostic utility of MRI in the painful wrist: when to reconsider advanced imaging in the pediatric patient. Pediatrics (Evanston) 137(Suppl 3):596–596A. https://doi.org/10.1542/peds.137.Supplement_3.596A

Hafezi-Nejad N, Carrino JA, Eng J, Blackmore C, Shores J, Lifchez SD, Farahani SJ, Demehri S (2016) Scapholunate interosseous ligament tears: diagnostic performance of 1.5T, 3T MRI, and MR arthrography – a systematic review and meta-analysis. Acad Radiol 23(9):1091–1103. https://doi.org/10.1016/j.acra.2016.04.006. Epub 2016 Jul 15. PMID: 27426979

Hauck RM, Skahen J 3rd, Palmer AK (1996) Classification and treatment of ulnar styloid nonunion. J Hand Surg Am 21(3):418–422. https://doi.org/10.1016/S0363-5023(96)80355-8. PMID: 8724472

Hunt TR 3rd. (2006) Degenerative and post-traumatic arthritis affecting the carpometacarpal joints of the fingers. Hand Clin 22(2):221–228. https://doi.org/10.1016/j.hcl.2006.02.004. PMID: 16701136

Iordache SD, Rowan R, Garvin GJ, Osman S, Grewal R, Faber KJ (2012) Prevalence of triangular fibrocartilage complex abnormalities on MRI scans of asymptomatic wrists. J Hand Surg Am 37(1):98–103. https://doi.org/10.1016/j.jhsa.2011.10.006. Epub 2011 Nov 30. PMID: 22129657

Jenkins NH, Mintowt-Czyz WJ, Fairclough JA (1987) Irreducible dislocation of the distal radioulnar joint. Injury 18(1):40–43. https://doi.org/10.1016/0020-1383(87)90384-6. PMID: 3440614

Jørgsholm P, Thomsen N, Besjakov J, Abrahamsson S, Björkman A (2016) MRI shows a high incidence of carpal fractures in children with posttraumatic radial-sided wrist tenderness. Acta Orthop 87(5):533–537. https://doi.org/10.1080/17453674.2016.1210940. Epub 2016 Jul 20. PMID: 27436058; PMCID: PMC5016915

Khalid M, Jummani Z, Kanagaraj K, Robinson D, Reed H (2006) Role of MRI in the diagnosis of occult wrist injury following foosh. J Hand Surg Br Vol 31:42–42. https://doi.org/10.1016/j.jhsb.2006.03.149

Kim JP, Park MJ (2008) Assessment of distal radioulnar joint instability after distal radius fracture: comparison of computed tomography and clinical examination results. J Hand Surg Am 33(9):1486–1492. https://doi.org/10.1016/j.jhsa.2008.05.017. PMID: 18984328

Kim S, Ward JP, Rettig ME (2012) Galeazzi fracture with volar dislocation of the distal radioulnar joint. Am J Orthop (Belle Mead NJ) 41(11):E152–E154. PMID: 23431520

Knirk JL, Jupiter JB (1986) Intra-articular fractures of the distal end of the radius in young adults. J Bone Joint Surg Am 68(5):647–659. PMID: 3722221

Kohyama S, Hara Y, Fukai R, Yamazaki M (2015) Subacute volar dislocation of the distal radioulnar joint without fracture: a case report and literature review. Trauma 17(3):229–234. https://doi.org/10.1177/1460408614560079

Kwon BC, Seo BK, Im HJ, Baek GH (2012) Clinical and radiographic factors associated with distal radioulnar joint instability in distal radius fractures. Clin Orthop Relat Res 470(11):3171–3179. https://doi.org/10.1007/s11999-012-2406-4. Epub 2012 Jun 6. PMID: 22669548; PMCID: PMC3462878

Langner I, Fischer S, Eisenschenk A, Langner S (2015) Cine MRI: a new approach to the diagnosis of scapholunate dissociation. Skeletal Radiol 44(8):1103–1110. https://doi.org/10.1007/s00256-015-2126-4. Epub 2015 Mar 12. PMID: 25761726

Lindau T, Aspenberg P (2002) The radioulnar joint in distal radial fractures. Acta Orthop Scand 73(5):579–588. https://doi.org/10.1080/000164702321022884. PMID: 12440504

Lo IK, MacDermid JC, Bennett JD, Bogoch E, King GJ (2001) The radioulnar ratio: a new method of quantifying distal radioulnar joint subluxation. J Hand Surg Am 26(2):236–243. https://doi.org/10.1053/jhsu.2001.22908. PMID: 11279569

Mack MG, Keim S, Balzer JO, Schwarz W, Hochmuth K, Windolf J, Vogl TJ (2003) Clinical impact of MRI in acute wrist fractures. Eur Radiol 13(3):612–617. https://doi.org/10.1007/s00330-002-1600-2. Epub 2002 Sep 11. PMID: 12594566

Malik AK, Pettit P, Compson J (2005) Distal radioulnar joint dislocation in association with elbow injuries. Injury 36(2):324–329. https://doi.org/10.1016/j.injury.2004.02.018. PMID: 15664598

May MM, Lawton JN, Blazar PE (2002) Ulnar styloid fractures associated with distal radius fractures: incidence and implications for distal radioulnar joint instability. J Hand Surg Am 27(6):965–971. https://doi.org/10.1053/jhsu.2002.36525. PMID: 12457345

McMurray D, Muralikuttan K (2008) Volar dislocation of the distal radio–ulnar joint without fracture: a case report and literature review. Inj Extra 39(11):352–355. https://doi.org/10.1016/j.injury.2008.06.013

Mespreuve M, Vanhoenacker F, Verstraete K (2015) Imaging findings of the distal radio-ulnar joint in trauma. J Belg Soc Radiol 99(1):1–20. https://doi.org/10.5334/jbr-btr.846. PMID: 30039059; PMCID: PMC6032773

Metz VM, Metz-Schimmerl SM, Yin Y (1997) Ligamentous instabilities of the wrist. Eur J Radiol 25(2):104–111. https://doi.org/10.1016/s0720-048x(97)00041-7. PMID: 9283838

Mino DE, Palmer AK, Levinsohn EM (1983) The role of radiography and computerized tomography in the diagnosis of subluxation and dislocation of the distal radioulnar joint. J Hand Surg Am 8(1):23–31. https://doi.org/10.1016/s0363-5023(83)80046-x. PMID: 6827048

Morrissy RT, Nalebuff EA (1979) Dislocation of the distal radioulnar joint: anatomy and clues to prompt diagnosis. Clin Orthop Relat Res 144:154–158. PMID: 535217

Mutimer J, Green J, Field J (2008) Comparison of MRI and wrist arthroscopy for assessment of wrist cartilage. J Hand Surg Eur Vol 33(3):380–382. https://doi.org/10.1177/1753193408090395. PMID: 18562375

Niacaris T, Ming BW, Lichtman DM (2015) Midcarpal instability: a comprehensive review and update. Hand Clin 31(3):487–493. https://doi.org/10.1016/j.hcl.2015.04.004. PMID: 26205710

Ochman S, Wieskötter B, Langer M, Vieth V, Raschke MJ, Stehling C (2017) High-resolution MRI (3T-MRI) in diagnosis of wrist pain: is diagnostic arthroscopy still necessary? Arch Orthop Trauma Surg 137(10):1443–1450. https://doi.org/10.1007/s00402-017-2747-2. Epub 2017 Aug 14. PMID: 28808768

Orbay J, Vernon L, Poirier S, Morales V, Cambo R, Mercer D (2021) Effect of ulnar head offset on distal radioulnar joint stability. J Hand Surg Am 46(9):816.e1–816.e7. https://doi.org/10.1016/j.jhsa.2020.12.014. Epub 2021 Mar 13. Erratum in: J Hand Surg Am. 2022 Jan;47(1):84. PMID: 33722471

Ozçelik A, Günal I, Köse N (2005) Stress views in the radiography of scapholunate instability. Eur J Radiol 56(3):358–361. https://doi.org/10.1016/j.ejrad.2005.06.011. Epub 2005 Jul 19. PMID: 16046094

Perlik PC, Guilford WB (1991) Magnetic resonance imaging to assess vascularity of scaphoid nonunions. J Hand Surg Am 16(3):479–484. https://doi.org/10.1016/0363-5023(91)90018-7. PMID: 1861031

Ramamurthy NK, Chojnowski AJ, Toms AP (2016) Imaging in carpal instability. J Hand Surg Eur Vol 41(1):22–34. https://doi.org/10.1177/1753193415610515. Epub 2015 Nov 19. PMID: 26586689

Rowan CH, Downing ND (2017) Trans-scaphoid perilunate fracture dislocation: 'notjust a scaphoid fracture'. BMJ Case Rep 2017:bcr2017221041. https://doi.org/10.1136/bcr-2017-221041. PMID: 28739625; PMCID: PMC5624016

Rubensson C, Johansson T, Adolfsson L (2018) Tensioning of the radioscaphocapitate and long radiolunate ligaments for dynamic radiocarpal instability. J Hand Surg Eur Vol 43(4):369–374. https://doi.org/10.1177/1753193418756805. Epub 2018 Feb 15. PMID: 29448916

Salter RB, Harris WR (1963) Injuries involving the epiphyseal plate. J Bone Joint Surg Am 45:108–115

Slattery D, Gohil S, Hogan G (2013) A case report and the literature review: volar dislocation of the DRUJ and stabilisation using mini-suture anchors. Eur J Orthop Surg Traumatol 23(Suppl 2):S203–S205. https://doi.org/10.1007/s00590-012-1157-y. Epub 2013 Jan 5. PMID: 23412303

Stuart PR, Berger RA, Linscheid RL, An KN (2000) The dorsopalmar stability of the distal radioulnar joint. J Hand Surg Am 25(4):689–699. https://doi.org/10.1053/jhsu.2000.9418. PMID: 10913210

Sulkers GSI, Strackee SD, Schep NWL, Maas M (2018) Wrist cineradiography: a protocol for diagnosing carpal instability. J Hand Surg Eur Vol 43(2):174–178. https://doi.org/10.1177/1753193417694820. Epub 2017 Mar 1. PMID: 28488457; PMCID: PMC5791518

Tanabe K, Nakajima T, Sogo E, Denno K, Horiki M, Nakagawa R (2011) Intra-articular fractures of the distal radius evaluated by computed tomography. J Hand Surg Am 36(11):1798–1803. https://doi.org/10.1016/j.jhsa.2011.08.021. Epub 2011 Oct 5. PMID: 21981830

Wechsler RJ, Wehbe MA, Rifkin MD, Edeiken J, Branch HM (1987) Computed tomography diagnosis of distal radioulnar subluxation. Skeletal Radiol 16(1):1–5. https://doi.org/10.1007/BF00349919. PMID: 3823954

Wolfe SW, Garcia-Elias M, Kitay A (2012) Carpal instability nondissociative. J Am Acad Orthop Surg 20(9):575–585. https://doi.org/10.5435/JAAOS-20-09-575. PMID: 22941800

Zancolli ER 3rd (2001) Localized medial triquetral-hamate instability: anatomy and operative reconstruction-augmentation. Hand Clin 17(1):83–96, vii. PMID: 11280162

Imaging Pitfalls

Contents

1 General

It cannot be stressed enough that standard views and MRI should always be evaluated together as one "unit". Subtle changes and alarm signals of both techniques may influence the choice of the technical approach, the (final) evaluation of the trauma, and the therapeutic choices.

2 Bone Marrow Oedema at MRI

Subtle anomalies are occasionally overlooked on standard views (Eriksen and Ringe 2012) (Fig. 1a). MRI is a very sensitive tool in the traumatic context thanks to the early detection of BMO. The discovery of obvious BMO (Fig. 1b), and in this case even a fine transverse fracture line (Bruno et al. 2019; Couzens et al. 2014) (Fig. 1c, d), may urge to re-review the standard views. The fracture line and a small cortical irregularity are confirmed in retrospect (Fig. 1a).

The pattern of the BMO may indicate the type of trauma. Narrow band-shaped oedema (Eriksen and Ringe 2012; Shabshin and Schweitzer 2009) traversing the carpus in a longitudinal direction (Fig. 2) indicates an axial trauma. Especially in medical expertise cases, it is important to be able to determine whether a specific trauma is indeed the cause of the radiological pathologic findings. In contrast to the normal standard views (Fig. 1a, b), MRI reveals a BMO running in a zig-zag longitudinal direction through the carpus (Fig. 3c), confirming a recent trauma. The route lines (Fig. 3d) can only be aligned in radial deviation (Boutin et al. 2013; Chaudhari et al. 2023; Li et al. 2022; Palmer et al. 1985) (Fig. 3e), which is compliant with the previously mentioned trauma at work.

M. Mespreuve, K. Waked, *MRI of the Wrist*, Medical Radiology,
https://doi.org/10.1007/978-3-031-63973-9_5

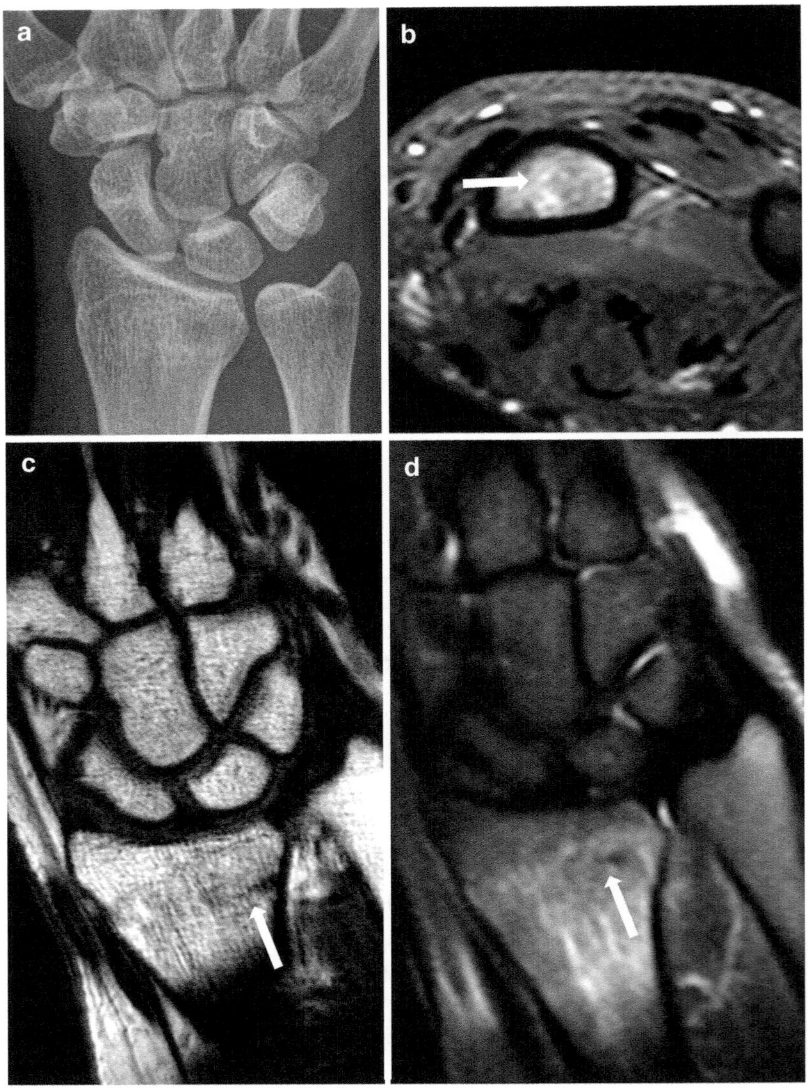

Fig. 1 Standard PA view (**a**); Ax T2-WI FS (**b**); Cor T1-WI (**c**); and Cor T2-WI FS. The standard PA view is considered normal (**a**). A BMO warning (**b**) leads to the discovery of a radius fracture (**c**, **d**)

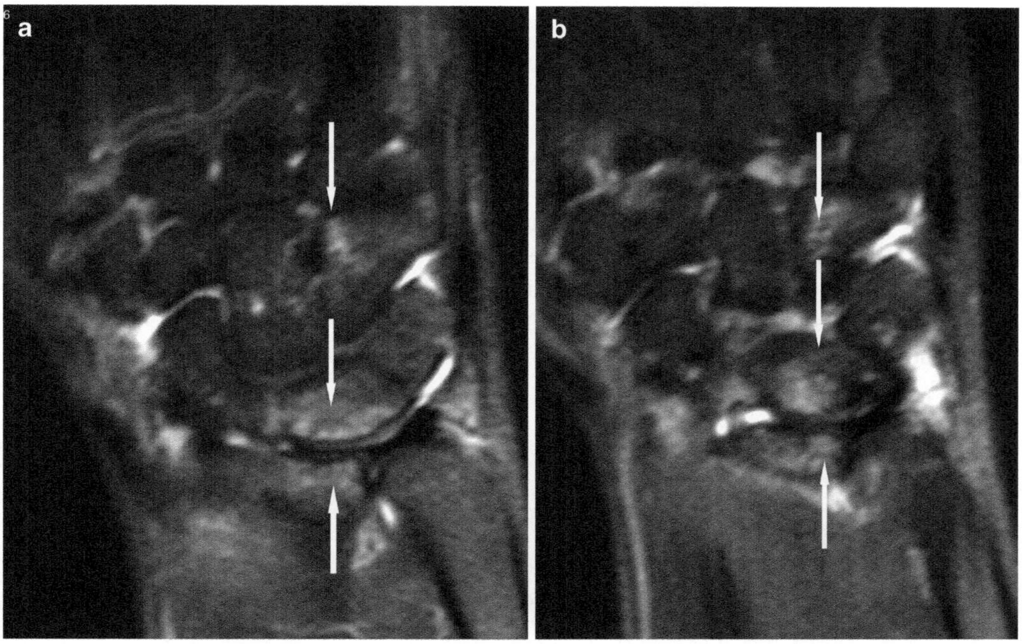

Fig. 2 Cor T2-WI FS (**a**, **b**). Narrow band-shaped oedema traversing R, L, and H in a longitudinal direction

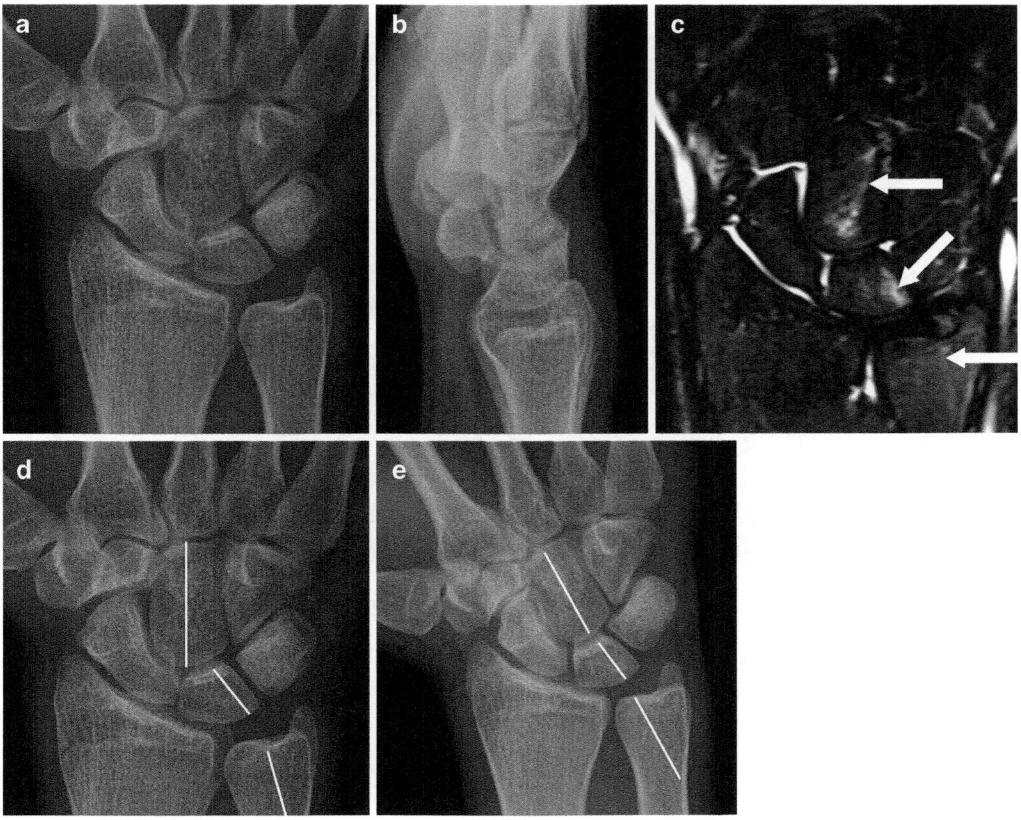

Fig. 3 Standard PA (**a**) and Lateral (**b**) views; Cor T2-WI FS; Standard PA view in neutral position (**d**) and in radial deviation (**e**). Normal standard views (**a**, **b**). MRI shows a longitudinal line-shaped oedema traversing C, L, and U in various directions (**c**). The oedema schematically drawn on a PA standard view (**d**) can only be aligned in radial deviation (**e**)

3 Soft Tissue Swelling and Fat Plane Erasure on Standard Views

Subtle anomalies on standard views should urge further evaluation of a trauma as well. A small fracture with cortical kink is noticed radially at the distal U (Fig. 4a, b). However, a serious swelling at some distance and next to the ulnar styloid was later diagnosed (Fig. 4c, d). MRI (Eriksen and Ringe 2012; Couzens et al. 2014; Matthews et al. 2019) at that time shows an oblique fracture Gaulke type 2c at the base of the styloid process with surrounding BMO (Fig. 4e, f). The ulnar insertion of the TFCC is lacerated as well (Fig. 4e, f).

Periosteal reaction at the waist of the scaphoid bone on a control standard view indicates a semi-recent trauma with fracture (Fig. 5a). MRI (Eriksen and Ringe 2012; Couzens et al. 2014) reveals a clear extensive and non-displaced S fracture with BMO (Fig. 5b–d).

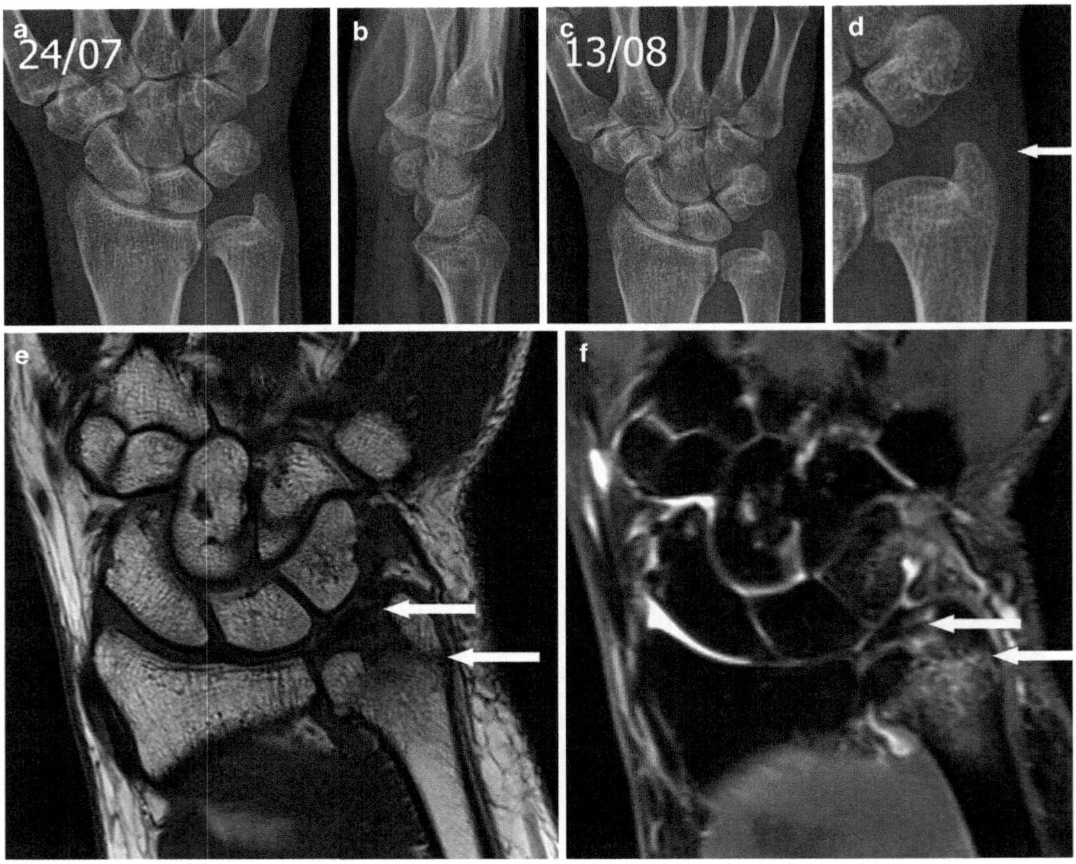

Fig. 4 Standard PA (**a**) and Lateral (**b**) views; control Standard PA (**c**) and Lateral (**d**) views; Cor T1-WI and T2-WI FS. Small fracture with cortical kink radially at the distal U (**a**, **b**). A swelling develops besides the ulnar styloid (**c**, **d**). An oblique fracture Gaulke type 2c of the styloid process (**e**, **f**) and a proximal tear of a Palmer IIb lesion of the TFCC is present (**e**, **f**)

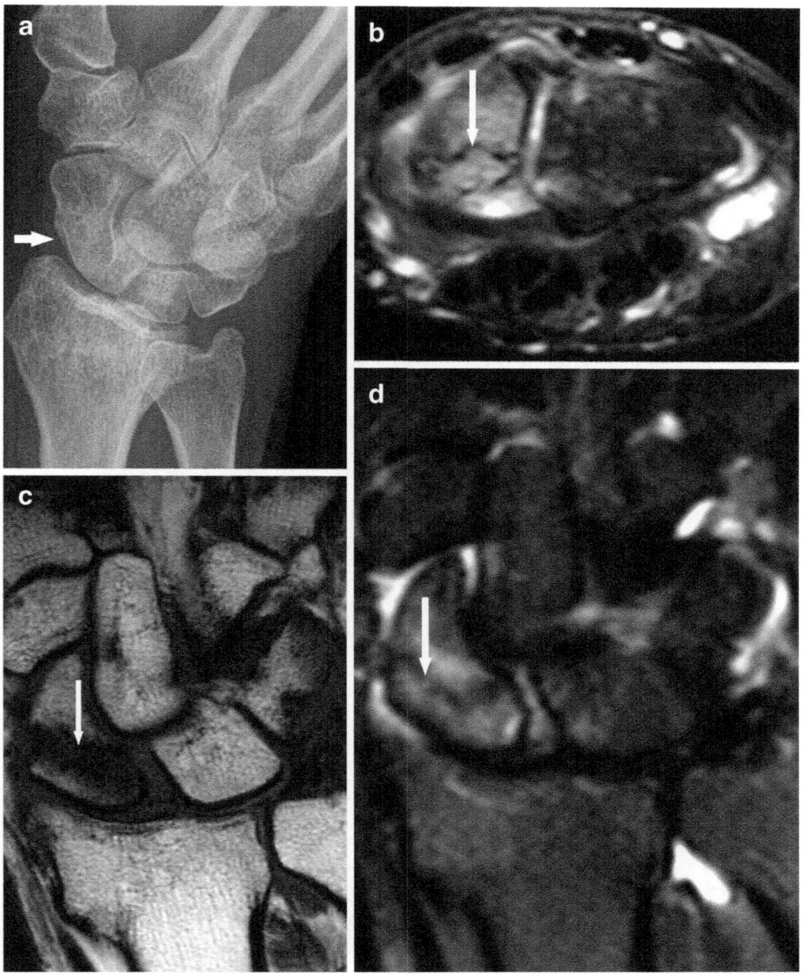

Fig. 5 Standard PA view (**a**); Ax T2-WI FS; Cor T1-WI (**c**); and T2-WI FS (**d**). Periosteal bone reaction at the S waist (**a**). S waist fracture with BMO (**b–d**)

An erased fat plane, especially at the S region, is an alarm sign which should encourage further investigation without delay. S fractures (Couzens et al. 2014; Shabshin and Schweitzer 2009; Demehri et al. 2016) are notorious for escaping from the first evaluation (Fig. 6a, b). Early diagnosis may be provided by MRI (Fig. 6c, d).

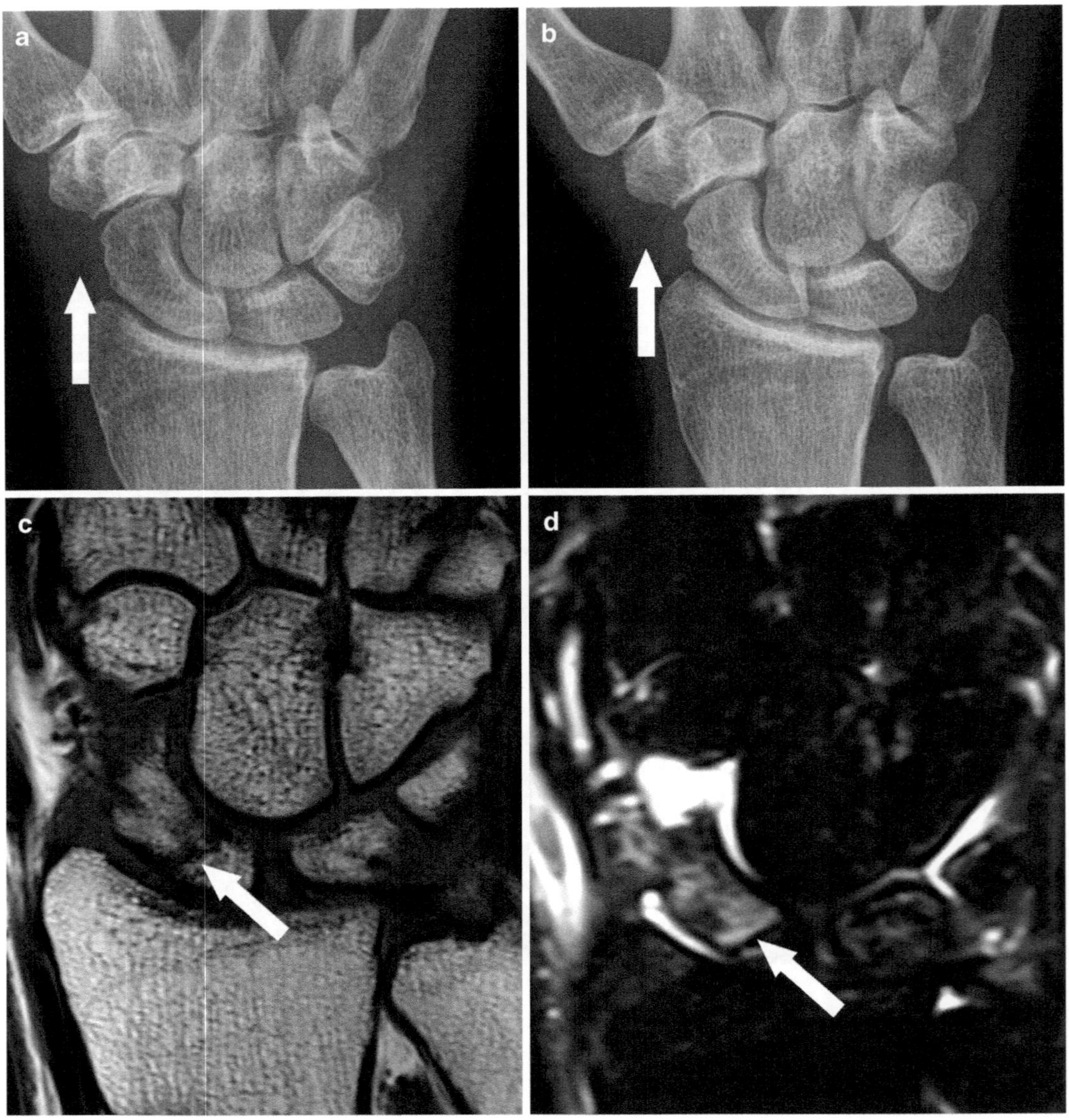

Fig. 6 Standard PA views (**a**, **b**); Cor T1-WI (**c**); and T2-WI FS (**d**). The peri S fat line is erased (**a**, **b**) due to a transverse S fracture with surrounding BMO (**c**, **d**)

4 Metal Artefact

Even in the presence of extensive osteosynthesis material (Fig. 7), MRI may yield a clear diagnosis and should be tried because the results are rather unpredictable (Stecco et al. 2019).

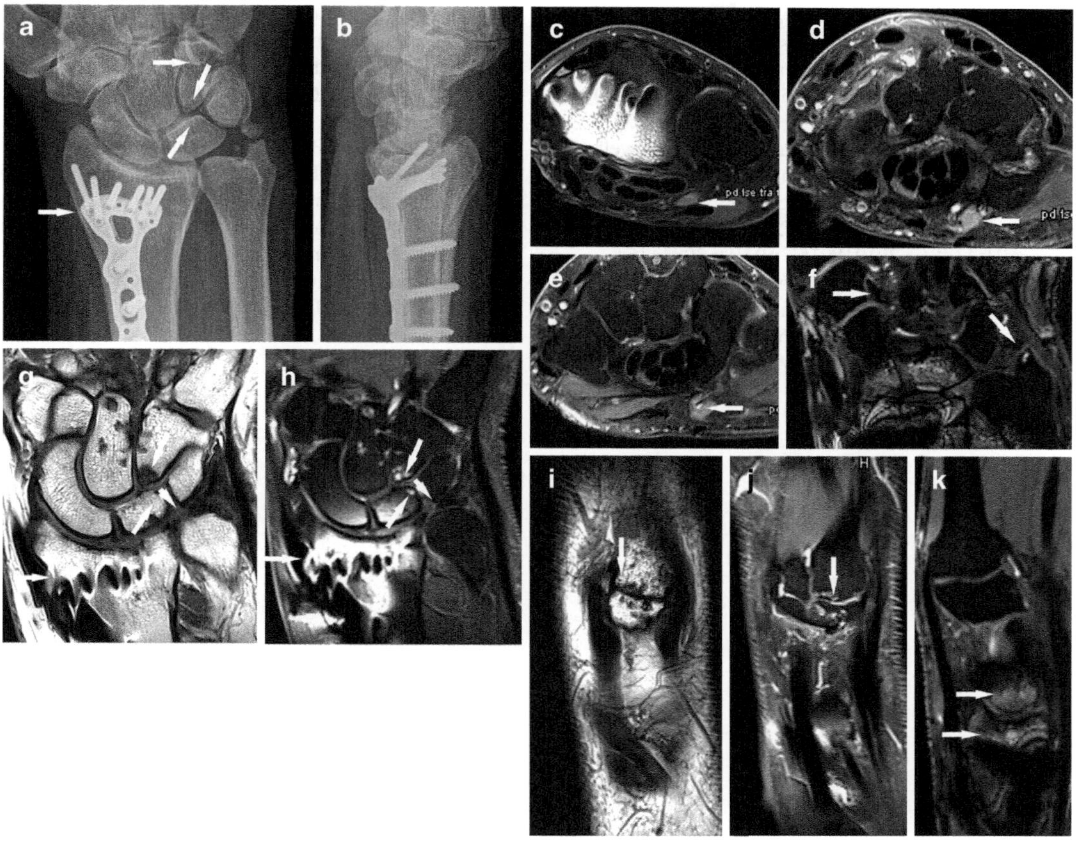

Fig. 7 Extensive presence of metal (**a**, **b**); post-traumatic positive ulnar variance (**a**); HLA and Viegas type 2 L (**a**, **g**, **h**); ulnar neuritis (**c**–**f**); large (neo-articulating) and small loose bone fragment at ulnar styloid (F); metal artefact (**g**, **h**, **k**); carpal boss with degenerative changes (**i**, **j**); degenerative TFCC II D (**g**, **h**)

References

Boutin RD, Buonocore MH, Immerman I, Ashwell Z, Sonico GJ, Szabo RM, Chaudhari AJ (2013) Real-time magnetic resonance imaging (MRI) during active wrist motion – initial observations. PLoS One 8(12):e84004. https://doi.org/10.1371/journal.pone.0084004. PMID: 24391865; PMCID: PMC3877133

Bruno F, Arrigoni F, Palumbo P, Natella R, Maggialetti N, Reginelli A, Splendiani A, Di Cesare E, Bazzocchi A, Guglielmi G, Masciocchi C, Barile A (2019) The acutely injured wrist. Radiol Clin North Am 57(5):943–955. https://doi.org/10.1016/j.rcl.2019.05.003. Epub 2019 Jun 26. PMID: 31351543

Chaudhari AJ, Lim Y, Cui SX, Bayne CO, Szabo RM, Boutin RD, Nayak KS (2023) Real-time MRI of the moving wrist at 0.55 tesla. Br J Radiol 96(1151):20230298. https://doi.org/10.1259/bjr.20230298. Epub 2023 Oct 11. PMID: 37750944; PMCID: PMC10607422

Couzens G, Daunt N, Crawford R, Ross M (2014) Positive magnetic resonance imaging findings in the asymptomatic wrist. ANZ J Surg 84(7–8):528–532. https://doi.org/10.1111/ans.12552. Epub 2014 Feb 26. PMID: 24612468

Demehri S, Hafezi-Nejad N, Morelli JN, Thakur U, Lifchez SD, Means KR, Eng J, Shores JT (2016) Scapholunate kinematics of asymptomatic wrists in comparison with symptomatic contralateral wrists using four-dimensional CT examinations: initial clinical experience. Skeletal Radiol 45(4):437–446. https://doi.org/10.1007/s00256-015-2308-0. Epub 2015 Dec 14. PMID: 26659662

Eriksen EF, Ringe JD (2012) Bone marrow lesions: a universal bone response to injury? Rheumatol Int 32(3):575–584. https://doi.org/10.1007/s00296-011-2141-2. Epub 2011 Sep 8. PMID: 21901347

Li J, Rath B, Hildebrand F, Eschweiler J (2022) Wrist bone motion during flexion-extension and radial-ulnar deviation: an MRI study. Life (Basel) 12(10):1458. https://doi.org/10.3390/life12101458. PMID: 36294894; PMCID: PMC9605103

Matthews GS, Kiani B, Wuertzer SD, Powell JA, Roller BL, Lenchik L, Torabi M (2019) MRI of the wrist: algorithmic approach for evaluating wrist pain. Radiographics 39(2):447–448. https://doi.org/10.1148/rg.2019180157. PMID: 30844354

Palmer AK, Werner FW, Murphy D, Glisson R (1985) Functional wrist motion: a biomechanical study. J Hand Surg Am 10(1):39–46. https://doi.org/10.1016/s0363-5023(85)80246-x. PMID: 3968403

Shabshin N, Schweitzer ME (2009) Age dependent T2 changes of bone marrow in pediatric wrist MRI. Skeletal Radiol 38(12):1163–1168. https://doi.org/10.1007/s00256-009-0752-4. Epub 2009 Aug 7. PMID: 19662404

Stecco A, Arioli R, Buemi F, Parziale G, Trisoglio A, Soligo E, Cerini P, Leigheb M, Brambilla M, Di Nardo G, Guzzardi G, Carriero A (2019) Overcoming metallic artefacts from orthopaedic wrist volar plating on a low-field MRI scanner. Radiol Med 124(5):392–399. https://doi.org/10.1007/s11547-018-0973-5. Epub 2018 Dec 17. PMID: 30560500

Ligament Injuries

Contents

1 Intrinsic Ligaments SL, LT, TFCC and Others

1.1 SL Ligament

The exact evaluation of this important intrinsic ligament remains challenging (Andersson et al. 2015; Bencardino and Rosenberg 2006; Boutry et al. 2005; Davis and Blankenbaker 2010; De Santis et al. 2021; Gilula 1979; Gilula and Weeks 1978; Girgis and Epstein 2000; Gitto et al. 2017; Lee et al. 2013a, 2017; Lee and Elfar 2015; Loredo et al. 2005; Mayfield 1984; Meyer 1991; Michelotti et al. 2018; Pulos and Bozentka 2015; Ringler 2013; Ringler and Murthy 2015). Obvious and large lesions may be shown indirectly by SL diastasis on standard views (Said et al. 2018) (Fig. 1a, b) or directly by US (Fig. 1c, d).

An extensive lesion of the SLL (Athlani et al. 2020; Buijze et al. 2011; Lok et al. 2014; Shahabpour et al. 2015) (Fig. 2a–c) does not always lead to changes in standard views (Couzens et al. 2014; Linscheid et al. 1983) (Fig. 2d, e). The additional MRI exam should always include T1 and T2-WI in order to not only evaluates the form and continuity of the SLL, but also the signal of the ligament on both sequences (Fig. 2a–c, f). The images need to cover the whole horseshoe-shaped ligament from dorsal to palmar (Hafezi-Nejad et al. 2016; Scheck et al. 1997) (Fig. 3). Fine images in at least two orthogonal directions show the extent of the SLL lesion (Fig. 4).

Controversially, extensive lesions at standard views do not always implicate a rupture of the SLL (Fig. 5).

M. Mespreuve, K. Waked, *MRI of the Wrist*, Medical Radiology,
https://doi.org/10.1007/978-3-031-63973-9_6

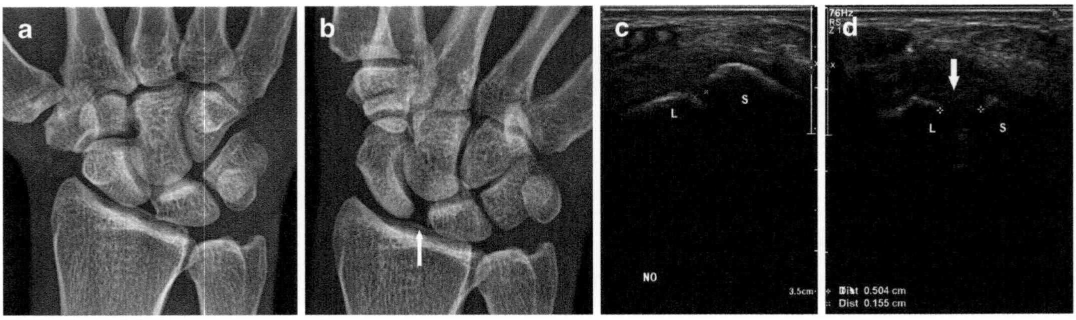

Fig. 1 Standard PA views in neutral position (**a**) and ulnar deviation (**b**); US Ax in neutral position (**c**) and ulnar deviation (**d**). The standard PA view is considered normal (**a**). Diastasis at the SL joint in ulnar deviation (**b**). US may be diagnostic in obvious lesions of the SLL with absence of the ligament (**c**) and SL diastasis in ulnar deviation (**d**)

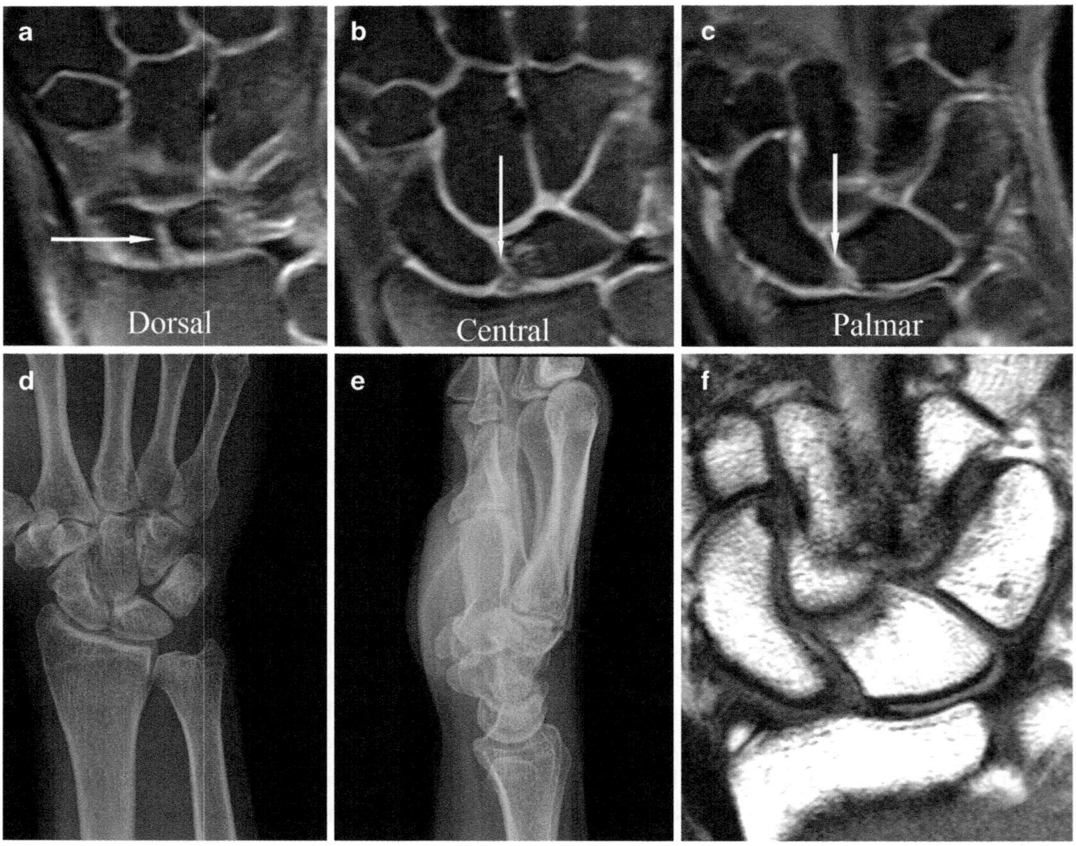

Fig. 2 Cor T2-WI FS (**a**, **c**); Standard PA (**d**) and lateral (**e**) views; Cor T1-WI (**f**). Extensive injury of the complete SLL (**a**, **c**), although the standard views are normal (**d**, **e**). Evaluation of the presence, form, and signal of the SLL on both T2 (**a**, **c**) and T1-WI (**f**) is mandatory

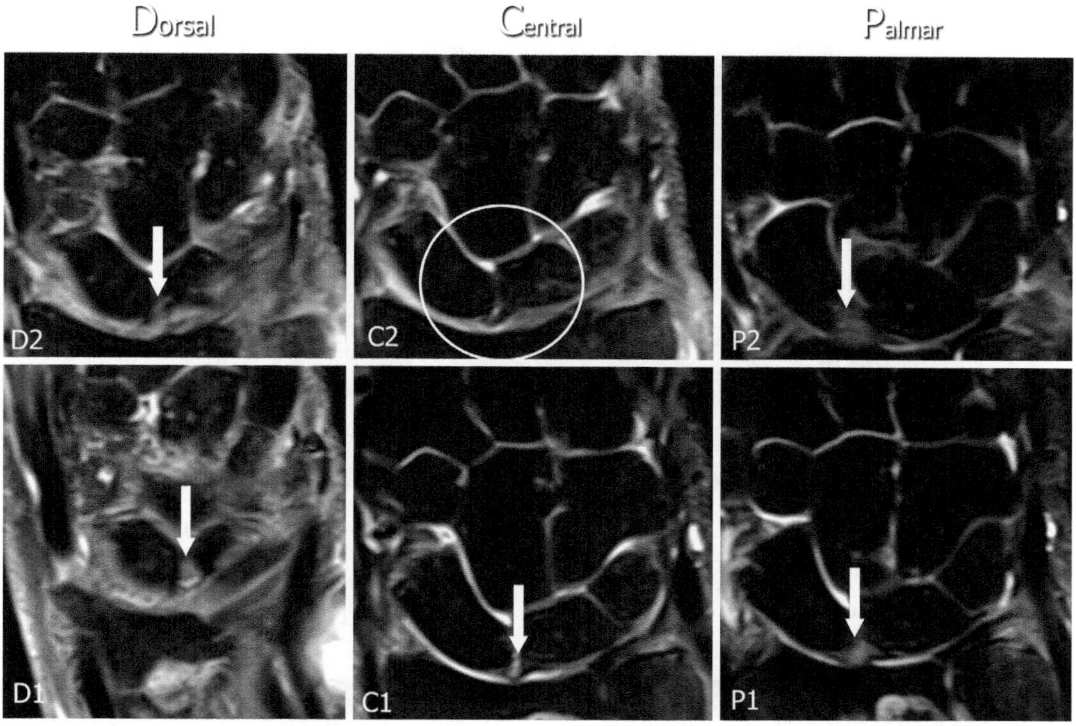

Fig. 3 Cor T2-WI FS (D-C-P). Thin images from dorsal (D1–2) over central (C1–2) to palmar (P1–2) are mandatory. The SLL shows a discontinuity of a part of the typical dorsal striation (D1–2), a central deformation (C1–2) and a diffuse focal signal increase

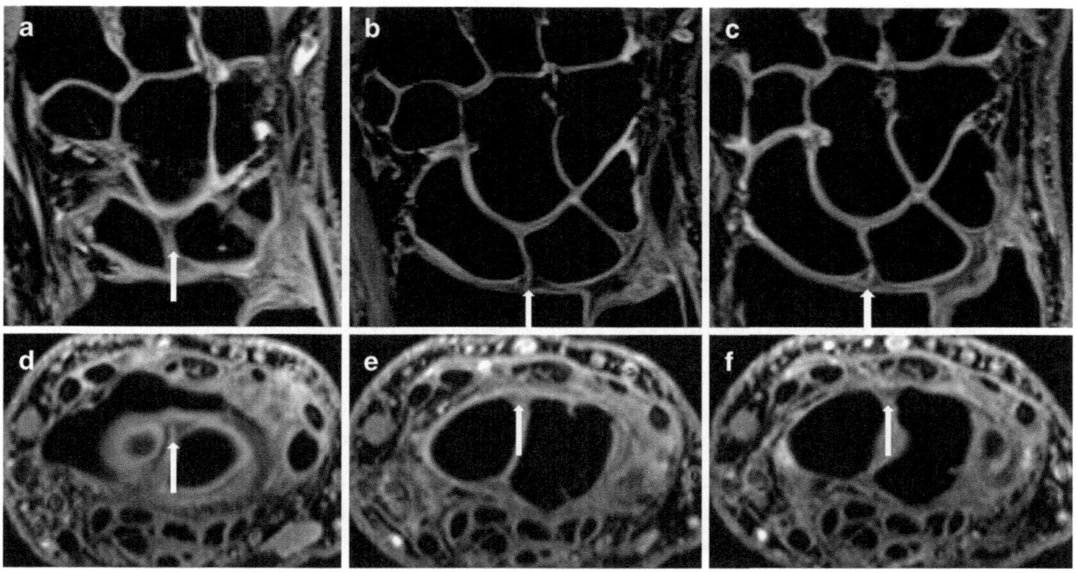

Fig. 4 Cor (**a**, **c**) and Ax (**d–f**) 3D GRE. Fine images in at least two orthogonal directions show the extent of the dorsocentral SLL lesion (**a–f**) with a small remnant of the most important dorsal part (**a**)

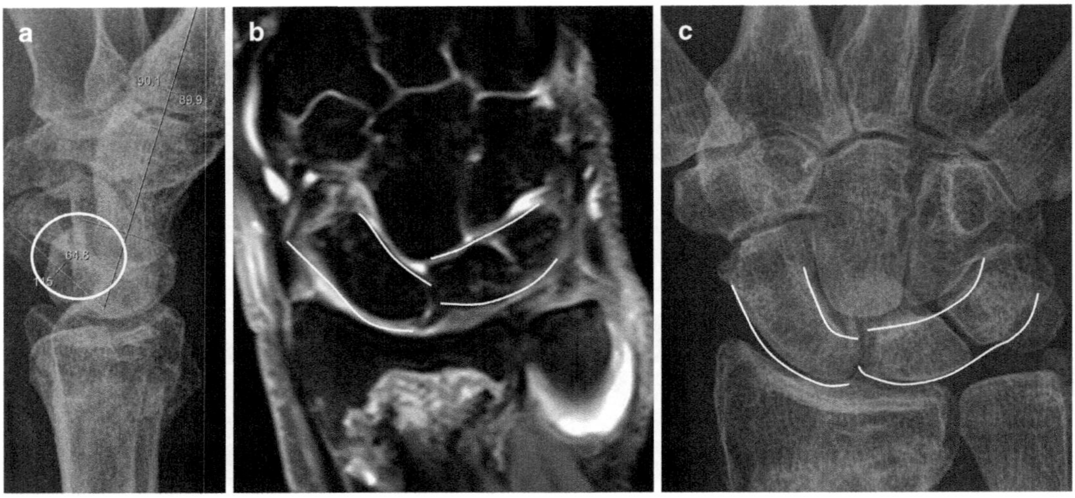

Fig. 5 Standard lateral view (**a**); Cor T2-WI FS (**b**) and Standard PA view (**c**). The SL angle is about 65° (possibly also influenced by the position of the R epiphysis) (**a**) after a semi-recent Pouteau fracture (**a**, **c**). There is a clear step off at the first and second line of Gilula (**b**, **c**) with diffuse hydrops at the main three wrist compartments. The SL is, however, continuous but deformed (**b**)

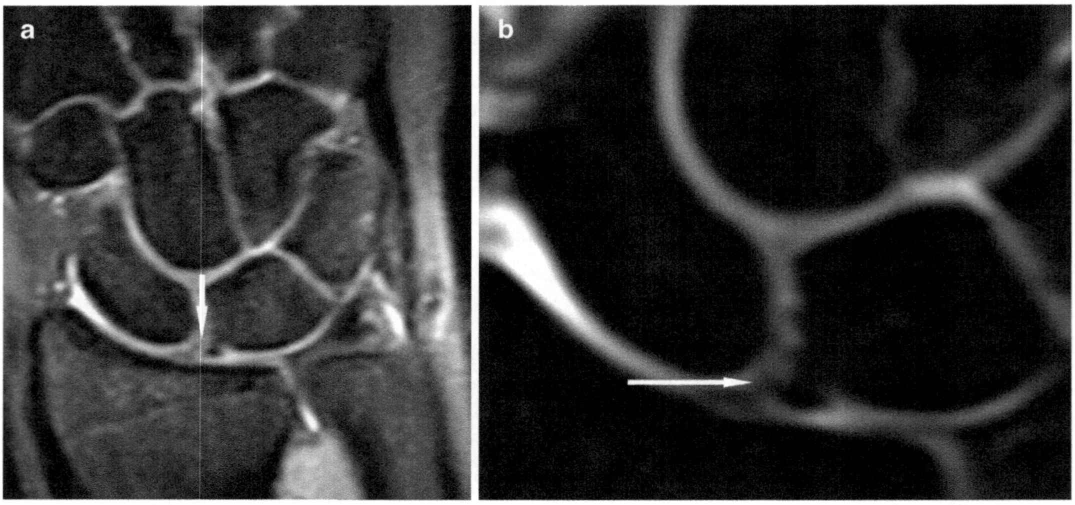

Fig. 6 Cor T2-WI FS (**a**) and 3D GRE (**b**). The SLL will preferably tear at the S side with an irregular delineation

The SLL tear will preferably appear and be looked for at the S side (Mania et al. 2022; Messina et al. 2013) (Fig. 6), as the attachment to the cortex of the L through Scharpey fibres is very firm. An indirect sign may be the presence of a dynamic diastasis at the SL space (Chan et al. 2019; Cheriex et al. 2017; Demehri et al. 2016) (Fig. 7a, b), which corresponds on MRI with a broadly widened SL space filled with fluid and an absent SL ligament (Fig. 7c, d). A standard PA view with clenched fist (Dornberger et al. 2015; Garcia-Elias et al. 2006; Linscheid 1984; Metz et al. 1993; Poznanski 1984; Ozçelik et al. 2005; Patel et al. 2015; Pliefke et al. 2008) may also show an indirect sign, known as the "vacuum phenomenon" (Fig. 8a). The SLL tear is directly shown (Fig. 8b). Juxta-articular BMO (Gornitzky and Carrigan 2016) may appear after a SLL tear (Fig. 9). In a later stage, subchondral cysts (Ramdhian-Wihlm et al. 2012) may appear

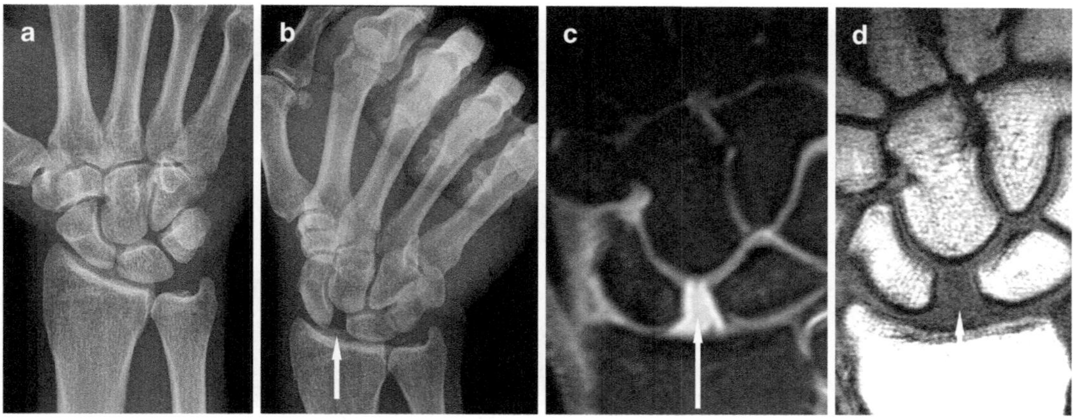

Fig. 7 Standard PA view (**a**) with clenched fist (**b**); Cor T2-WI FS (**c**) and T1-WI (**d**). Dynamic diastasis at the SL space (**a**, **b**). The SL pace is broadly widened, filled with fluid and the ligament is absent (**c**, **d**)

Fig. 8 Standard PA view with clenched fist (**a**); Cor 2D GRE (**b**). Dynamic diastasis at the SL space with a vacuum phenomenon (**a**). The SLL is torn (**b**)

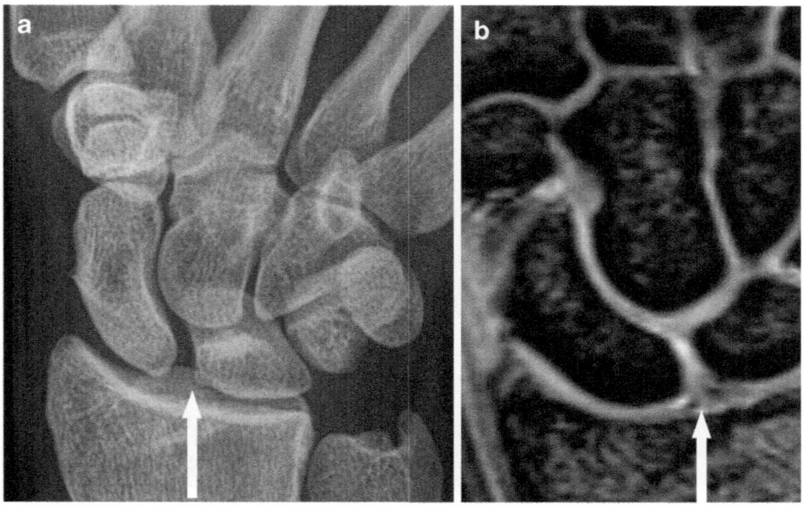

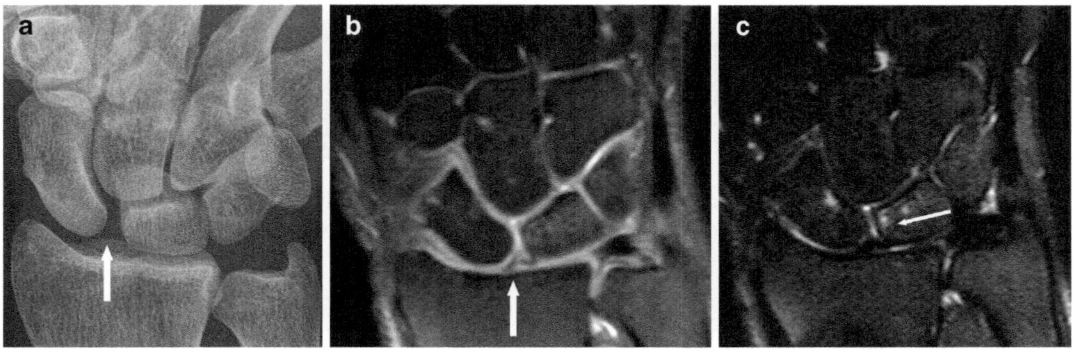

Fig. 9 Standard PA view with clenched fist (**a**); Cor PD WI (**b**) and T2WI-FS (**c**). Dynamic diastasis at the SL space (**a**) with a laceration of the SLL (**b**). Juxta-articular BMO at the L side (**c**)

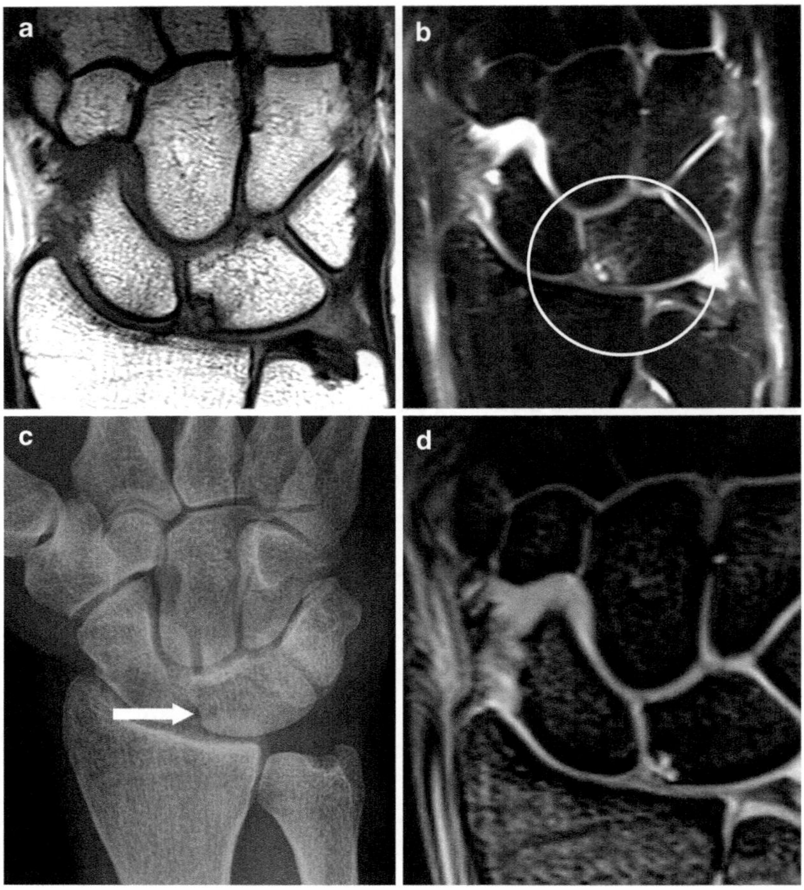

Fig. 10 Cor T1-WI (**a**) and T2-WI FS (**b**); Standard PA view (**c**) and Cor 2D GRE (**d**). At the insertion of the torn SLL on the L, subchondral cysts appear, surrounded by BMO (**a**, **b**). Even on standard views, the small cysts with discrete sclerosis at the borders are visible (**c**) and are sharply delineated on MRI (**d**)

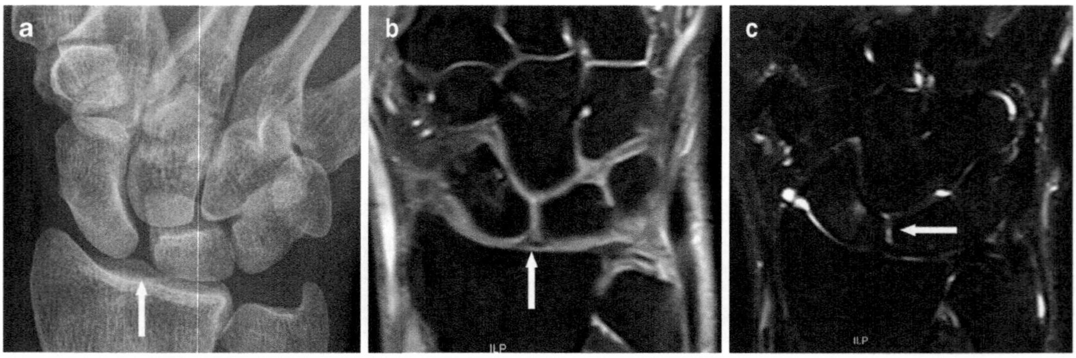

Fig. 11 Standard PA view with clenched fist (**a**), Cor PD-WI (**b**), and Cor T2-WI FS (**c**). SL diastasis (**a**). Only a discrete signal increase remains at tip of the SLL (**b**) and a small amount of fluid in the SL joint space (**c**). The BMO has regressed completely (**c** versus Fig. 9c)

at the insertion of the torn SLL, mostly on the L side, surrounded by BMO (Fig. 10a, b). Even on standard views, the small cysts with discrete sclerosis at the borders may be visible (Fig. 10c) and are sharply delineated on MRI (Fig. 10d). Dynamic diastasis (Abou Arab et al. 2018; Dao et al. 2004; Grunz et al. 2021; Langner et al. 2015; Ramamurthy et al. 2016; Shaw et al. 2019; Sulkers et al. 2014) at the SSL joint space (Fig. 11a) remains due to an elongation of the

SLL with very subtle signal changes of the SLL (Fig. 11b) and a discrete amount of fluid in the SL joint space with complete regression of the BMO (Fig. 11c versus Fig. 9c). SLL tears may or may not change (Garcia-Elias 2008) after an indefinite period of time. Besides the regression of the oedema, small tears often remain unchanged (Fig. 12). On the contrary, large SLL tears may be replaced by broad, ill defined, heterogenous scar tissue (Fig. 13).

MRI should always be considered as the first examination in order to evaluate the form, signal, and continuity of the SLL. MRA (Fig. 14) may be added in a second stage to evaluate very spe-

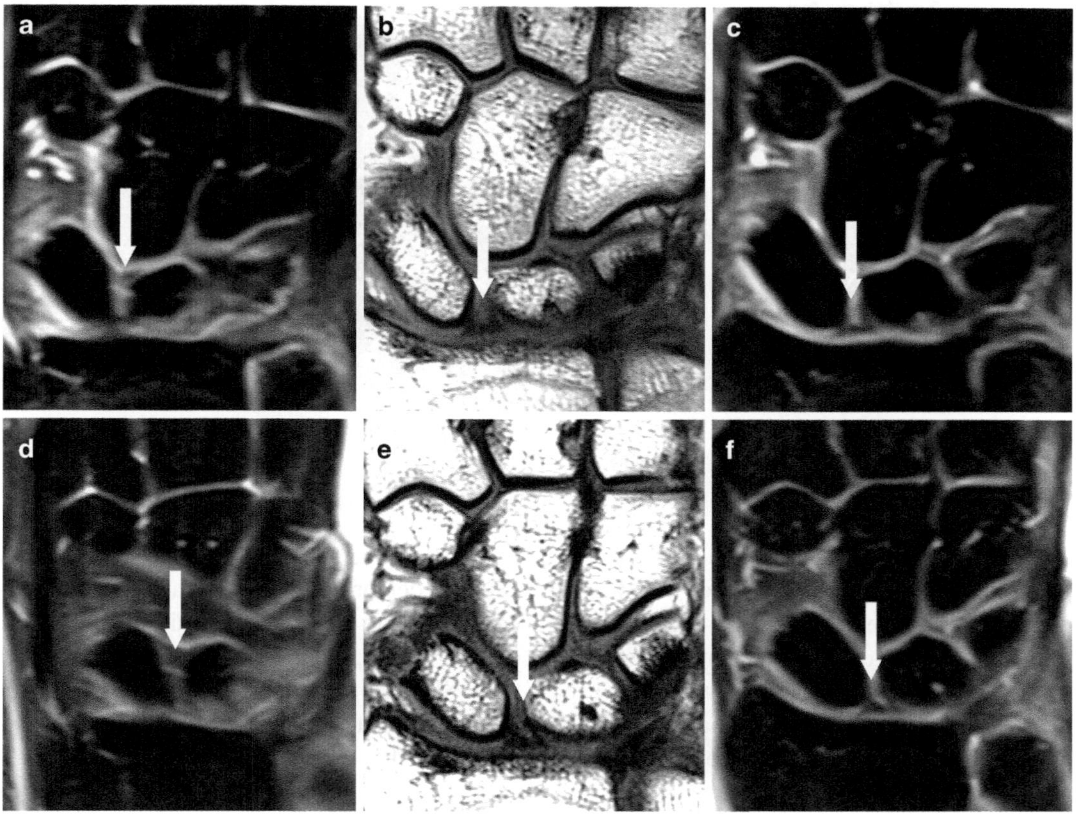

Fig. 12 Cor PD-WI (**a**, **d**), T1WI (**b**, **e**), and T2-WI FS (**c**, **f**). The aspect of this SLL tear (**a**, **c**) almost does not change over a period of 10 months (**d–f**). Posteriorly, there is a reduction of the limited oedema (**a**, **d**)

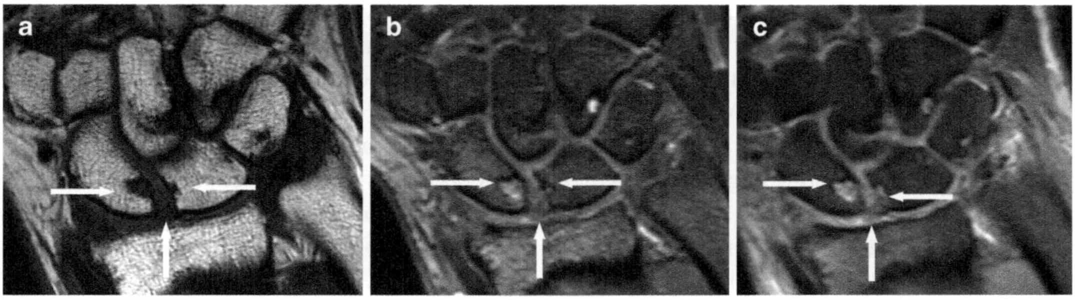

Fig. 13 Cor T1WI (**a**), 2D GRE (**b**), and T2-WI FS (**c**). The SLL is replaced by a broad, ill defined, heterogenous band of scar tissue with adjacent subchondral cysts (S and L)

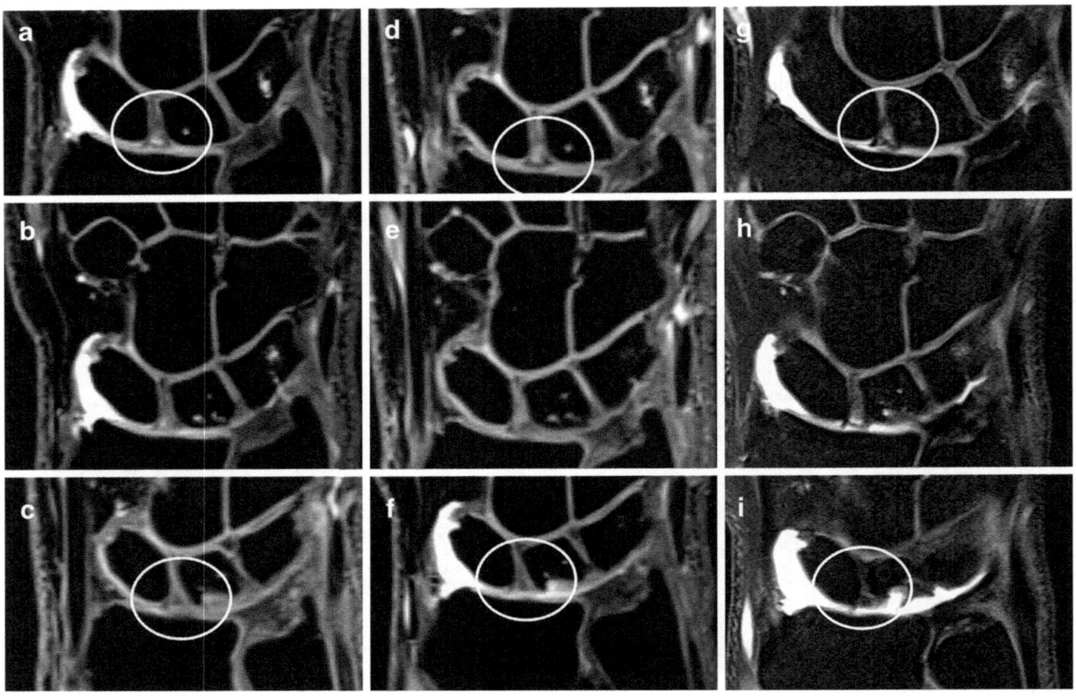

Fig. 14 Cor 3D GRE (**a–f**) and T1-WI FS (**g–i**). MRA (RC injection) shows no contrast leakage from the RC into de MC joint in fine 3D GRE, nor in T1-WI FS images

cific problems. False negative results are possible in case of an external continuity of the SL ligament (Fig. 14), due to significant—but internally limited—damage of the ligament, fibrous scar formation, local synovial proliferation, or even the valve phenomenon. The signal alteration is also less obvious (T1-WI FS) or less reliable (GRE). If only one compartment is injected, midcarpal arthrography should be preferred as this generally results in the best evaluations.

Arthrosynovial cysts are very frequently associated with SLL tears. They are also often the first sign of a SLL lesion and mainly detected by US (Fig. 15). The most frequent cysts are located superficially, between the tendons of the extensor compartment II (ecl, ecb) and IV (ed) (Fig. 15a). The stalk needs to be demonstrated until the SL joint (Fig. 15b). In detecting large cysts (Fig. 16), MRI does not have an advantage over US. However, small cysts are more likely to be discovered by MRI due to their obvious bright signal and the underlying SLL tear may be demonstrated as well (Fig. 17). In addition, the trajectory of the (fine and tortuous) stalks (Fig. 18) is easier to demonstrate on MRI (and to communicate visually to the clinician). This is certainly the case for radio-palmar cysts (Fig. 19), associated with SL lesions. The cysts develop and run through the space of Poirrier and surface just distal from the pronator quadratus (Fig. 19a). Proximal expansion may be superficial (Fig. 19b) and/or deep of the pronator quadratus (Fig. 19c).

Detecting a tear of the strong SLL tear should spontaneously trigger a search for associated lesions. A bony erosion of the adjacent carpal bones may develop over time (Fig. 20). A similar image may be found in RA (Fig. 21a, b), but additional series with contrast will clearly define the aetiology (Fig. 21c). SLL tears may exist alongside S fractures (Fig. 22). A tear of the LTL may coexist as well (Figs. 22b, c and 23). Despite these important lesions, the mobility in ulnar and radial deviation may initially remain quite normal (Fig. 23e, f). Associated extrinsic ligament lesions have to be excluded (Fig. 24) in order to obtain a complete diagnosis, in function of the

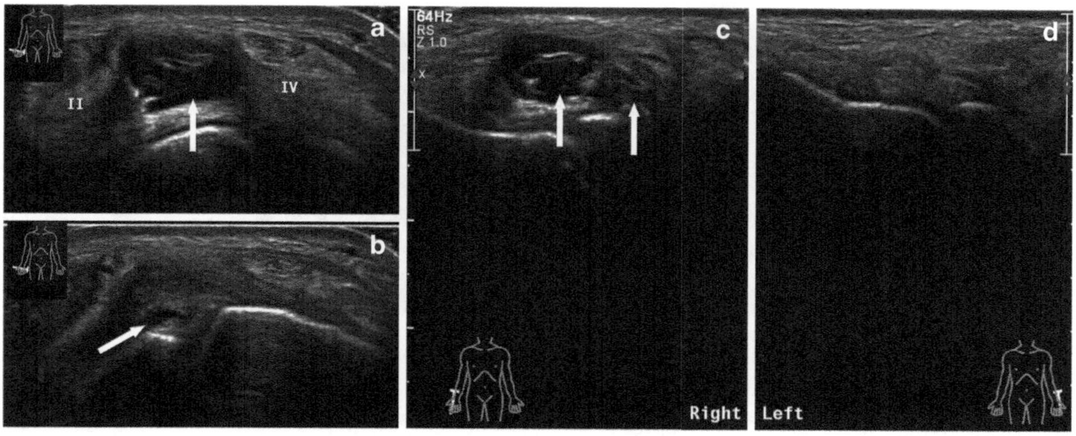

Fig. 15 US transverse (**a**, **b**), sagittal at pathological (**c**) and normal side (**d**). US reveals an arthrosynovial cyst at the dorsal side between the tendons of the II and IV extensor compartments (**a**). In the depth, the stalk is followed to the SL space (**b**). Comparative imaging (**c**, **d**) shows the bilobular cyst at the right side, posteriorly from the C and L (**c**)

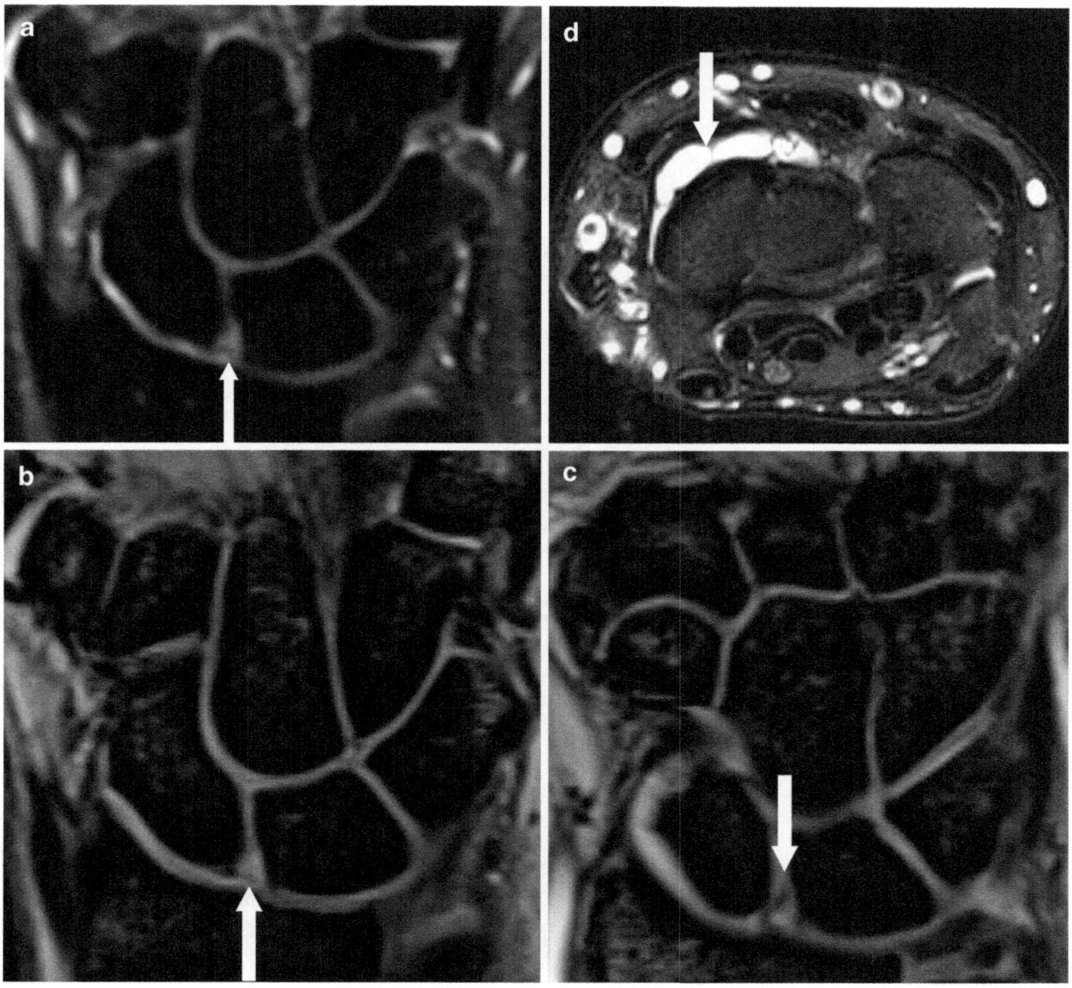

Fig. 16 Cor 2D GRE (**a**, **c**) and Ax T2-WI FS. Extensive SLL tear (**a**, **c**) with large deep dorsal ASC (**d**)

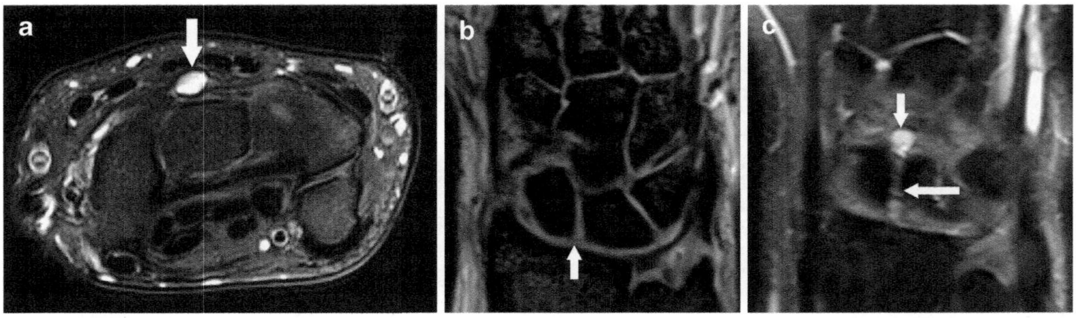

Fig. 17 Ax T2-WI FS; Cor 2D GRE (**b**) and T2-WI FS (**c**). Small cyst dorsal from the torn SLL

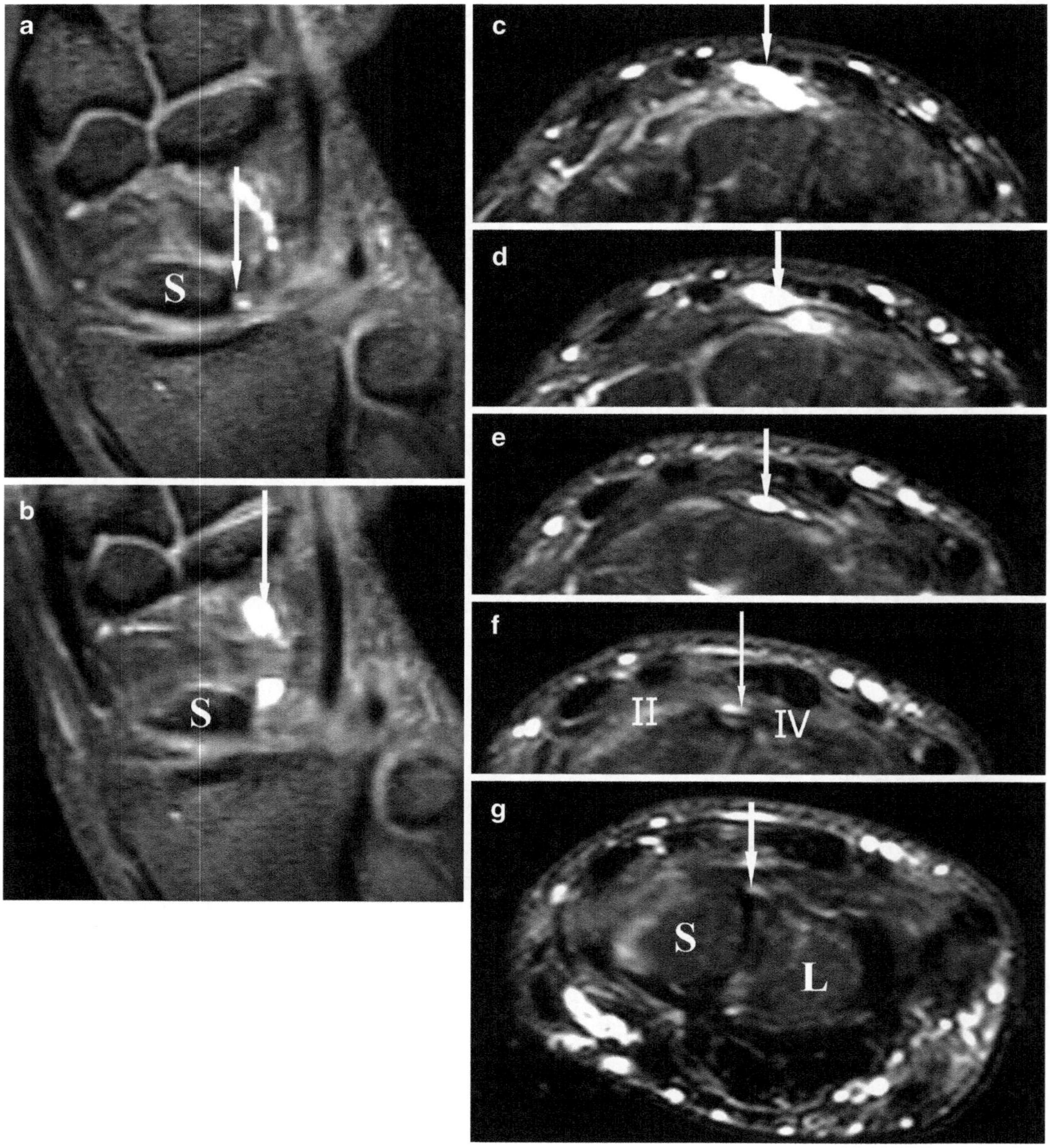

Fig. 18 Cor (**a**, **b**) and Ax T2-WI FS (**c**–**g**). Small ASC dorsally of the SLL with illustration of the trajectory of the stalk until the SLL

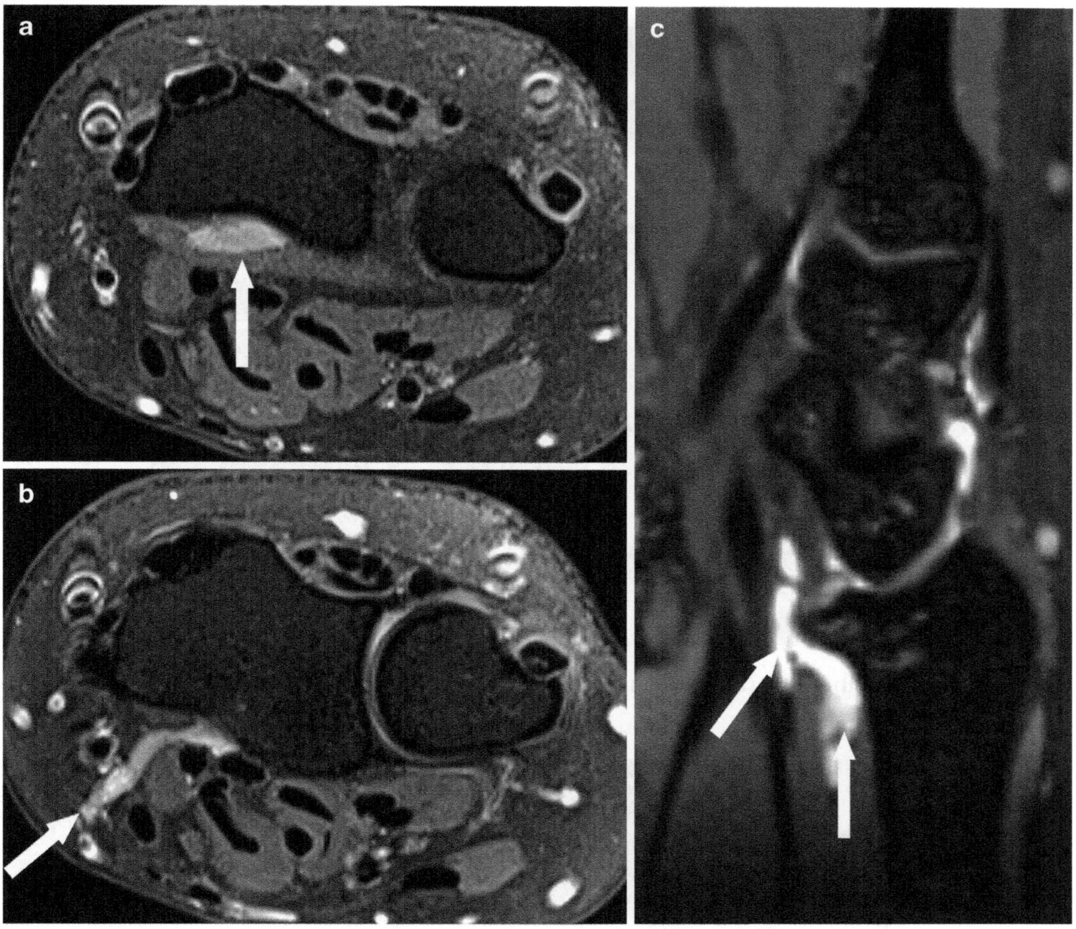

Fig. 19 Ax T2-WI FS (**a**, **b**) and Sag 3D GRE (**c**). ASC at the radio-palmar region

evaluation of the importance of the trauma and to guide the therapy. Even a pseudarthrosis may be associated with a SLL tear (Fig. 25). Accompanying traumatic TFCC tears (Fig. 26) may appear more obviously.

Early diagnosis of a SLL tear is important. Careful analysis of "normal" standard views (Fig. 27a, b) should avoid the further evolution of the S rotatory subluxation (Gelberman et al. 2001). Signet ring sign (Fig. 27c), an increased SL angle (Fig. 27d) and widening of the SL space in ulnar deviation (Fig. 27e) are obvious red alert signs in the early stage after trauma. Further increase of the signet ring sign (Fig. 27f), the SL angle (Fig. 27g) and of the widening of the SL space, even in neutral position (Fig. 27h), has to be avoided through early treatment. Treatment failure may otherwise lead to a carpal collapse with reduced height, resulting from proximal migration of the C (Fig. 27f) and thinning of the midcarpal cartilage (Fig. 27i–l) with surrounding BMO between S and C (Fig. 27i–k).

Standard views may give some idea about the post-operative status (Michelotti et al. 2018; Del Piñal 2013; Szabo 2008), depending on the technique used (Fig. 28). In case of the use of plugs, they should be continuous and fixed in the bone without apparent (sclerotic outlined) radiolucency around (Fig. 28b). However, increase of the SL angle (Fig. 28b) and the SL diastasis (Fig. 28c) are highly suspicious for (internal) rupture and/or elongation. The continuity of a

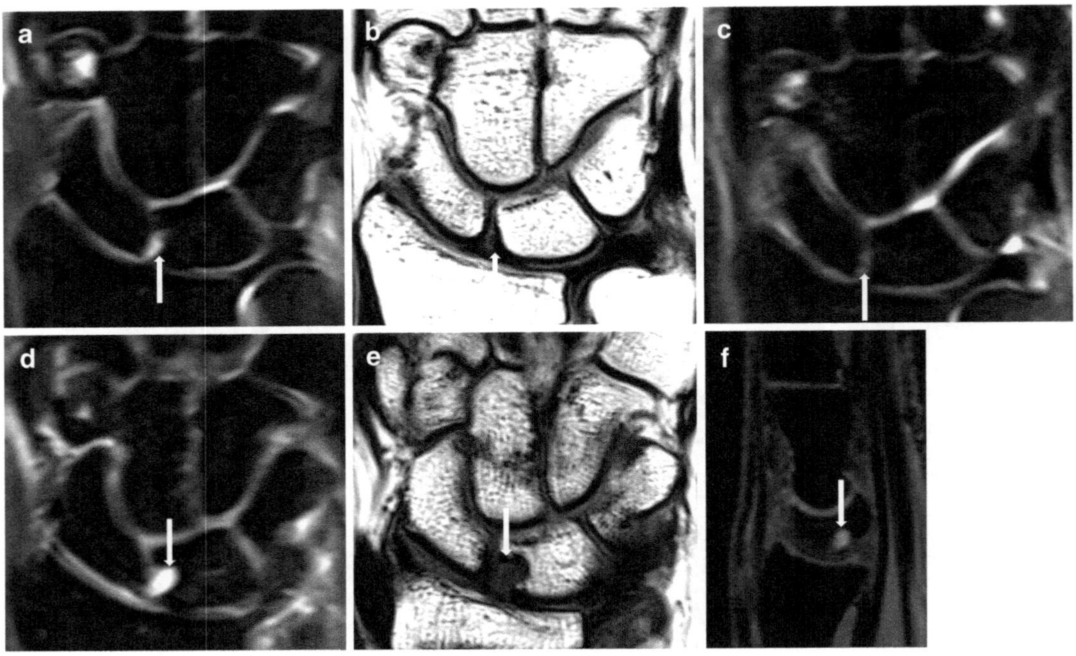

Fig. 20 Cor T2-WI (**a**, **d**), T1-WI (**b**, **e**), Cor (**c**) and Sag (**f**) T2-WI FS. SLL tear (**a**, **c**) with L bone erosion (**d–f**)

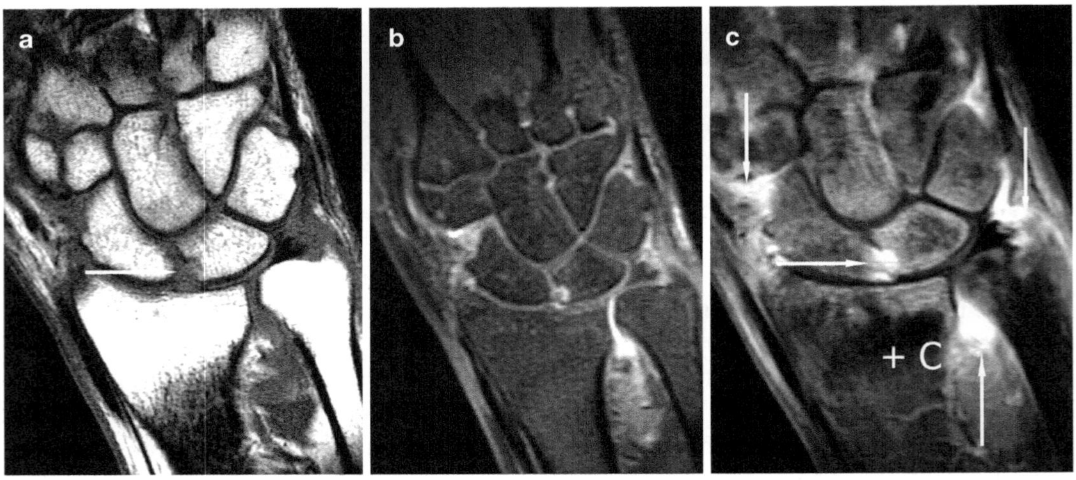

Fig. 21 Cor T1-WI (**a**), T2-WI FS (**b**), and T1-WI FS with contrast (**c**). SLL "lesion" with lunate erosion (**a**, **b**). CE at the SLL, the adjacent erosion, and the diffuse synovial proliferations as at diffuse bony (oedema) regions in RA

fixed external ligamentous reconstruction as well as the scar tissue between S and L may be delineated on MRI. However, due to artefact, postoperative sequels and signal alterations, and a variable aspect of the scar formation, the interpretation remains doubtful (Fig. 29).

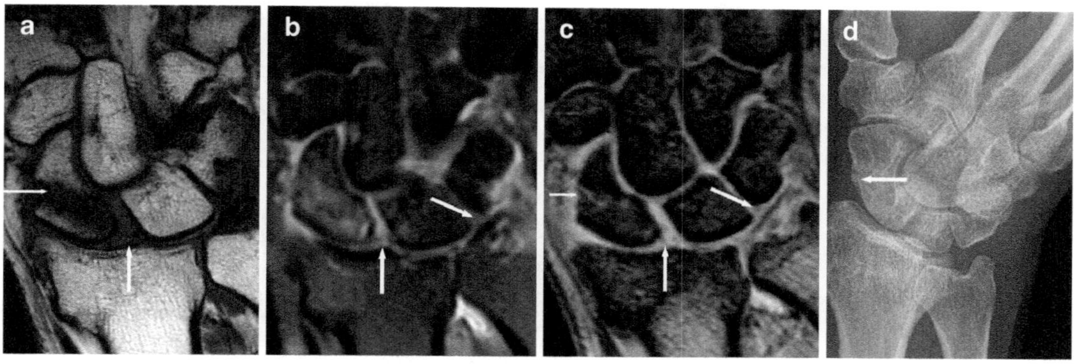

Fig. 22 Cor T1-WI (**a**), T2-WI (**b**), 2D GRE (**c**), and Standard PA view. SLL tear (**a**, **c**), fracture of the S (**a**, **d**) with already callus formation (**d**), and LTL tear (**b**, **c**)

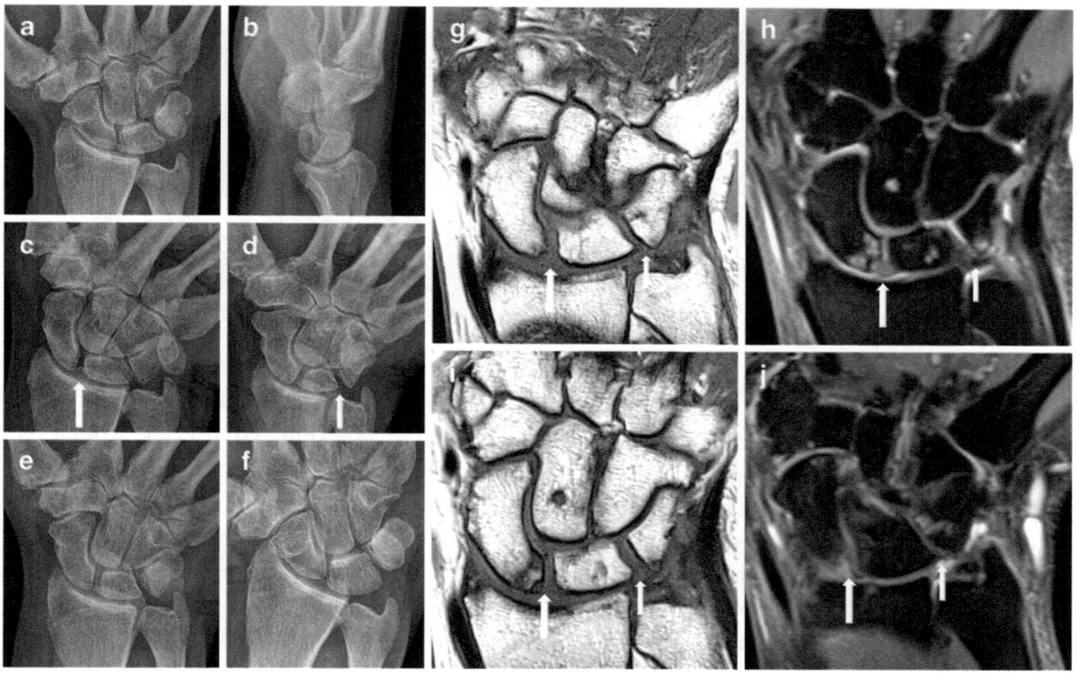

Fig. 23 Standard PA (**a**), Lateral (**b**), Slightly oblique with clenched fist (**c**, **d**), PA with ulnar (**e**) and radial deviation (**f**) views; Cor T1-WI (**g**, **i**) and T2-WI FS (**h**, **j**). Normal standard PA and Lateral view (**a**, **b**) with diastasis SL (**c**) and LT (**d**). Mobility is not significantly reduced (**e**, **f**). Both ligaments SLL and LTL are torn with adjacent BMO (**g**–**j**)

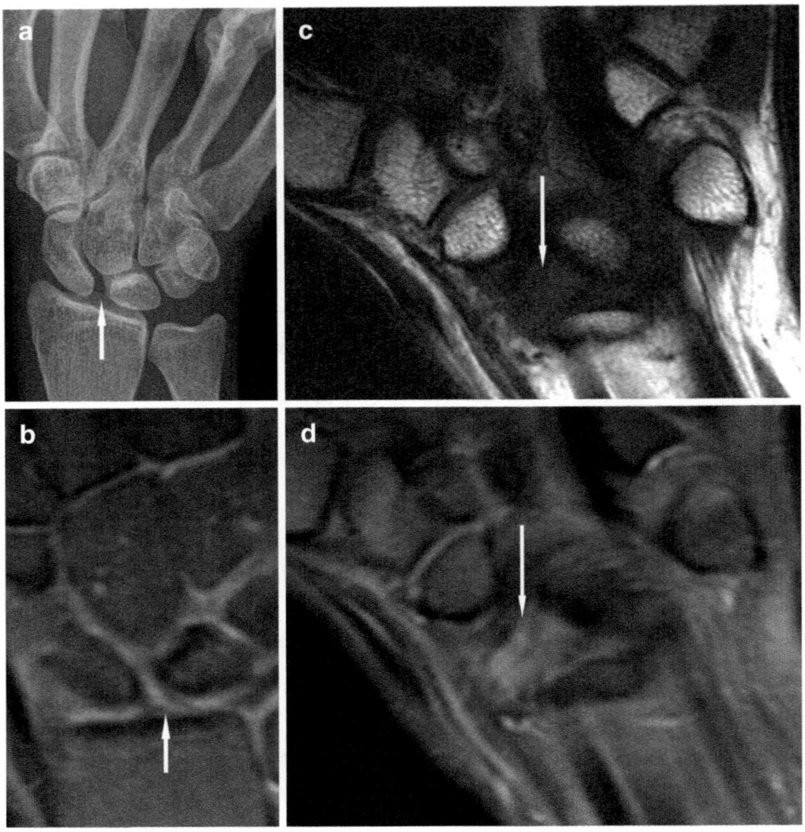

Fig. 24 Standard PA view with clenched fist (**a**); Cor T2-WI FS (**b**), T1-WI (**c**), and PD-WI (**d**). Diastasis SL (**a**) due to a SLL tear (**b**). Associated laceration of the radial part of the palmar V with oedema and erasure of the striated pattern (**c**, **d**)

1.2 LT Ligament

A lesion of this even smaller intrinsic ligament may be strongly suspected on standard PA views. Indirect signs (Devilliers Minnaar 1952; Shin et al. 2000), such as sclerotic margins at the LT joint (Fig. 30a), indicate a reaction to the abnormal mobility. The additional MRI exam (Figs. 30b, c and 31) should always include T1 and T2-WI in order to not only evaluates the form and continuity of the LTL, but also the signal of the ligament on both sequences. The images need to cover the whole horseshoe-shaped ligament from dorsal to palmar. Fine images in at least two orthogonal directions may show the extent of the LTL lesion (Fig. 31). The LTL tear is observed on MRI (Ritt et al. 1998) (Figs. 30b and 31), as is the juxta-articular BMO (Figs. 30c and 31a–c, f). The ligament is mostly torn at the L side (Fig. 31b, c). The palmar part of the LTL is the most important one (Fig. 31d–e). As the ligament is small, MRI will miss more lesions of this intrinsic ligament and MRA or CTA (Fig. 32) will be needed to make a definite diagnosis (Fig. 32).

The significance of an isolated LTL tear is still debated (Garn et al. 1971). Some authors state the need for an additional lesion of the extrinsic palmar radiolunotriquetral ligament for the LTL lesion to be significant. The classically associated VISI appears after an LTL tear with a palmar radiolunotriquetral and a dorsal radiotriquetral ligament tear. The coexistence with a SLL tear (Wolfe et al. 2012) has already been mentioned as well (Fig. 23). Other (bony) lesions may also be detected (Fig. 32c–e).

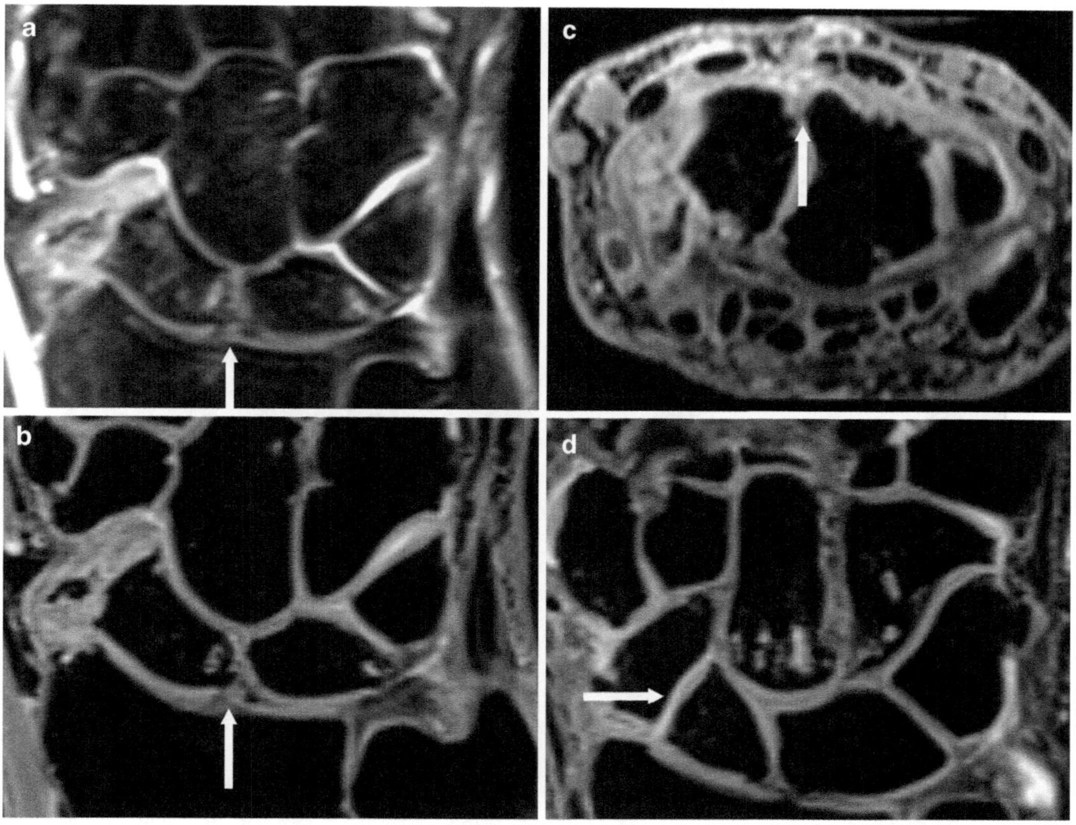

Fig. 25 Cor T2-WI FS (**a**); Cor (**b**, **d**) and Ax 3D GRE (**c**). Clear old SLL tear (**a**, **c**) with a hazardous discovery of a S pseudarthrosis

1.3 TFCC

TFCC (Luetkens et al. 2021; Magee 2009; Mannil et al. 2016; Matthews et al. 2019; Mikić 1989; Nakamura et al. 2001a; Oneson et al. 1997; Yoshioka et al. 2007) stands for triangular fibrocartilage complex, meaning that this structure is a unit of multiple and quite different parts. The location of the tear—most classically central (Mespreuve et al. 2015; Spies et al. 2022; Wang et al. 2023; Watanabe et al. 2010)—and its extent (Anderson et al. 2008; Iordache et al. 2012; Lindau et al. 2000; Chong and Kandathil 2013) (Fig. 33) are evaluated on at least two perpendicular images, usually coronal (Fig. 33a) and axial (Fig. 33b). A frequent pitfall on the first one is the brighter signal of the small zone of cartilage adjacent to the sigmoid notch (Nevalainen et al. 2023) (Fig. 33a), which should not be mistaken for a tear.

The traumatic tears are classified using the Palmer classification (Palmer 1989, 1990; Palmer and Werner 1981; Palmer et al. 1985; Zhan et al. 2020; Zlatkin and Rosner 2006) (Fig. 34). A type I A tear (Fig. 33) may be very subtle and/or oblique (Fig. 35). Accompanying fluid in the DRUJ should be an alert sign (Figs. 33a and 35). A small high signal zone in the TFC on GRE (Fig. 36a) needs to be considered with caution and wrist arthrography (always combined with MRA or CTA) may be needed for the definite diagnosis (Fig. 36b). The forceful contrast injection may open a "valve" lesion with only a small step off in case of a I A type TFFC lesion (Fig. 37).

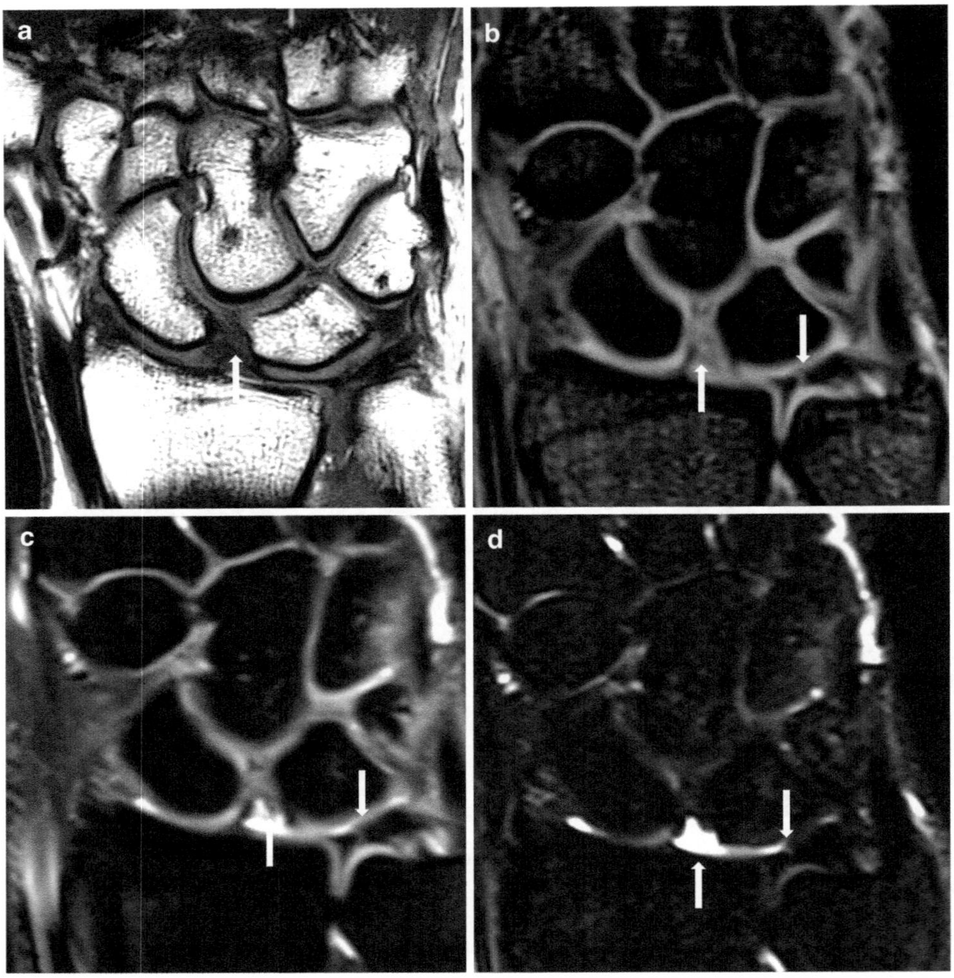

Fig. 26 Cor T2-WI FS (**a**); Cor 2D GRE (**b**), T2-WI FS (**c**), and 3D GRE (**d**). SLL tear (A-D) with diastasis and a TFCC tear Palmer type I A (B-D)

A type I B consists of an avulsion fracture of the double ulnar attachment (Fig. 38). More extended lesions (Fig. 39) may include a (sub) luxation of the disc (Figs. 39a and 40), laceration with tenosynovitis (Fig. 39e), and luxation (Fig. 39f) of the ECU, and a posterior ulna luxation (Fig. 40). A (large) arthrosynovial cyst (Fig. 41) may develop at the palmar side (Fig. 41c–e), starting from the region of the tear (Fig. 41b–d). This cyst should not be confused with a fluid accumulation extending between the meniscus homologue and the TFCC to the prestyloid recessus of the RC joint (Fig. 42a). A well delineated peritendinous cyst without stalk (Fig. 42b) of the ECU may also be confusing in this small region.

A rare, isolated lesion of the ulno-lunar and ulno-triquetral ligaments is categorized as type I C (Fig. 43). As these are very small structures and since these lesions are frequently associated with other "close vicinity" lesions (TFC; LT) (Fig. 44), the diagnosis is not always obvious, even with prominent hydrops.

The Palmer type I D lesion is the most exceptional one, touching the TFC at the ulnar border of the cartilage of the sigmoid notch (Fig. 45).

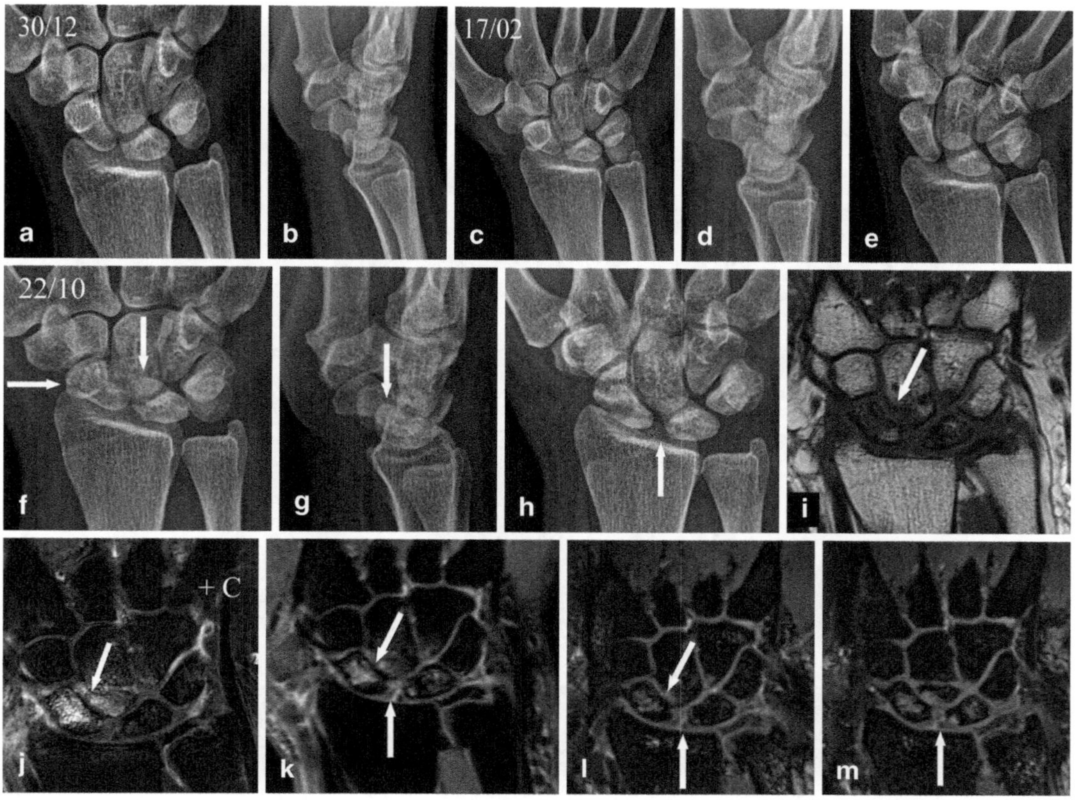

Fig. 27 Standard AP (**a**, **c**, **f**) with clenched fist (**e**, **h**) and Lateral (**b**, **d**, **g**) views; Cor T1-WI (**i**) with contrast (**j**), T2-WI FS (**k**), and 3D GRE (**l**, **m**). "Normal" standard views (**a**, **b**). Signet ring sign (**c**), increased SL angle (**d**) and widening of the SL space in ulnar deviation (**e**). Further increase of the signet ring sign (**f**), the SL angle (**g**) and of the widening of the SL space now even in neutral position (**h**). The C starts to migrate proximally (**f**). The midcarpal cartilage is thinned (**i**–**l**) with BMO between S and C (**i**–**k**). The SLL is torn (**k**–**m**) with SL diastasis

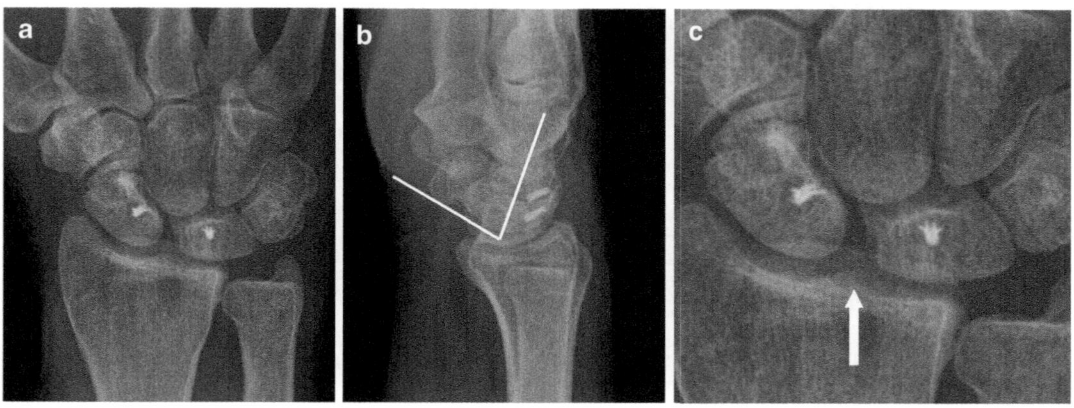

Fig. 28 Standard PA (**a**, **c**) and Lateral (**b**) views (**b**). Radio-opaque plugs indicating a reconstruction of the ligament (**a**, **c**). The SL angle remains about 80° (**b**). The SL diastasis is still present (**c**)

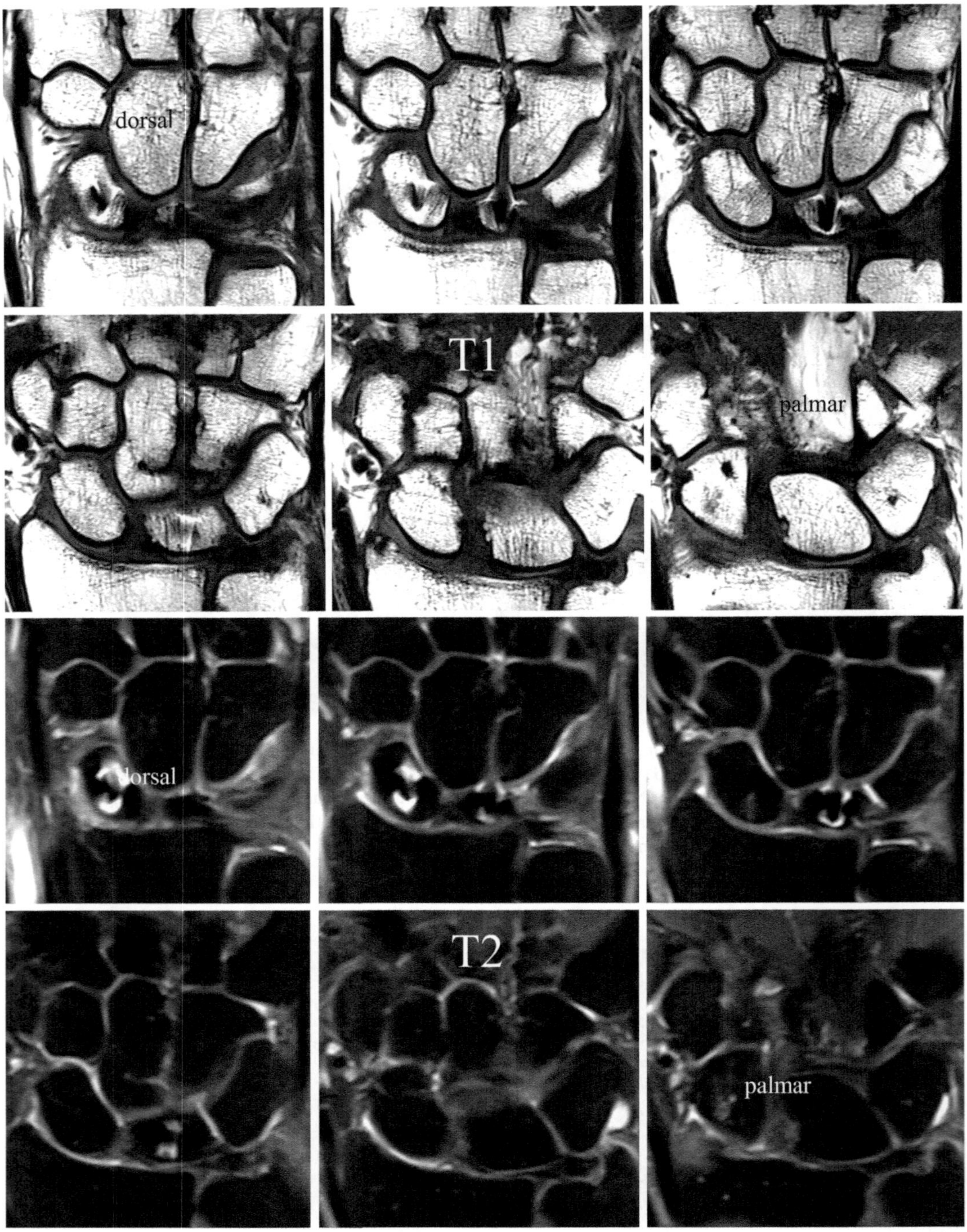

Fig. 29 Cor T1-WI and T2-WI FS from dorsal to palmar. The externally fixed ligamentous reconstruction and the scar tissue between S and L may be delineated

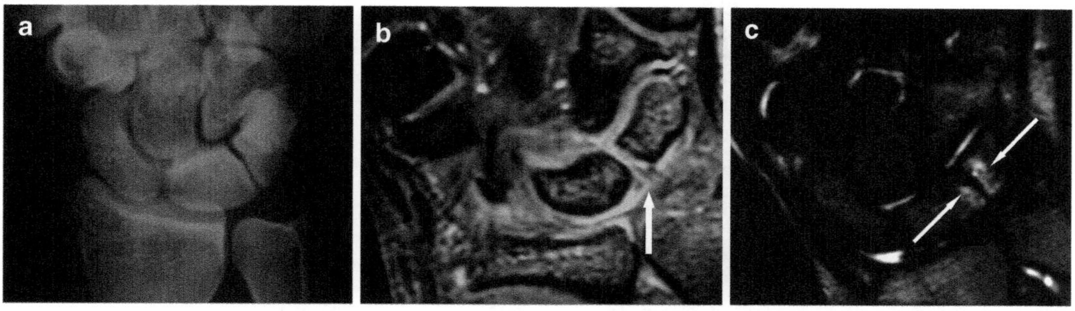

Fig. 30 Standard PA view (**a**); Cor 2D GRE (**b**); and T2-WI FS (**c**). Sclerotic borders at the LT joint (**a**). A tear of the LTL (**b**) is accompanied by BMO at the borders of the LT joint

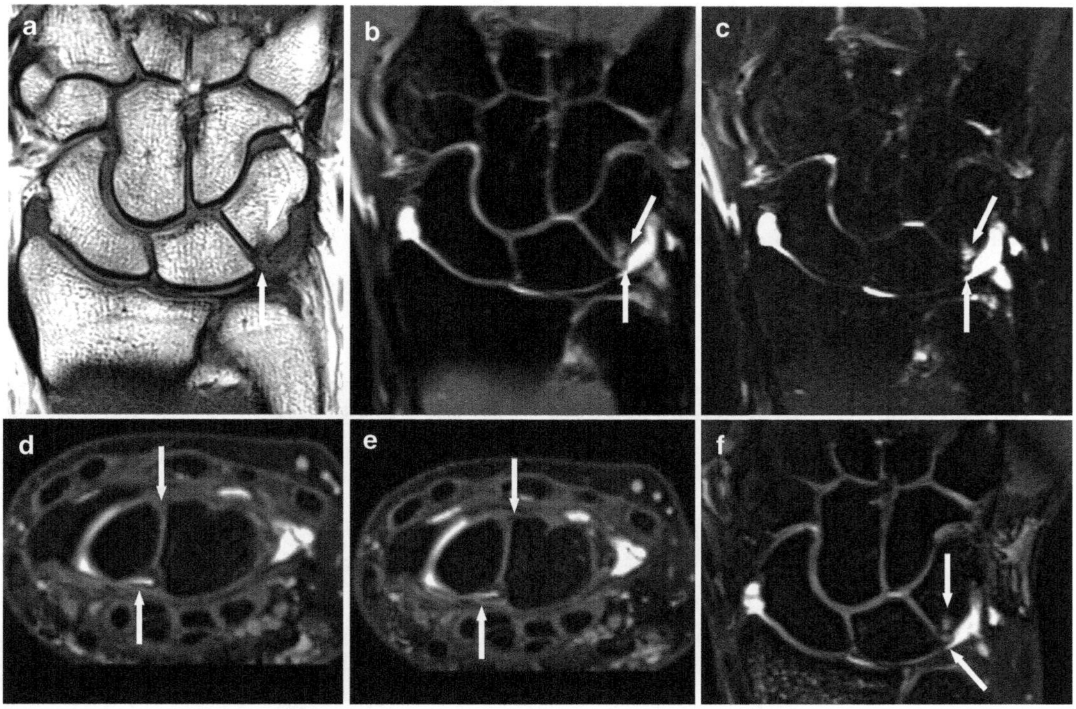

Fig. 31 Cor T1WI (**a**) and T2-WI FS (**b**, **c**), Ax (**d**, **e**) and Cor (**f**) 3D GRE. LTL tear (**a–f**) with BMO at the L side (**b**, **c**, **f**). The dorsal part is not delineable (**d**, **e**) and the palmar part shows an internal high signal (**d**, **e**)

Other components, such as the distal radioulnar ligaments (Ekenstam and Hagert 1985; Kim and Park 2008; Kim et al. 2012; Morrissy and Nalebuff 1979; Slattery et al. 2013; Reghunath et al. 2022) of the TFCC, may also rupture after (sub)luxation at the DRUJ (Adams and Berger 2002; Carlsen et al. 2010; Lo et al. 2001; May et al. 2002; McMurray and Muralikuttan 2008; Mikic 1995; Mino et al. 1983; Orbay et al. 2021; Rijal et al. 2023; Stuart et al. 2000; Viegas et al. 1990; Wechsler et al. 1987; Zannou et al. 2015) (Figs. 46 and 47). Traumatic sequels may be obvious (Fig. 46a, b) with a rupture of the rul (Gillis et al. 2019;

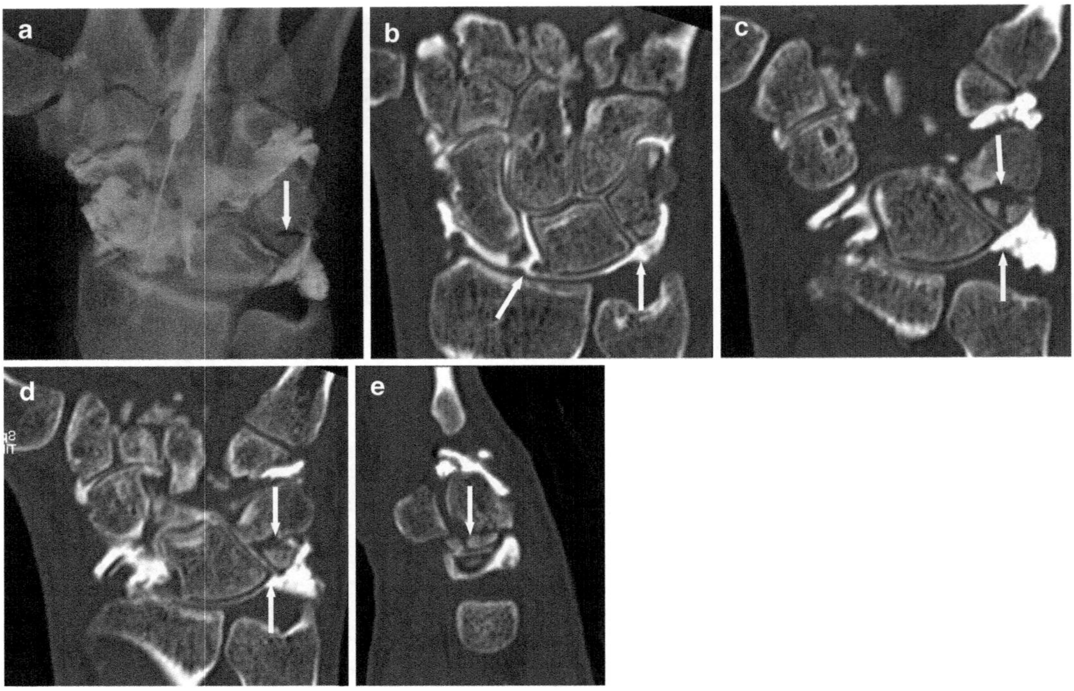

Fig. 32 Wrist arthrography (RC injection) (**a**); Cor (**b–d**) and Sag (**e**) CT images. Small LTL (**a–d**) and SLL (**b**) tear with an old fracture of the Tri (**c–e**)

Fig. 33 Cor PD WI (**a**) and Ax T2-WI FS (**b**). Central tear of the TFCC (Palmer type I A)

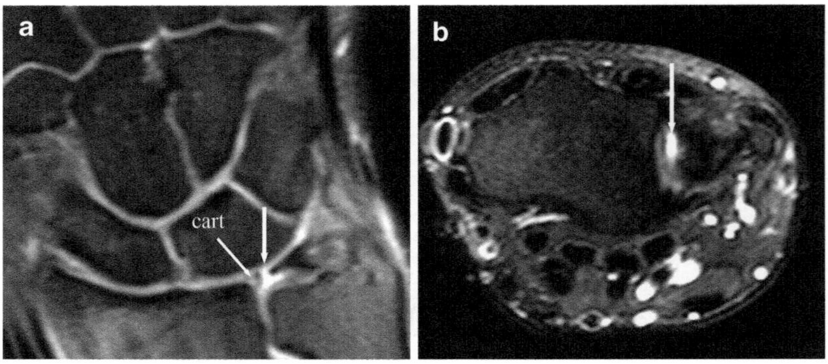

TRAUMATIC:
I A : central perforation of the TFC
I B : traumatic ulnar avulsion
I C : tear of the ulno-lunar and ulno-triquetral ligaments
I D : radial avulsion

Fig. 34 Palmer classification of traumatic TFCC lesions

Mulford and Axelrod 2007; Mulford et al. 2010; Nakamura 2012; Verhiel et al. 2022) (Fig. 46c). (Restored) normal relation at the DRUJ, however, may hide a clear lesion of the rul (Fig. 47c–e). The impression of the cortex that may remain after an anterior U luxation at the DRUJ is known as the second ulnar groove sign (Mespreuve and Coenen 2017) (Fig. 48).

1.4 Others

The isolated rupture (Lichtman and Wroten 2006; Nakamura et al. 2001b; Theumann et al. 2002; Zancolli 2001; Zancolli et al. 1987) of the sca-

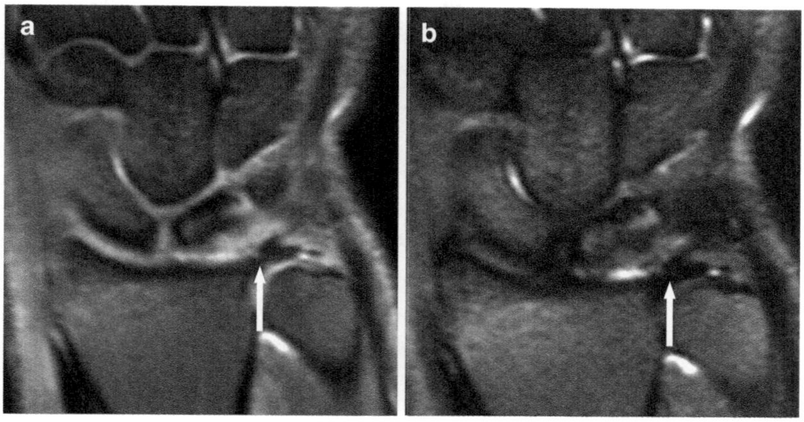

Fig. 35 Cor T2-WI FS (**a**, **b**). Palmer type I A TFCC tear with hydrops at the DRUJ

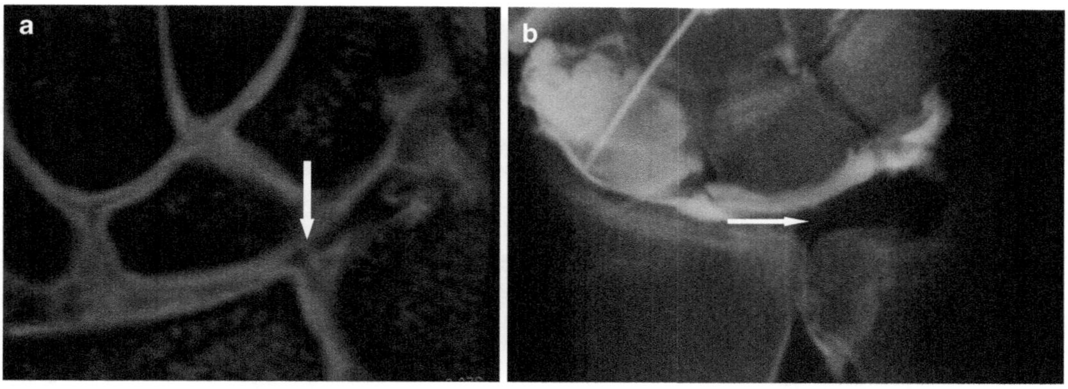

Fig. 36 Cor 2D GRE (**a**) and wrist arthrography (RC injection) (**b**). Palmer type I A slit-like TFCC tear with contrast leakage to the DRUJ

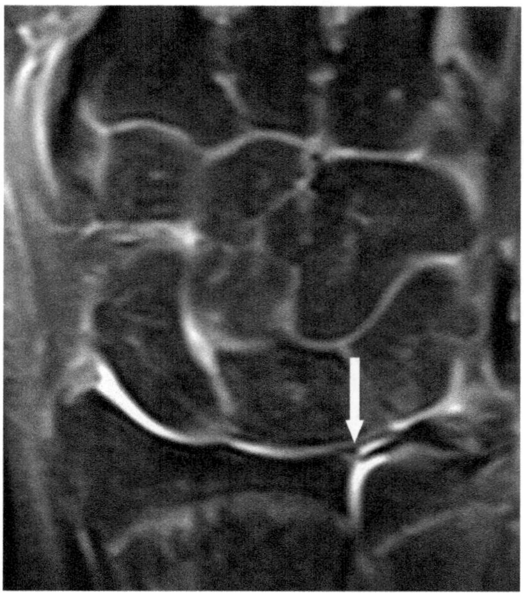

Fig. 37 Cor T1-WI FS wrist arthrography (RC injection). Palmer type I A slit-like TFCC tear with contrast leakage to the DRUJ and small step off

photrapezial ligament (Fig. 49a, b) is a very rare finding. Here also, an arthrosynovial cyst may develop (Fig. 49c).

1.5 General

Notice that, in general, even with the best MRI techniques used, some lesions of the ligaments will go unnoticed (Fig. 50a, b). The wrist arthrography (Cerezal et al. 2005; De Filippo et al. 2010; Lee et al. 2013b; Moneim and Omer 1983; Moser et al. 2007; Scheck et al. 1999; Schmid et al. 2005; Schmitt et al. 2003; Theumann et al. 2001, 2006; Zanetti et al. 1997)—always completed with CTA or MRA—remains a very valuable additional technique to exclude thin lesions (Fig. 50c) in case of clinical doubt.

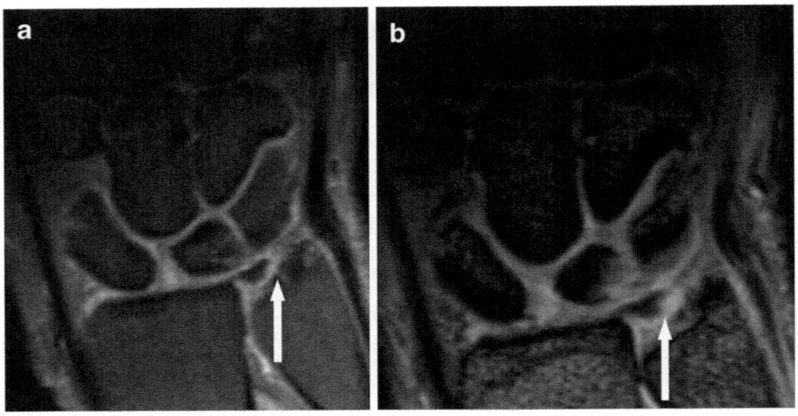

Fig. 38 Cor T2-WI FS (**a**) and 2D GRE (**b**). Palmer type I B tear of the TFCC (note: also a SL tear with diastasis)

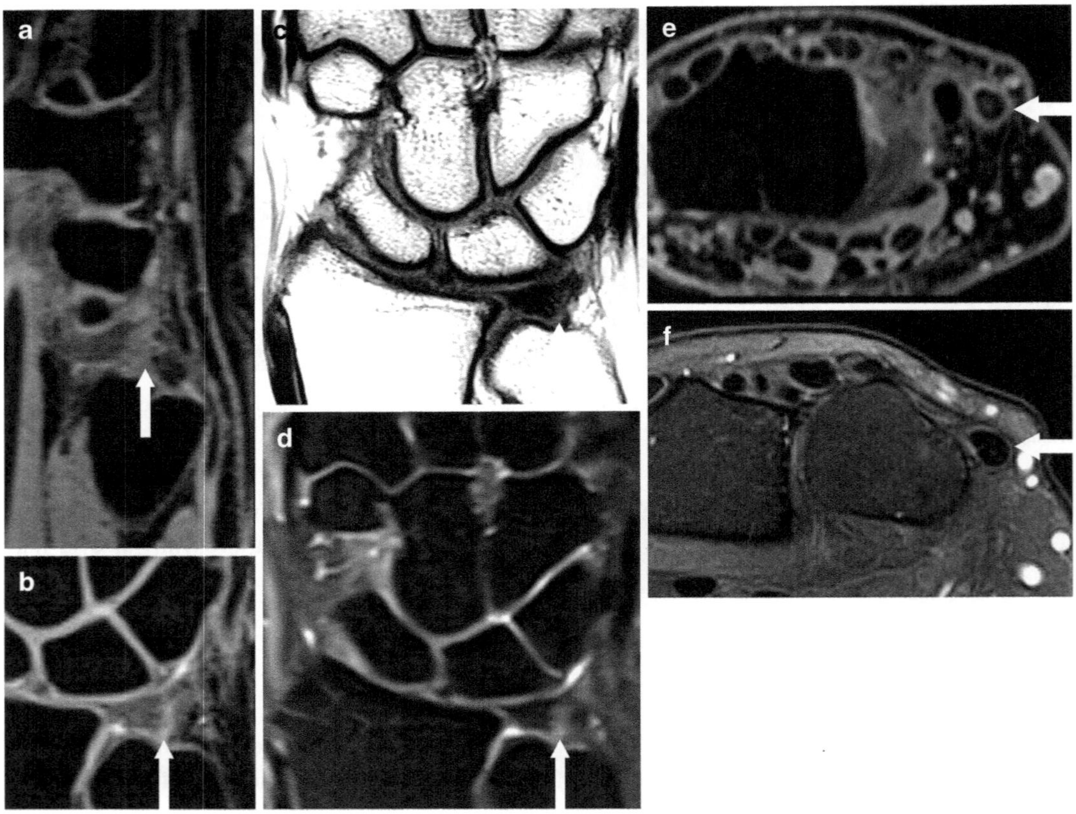

Fig. 39 Sag (**a**) and Cor (**b**) 3D GRE; Cor T1-WI (**c**) and T2-WI FS (**d–f**), Ax 3D GRE (**e**) and T2-WI FS (**f**). Palmer type I B tear of the TFCC (**a–d**) with extension in the anteriorly subluxated disc (**a**), tenosynovitis of the ECU (**e**), and luxation of the ECU tendon (**f**)

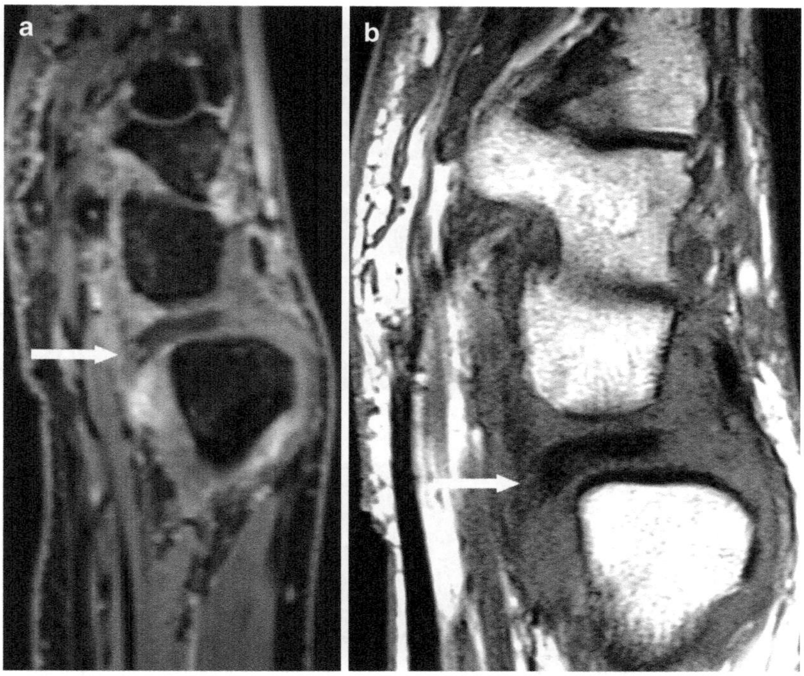

Fig. 40 Sag 3D GRE (**a**) and T1-WI (**b**). Anteriorly luxated disc with posterior U displacement

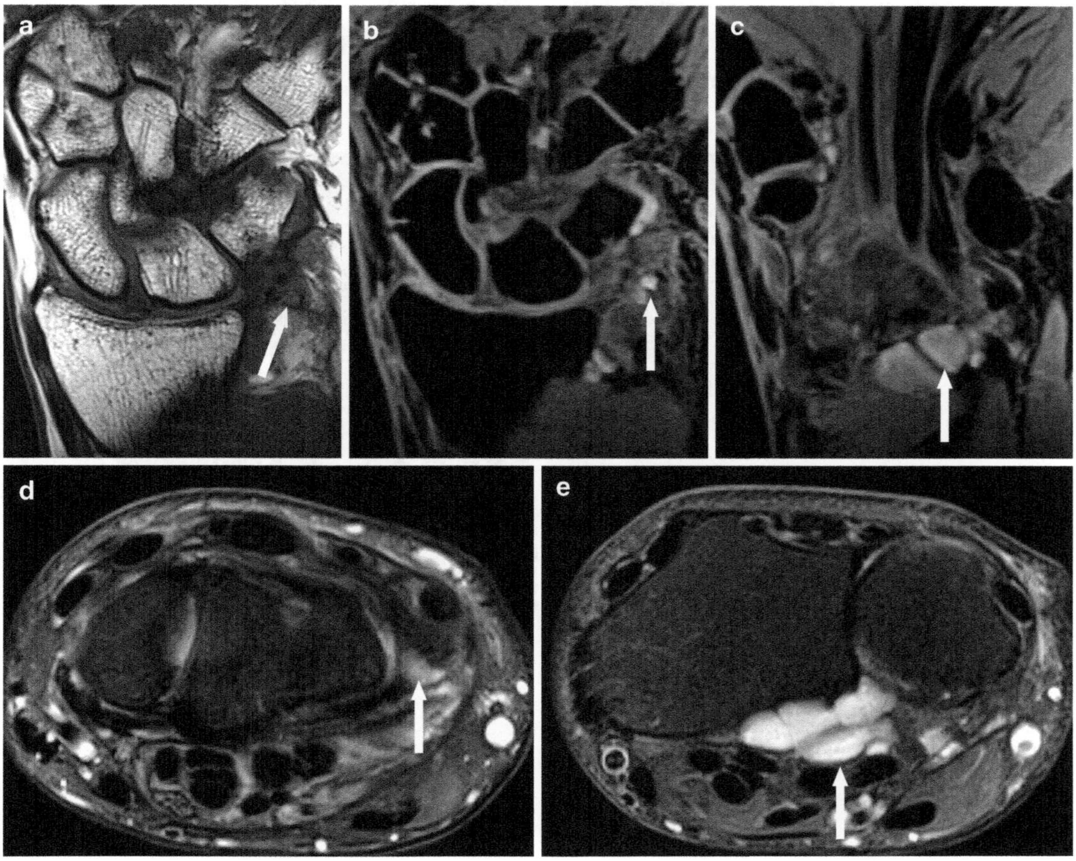

Fig. 41 Cor T1-WI (**a**) and 3D GRE (**b**, **c**); Ax T2-WI FS (**d**, **e**). Palmer type I B tear of the TFCC (**a**, **b**) with large arthrosynovial cyst at the palmar side (**c**–**e**) starting from the region of the tear (**b**–**d**)

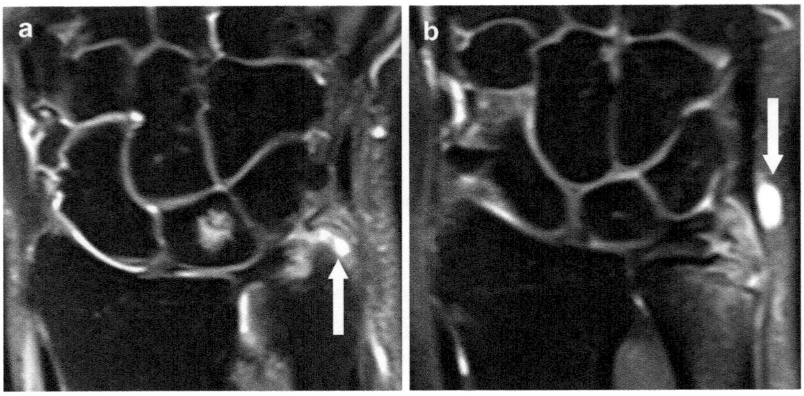

Fig. 42 Cor T2-WI FS. Prestyloid recessus filled with fluid (**a**) and peritendinous cyst of the ECU (**b**)

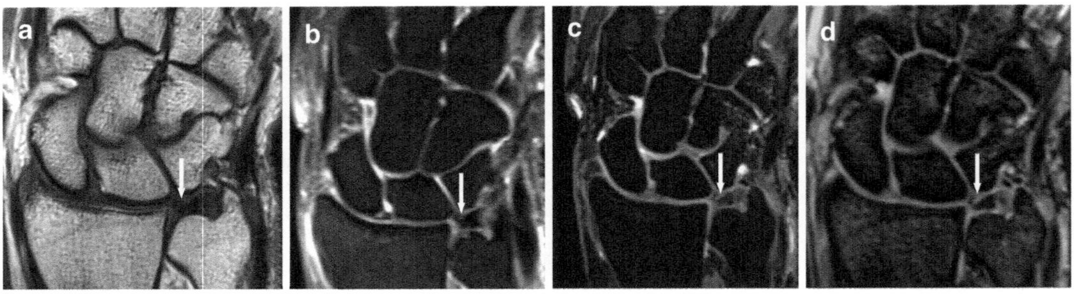

Fig. 43 Cor T1-WI FS (**a**); T2-WI FS (**b**); 3D GRE (**c**), and 2d GRE (**d**). An isolated Palmer type I C lesion of the TFCC with deformed ulno-lunate and ruptured ulno-triquetral ligament

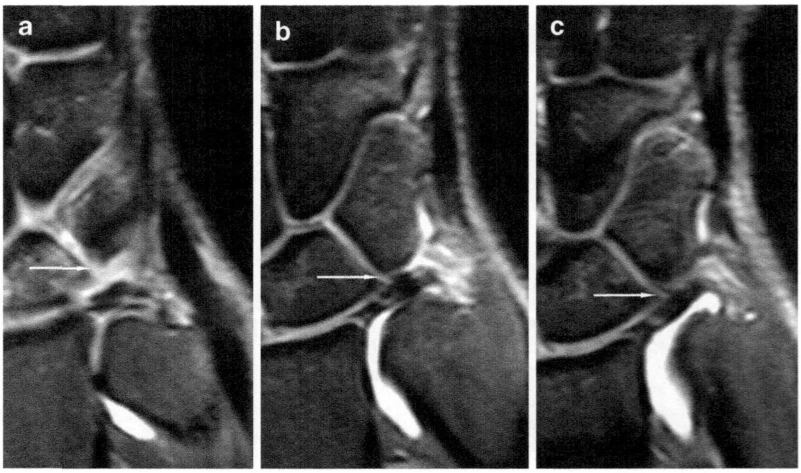

Fig. 44 T2-WI FS (**a–c**). Probable lesion Palmer I C type with LT and I A TFCC lesions with prominent tri-compartmental hydrops

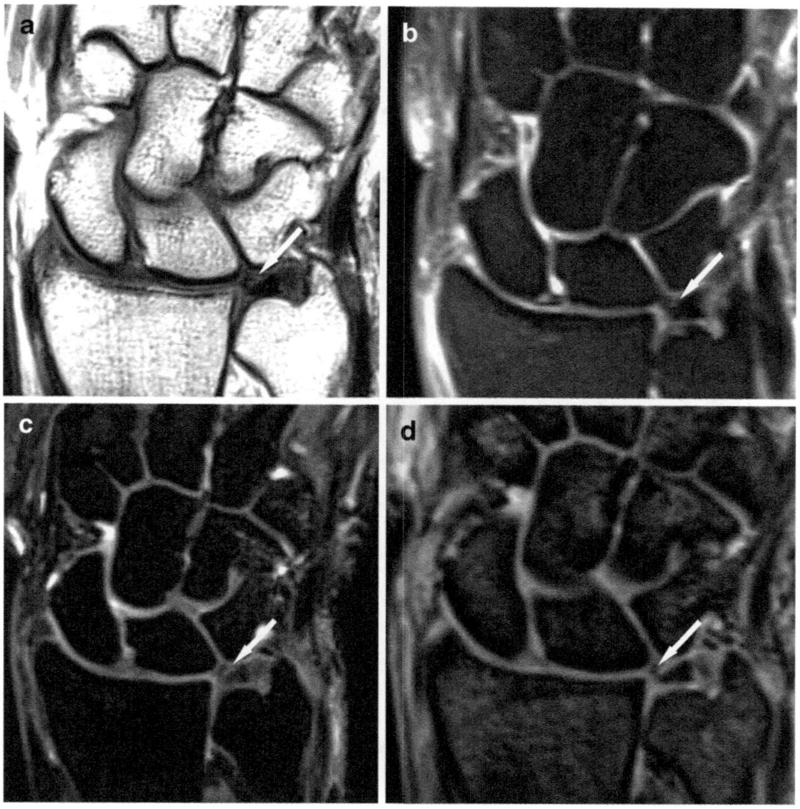

Fig. 45 Cor T1-WI FS (**a**); T2-WI FS (**b**, **c**); and 2D GRE (**d**). Palmer type I D lesion of the TFCC

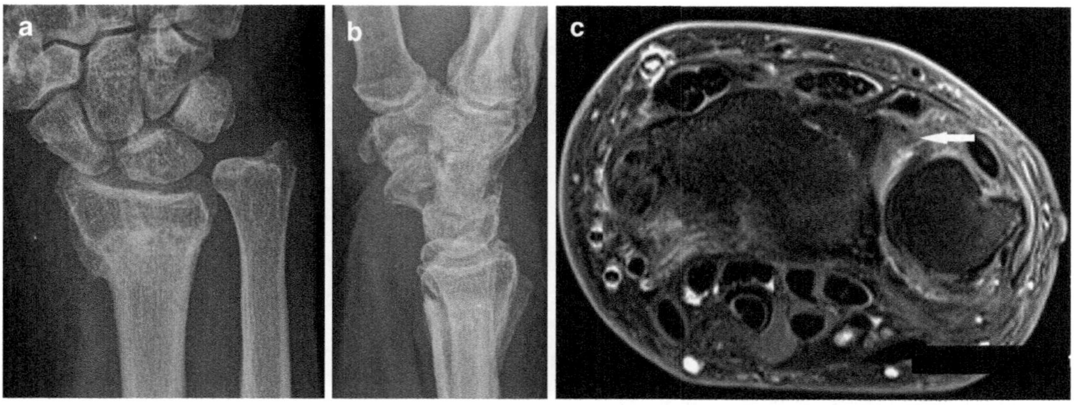

Fig. 46 Standard PA (**a**) and Lateral (**b**) views; Ax T2- WI FS (**c**). Sequel of an impacted Pouteau fracture with radial shortening and distal luxation of the ulnar head (**a**, **b**). Rupture of the dorsal rul (**c**)

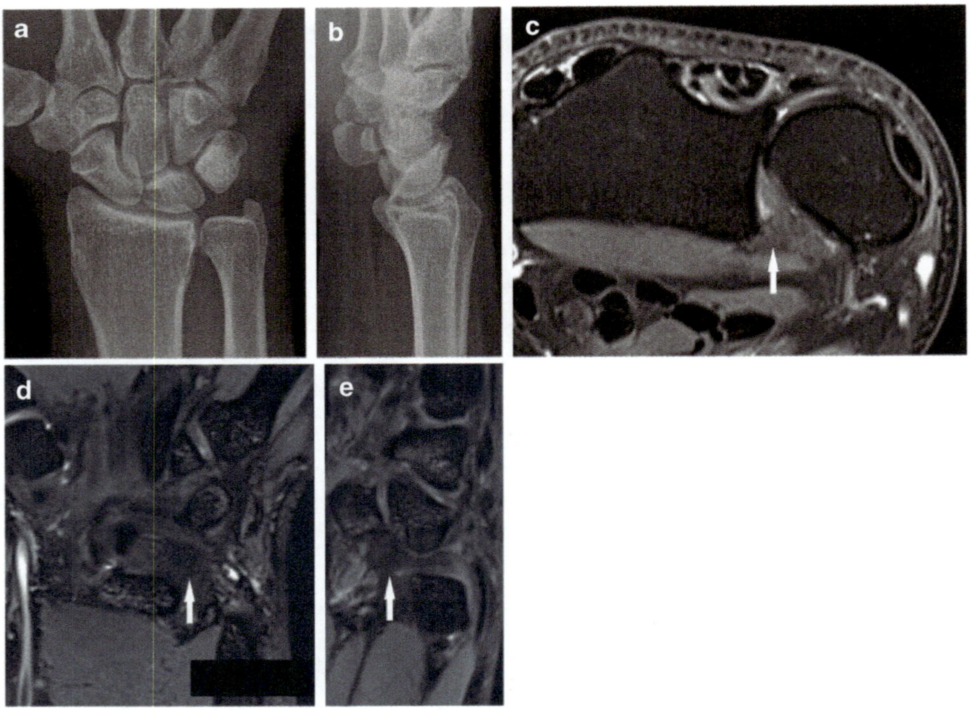

Fig. 47 Standard PA (**a**) and Lateral (**b**) views; (**c**) Cor (**d**) and Sag (**e**) 3D GRE. Reduced posterior U luxation with normal standard views (**a, b**). Rupture of the palmar rul with scar formation (**c–e**)

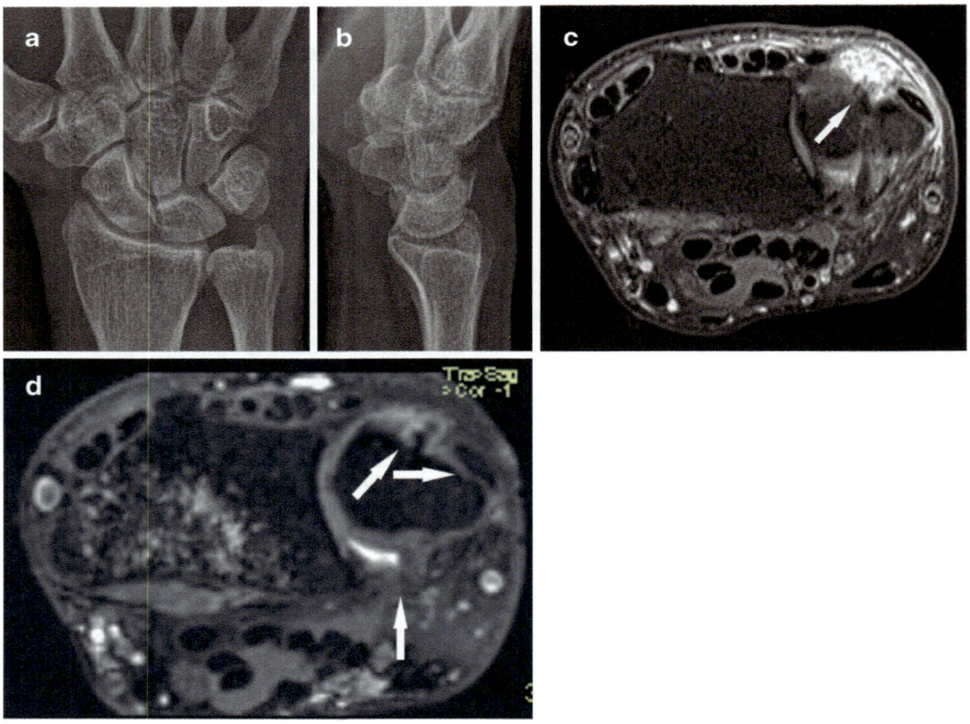

Fig. 48 Standard PA (**a**) and Lateral (**b**) views; Ax T2-WI FS (**c, d**). Sequels of a reduced anterior U luxation with a second ulnar groove sign (**c, d**) antero-radial form the ECU groove (**d**) and rupture of the palmer rul (**d**)

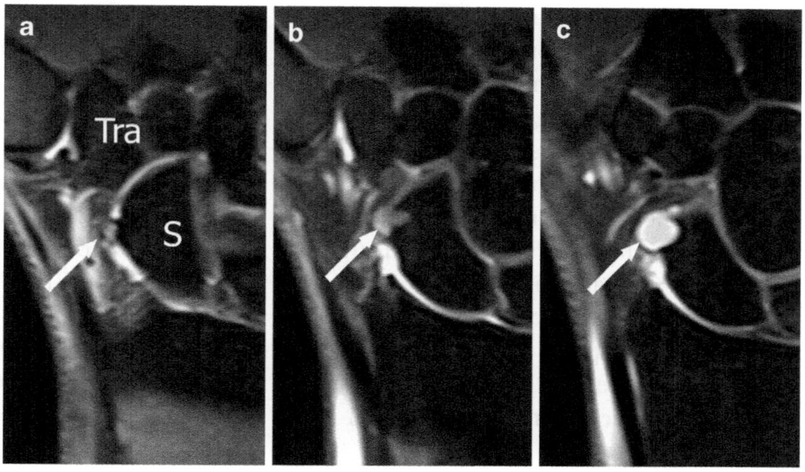

Fig. 49 Cor T2-WI FS (**a**, **c**). Sequels a rupture of the scaphotrapezial ligament (**a**, **b**) with small cyst formation (**c**)

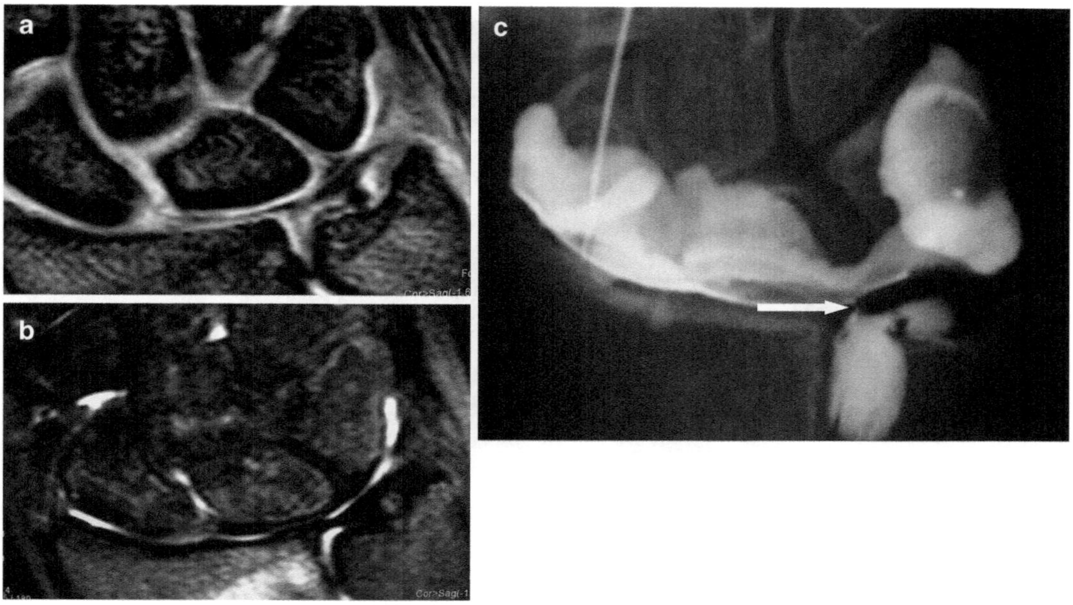

Fig. 50 Cor 3d GRE (**a**) and T2-WI FS (**b**); wrist arthrography (RC joint injection). MRI reveals no lesion, but there is a small hydrops at the DRUJ. A very thin Palmer type I A lesion of the TFCC (**c**) is obvious

2 Extrinsic Ligaments

2.1 Palmar

The exact evaluation of these important multidirectional ligaments remains even more challenging (Andersson et al. 2015; Bencardino and Rosenberg 2006; Boutry et al. 2005; Davis and Blankenbaker 2010; Gilula and Weeks 1978; Girgis and Epstein 2000; Gitto et al. 2017; Lee and Elfar 2015; Loredo et al. 2005; Mayfield 1984; Pulos and Bozentka 2015; Ringler 2013; Ringler and Murthy 2015; Lacelli et al. 2008; Manley et al. 2013), also due to their anatomical location in the capsule (Zdravkovic et al. 1994). This makes arthrography also less suitable (Sennwald et al. 1994; Shahabpour et al. 2011).

At the radial component of the palmar V, composed of the radioscaphocapitate and the radiolunotriquetral ligament, the striped aspect is erased and replaced by a higher and more homogenous signal (Figs. 51a, b and 54a), eventually with small cystic components (Figs. 51c and 54a). Elongation and/or partial tears give rise to oedema between the low signal striations and/or with partial rupture of the low signal stripes (Fig. 52), respectively. A bony detachment may accompany the ligamentous lesion (Fig. 53). More frequently, a periosteal stripping at the carpal attachments results in focal BMO (Fig. 54b, c).

The ulnar component of the palmar V (capitate-triquetral ligament) (Figs. 55, 56, and 57) rarely lacerates but—if extensive enough—it may lead to ulnar midcarpal instability (Anderson et al. 2008; Niacaris et al. 2015).

(Diffuse) destruction of an extrinsic ligament should always be differentiated from destruction through infiltration by rheumatoid arthritis (Ochman et al. 2017) (Fig. 58).

The indirect effect of the palmar extrinsic ligaments in trauma may result in a manually non-reducible anterior luxation of the lunate, trapped in the space of Poirier between the rsc and rlt ligament (Fig. 59). In addition, the hump back

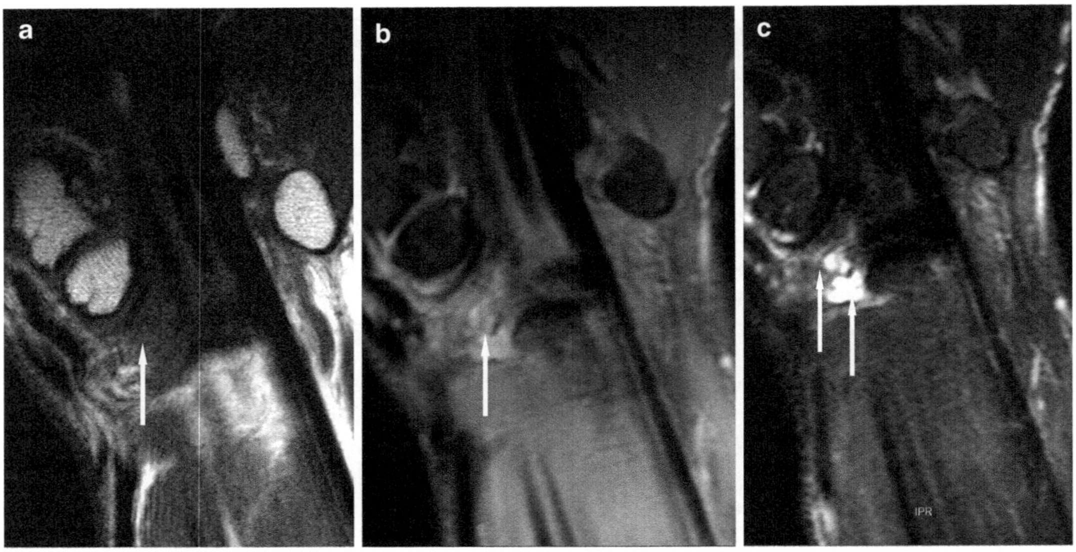

Fig. 51 Cor T1-WI (**a**); PD WI (**b**); and T2-WI FS (**c**). Tear at the radial part of the Palmar V (rsc and rlt)

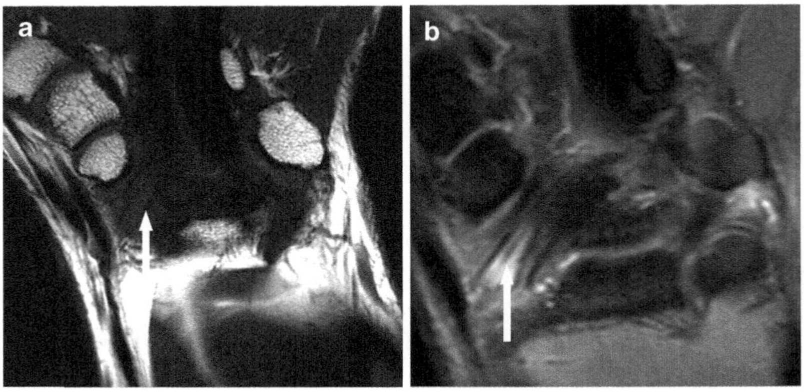

Fig. 52 Cor T1-WI (**a**) and PD WI (**b**). Oedema between the low signal stripes at the radial part of the Palmar V

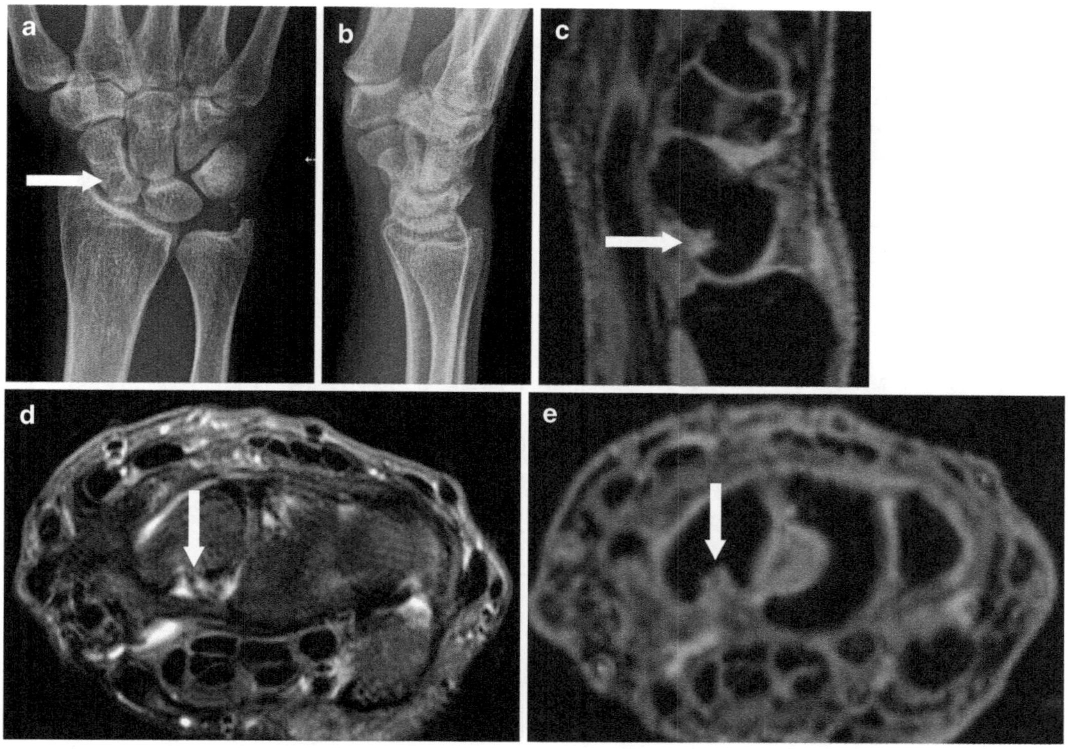

Fig. 53 Standard PA (**a**) and lateral (**b**) views; Cor 3D GRE (**c**); Ax T2-WI FS (**d**); and 3D GRE (**e**). A small translucency at the S (S) corresponds to a palmar, small broken S bone fragment (**c**–**e**) at the insertion point of the palmar V (**d**, **e**), which shows a higher signal zone (**d**)

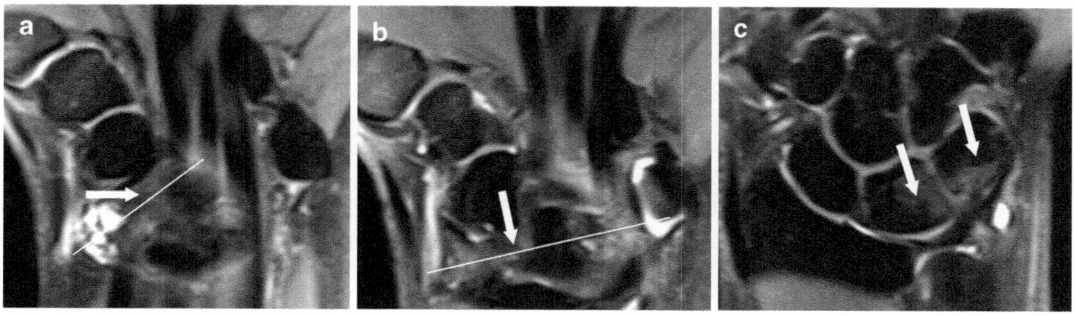

Fig. 54 Cor PD WI (**a**, **c**). Higher signal with cyst formation along the trajectory of the rsc (**a**). Focal BMO along the trajectory of the rlt (**b**, **c**) due to periosteal stripping

deformity of the S after trauma (Fig. 60) is the result of the ligaments of the ulnar palmar V (rsc and rlt). The proximal part of the S tilts backward with the lunate (Fig. 60a, b), while the distal part has a natural tendency to tilt in the palmar direction (Fig. 60b) around the ligaments at the waist of the S (Fig. 60c).

2.2 Dorsal

The same pattern as in the palmar ligaments will appear at the dorsal ligaments (Fig. 61) after a tear and/or an elongation (Özkan et al. 2019). An extreme elongation (Fig. 62a, b) combined with a palmar ligament lesion may lead to an ulnar

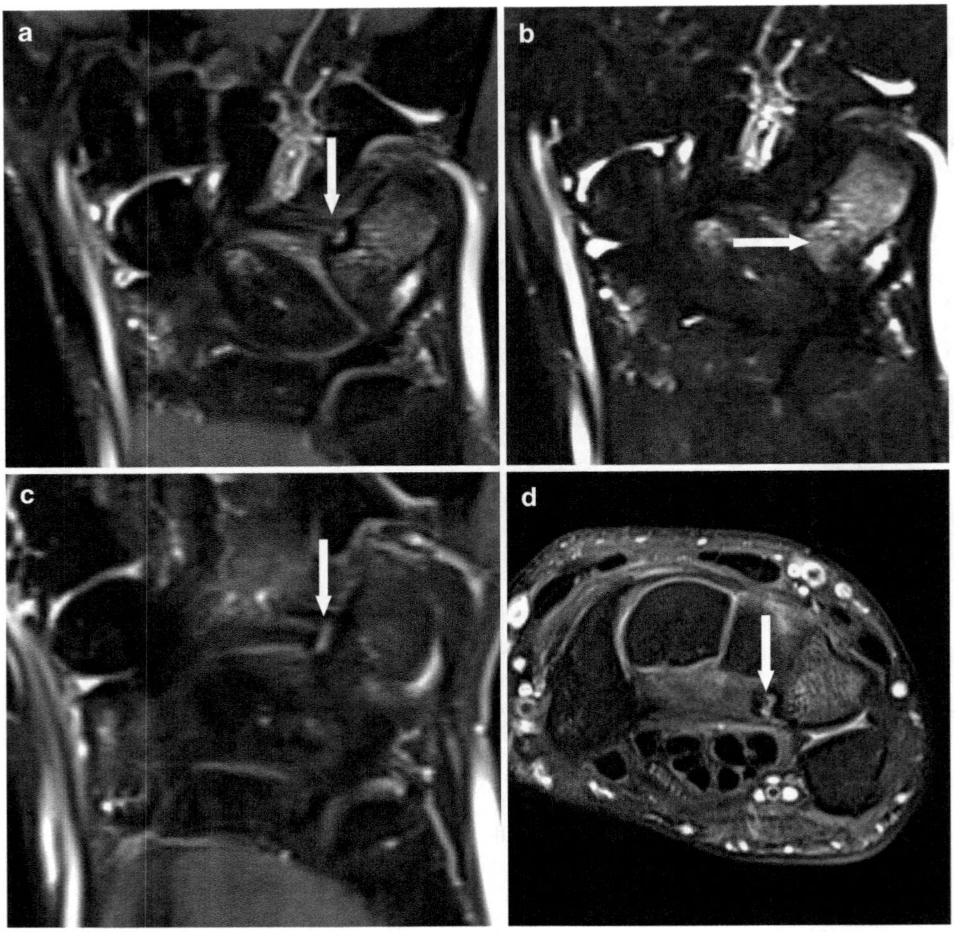

Fig. 55 Cor (**a–c**) and Ax (**d**) T2-WI FS. Laceration at the triquetral insertion of the ligament between C and Tri and extensive post-traumatic BMO at the Tri

translation (Metz et al. 1997) of the whole carpus (Fig. 62c, d). On the other hand, also an (old) fracture of the common triquetral insertion of the dorsal ligaments (Rubensson et al. 2018; Schmitt et al. 2006; Sulkers et al. 2018; Viegas et al. 1995; Theumann et al. 2003) (Fig. 63) may result in ulnar translation on the long term.

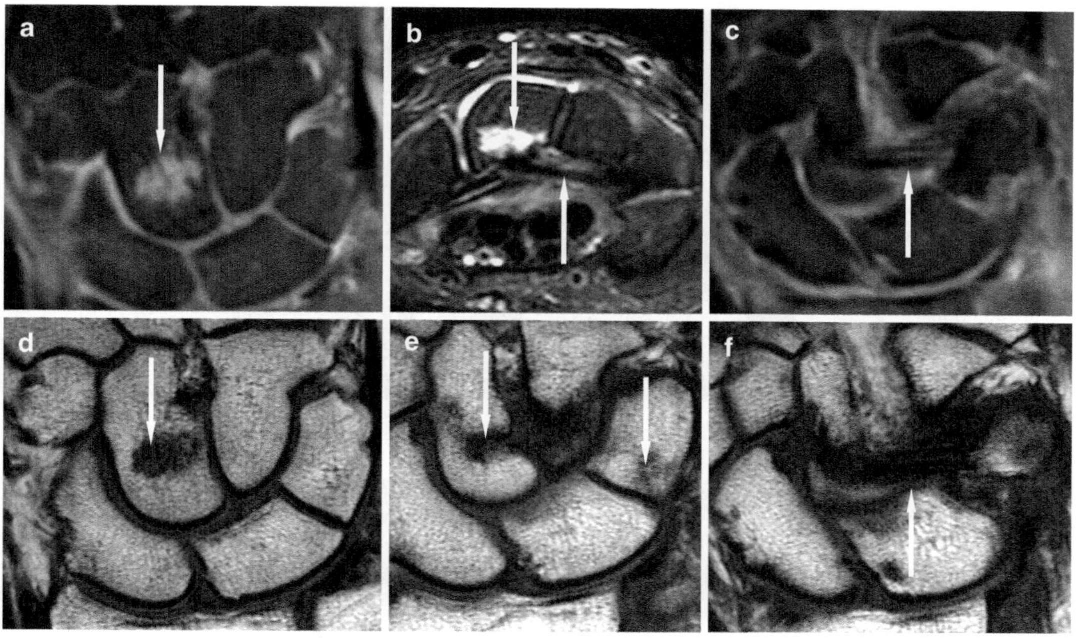

Fig. 56 Cor (**a**, **c**) and Ax (**b**) T2-WI FS; Cor T1-WI (**d**–**f**). Periosteal stripping at the C (**a**, **b**, **d**, **e**) and the Tri (**e**) with an intact ligament (**b**, **f**) between C and Tri

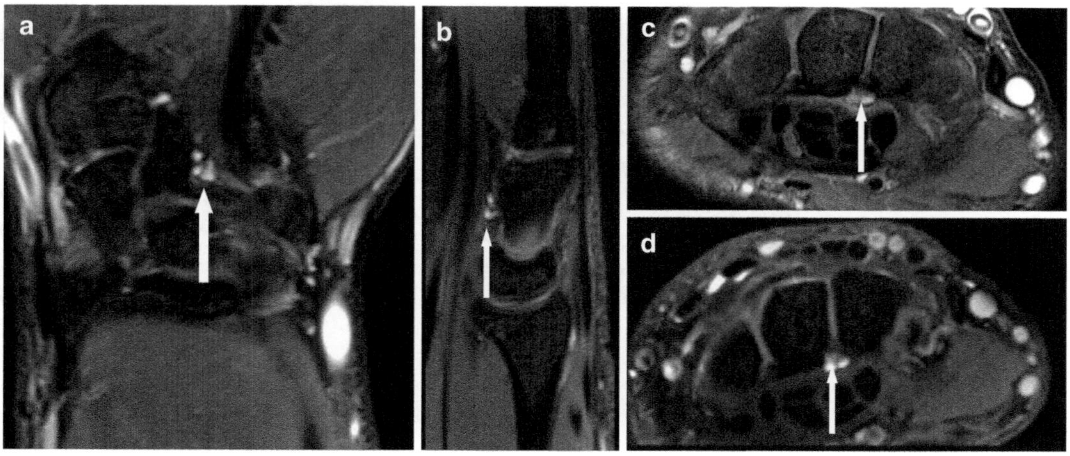

Fig. 57 Cor (**a**) and Sag (**b**) 3D GRE; Ax T2-WI FS (**c**); and 3D GRE (**d**). Small laceration of the distal part of the ligament between the C and Tri with small internal cystic formations, probably not significant/extensive enough

Fig. 58 Cor T1-WI (**a**) and T1-WI FS with contrast (**b**). Extensive infiltration and destruction of the palmar ligaments (**a**) with diffuse CE (**b**) due to RA (**a, b**). The hydrops of the Tri-P joint and the CMC I joint with adjacent bone erosion (**b**) are additional arguments in favour of RA

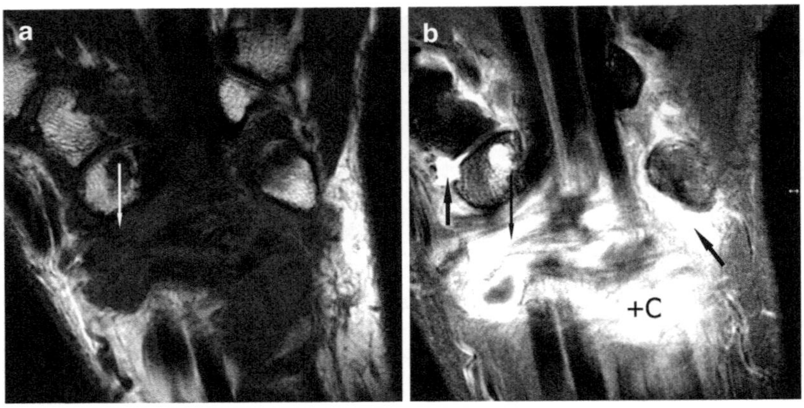

Fig. 59 Standard Lateral (**a**) and PA (**b**) view; T2-WI FS (**c**). The lunate bone is luxated through the space of Poirier between the palmar rsc and rlt ligament

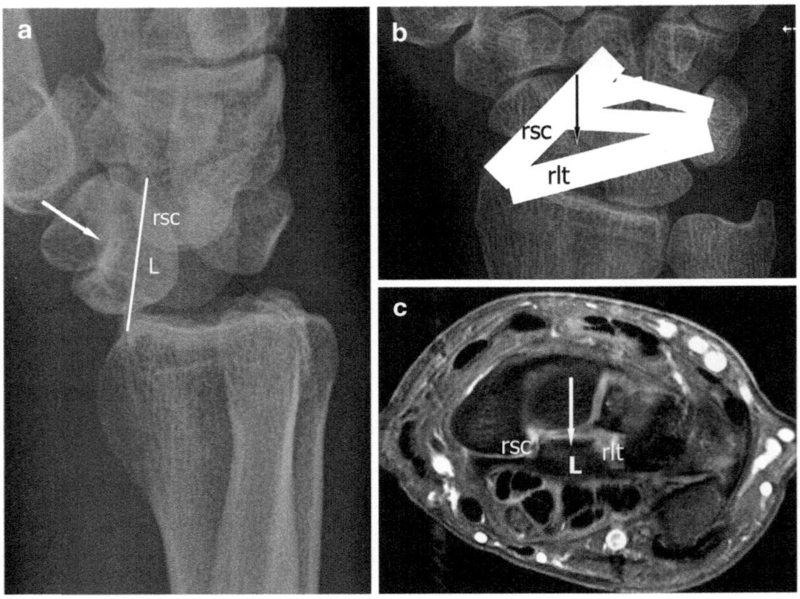

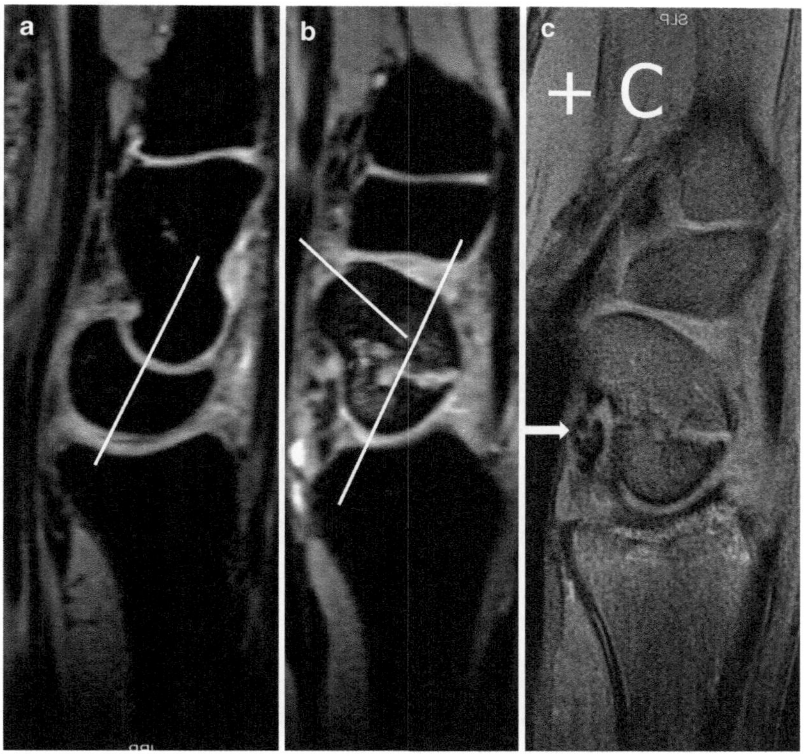

Fig. 60 Sag 3D GRE (**a**, **b**) and T1-WI FS with CE (**c**). The post-traumatic hump-back deformity of the S around the ulnar palmar V components (rsc and rlt) at the S waist

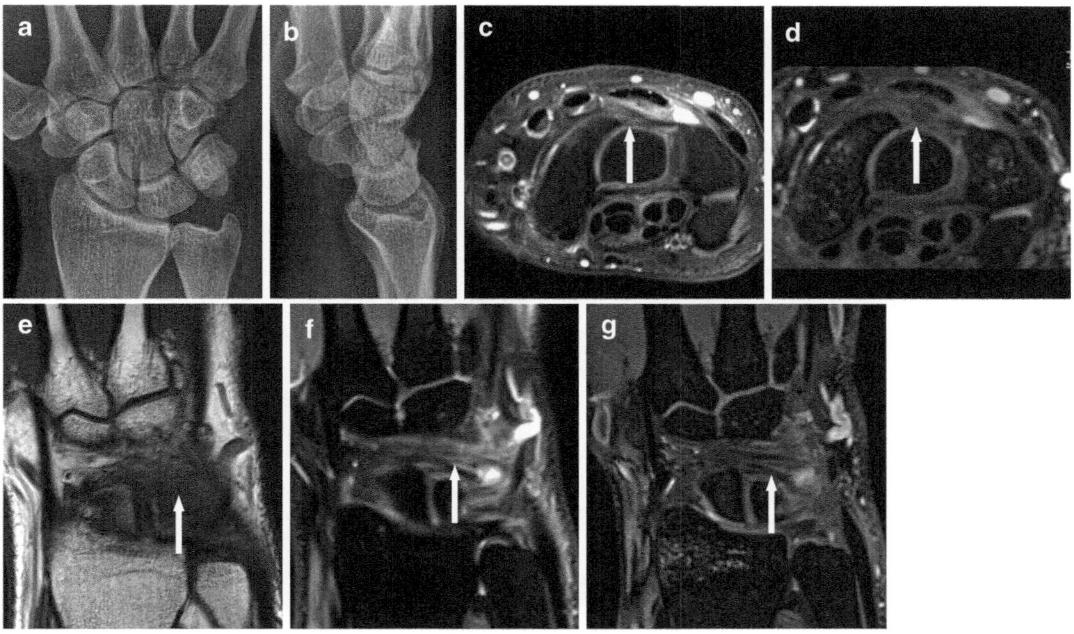

Fig. 61 Standard PA (**a**) and Lateral (**b**) views; Ax T2-WI FS (**c**) and 3D GRE (**d**); Cor T1-WI (**e**), T2-WI FS (**f**), and 3D GRE (**g**). The dorsal intercarpal ligament shows a higher signal infiltration with partial erasure of the longitudinal low signal stripes (**c**–**g**) and a periosteal stripping at the Tri side (**d**, **f**, **g**)

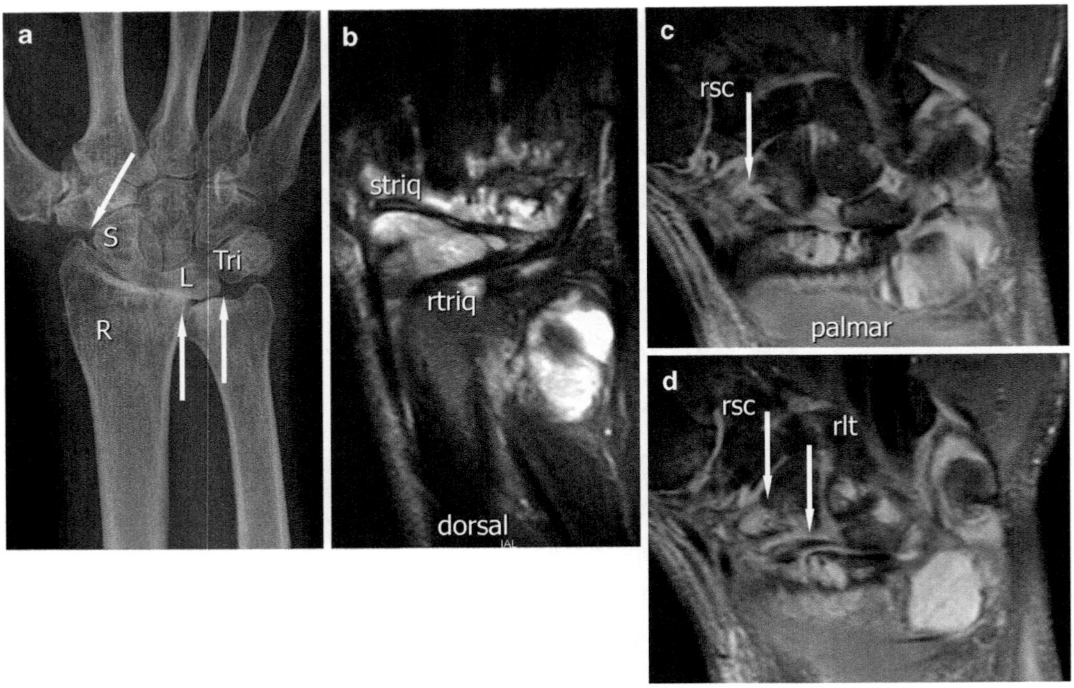

Fig. 62 Standard PA view (**a**); Cor T2-WI FS (**b**); and PD WI (**c**, **d**). The whole carpus is translated (type 1) to the ulnar side with an extensively degenerative RC joint (**a**). The dorsal ligaments are continuous, but elongated, flaccid, and deformed (**b**). The palmar ligaments are affected in the same way (**c**, **d**), all suggesting an old traumatic lesion

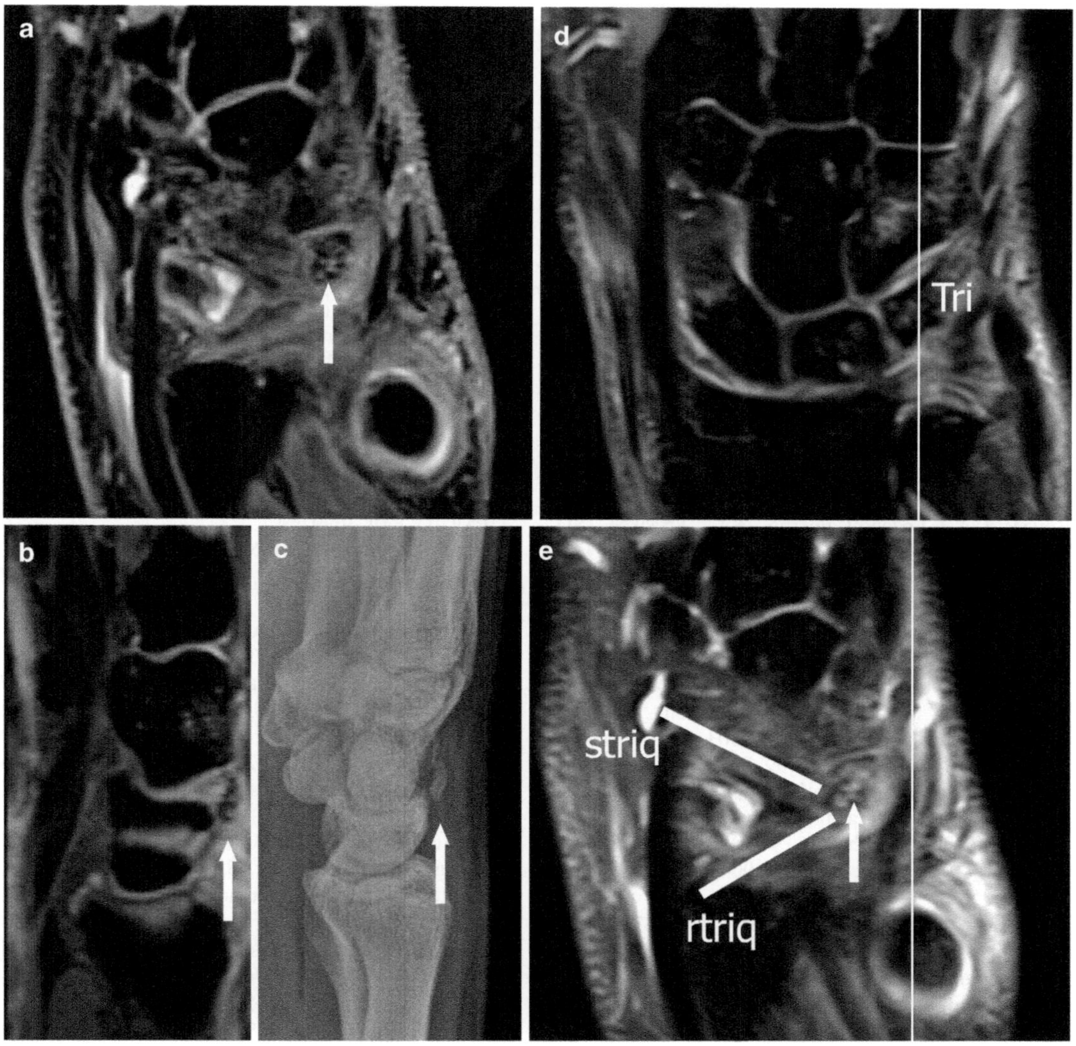

Fig. 63 Cor (**a**) and Sag (**b**) 3D GRE; Standard lateral view (**c**); Cor T2-WI FS (**d**, **e**). A small fragment posteriorly of the proximal carpal row (**a**, **c**) corresponds with a fracture at the dorsal side of the triquetral bone (**c**). The fragment and the depicted attached ligaments (S Triq and R Triq) are displaced radially versus the white line through the normal position (**d**, **e**) on the more dorsal image (**e**)

References

Abou Arab W, Rauch A, Chawki MB, Dap F, Dautel G, Blum A, Gondim Teixeira PA (2018) Scapholunate instability: improved detection with semi-automated kinematic CT analysis during stress manoeuvres. Eur Radiol 28(10):4397–4406. https://doi.org/10.1007/s00330-018-5430-2. Epub 2018 Apr 30. PMID: 29713765

Adams BD, Berger RA (2002) An anatomic reconstruction of the distal radioulnar ligaments for post-traumatic distal radioulnar joint instability. J Hand Surg Am 27(2):243–251. https://doi.org/10.1053/jhsu.2002.31731. PMID: 11901383

Anderson ML, Skinner JA, Felmlee JP, Berger RA, Amrami KK (2008) Diagnostic comparison of 1.5 Tesla and 3.0 Tesla preoperative MRI of the wrist in patients with ulnar-sided wrist pain. J Hand Surg Am 33(7):1153–1159. https://doi.org/10.1016/j.jhsa.2008.02.028. PMID: 18762112

Andersson JK, Andernord D, Karlsson J, Fridén J (2015) Efficacy of magnetic resonance imaging and clinical tests in diagnostics of wrist ligament injuries: a systematic review. Arthroscopy 31(10):2014–20.e2. https://doi.org/10.1016/j.arthro.2015.04.090. Epub 2015 Jun 18. PMID: 26095820.

Athlani L, Rouizi K, Granero J, Hossu G, Blum A, Dautel G, Gondim Teixeira PA (2020) Assessment of scapholunate instability with dynamic computed tomography. J Hand Surg Eur Vol 45(4):375–382. https://doi.org/10.1177/1753193419893890. Epub 2019 Dec 16. PMID: 31842675

Bencardino JT, Rosenberg ZS (2006) Sports-related injuries of the wrist: an approach to MRI interpretation. Clin Sports Med 25(3):409–432. https://doi.org/10.1016/j.csm.2006.02.007, vi. PMID: 16798135

Boutry N, Lapegue F, Masi L, Claret A, Demondion X, Cotten A (2005) Ultrasonographic evaluation of normal extrinsic and intrinsic carpal ligaments: preliminary experience. Skeletal Radiol 34(9):513–521. https://doi.org/10.1007/s00256-005-0929-4. Epub 2005 Jul 12. PMID: 16010593

Buijze GA, Lozano-Calderon SA, Strackee SD, Blankevoort L, Jupiter JB (2011) Osseous and ligamentous scaphoid anatomy: part I. A systematic literature review highlighting controversies. J Hand Surg Am 36(12):1926–1935. https://doi.org/10.1016/j.jhsa.2011.09.012. Epub 2011 Nov 3. PMID: 22051230

Carlsen BT, Dennison DG, Moran SL (2010) Acute dislocations of the distal radioulnar joint and distal ulna fractures. Hand Clin 26(4):503–516. https://doi.org/10.1016/j.hcl.2010.05.009. PMID: 20951900

Cerezal L, Abascal F, García-Valtuille R, Del Piñal F (2005) Wrist MR arthrography: how, why, when. Radiol Clin North Am 43(4):709–731. https://doi.org/10.1016/j.rcl.2005.02.004, viii. PMID: 15893533

Chan K, Vutescu ES, Wolfe SW, Lee SK (2019) Radiographs detect dorsal scaphoid translation in scapholunate dissociation. J Wrist Surg 8(3):186–191. https://doi.org/10.1055/s-0038-1677536. Epub 2019 Jan 18. PMID: 31192038; PMCID: PMC6546485

Cheriex KCAL, Sulkers GSI, Terra MP, Schep NWL, van Aard BJPL, Strackee SD (2017) Scapholunate dissociation; diagnostics made easy. Eur J Radiol 92:45–50. https://doi.org/10.1016/j.ejrad.2017.04.015. Epub 2017 Apr 25. PMID: 28624019

Chong C, Kandathil JC (2013) MR imaging of TFCC, what every radiologist need to know. Eur Congr Radiol:poster C-1841. https://doi.org/10.1594/ecr2013/C-1841

Couzens G, Daunt N, Crawford R, Ross M (2014) Positive magnetic resonance imaging findings in the asymptomatic wrist. ANZ J Surg 84(7–8):528–532. https://doi.org/10.1111/ans.12552. Epub 2014 Feb 26. PMID: 24612468

Dao KD, Solomon DJ, Shin AY, Puckett ML (2004) The efficacy of ultrasound in the evaluation of dynamic scapholunate ligamentous instability. J Bone Joint Surg Am 86(7):1473–1478. https://doi.org/10.2106/00004623-200407000-00016. PMID: 15252095

Davis KW, Blankenbaker DG (2010) Imaging the ligaments and tendons of the wrist. Semin Roentgenol 45(3):194–217. https://doi.org/10.1053/j.ro.2009.12.005. PMID: 20483115

De Filippo M, Pogliacomi F, Bertellini A, Araoz PA, Averna R, Sverzellati N, Ingegnoli A, Corradi M, Costantino C, Zompatori M (2010) MDCT arthrography of the wrist: diagnostic accuracy and indications. Eur J Radiol 74(1):221–225. https://doi.org/10.1016/j.ejrad.2009.01.023. Epub 2009 Feb 23. PMID: 19233582

De Santis S, Cozzolino R, Luchetti R, Cazzoletti L (2021) Comparison between MRI and arthroscopy of the wrist for the assessment of posttraumatic lesions of intrinsic ligaments and the triangular fibrocartilage complex. J Wrist Surg 11(1):28–34. https://doi.org/10.1055/s-0041-1729757. PMID: 35127261; PMCID: PMC8807093

Del Piñal F (2013) Arthroscopic volar capsuloligamentous repair. J Wrist Surg 2(2):126–128. https://doi.org/10.1055/s-0033-1343016. PMID: 24436804; PMCID: PMC3699269

Demehri S, Hafezi-Nejad N, Morelli JN, Thakur U, Lifchez SD, Means KR, Eng J, Shores JT (2016) Scapholunate kinematics of asymptomatic wrists in comparison with symptomatic contralateral wrists using four-dimensional CT examinations: initial clinical experience. Skeletal Radiol 45(4):437–446. https://doi.org/10.1007/s00256-015-2308-0. Epub 2015 Dec 14. PMID: 26659662

Devilliers Minnaar AB (1952) Congenital fusion of the lunate and triquetral bones in the South African Bantu. J Bone Joint Surg Br 34-B(1):45–48. https://doi.org/10.1302/0301-620X.34B1.45. PMID: 12999869

Dornberger JE, Rademacher G, Mutze S, Eisenschenk A, Stengel D (2015) Accuracy of simple plain radiographic signs and measures to diagnose acute scapholunate ligament injuries of the wrist. Eur Radiol 25(12):3488–3498. https://doi.org/10.1007/s00330-015-3776-2. Epub 2015 May 17. PMID: 25981221

Ekenstam F, Hagert CG (1985) Anatomical studies on the geometry and stability of the distal radio ulnar joint. Scand J Plast Reconstr Surg 19(1):17–25. https://doi.org/10.3109/02844318509052861. PMID: 4023639

Garcia-Elias M (2008) The non-dissociative clunking wrist: a personal view. J Hand Surg Eur Vol 33(6):698–711. https://doi.org/10.1177/1753193408090148. Epub 2008 Oct 20. PMID: 18936125

Garcia-Elias M, Lluch AL, Stanley JK (2006) Three-ligament tenodesis for the treatment of scapholunate dissociation: indications and surgical technique. J Hand Surg Am 31(1):125–134. https://doi.org/10.1016/j.jhsa.2005.10.011. PMID: 16443117

Garn SM, Frisancho AR, Poznanski AK, Schweitzer J, McCann MB (1971) Analysis of triquetral-lunate fusion. Am J Phys Anthropol 34(3):431–433. https://doi.org/10.1002/ajpa.1330340313. PMID: 5120558

Gelberman RH, Cooney WP 3rd, Szabo RM (2001) Carpal instability. Instr Course Lect 50:123–134. PMID: 11372306

Gillis JA, Soreide E, Khouri JS, Kadar A, Berger RA, Moran SL (2019) Outcomes of the Adams-Berger ligament reconstruction for the distal radioulnar joint instability in 95 consecutive cases. J Wrist Surg 8(4):268–275. https://doi.org/10.1055/s--0039-1685235. Epub 2019 Apr 22. PMID: 31404256; PMCID: PMC6685731

Gilula LA (1979) Carpal injuries: analytic approach and case exercises. AJR Am J Roentgenol 133(3):503–517. https://doi.org/10.2214/ajr.133.3.503. PMID: 111512

Gilula LA, Weeks PM (1978) Post-traumatic ligamentous instabilities of the wrist. Radiology 129(3):641–651. https://doi.org/10.1148/129.3.641. PMID: 725039

Girgis WS, Epstein RE (2000) Magnetic resonance imaging of the hand and wrist. Semin Roentgenol 35(3):286–296. https://doi.org/10.1053/sroe.2000.7339. PMID: 10939130

Gitto S, Messina C, Mauri G, Aliprandi A, Sardanelli F, Sconfienza LM (2017) Dynamic high-resolution ultrasound of intrinsic and extrinsic ligaments of the wrist: how to make it simple. Eur J Radiol 87:20–35. https://doi.org/10.1016/j.ejrad.2016.12.002. Epub 2016 Dec 5. PMID: 28065372

Gornitzky AL, Carrigan RB (2016) The diagnostic utility of MRI in the painful wrist: when to reconsider advanced imaging in the pediatric patient. Pediatrics (Evanston) 137(Suppl 3):596–596A. https://doi.org/10.1542/peds.137.Supplement_3.596A

Grunz JP, Gietzen CH, Grunz K, Bley T, Schmitt R (2021) Imaging of carpal instabilities. Rofo 193(2):139–150. https://doi.org/10.1055/a-1219-8158. English. Epub 2020 Sep 3. PMID: 32882727

Hafezi-Nejad N, Carrino JA, Eng J, Blackmore C, Shores J, Lifchez SD, Farahani SJ, Demehri S (2016) Scapholunate interosseous ligament tears: diagnostic performance of 1.5T, 3T MRI, and MR arthrography-a systematic review and meta-analysis. Acad Radiol 23(9):1091–1103. https://doi.org/10.1016/j.acra.2016.04.006. Epub 2016 Jul 15. PMID: 27426979

Iordache SD, Rowan R, Garvin GJ, Osman S, Grewal R, Faber KJ (2012) Prevalence of triangular fibrocartilage complex abnormalities on MRI scans of asymptomatic wrists. J Hand Surg Am 37(1):98–103. https://doi.org/10.1016/j.jhsa.2011.10.006. Epub 2011 Nov 30. PMID: 22129657

Kim JP, Park MJ (2008) Assessment of distal radioulnar joint instability after distal radius fracture: comparison of computed tomography and clinical examination results. J Hand Surg Am 33(9):1486–1492. https://doi.org/10.1016/j.jhsa.2008.05.017. PMID: 18984328

Kim S, Ward JP, Rettig ME (2012) Galeazzi fracture with volar dislocation of the distal radioulnar joint. Am J Orthop (Belle Mead NJ) 41(11):E152–E154. PMID: 23431520

Lacelli F, Muda A, Sconfienza LM, Schettini D, Garlaschi G, Silvestri E (2008) High-resolution ultrasound anatomy of extrinsic carpal ligaments. Radiol Med 113(4):504–516. https://doi.org/10.1007/s11547-008-0269-2. English, Italian. Epub 2008 May 20. PMID: 18493830

Langner I, Fischer S, Eisenschenk A, Langner S (2015) Cine MRI: a new approach to the diagnosis of scapholunate dissociation. Skeletal Radiol 44(8):1103–1110. https://doi.org/10.1007/s00256-015-2126-4. Epub 2015 Mar 12. PMID: 25761726

Lee DJ, Elfar JC (2015) Carpal ligament injuries, pathomechanics, and classification. Hand Clin 31(3):389–398. https://doi.org/10.1016/j.hcl.2015.04.011. PMID: 26205700; PMCID: PMC4514919

Lee YH, Choi YR, Kim S, Song HT, Suh JS (2013a) Intrinsic ligament and triangular fibrocartilage complex (TFCC) tears of the wrist: comparison of isovolumetric 3D-THRIVE sequence MR arthrography and conventional MR image at 3 T. Magn Reson Imaging 31(2):221–226. https://doi.org/10.1016/j.mri.2012.06.024. Epub 2012 Sep 7. PMID: 22959873

Lee RK, Ng AW, Tong CS, Griffith JF, Tse WL, Wong C, Ho PC (2013b) Intrinsic ligament and triangular fibrocartilage complex tears of the wrist: comparison of MDCT arthrography, conventional 3-T MRI, and MR arthrography. Skeletal Radiol 42(9):1277–1285. https://doi.org/10.1007/s00256-013-1666-8. Epub 2013 Jun 28. PMID: 23812413

Lee RK, Griffith JF, Ng AW, Law EK, Tse WL, Wong CW, Ho PC (2017) Intrinsic carpal ligaments on MR and multidetector CT arthrography: comparison of axial and axial oblique planes. Eur Radiol 27(3):1277–1285. https://doi.org/10.1007/s00330-016-4436-x. Epub 2016 Jun 10. PMID: 27287482

Lichtman DM, Wroten ES (2006) Understanding midcarpal instability. J Hand Surg Am 31(3):491–498. https://doi.org/10.1016/j.jhsa.2005.12.014. PMID: 16516747

Lindau T, Adlercreutz C, Aspenberg P (2000) Peripheral tears of the triangular fibrocartilage complex cause distal radioulnar joint instability after distal radial fractures. J Hand Surg Am 25(3):464–468. https://doi.org/10.1053/jhsu.2000.6467. PMID: 10811750

Linscheid RL (1984) Scapholunate ligamentous instabilities (dissociations, subdislocations, dislocations). Ann Chir Main 3(4):323–330. https://doi.org/10.1016/s0753-9053(84)80008-3. English, French. PMID: 6397152

Linscheid RL, Dobyns JH, Beckenbaugh RD, Cooney WP 3rd, Wood MB (1983) Instability patterns of the wrist. J Hand Surg Am 8(5 Pt 2):682–686. https://doi.org/10.1016/s0363-5023(83)80246-9. PMID: 6630949

Lo IK, MacDermid JC, Bennett JD, Bogoch E, King GJ (2001) The radioulnar ratio: a new method of quantifying distal radioulnar joint subluxation. J Hand Surg Am 26(2):236–243. https://doi.org/10.1053/jhsu.2001.22908. PMID: 11279569

Lok RL, Griffith JF, Ng AW, Wong CW (2014) Imaging of radial wrist pain. Part II: pathology. Skeletal Radiol 43(6):725–743. https://doi.org/10.1007/s00256-014-1826-5. Epub 2014 Feb 14. PMID: 24522772

Loredo RA, Sorge DG, Garcia G (2005) Radiographic evaluation of the wrist: a vanishing art. Semin Roentgenol 40(3):248–289. https://doi.org/10.1053/j.ro.2005.01.014. PMID: 16060116

Luetkens KS, Laas SF, Haßler S, Gassenmaier T, Gietzen CH, Christopoulos G, Huflage H, Kunz AS, Bley

TA, Schmitt R, Grunz JP (2021) Contrast-enhanced MRI of the wrist: intravenous application of gadolinium improves diagnosis in ulnar-sided injuries of the TFCC. Eur J Radiol 143:109901. https://doi.org/10.1016/j.ejrad.2021.109901. Epub 2021 Aug 10. PMID: 34392004

Magee T (2009) Comparison of 3-T MRI and arthroscopy of intrinsic wrist ligament and TFCC tears. AJR Am J Roentgenol 192(1):80–85. https://doi.org/10.2214/AJR.08.1089. PMID: 19098183

Mania S, Boudabbous S, Delattre BMA, Lamy C, Beaulieu JY (2022) Anatomical and radiological description of ligament insertions on the radial aspect of the scaphoid bone. Hand Surg Rehabil 41(4):445–451. https://doi.org/10.1016/j.hansur.2022.05.008. Epub 2022 May 31. PMID: 35660467

Manley M, Boardman M, Goitz RJ (2013) The carpal insertions of the transverse carpal ligament. J Hand Surg Am 38(4):729–732. https://doi.org/10.1016/j.jhsa.2013.01.015. PMID: 23537443

Mannil L, Martin W, Dahmen J, Witte T, Juten PG, Deneken F, Räder M, Homann HH (2016) Arthroscopic treatment for ulnar-sided TFCC-tears. Eur J Trauma Emerg Surg 42(1):29–35. https://doi.org/10.1007/s00068-015-0593-x. Epub 2015 Nov 13. PMID: 26566794

Matthews GS, Kiani B, Wuertzer SD, Powell JA, Roller BL, Lenchik L, Torabi M (2019) MRI of the wrist: algorithmic approach for evaluating wrist pain. Radiographics 39(2):447–448. https://doi.org/10.1148/rg.2019180157. PMID: 30844354

May MM, Lawton JN, Blazar PE (2002) Ulnar styloid fractures associated with distal radius fractures: incidence and implications for distal radioulnar joint instability. J Hand Surg Am 27(6):965–971. https://doi.org/10.1053/jhsu.2002.36525. PMID: 12457345

Mayfield JK (1984) Patterns of injury to carpal ligaments. A spectrum. Clin Orthop Relat Res 187:36–42. PMID: 6744735

McMurray D, Muralikuttan K (2008) Volar dislocation of the distal radio–ulnar joint without fracture: a case report and literature review. Inj Extra 39(11):352–355. https://doi.org/10.1016/j.injury.2008.06.013

Mespreuve M, Coenen L (2017) The "second ulnar groove", a MRI sign suggesting a previous palmar luxation of the ulna at the distal radioulnar joint. Eur J Radiol 96:50–54. https://doi.org/10.1016/j.ejrad.2017.09.009. Epub 2017 Sep 20

Mespreuve M, Vanhoenacker F, Verstraete K (2015) Imaging findings of the distal radio-ulnar joint in trauma. J Belg Soc Radiol 99(1):1–20. https://doi.org/10.5334/jbr-btr.846. PMID: 30039059; PMCID: PMC6032773

Messina JC, Van Overstraeten L, Luchetti R, Fairplay T, Mathoulin CL (2013) The EWAS classification of scapholunate tears: an anatomical arthroscopic study. J Wrist Surg 2(2):105–109. https://doi.org/10.1055/s-0033-1345265. PMID: 24436801; PMCID: PMC3699273

Metz VM, Schimmerl SM, Gilula LA, Viegas SF, Saffar P (1993) Wide scapholunate joint space in lunotriquetral coalition: a normal variant? Radiology 188(2):557–559. https://doi.org/10.1148/radiology.188.2.8327715. PMID: 8327715

Metz VM, Metz-Schimmerl SM, Yin Y (1997) Ligamentous instabilities of the wrist. Eur J Radiol 25(2):104–111. https://doi.org/10.1016/s0720-048x(97)00041-7. PMID: 9283838

Meyer S (1991) Radiographic evaluation of wrist trauma. Semin Roentgenol 26(4):300–317. https://doi.org/10.1016/0037-198x(91)90028-m. PMID: 1745909

Michelotti BF, Mathews A, Chung KC (2018) Appropriateness of the use of MRI in the diagnosis and treatment of wrist ligamentous injury. Plast Reconstr Surg 141(2):410–419. https://doi.org/10.1097/PRS.0000000000004023

Mikić ZD (1989) Detailed anatomy of the articular disc of the distal radioulnar joint. Clin Orthop Relat Res 245:123–132. PMID: 2752612

Mikic ZD (1995) Treatment of acute injuries of the triangular fibrocartilage complex associated with distal radioulnar joint instability. J Hand Surg Am 20(2):319–323. https://doi.org/10.1016/S0363-5023(05)80033-4. PMID: 7775777

Mino DE, Palmer AK, Levinsohn EM (1983) The role of radiography and computerized tomography in the diagnosis of subluxation and dislocation of the distal radioulnar joint. J Hand Surg Am 8(1):23–31. https://doi.org/10.1016/s0363-5023(83)80046-x. PMID: 6827048

Moneim MS, Omer GE (1983) Wrist arthrography in acute carpal injuries. Orthopedics 6(3):299–306. https://doi.org/10.3928/0147-7447-19830301-02. PMID: 24822757

Morrissy RT, Nalebuff EA (1979) Dislocation of the distal radioulnar joint: anatomy and clues to prompt diagnosis. Clin Orthop Relat Res 144:154–158. PMID: 535217

Moser T, Dosch JC, Moussaoui A, Dietemann JL (2007) Wrist ligament tears: evaluation of MRI and combined MDCT and MR arthrography. AJR Am J Roentgenol 188(5):1278–1286. https://doi.org/10.2214/AJR.06.0288. PMID: 17449771

Mulford JS, Axelrod TS (2007) Traumatic injuries of the distal radioulnar joint. Orthop Clin North Am 38(2):289–297. https://doi.org/10.1016/j.ocl.2007.03.007, vii. PMID: 17560410

Mulford JS, Jansen S, Axelrod TS (2010) Isolated volar distal radioulnar joint dislocation. J Trauma 68(1):E23–E25. https://doi.org/10.1097/TA.0b013e3181568db2. PMID: 20065743

Nakamura T (2012) Anatomy and biomechanics of the distal radioulnar joint (DRUJ). In: Arthroscopic management of ulnar pain. Springer, Berlin/Heidelberg, pp 15–23. https://doi.org/10.1007/978-3-642-30544-3_2

Nakamura T, Takayama S, Horiuchi Y, Yabe Y (2001a) Origins and insertions of the triangular fibrocartilage complex: a histological study. J Hand Surg Br 26(5):446–454. https://doi.org/10.1054/jhsb.2001.0562. PMID: 11560427

Nakamura K, Patterson RM, Viegas SF (2001b) The ligament and skeletal anatomy of the second through fifth carpometacarpal joints and adjacent structures. J Hand Surg Am 26(6):1016–1029. https://doi.org/10.1053/jhsu.2001.26329. PMID: 11721245

Nevalainen MT, Zoga AC, Rivlin M, Morrison WB, Roedl JB (2023) Extensor carpi ulnaris tendon pathology and ulnar styloid bone marrow edema as diagnostic markers of peripheral triangular fibrocartilage complex tears on wrist MRI: a case-control study. Eur Radiol 33(5):3172–3177. https://doi.org/10.1007/s00330-023-09446-x. Epub 2023 Feb 21. PMID: 36809434; PMCID: PMC10121535

Niacaris T, Ming BW, Lichtman DM (2015) Midcarpal instability: a comprehensive review and update. Hand Clin 31(3):487–493. https://doi.org/10.1016/j.hcl.2015.04.004. PMID: 26205710

Ochman S, Wieskötter B, Langer M, Vieth V, Raschke MJ, Stehling C (2017) High-resolution MRI (3T-MRI) in diagnosis of wrist pain: is diagnostic arthroscopy still necessary? Arch Orthop Trauma Surg 137(10):1443–1450. https://doi.org/10.1007/s00402-017-2747-2. Epub 2017 Aug 14. PMID: 28808768

Oneson SR, Timins ME, Scales LM, Erickson SJ, Chamoy L (1997) MR imaging diagnosis of triangular fibrocartilage pathology with arthroscopic correlation. AJR Am J Roentgenol 168(6):1513–1518. https://doi.org/10.2214/ajr.168.6.9168716. PMID: 9168716

Orbay J, Vernon L, Poirier S, Morales V, Cambo R, Mercer D (2021) Effect of ulnar head offset on distal radioulnar joint stability. J Hand Surg Am 46(9):816.e1–816.e7. https://doi.org/10.1016/j.jhsa.2020.12.014. Epub 2021 Mar 13. Erratum in: J Hand Surg Am. 2022 Jan;47(1):84. PMID: 33722471

Ozçelik A, Günal I, Köse N (2005) Stress views in the radiography of scapholunate instability. Eur J Radiol 56(3):358–361. https://doi.org/10.1016/j.ejrad.2005.06.011. Epub 2005 Jul 19. PMID: 16046094

Özkan S, Kheterpal A, Palmer WE, Chen NC (2019) Dorsal extrinsic ligament injury and static scapholunate diastasis on magnetic resonance imaging scans. J Hand Surg Am 44(8):641–648. https://doi.org/10.1016/j.jhsa.2019.03.003. Epub 2019 Apr 29. PMID: 31047744

Palmer AK (1989) Triangular fibrocartilage complex lesions: a classification. J Hand Surg Am 14(4):594–606. https://doi.org/10.1016/0363-5023(89)90174-3. PMID: 2666492

Palmer AK (1990) Triangular fibrocartilage disorders: injury patterns and treatment. Arthroscopy 6(2):125–132. https://doi.org/10.1016/0749-8063(90)90013-4. PMID: 2363780

Palmer AK, Werner FW (1981) The triangular fibrocartilage complex of the wrist – anatomy and function. J Hand Surg Am 6(2):153–162. https://doi.org/10.1016/s0363-5023(81)80170-0. PMID: 7229292

Palmer AK, Werner FW, Murphy D, Glisson R (1985) Functional wrist motion: a biomechanical study. J Hand Surg Am 10(1):39–46. https://doi.org/10.1016/s0363-5023(85)80246-x. PMID: 3968403

Patel RM, Kalainov DM, Chilelli BJ, Makowiec RL (2015) Comparisons of three radiographic views in assessing for scapholunate instability. Hand (N Y) 10(2):233–238. https://doi.org/10.1007/s11552-014-9695-x. PMID: 26034436; PMCID: PMC4447670

Pliefke J, Stengel D, Rademacher G, Mutze S, Ekkernkamp A, Eisenschenk A (2008) Diagnostic accuracy of plain radiographs and cineradiography in diagnosing traumatic scapholunate dissociation. Skeletal Radiol 37(2):139–145. https://doi.org/10.1007/s00256-007-0410-7. Epub 2007 Nov 16. PMID: 18087747

Poznanski AK (1984) The hand in radiologic diagnosis: with gamuts and pattern profiles, 2nd edn. Saunders Company, Philadephia, p 138

Pulos N, Bozentka DJ (2015) Carpal ligament anatomy and biomechanics. Hand Clin 31(3):381–387. https://doi.org/10.1016/j.hcl.2015.04.007. PMID: 26205699

Ramamurthy NK, Chojnowski AJ, Toms AP (2016) Imaging in carpal instability. J Hand Surg Eur Vol 41(1):22–34. https://doi.org/10.1177/1753193415610515. Epub 2015 Nov 19. PMID: 26586689

Ramdhian-Wihlm R, Le Minor JM, Schmittbuhl M, Jeantroux J, Mahon PM, Veillon F, Dosch JC, Dietemann JL, Bierry G (2012) Cone-beam computed tomography arthrography: an innovative modality for the evaluation of wrist ligament and cartilage injuries. Skeletal Radiol 41(8):963–969. https://doi.org/10.1007/s00256-011-1305-1. Epub 2011 Nov 8. PMID: 22064983

Reghunath A, Singh DK, Aggarwal A, Babbar N, Choudhary R, Surya S (2022) MRI and MR arthrography imaging of the pathologies of the wrist: a pictorial essay. J Clin Diagn Res 16(12):TE01–TE07. https://doi.org/10.7860/JCDR/2022/59277.17323

Rijal L, Sagar G, Ansari T et al (2023) Isolated volar dislocation of distal radioulnar joint: rarely occurring, commonly missed. Eur Orthop Traumatol 3:151–154. https://doi.org/10.1007/s12570-012-0104-z

Ringler MD (2013) MRI of wrist ligaments. J Hand Surg Am 38(10):2034–2046. https://doi.org/10.1016/j.jhsa.2013.02.042. Epub 2013 May 6. PMID: 23660198

Ringler MD, Murthy NS (2015) MR imaging of wrist ligaments. Magn Reson Imaging Clin N Am 23(3):367–391. https://doi.org/10.1016/j.mric.2015.04.007. PMID: 26216769

Ritt MJ, Bishop AT, Berger RA, Linscheid RL, Berglund LJ, An KN (1998) Lunotriquetral ligament properties: a comparison of three anatomic subregions. J Hand Surg Am 23(3):425–431. https://doi.org/10.1016/S0363-5023(05)80460-5. PMID: 9620183

Rubensson C, Johansson T, Adolfsson L (2018) Tensioning of the radioscaphocapitate and long radiolunate ligaments for dynamic radiocarpal instability. J Hand Surg Eur Vol 43(4):369–374. https://doi.org/10.1177/1753193418756805. Epub 2018 Feb 15. PMID: 29448916

Said J, Baker K, Fernandez L, Komatsu DE, Gould E, Hurst LC (2018) The optimal location to measure scapholunate diastasis on screening radiographs. Hand (N Y) 13(6):671–677. https://doi.org/10.1177/1558944717729219. Epub 2017 Sep 6. PMID: 28877592; PMCID: PMC6300175

Scheck RJ, Kubitzek C, Hierner R, Szeimies U, Pfluger T, Wilhelm K, Hahn K (1997) The scapholunate interosseous ligament in MR arthrography of the wrist: correlation with non-enhanced MRI and wrist arthroscopy. Skeletal Radiol 26(5):263–271. https://doi.org/10.1007/s002560050233. PMID: 9194225

Scheck RJ, Romagnolo A, Hierner R, Pfluger T, Wilhelm K, Hahn K (1999) The carpal ligaments in MR arthrography of the wrist: correlation with standard MRI and wrist arthroscopy. J Magn Reson Imaging 9(3):468–474. https://doi.org/10.1002/(sici)1522-2586(199903)9:3<468::aid-jmri16>3.0.co;2-t. PMID: 10194719

Schmid MR, Schertler T, Pfirrmann CW, Saupe N, Manestar M, Wildermuth S, Weishaupt D (2005) Interosseous ligament tears of the wrist: comparison of multi-detector row CT arthrography and MR imaging. Radiology 237(3):1008–1013. https://doi.org/10.1148/radiol.2373041450. PMID: 16304116

Schmitt R, Christopoulos G, Meier R, Coblenz G, Fröhner S, Lanz U, Krimmer H (2003) Direkte MR-Arthrographie des Handgelenks im Vergleich zur Arthroskopie: Eine prospektive Studie an 125 Patienten [Direct MR arthrography of the wrist in comparison with arthroscopy: a prospective study on 125 patients]. Rofo 175(7):911–919. https://doi.org/10.1055/s-2003-40434. German. PMID: 12847645

Schmitt R, Froehner S, Coblenz G, Christopoulos G (2006) Carpal instability. Eur Radiol 16(10):2161–2178. https://doi.org/10.1007/s00330-006-0161-1. Epub 2006 Mar 1. PMID: 16508768

Sennwald GR, Zdravkovic V, Oberlin C (1994) The anatomy of the palmar scaphotriquetral ligament. J Bone Joint Surg Br 76(1):147–149. PMID: 8300661

Shahabpour M, De Maeseneer M, Pouders C, Van Overstraeten L, Ceuterick P, Fierens Y, Goubau J, De Mey J (2011) MR imaging of normal extrinsic wrist ligaments using thin slices with clinical and surgical correlation. Eur J Radiol 77(2):196–201. https://doi.org/10.1016/j.ejrad.2010.05.043. PMID: 20599335

Shahabpour M, Staelens B, Van Overstraeten L, De Maeseneer M, Boulet C, De Mey J, Scheerlinck T (2015) Advanced imaging of the scapholunate ligamentous complex. Skeletal Radiol 44(12):1709–1725. https://doi.org/10.1007/s00256-015-2182-9. Epub 2015 Jul 30. PMID: 26219592

Shaw CB, Foster BH, Borgese M, Boutin RD, Bateni C, Boonsri P, Bayne CO, Szabo RM, Nayak KS, Chaudhari AJ (2019) Real-time three-dimensional MRI for the assessment of dynamic carpal instability. PLoS One 14(9):e0222704. https://doi.org/10.1371/journal.pone.0222704. PMID: 31536561; PMCID: PMC6752861

Shin AY, Battaglia MJ, Bishop AT (2000) Lunotriquetral instability: diagnosis and treatment. J Am Acad Orthop Surg 8(3):170–179. https://doi.org/10.5435/00124635-200005000-00004. PMID: 10874224

Slattery D, Gohil S, Hogan G (2013) A case report and the literature review: volar dislocation of the DRUJ and stabilisation using mini-suture anchors. Eur J Orthop Surg Traumatol 23(Suppl 2):S203–S205. https://doi.org/10.1007/s00590-012-1157-y. Epub 2013 Jan 5. PMID: 23412303

Spies CK, Unglaub F, Bruckner T, Müller L, Eysel P, Rau J (2022) Diagnostic accuracy of wrist MRI in comparison to wrist arthroscopy regarding TFCC lesions in clinical practice. Arch Orthop Trauma Surg 142(5):879–885. https://doi.org/10.1007/s00402-021-04329-6. Epub 2022 Jan 10. PMID: 35006371

Stuart PR, Berger RA, Linscheid RL, An KN (2000) The dorsopalmar stability of the distal radioulnar joint. J Hand Surg Am 25(4):689–699. https://doi.org/10.1053/jhsu.2000.9418. PMID: 10913210

Sulkers GS, Schep NW, Maas M, van der Horst CM, Goslings JC, Strackee SD (2014) The diagnostic accuracy of wrist cineradiography in diagnosing scapholunate dissociation. J Hand Surg Eur Vol 39(3):263–271. https://doi.org/10.1177/1753193413489056. Epub 2013 May 22. PMID: 23697681

Sulkers GSI, Strackee SD, Schep NWL, Maas M (2018) Wrist cineradiography: a protocol for diagnosing carpal instability. J Hand Surg Eur Vol 43(2):174–178. https://doi.org/10.1177/1753193417694820. Epub 2017 Mar 1. PMID: 28488457; PMCID: PMC5791518

Szabo RM (2008) Scapholunate ligament repair with capsulodesis reinforcement. J Hand Surg Am 33(9):1645–1654. https://doi.org/10.1016/j.jhsa.2008.08.016. PMID: 18984352

Theumann N, Favarger N, Schnyder P, Meuli R (2001) Wrist ligament injuries: value of post-arthrography computed tomography. Skeletal Radiol 30(2):88–93. https://doi.org/10.1007/s002560000302. PMID: 11310205

Theumann NH, Pfirrmann CW, Chung CB, Antonio GE, Trudell DJ, Resnick D (2002) Ligamentous and tendinous anatomy of the intermetacarpal and common carpometacarpal joints: evaluation with MR imaging and MR arthrography. J Comput Assist Tomogr 26(1):145–152. https://doi.org/10.1097/00004728-200201000-00026. PMID: 11801922

Theumann NH, Pfirrmann CW, Antonio GE, Chung CB, Gilula LA, Trudell DJ, Resnick D (2003) Extrinsic carpal ligaments: normal MR arthrographic appearance in cadavers. Radiology 226(1):171–179. https://doi.org/10.1148/radiol.2261011715. PMID: 12511687

Theumann NH, Etechami G, Duvoisin B, Wintermark M, Schnyder P, Favarger N, Gilula LA (2006) Association between extrinsic and intrinsic carpal ligament injuries at MR arthrography and carpal instability at radiography: initial observations. Radiology 238(3):950–957. https://doi.org/10.1148/radiol.2383050013. Epub 2006 Jan 19. PMID: 16424247

Verhiel SHWL, Blackburn J, Ritt MJPF, Simeone FJ, Chen NC (2022) MRI findings in patients undergoing triangular fibrocartilage complex repairs versus patients without ulnar-sided wrist pain. Hand (N Y) 17(3):483–490. https://doi.org/10.1177/1558944720937369. Epub 2020 Jul 19. PMID: 32686539; PMCID: PMC9112747

Viegas SF, Pogue DJ, Patterson RM, Peterson PD (1990) Effects of radioulnar instability on the radiocarpal joint: a biomechanical study. J Hand Surg Am 15(5):728–732. https://doi.org/10.1016/0363-5023(90)90144-g. PMID: 2229967

Viegas SF, Patterson RM, Ward K (1995) Extrinsic wrist ligaments in the pathomechanics of ulnar translation instability. J Hand Surg Am 20(2):312–318. https://doi.org/10.1016/S0363-5023(05)80032-2. PMID: 7775776

Wang Z, Chen S, Liu B, Qian Z, Zhu J, Wang Q (2023) Abnormal MRI signal intensity of the triangular fibrocartilage complex in asymptomatic wrists. J Hand Surg Eur Vol 48(4):326–332. https://doi.org/10.1177/17531934221141986. Epub 2022 Dec 8. PMID: 36482744

Watanabe A, Souza F, Vezeridis PS, Blazar P, Yoshioka H (2010) Ulnar-sided wrist pain. II. Clinical imaging and treatment. Skeletal Radiol 39(9):837–857. https://doi.org/10.1007/s00256-009-0842-3. Epub 2009 Dec 10. PMID: 20012039; PMCID: PMC2904904

Wechsler RJ, Wehbe MA, Rifkin MD, Edeiken J, Branch HM (1987) Computed tomography diagnosis of distal radioulnar subluxation. Skeletal Radiol 16(1):1–5. https://doi.org/10.1007/BF00349919. PMID: 3823954

Wolfe SW, Garcia-Elias M, Kitay A (2012) Carpal instability nondissociative. J Am Acad Orthop Surg 20(9):575–585. https://doi.org/10.5435/JAAOS-20-09-575. PMID: 22941800

Yoshioka H, Tanaka T, Ueno T, Carrino JA, Winalski CS, Aliabadi P, Lang P, Weissman BN (2007) Study of ulnar variance with high-resolution MRI: correlation with triangular fibrocartilage complex and cartilage of ulnar side of wrist. J Magn Reson Imaging 26(3):714–719. https://doi.org/10.1002/jmri.21084. PMID: 17729368

Zancolli ER 3rd (2001) Localized medial triquetral-hamate instability: anatomy and operative reconstruction-augmentation. Hand Clin 17(1):83–96, vii. PMID: 11280162

Zancolli EA, Ziadenberg C, Zancolli E Jr (1987) Biomechanics of the trapeziometacarpal joint. Clin Orthop Relat Res 220:14–26. PMID: 3594983

Zanetti M, Bräm J, Hodler J (1997) Triangular fibrocartilage and intercarpal ligaments of the wrist: does MR arthrography improve standard MRI? J Magn Reson Imaging 7(3):590–594. https://doi.org/10.1002/jmri.1880070322. PMID: 9170047

Zannou RS, Rezzouk J, Ruijs AC (2015) Non-reducible palmar dislocation of the distal radioulnar joint. Case Rep Plast Surg Hand Surg 2(2):43–45. https://doi.org/10.3109/23320885.2015.1026348. Epub 2015 Mar 23. PMID: 26158121; PMCID: PMC4467246

Zdravkovic V, Sennwald GR, Fischer M, Jacob HA (1994) The palmar wrist ligaments revisited, clinical relevance. Ann Chir Main Memb Super 13(5):378–382. https://doi.org/10.1016/s0753-9053(05)80078-x. PMID: 7531477

Zhan H, Bai R, Qian Z, Yang Y, Zhang H, Yin Y (2020) Traumatic injury of the triangular fibrocartilage complex (TFCC)-a refinement to the Palmer classification by using high-resolution 3-T MRI. Skeletal Radiol 49(10):1567–1579. https://doi.org/10.1007/s00256-020-03438-4. Epub 2020 May 5. PMID: 32372253

Zlatkin MB, Rosner J (2006) MR imaging of ligaments and triangular fibrocartilage complex of the wrist. Radiol Clin North Am 44(4):595–623. https://doi.org/10.1016/j.rcl.2006.04.010, ix. PMID: 16829252

Post-Operative Lesions

Contents

1 General

Traumatic lesions are often repaired by surgery. As a huge variety of interventions with (personal) variants exists, it is crucial to be informed about the type of surgery, the prosthesis and materials chosen, and the appraoch used. Comparison with the pre-operative MRI—if available—is also highly recommended as signals and forms may have changed previously due to the trauma.

2 Bone

Some (older) silicone prosthesis of the lunate bone are fixed with a stalk in the adjacent triquetral bone (Fig. 1). Rupture of the stalk (Fig. 1a) results in a dorsal tilt of the L that also becomes prominent in the carpal tunnel (Fig. 1b, c) and compresses the adjacent soft tissues (Fig. 1b). Even with the (L, Tra) prosthesis perfectly in place, surrounding reactive synovitis, BMO, and erosions may develop (Figs. 2 and 3).

Unfortunately, complex or repeated surgery (Fig. 4a–e) may render the interpretation of signals on MRI, especially on T2-WI, very risky (Fig. 4f, g) due to artefacts, scar formation, and tissue signal alterations. However, an unsuspected pathology (tenosynovitis) may also arise (Fig. 4f, g) at unusual places (secondary degenerative changes) (Fig. 5).

The (Tra) prosthesis itself may luxate (Fig. 6) and become palpable or even visible as a mass (at the base of the thumb).

After arthrodesis, the evaluation of the adjacent joint spaces is much more thorough with 3D evaluation and the presence of BMO may be confirmed or excluded (Fig. 7).

M. Mespreuve, K. Waked, *MRI of the Wrist*, Medical Radiology,
https://doi.org/10.1007/978-3-031-63973-9_7

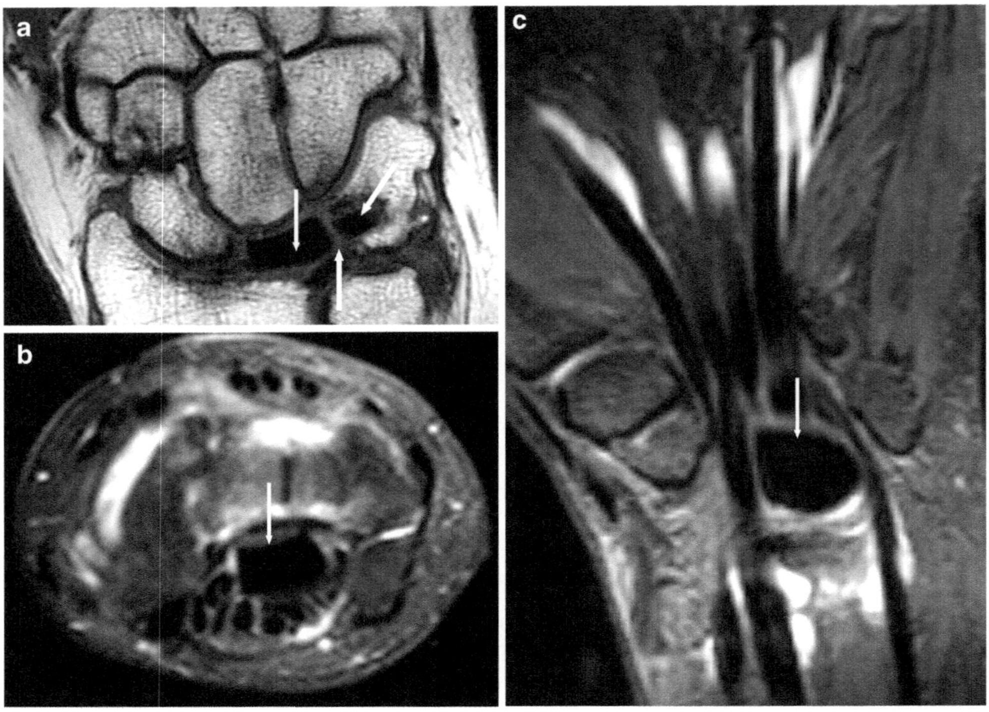

Fig. 1 Cor T1-WI (**a**); Ax (**b**) and Cor (**c**) T2-WI FS. Broken fixation stalk (**a**) in the Tri (**a**) of the L prosthesis (**a**–**c**). Prominence of the L in the carpal tunnel (**b**, **c**) with compression of the content and resulting tenosynovitis

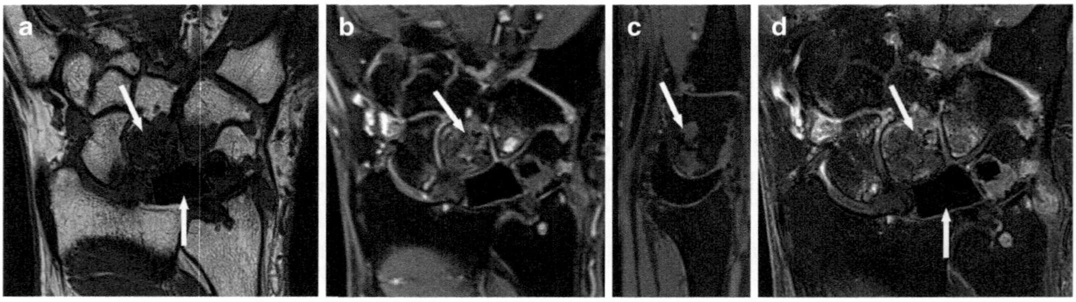

Fig. 2 Cor T1-WI (**a**) and T2-WI FS (**b**); Sag 3D GRE (**c**); Cor T1-WI FS after CE. Reactive synovitis, BMO, and small erosions (**a**–**d**) around the L prosthesis (**a**, **d**)

In case of healed extensive traumatic lesions, and certainly in expert cases, additional MRI is mandatory. A "completely healed" saw injury (Fig. 8a, b) shows barely any BMO visible at and around the saw trajectory (C). However, the fossa for the L is impacted and very irregular (Fig. 8c, e). Small secondary synovial osteochondromatosis fragments are detected in the RC joint space (Fig. 8d). Chondromalacia is already present at the RC (Fig. 8e), the C-L (Fig. 8f), and the CMC-II (Fig. 8g) joint. There is also a rupture of the SLL, LTL, and the TFCC (Fig. 8h).

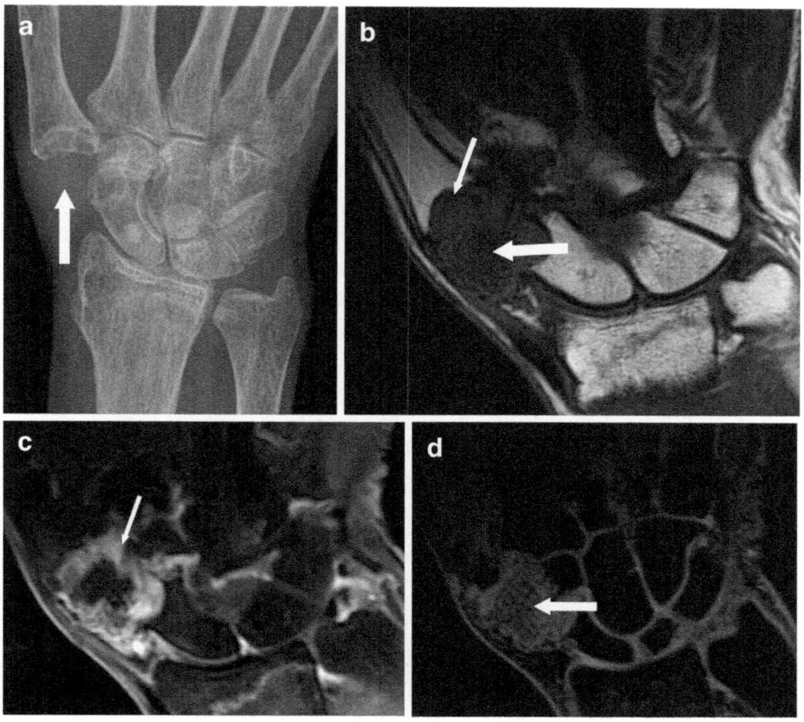

Fig. 3 Standard PA view (**a**); Cor T1-WI (**b**) with FS after CE (**c**) and 3D GRE (**d**). Tra resection arthroplasty. Secondary proximal migration of the first MC and erosions at the surrounding bones (**a**). The prosthetic element is clearly identified (**b**, **d**) with surrounding reactive synovial (**b**, **d**) enhancing (**c**) proliferation

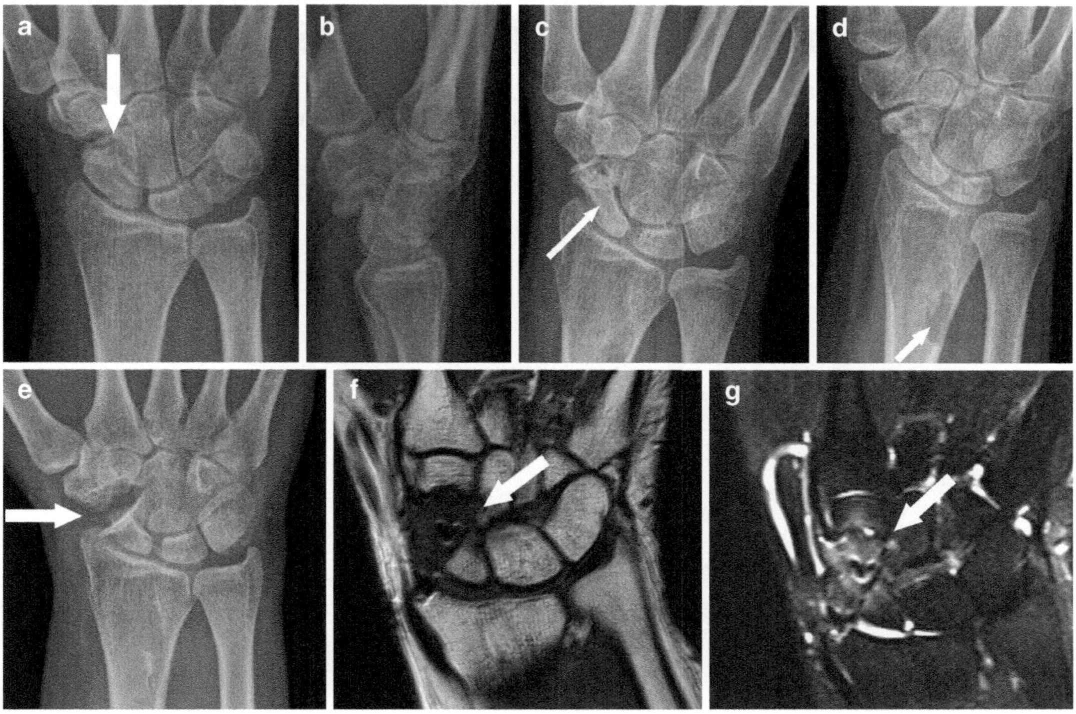

Fig. 4 Standard PA (**a**) and lateral (**b**) views; standard PA view after bone graft (**c**), follow up (**d**), and after partial resection with Marlex arthroplasty (**e**); Cor T1-WI (**f**); and T2-WI FS (**g**). S malunion (**a**, **b**) resulted in a fixation by a bone graft (**c**). A pseudarthrosis develops with normal aspect at the grafting site (**d**). A partial distal S resection with a Marlex mesh interposed (**f**, **g**). Extensive tenosynovitis at extensor compartment I (**f**, **g**)

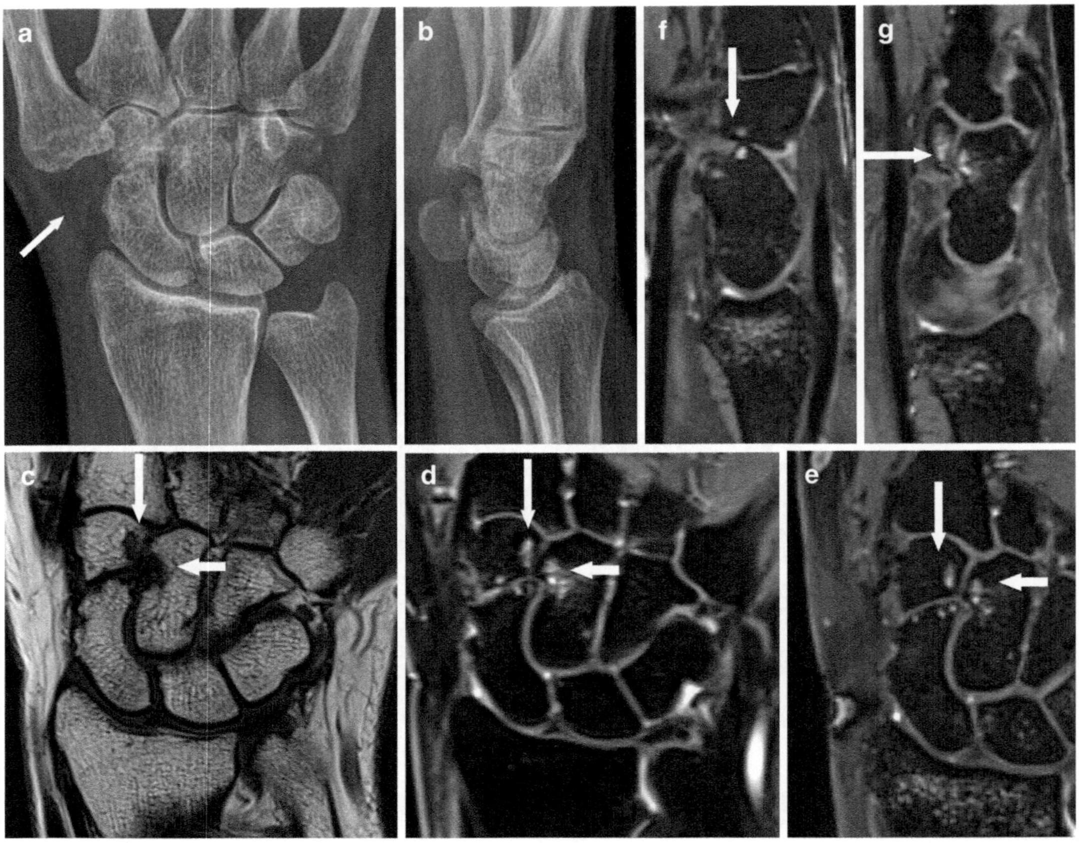

Fig. 5 Standard PA (**a**) and Lateral (**b**) views; Cor T1-WI (**c**), T2-WI FS (**d**), and 3D GRE (**e**); Sag 3D GRE (**f**, **g**). Tra resection arthroplasty (**a**, **b**). Secondary degenerative subchondral cysts appear at the tra-S (**c–f**) and tra-C joint (**c–e**, **g**)

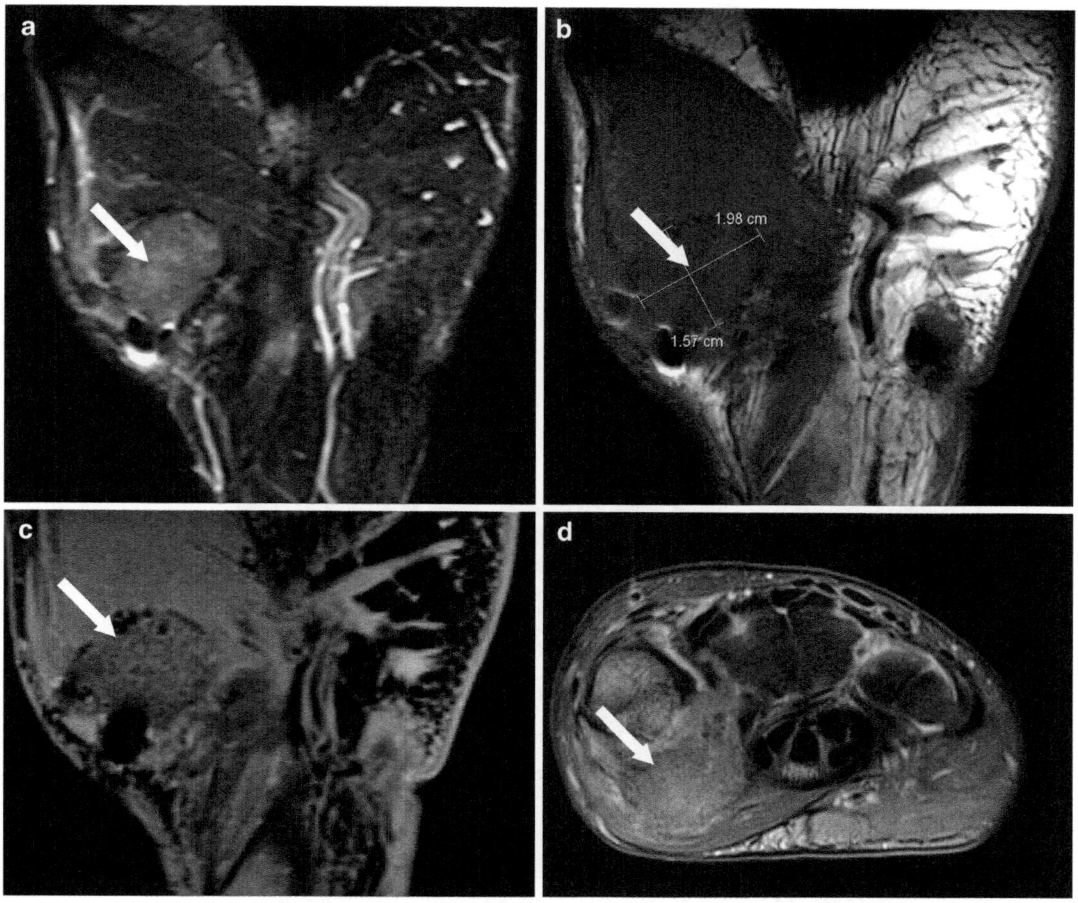

Fig. 6 Cor T2-WI FS (**a**), T1-WI (**b**) and 3D GRE (**c**); Ax T2-WI FS (**d**). Luxated Tra prosthesis

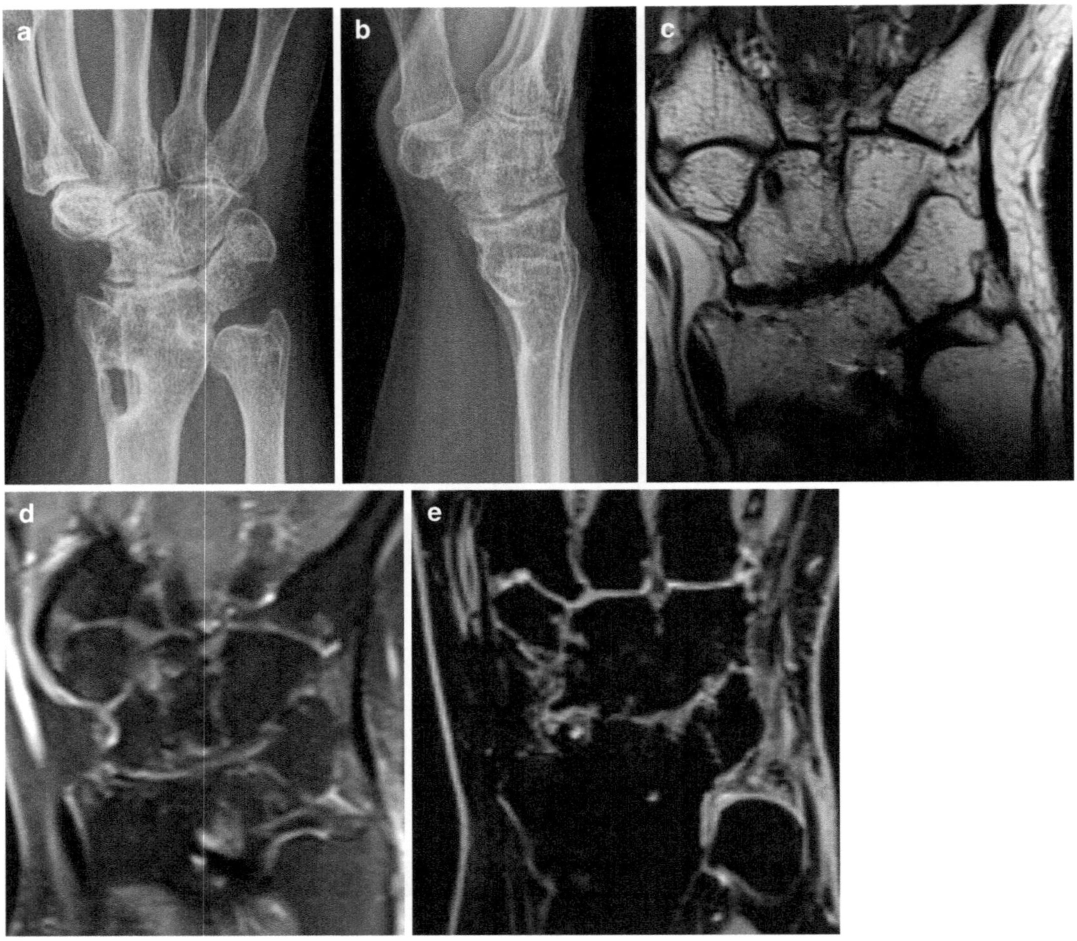

Fig. 7 Standard PA (**a**) and Lateral (**b**) views; Cor T1-WI (**c**), T2-WI FS (**d**), and 3D GRE (**e**). Radiocarpal arthrodesis (**a**, **b**) with degenerative changes at the very irregular MC joint without BMO (**c**–**e**)

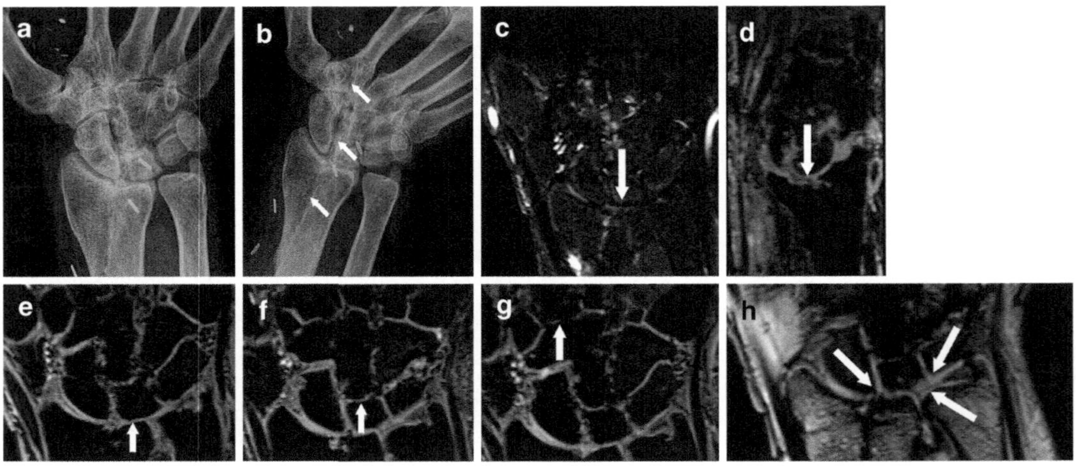

Fig. 8 Standard PA (**a**) and oblique (**b**) views; Sag (**c**) and Cor (**e**–**g**) 3D GRE; 2D GRE (**h**). "Completely healed" saw injury (**a**, **b**) with barely any residual BMO (**c**). Impacted and irregular fossa for the L (**c**–**e**). Small chondromatosis (**d**). Diffuse chondromalacia RC (**e**), C-L (**f**) and CMC-II (**g**). SL, LT, and TFCC lesion (**h**)

3 Ligaments

After SLL repair (Del Piñal 2013; Szabo 2008) with plug fixation of a tendinous fragment (Fig. 9), there remains a rotatory subluxation of the S, diastasis of the S, proximal migration of the C with reduced carpal height, and OA at the CL joint (Fig. 9a). The SL angle is increased (DISI configuration) as well (Fig. 9b). Mobility views show an absent radial (Fig. 9c) and ulnar (Fig. 9d) deviation. Additionally, no low signal ligamentous reconstruction is observed at the SL joint space (Fig. 9e, f). There are subcortical cysts at the C-L joint with BMO around and total loss of the cartilage (Fig. 9e–g). Postoperative MRI (and even MRA) evaluation of the SLL remains daring and should also include the reevaluation of all the previous (radiological) documents. Indirect signs of a pre-traumatic existing SLL lesion (Fig. 10a–e) with probably only a small more recent component (Fig. 10h–i) may explain the failure of the pinning (Fig. 10f, g).

After LT arthrodesis (Wharton and Ahearne 2021), the RD and UD are absent (Fig. 11) without apparent bony nor joint anomalies. At the LT arthrodesis, and as well at and around the wrist, the signals are normal on all sequences and there is a perfect consolidation in a correct position (Fig. 12). Pseudarthrosis, fracture, residual BMO, and/or poor alignment are all excluded. Additional evaluation of the capsule (IA adhesions? Retraction?) is mandatory by MR/CT-arthrography.

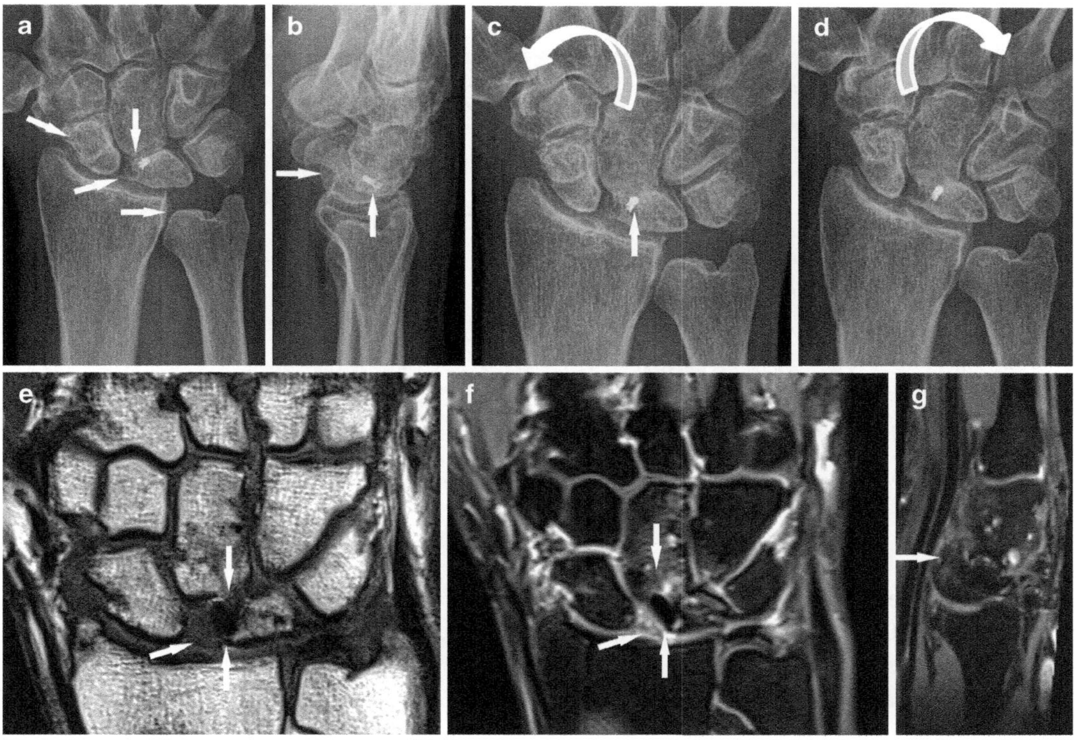

Fig. 9 Standard PA (**a**), lateral (**b**), and mobility (**c**, **d**) views; Cor T1-WI (**e**) and T2-WI FS (**f**); Sag 3D GRE (**g**). After SLL repair (plug fixation), there is a rotatory subluxation of the S; diastasis SL; a proximal migration of the C with midcarpal OA (**a**); and a DISI configuration (**b**). Almost absent radial (**c**) and ulnar (**d**) deviation. No low signal ligamentous reconstruction in the SL joint space (**e**, **f**). BMO around the C-L joint with absent cartilage and subchondral cysts (**f**, **g**)

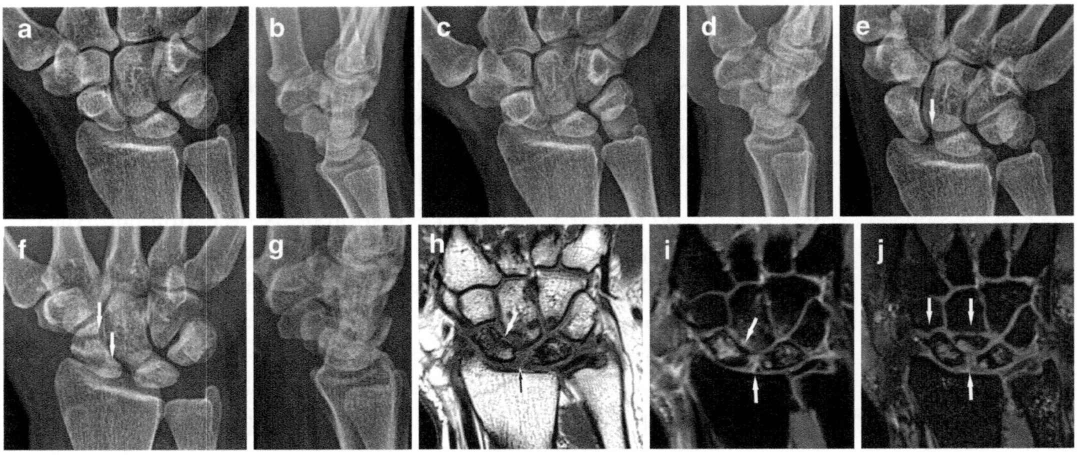

Fig. 10 Standard PA and Lateral views before (**a**, **B**) and after (**c**, **d**) trauma with clenched fist view (**e**) view, and after removal of pins (**f**, **g**); Cor T1-WI (**h**), and 3D GRE (**i**, **j**). Increased SL angle before (**a**, **b**) and after (**c**, **d**) trauma with dynamic SL diastasis (**e**). SL diastasis (**f**) in neutral position after double pin fixation (**f**, **j**) with a slightly increased SL angle (**g**). Proximally moved C with C-L chondromalacia (**f**, **h**, **i**). Clearly visible trajectory of the pins (**f**, **j**). The SLL shows an (old?) extended tear (**h–j**) with possibly a more recent component (**i**)

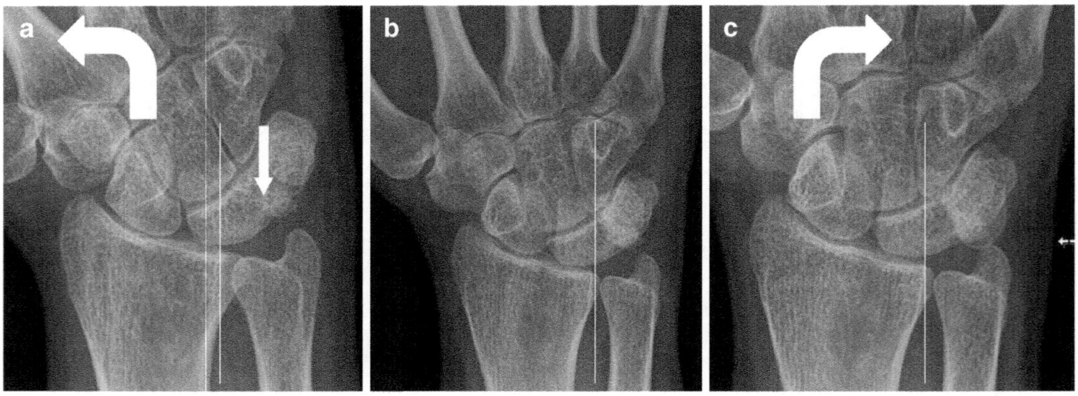

Fig. 11 Standard PA views in radial (**a**), neutral (**b**), and ulnar (**c**) deviation. LT arthrodesis without mobility in radial nor ulnar deviation

After debridement of a central tear at the disc of the TFCC (Mikic 1995), a large central defect is noticed without further anomalies (Fig. 13). Clinical information is also crucial in order to differentiate from a large (degenerative) TFCC tear, mostly accompanied by other anomalies.

The evaluation of an extrinsic ligament reconstruction needs extensive exploration in all 3D directions. Only indirect signs, such as a drill hole (Fig. 14a), are noticed on a standard view. Metal artefacts are observed at the fixation points, and they may be hidden (Fig. 14b, c). The trajectory of the reconstruction and the continuity of the used tendon (Fig. 15) are demonstrated in a detailed way. Comparison with the pre-operative MRI is very useful (Fig. 16).

Even complex reconstructions can be evaluated by MRI. On standard views (Fig. 17) only the drill holes are obvious after a DRUJ stabiliza-

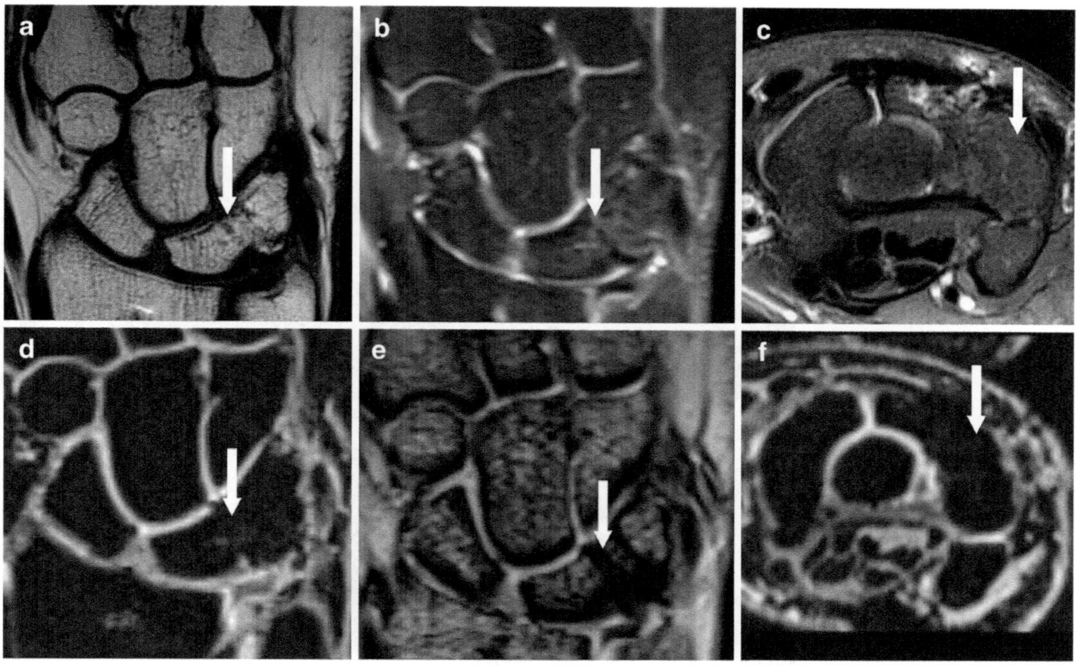

Fig. 12 Cor T1-WI (**a**); Cor (**b**) and Ax (**c**) T2-I FS; Cor 3D (**d**) and 2D (**e**) GRE; Ax 3D GRE (**f**). Normal consolidated LT arthrodesis in all directions and on all sequences

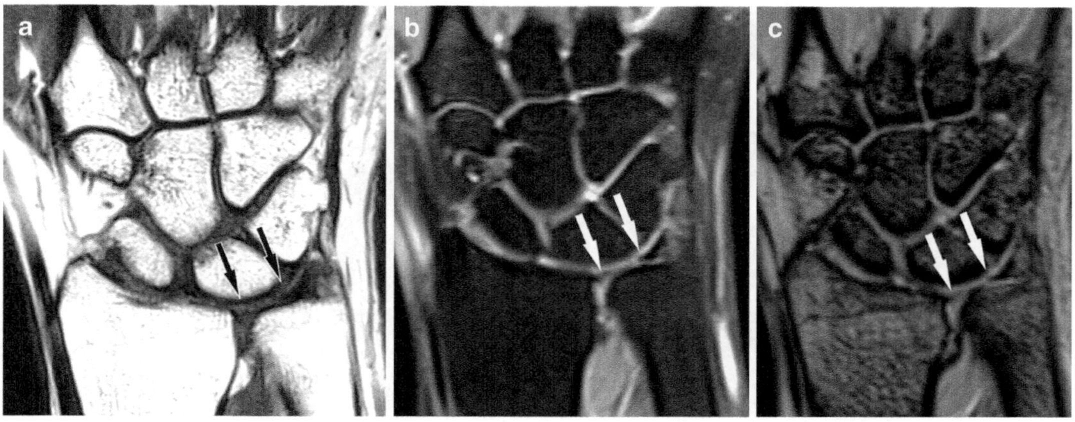

Fig. 13 Cor T1-WI (**a**); Cor 3D (**b**) and 2D (**c**) GRE. Normal status after TFCC central tear debridement with large central defect in the TFC

tion by a modified Adams-Berger technique (Gillis et al. 2019) with plug (Fig. 17-green loop). Part of the extensor retinaculum or the palmaris longus muscle is used for this fixation. The radial (Fig. 18) as well as the ulnar (Fig. 19) component are evaluated in the three dimensions to determine the continuity. The signal (Figs. 18a and 19e) of the reconstruction ideally should remain low and homogenous, but (bone and metal) artefacts may interfere.

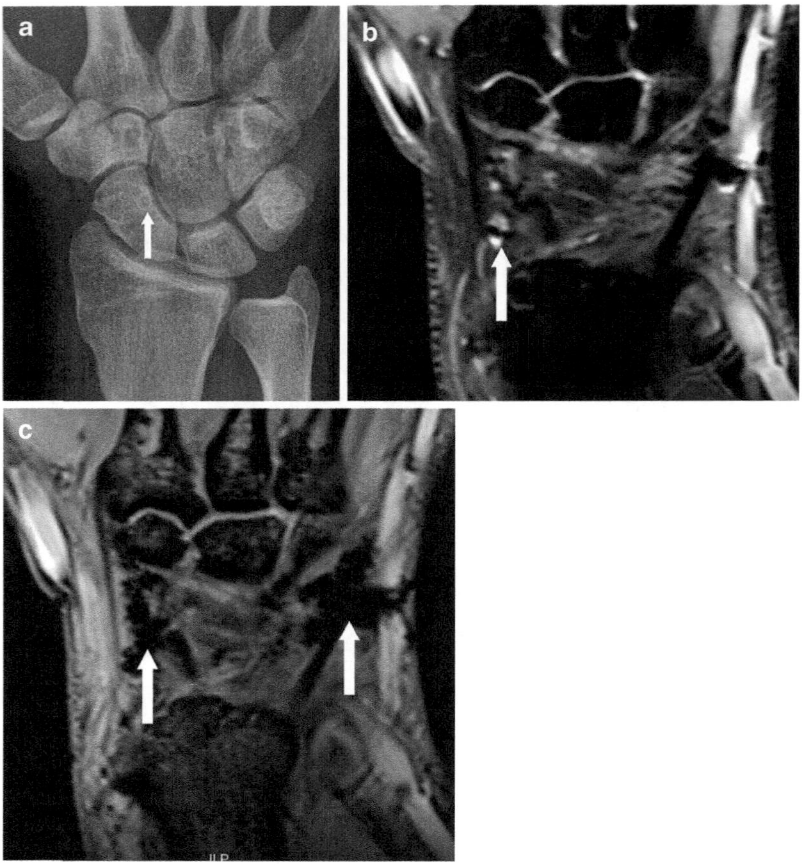

Fig. 14 Standard PA view (**a**); Cor T2-WI FS (**b**) and 2D GRE (**c**). Normal status after dorsal S-Tri extrinsic ligament reconstruction. Drill hole in the S (**a**). Metal artefacts at S and Tri (**b**, **c**)

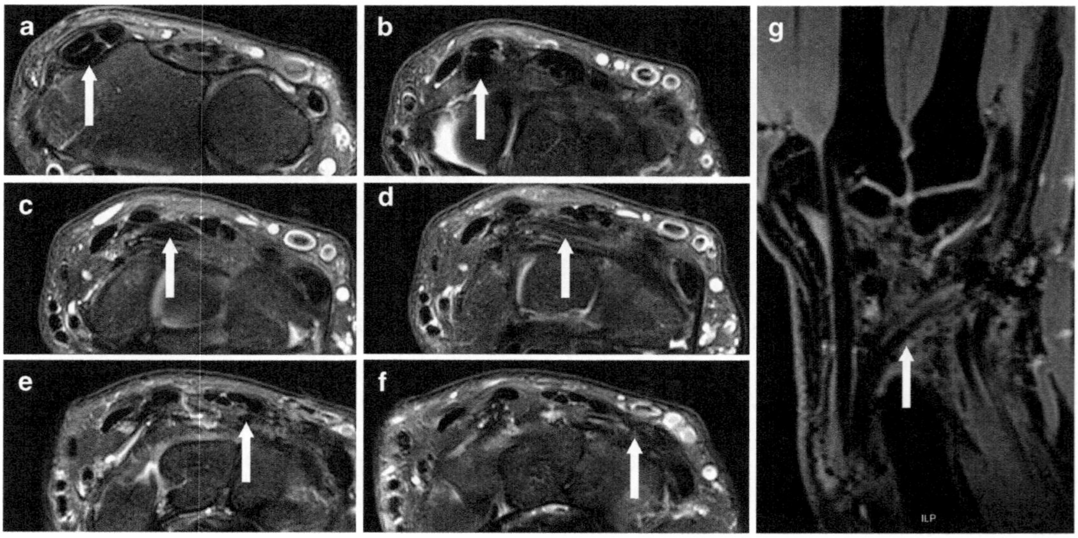

Fig. 15 Ax T2-WI FS (**a–f**) and 2D GRE (**g**). Normal status after dorsal R-Tri extrinsic ligament reconstruction with brachioradialis tendon Continuous trajectory of the tendon

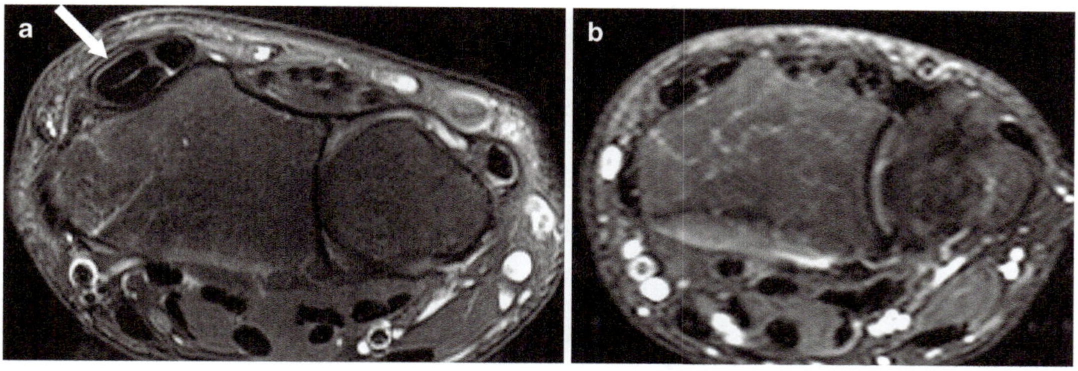

Fig. 16 Ax T2-WI FS after surgery (**a**) compared to the pre-operative status (**b**). "Accessory" tendon in the region of the second extensor compartment (**a**) and previous "normal" status (**b**)

Fig. 17 Standard PA (**a**) and Lateral (**b**) views. Normal status after a DRUJ stabilization by a modified Adams-Berger (red) technique with plug (green). Trajectory of the reconstructions marked on the PA view

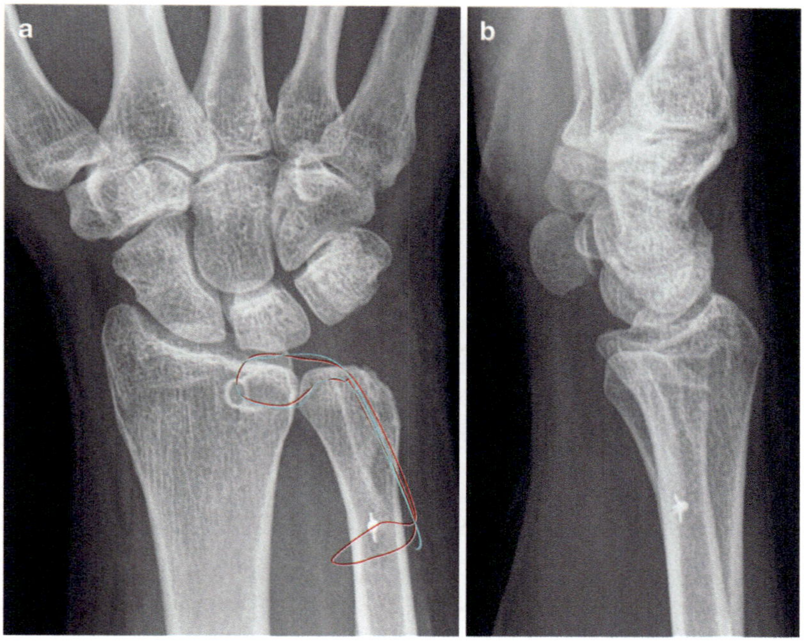

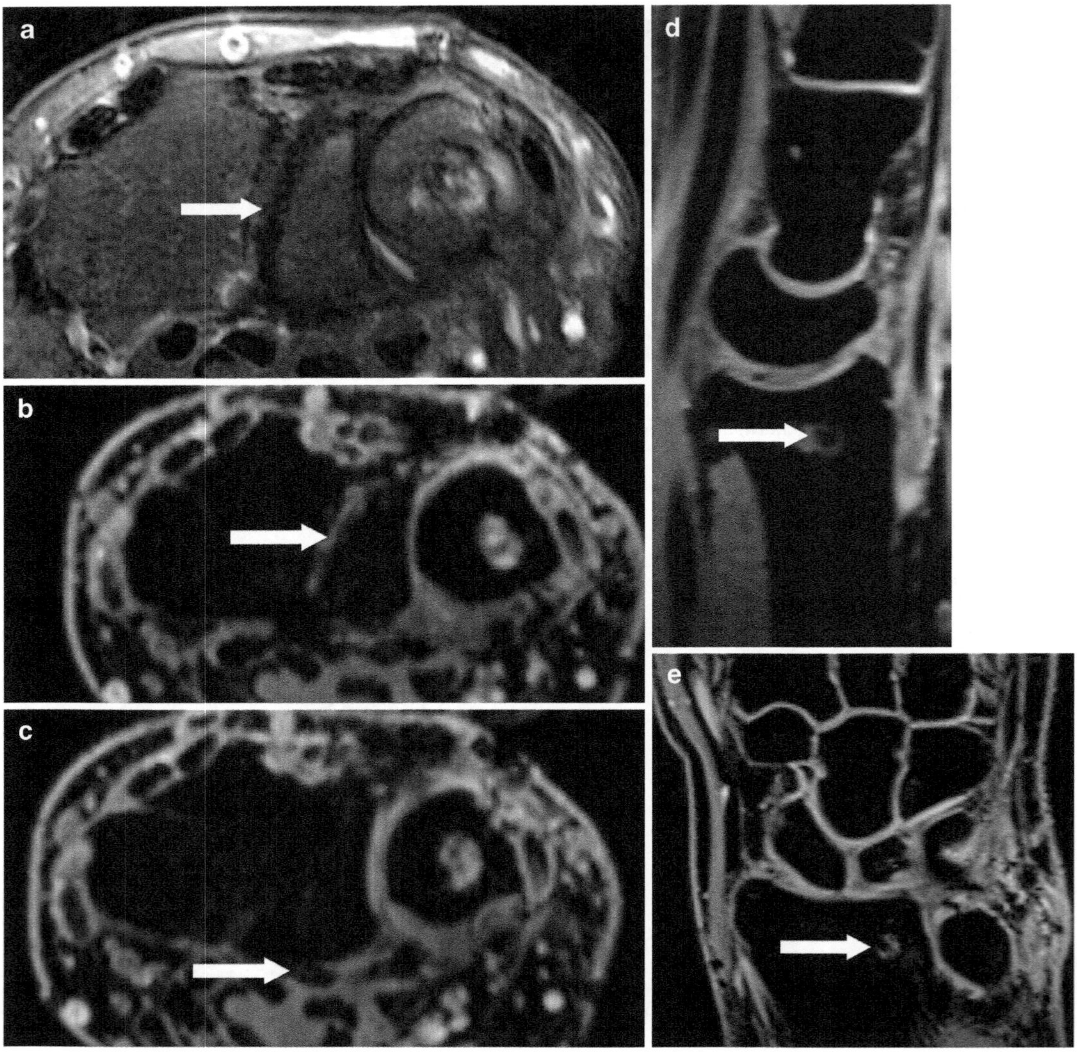

Fig. 18 Ax T2-WI FS (**a**); Ax (**b**, **c**), Sag (**d**), and Cor (**c**) 3D GRE. Normal status (radial part) after a DRUJ stabilization by a modified Adams-Berger technique with plug. The continuity of the tendon in the tunnel can be illustrated in 3D (**a**–**e**). The signals remain low and even (**a**)

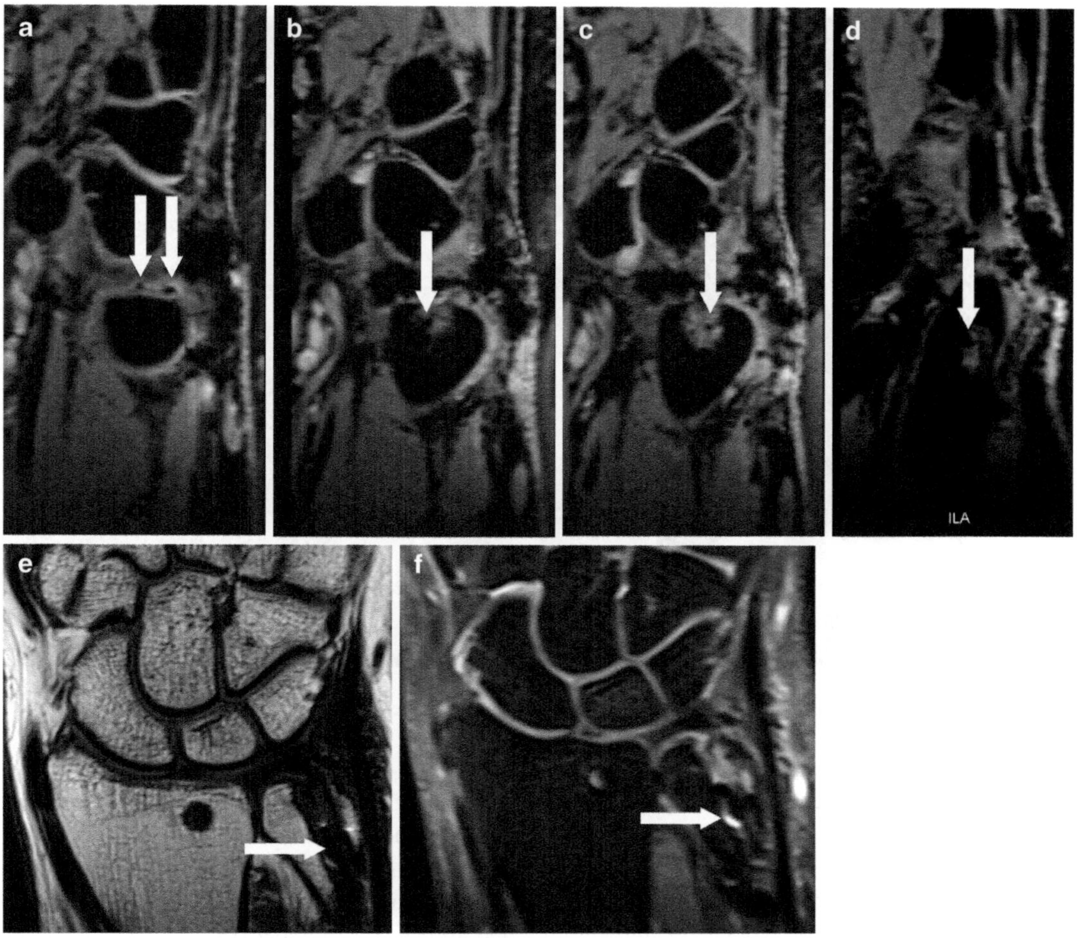

Fig. 19 Sag 3D GRE (**a–d**); Cor T1-WI (**e**); and 3D GRE (**f**). Normal status (ulnar part) after a DRUJ stabilization by a modified Adams-Berger technique with plug. The continuity of the tendon in the tunnel can be illustrated in 3D (**a–f**). The signals remain low and even (**e**)

4 Others

Unexpected iatrogenic pathology may appear after surgery (Cuono and Watson 1979; D'Agostino et al. 2011; Perlik and Guilford 1991; Yaghoubian et al. 2001). After a TFCC repair, a local kink in the ulnar artery (Fig. 20) is found compatible with the ulnar pain after intensive effort and disappearing after a rather short time.

After a trans DRUJ fixation with double pinning in a R and U fracture (Fig. 21), a significant dissection of the ECU with tendinitis (Fig. 21b–d) is observed. However, crepitations were not observed.

The postoperative clinical evaluation may reveal remaining complaints, other than the preoperative ones. Ulnar sided pain and DRUJ instability are initially related to a reduced and fixed luxation of the ECU and a dorsal subluxation of

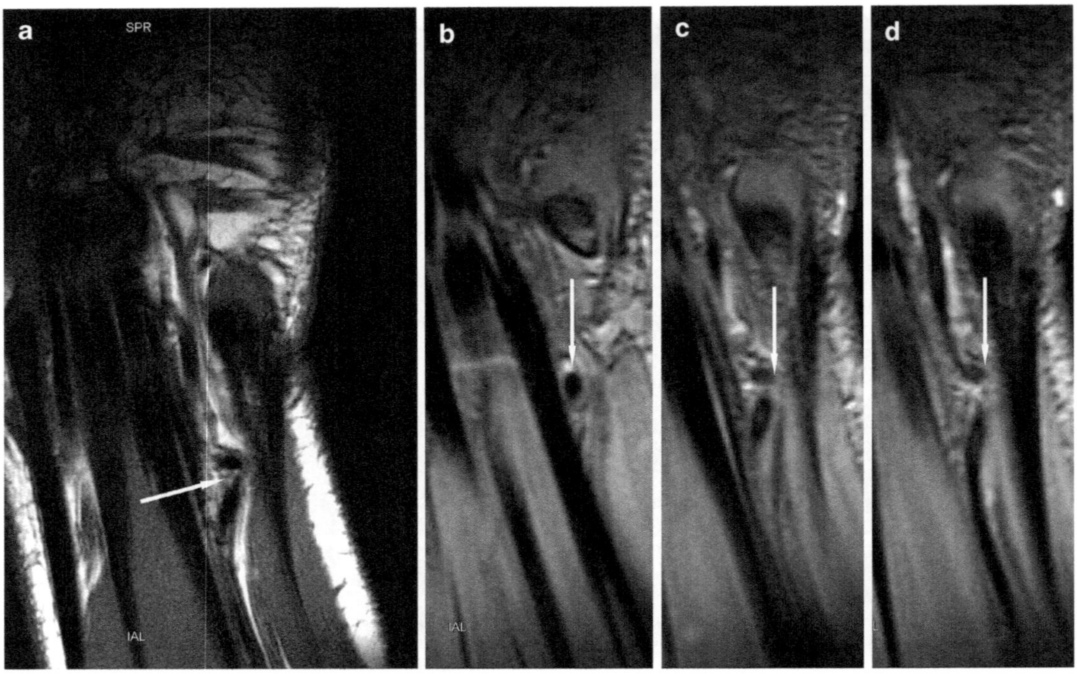

Fig. 20 Cor T1-WI (**a**); Cor T2-WI FS (**b–d**). Kink of the ulnar artery after TFCC repair

the U (Fig. 22a–c). However, midcarpal crepitations and laxity may eventually emerge. No abnormalities on the additional triple wrist arthrography (Fig. 22d-f) are found. A midcarpal stress view on the contrary shows a subluxation of the C versus the L, compatible with a capitatolunate instability to the posterior side (CLIP) as the head of the C moves beyond the orthogonal midline of the L (Fig. 22g, h).

An ECU luxation is surgically reduced and fixed with a small screw (Fig. 23a, b). The ECU tendon in then placed into the sulcus (Fig. 23c). The idea at first glance of a "tenosynovitis of the ECU" image is in reality due to a metal artefact (Fig. 23d) next to the ECU tendon.

Tendon continuity, internal signal, position, and eventually fluid in the sheath can be evaluated after repair of a tear (Fig. 24). The location, aspect, and extent of scar tissue are demonstrated (Fig. 24a, e). Any postoperative fluid collection may also be demonstrated.

During surgical resection of an arthrosynovial cyst, tying of the stalk is recommended. However, recurrence of a (symptomatic) swelling and cyst formation is frequent (approximately 30%) (Fig. 25).

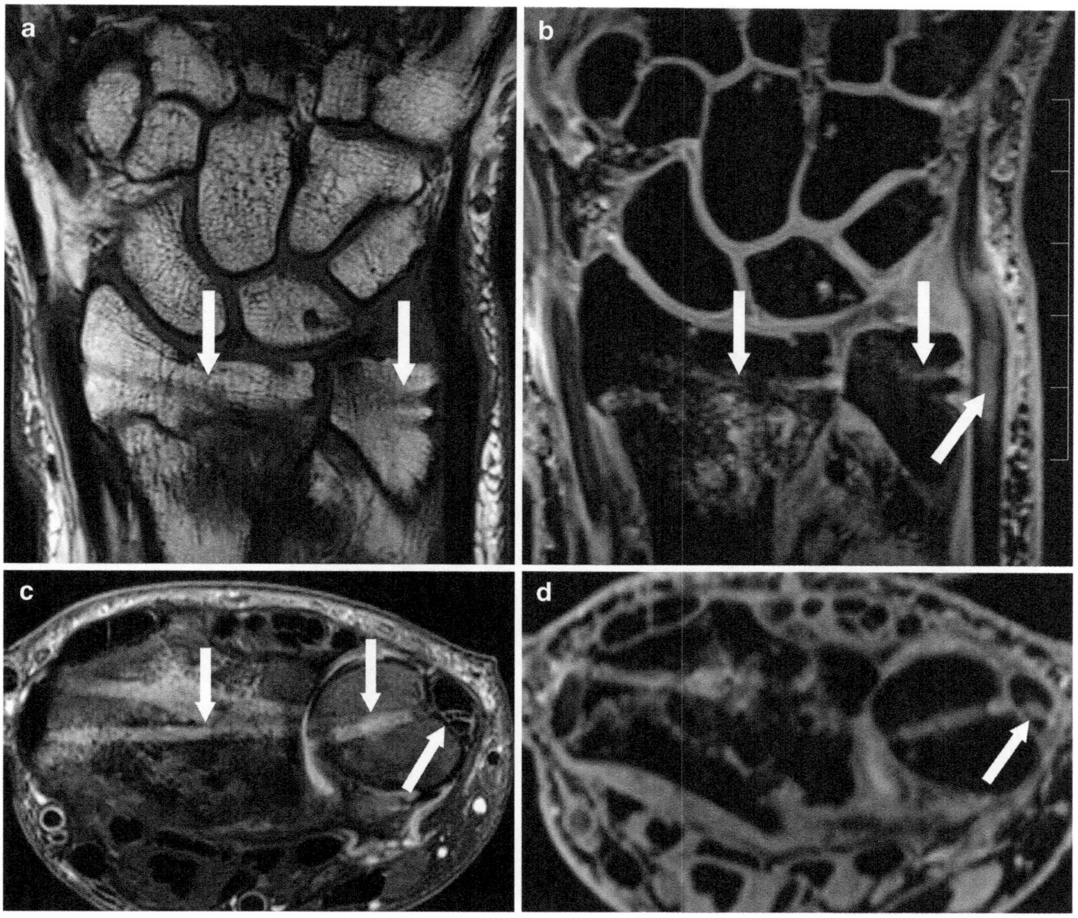

Fig. 21 Cor T1-WI (**a**) and T2-WI FS (**b**); Ax T2-WI FS (**c**); and 3D GRE (**d**). Old trajectory of two fixation pins (**a–d**) through R and U with splitting of the ECU tendon and tendonitis (**b–d**)

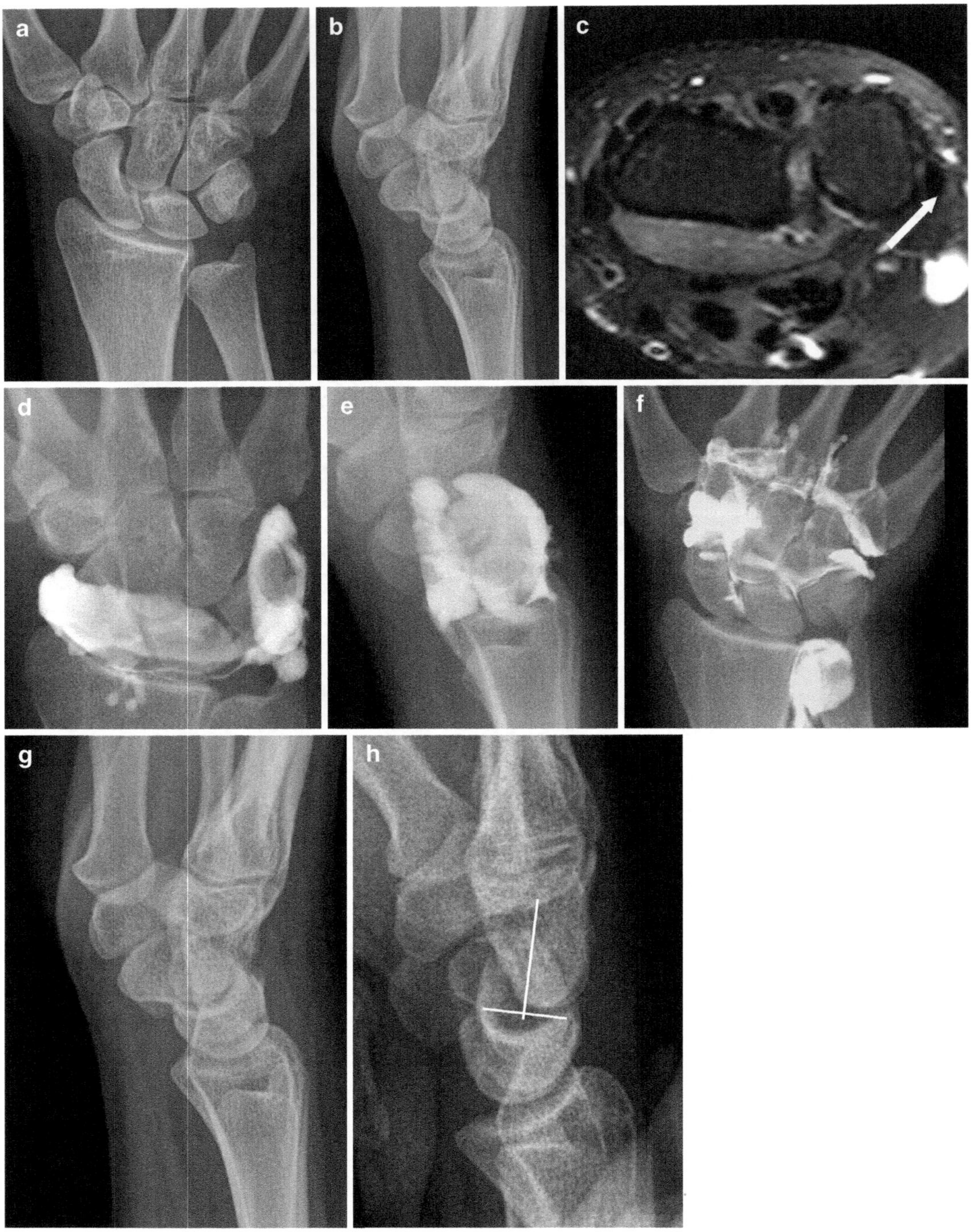

Fig. 22 Standard PA (**a**) and Lat (**b**) views; Ax T2-WI FS (**c**); Triple wrist arthrography: RC joint (**d–e**) and midcarpal- DRU joints (**f**); Midcarpal lateral neutral (**g**); and dorsal stress view (**h**). Negative ulnar variance (**a**), but no other abnormalities on standard views (**a, b**). A luxation of the ECU (**c**) and a dorsal subluxation of the U are reduced and fixed. No abnormalities demonstrated on the triple wrist arthrography (**d–f**). Midcarpal stress view shows a CLIP (**g, h**)

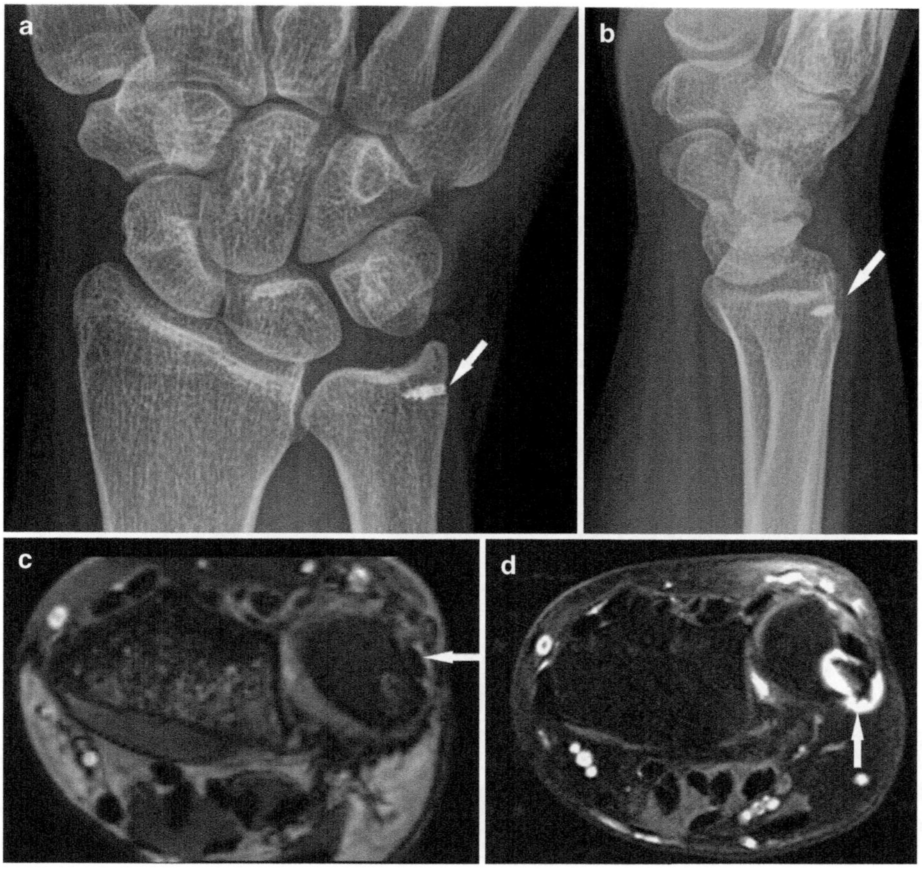

Fig. 23 Standard PA (**a**) and lateral (**b**) views; Ax 2D GRE (**c**); and T2-WI FS (**d**). The ECU luxation was reduced and fixed with a small screw (**a**, **b**). The ECU tendon in in the sulcus (**c**). "Tenosynovitis of the ECU" due to metal artefact (**d**)

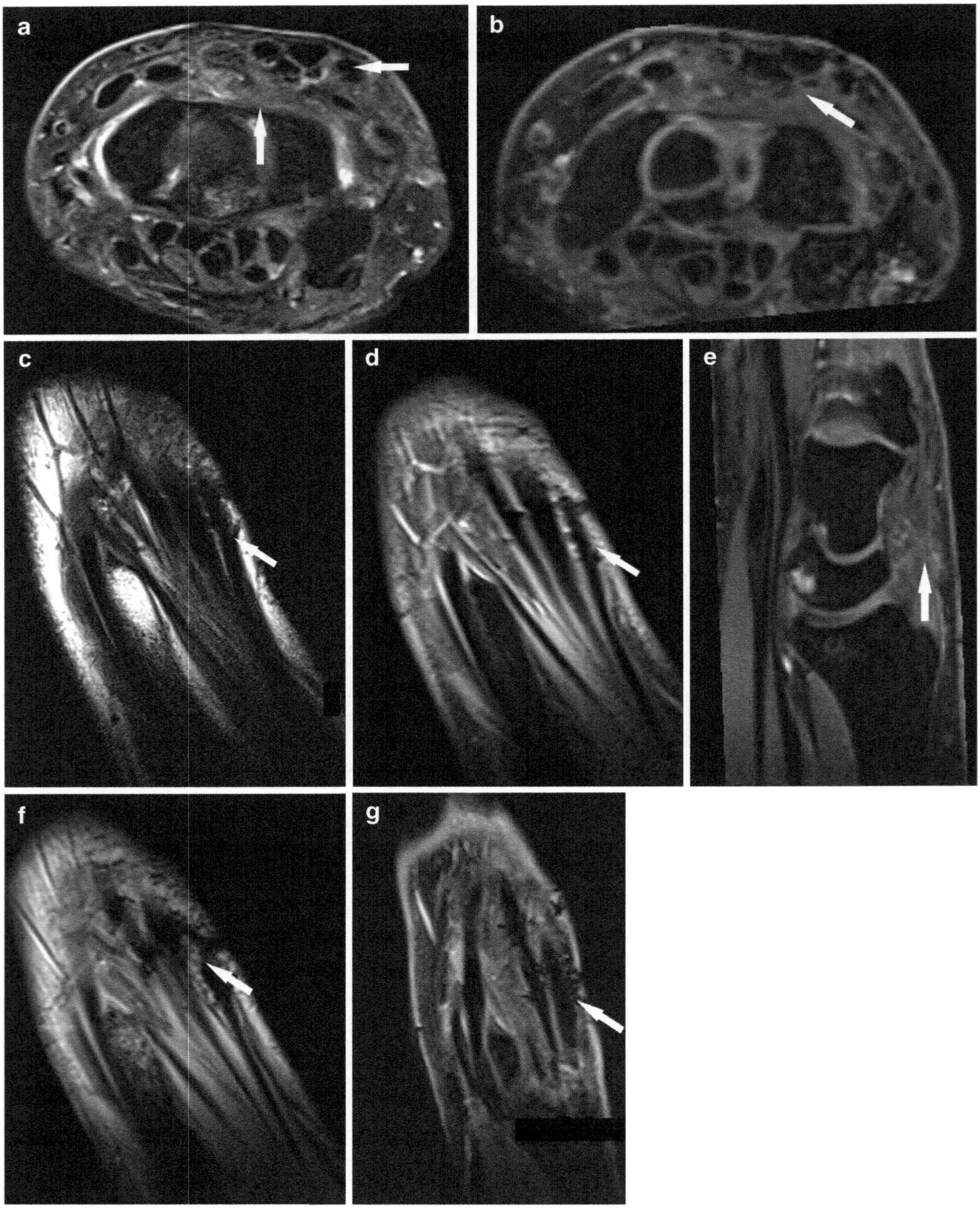

Fig. 24 Ax T2-WI FS (**a**) and 3D GRE (**b**); Cor T1-WI (**c**) and T2-WI FS (**d**); Sag 3D GRE (**e**); Cor 2D GRE (**f**, **g**). The continuity of the ruptured epl (III) and ed. (IV) is repaired (**a**). The tendons are displaced in ulnar direction (**b**–**g**) with surrounding small metal artefacts (**f**, **g**). A heterogenous higher signal scar tissue area is present dorsally of the carpus (**a**, **e**)

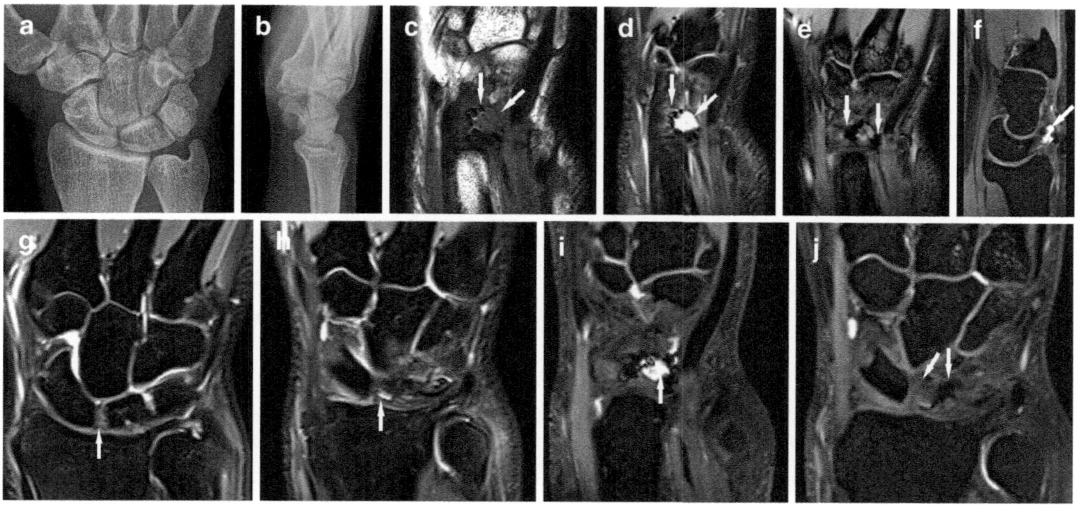

Fig. 25 Standard PA and Lateral views (**a**, **b**); Cor T1-WI (**c**), T2-WI FS and 3D GRE (**e**); Sag 3D GRE (**f**); Cor T2-WI FS (**g–i**); and 3D GRE (**j**). After successful surgery of a dorsal ASC, a symptomatic swelling reappeared due to an ASC (**c–f**) with adjacent postoperative metal artefacts (**e**, **j**). A small tear at the central part of the SLL (**g**, **h**) is present at the base of the ASC (**f**, **h**, **i**)

References

Cuono CB, Watson HK (1979) The carpal boss: surgical treatment and etiological considerations. Plast Reconstr Surg 63(1):88–93. PMID: 432327

D'Agostino P, Townley WA, Le Viet D, Roulot E (2011) Oblique ulnar styloid osteotomy – a treatment for ulnar styloid impaction syndrome. J Hand Surg Am 36(11):1785–1789. https://doi.org/10.1016/j.jhsa.2011.07.023. Epub 2011 Oct 5. PMID: 21975097

Del Piñal F (2013) Arthroscopic volar capsuloligamentous repair. J Wrist Surg 2(2):126–128. https://doi.org/10.1055/s-0033-1343016. PMID: 24436804; PMCID: PMC3699269

Gillis JA, Soreide E, Khouri JS, Kadar A, Berger RA, Moran SL (2019) Outcomes of the Adams-Berger ligament reconstruction for the distal radioulnar joint instability in 95 consecutive cases. J Wrist Surg. 8(4):268–275. https://doi.org/10.1055/s--0039-1685235. Epub 2019 Apr 22. PMID: 31404256; PMCID: PMC6685731

Mikic ZD (1995) Treatment of acute injuries of the triangular fibrocartilage complex associated with distal radioulnar joint instability. J Hand Surg Am 20(2):319–323. https://doi.org/10.1016/S0363-5023(05)80033-4. PMID: 7775777

Perlik PC, Guilford WB (1991) Magnetic resonance imaging to assess vascularity of scaphoid nonunions. J Hand Surg Am 16(3):479–484. https://doi.org/10.1016/0363-5023(91)90018-7. PMID: 1861031

Szabo RM (2008) Scapholunate ligament repair with capsulodesis reinforcement. J Hand Surg Am 33(9):1645–1654. https://doi.org/10.1016/j.jhsa.2008.08.016. PMID: 18984352

Wharton RMH, Ahearne D (2021) Bilateral STT arthrodesis in a young patient with occult proximal row coalition. J Wrist Surg 11(6):546–549. https://doi.org/10.1055/s-0041-1740137. PMID: 36504535; PMCID: PMC9731740

Yaghoubian R, Goebel F, Musgrave DS, Sotereanos DG (2001) Diagnosis and management of acute fracture-dislocation of the carpus. Orthop Clin North Am 32(2):295–305. https://doi.org/10.1016/s0030-5898(05)70250-9, viii. PMID: 11331542

Part III

Section on Non-Traumatic Pathology

Avascular Necrosis

Contents

1 General

A lack of blood supply may result in avascular necrosis of a carpal bone. The carpal bones are rarely affected, with the exception of two carpal bones: (the proximal pole of) the lunate* (Kienbock) (Arnaiz et al. 2014) and the scaphoid (post-traumatic or Preiser) (Abascal et al. 2001; Gelberman et al. 1986). These two carpal bones are most susceptible to AVN due to the unique vascular supply [the nurturing artery is at the distal end of the bone and the proximal pole is solely dependent on the intraosseous retrograde blood supply) (Table 1)], their position in the carpus and their large cartilage surface. Besides traumatic AVN, repetitive motion trauma seems to be the most causal factor (leaving aside some predisposing factors, such as gout, peripheral vasculopathy in diabetics, lupus, haemoglobinopathy, steroids, renal transplant, alcohol, hyperbaric conditions, and radiotherapy), followed by intense manual labour and subsequent micro traumata. The dominant hand is mostly affected in the latter. In case of a fracture of the scaphoid, the risk of AVN is the highest for fractures close to the proximal pole, i.e. the pole furthest from the distal entering point of the nurturing artery

Table 1 Blood supply type of the carpal bones as described by Gelderman and Gross (1986)

3 types of blood supply	
1.	Unique blood vessel: scaphoid, capitate, and lunate* bone
2.	Two arteries with an interosseus anastomosis: trapezial, triquetral, pisiform, and lunate* bone
3.	Two arteries without an interosseus anastomosis: trapezoidal and hamate bone

M. Mespreuve, K. Waked, *MRI of the Wrist*, Medical Radiology,
https://doi.org/10.1007/978-3-031-63973-9_8

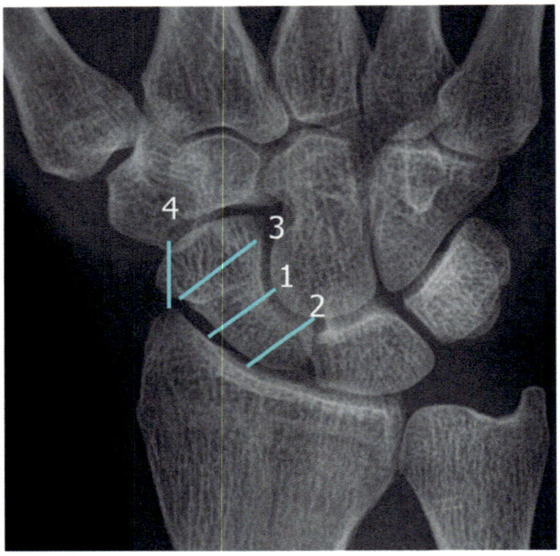

Fig. 1 Fractures at (1) the waist (80%) and (2) the proximal pole (10%) are responsible for 30% of the carpal bone AVN. The distal pole (3) and tuberculum (4) fractures are generally not involved

(Fig. 1). Caffey's disease (infantile cortical hyperostosis) should be considered if multiple carpal bones are involved in a young child.

2 MRI Findings

The different signal changes in the affected carpal bone vary depending on the phase of AVN (Lichtman et al. 2010). Table 2 summarises a practical MRI approach to the different stages, based on the original Lichtman classification on standard views for AVN of the lunate bone.

To evaluate the extent of AVN, basic T1-WI and T2-WI FS sequences should always be supplemented with CE series in at least two dimensions (Figs. 2 and 3). More anatomical detail is provided by 3D GRE (Fig. 3).

Basically, the "normal, dense bone" (Fig. 4a, b) will display a low marrow signal on T1-WI (Fig. 4c, e, f). In the oedematous phase, the T2-WI FS will disclose a high signal BMO (Fig. 4d). The radiologist should be attentive for a potential early revascularisation, which may show a similar high signal on T2-WI FS. By contrast, if the signal on the T2-WI FS is low, the presence of CE reflects fibrosis (Fig. 4e versus Fig. 4g) and absence of CE reflects necrosis (Fig. 4f versus Fig. 4h). Viable bone enhances the signal due to a reactive hyperaemia.

Phase 0 of AVN with normal standard views (Fig. 5a, b) may show a pathognomonic subcortical hypo-intense line (Figs. 5c, d and 7a, d), mostly visible on T1-WI, corresponding to a stress fracture.

Phase 1 with still normal standard views (Figs. 6a and 7c) additionally exhibits areas of (Fig. 6b) or diffuse BMO (7D-E). Even during adolescence in young top athletes, AVN of the L rarely manifests itself (Fig. 8). CE is uniform in the affected carpal bone (Fig. 9).

Phase 2 AVN shows a contour deformation of the L, typically at the proximal-radial side (Fig. 10a). The SI is low on T1-WI (Figs. 10b, 11a, b, and 12c, d) and T2-WI (Figs. 10c and 12e). CE is inhomogeneous or absent (Figs. 10d and 12f, g). The cortical deformation may be subtle (Fig. 11c) and is best appreciated on 3D GRE.

Phase 3 (A for the L and B for the S) involves collapse and fragmentation of the carpal or lunate bone (Figs. 13 and 14). 3D GRE is preferred to illustrate fragmentation (Fig. 13e), but CT may be needed to either confirm (Fig. 13f, g) it or rule it out. In the collapse phase of the S, a rotatory subluxation (Fig. 14a) and a widening of the SL joint (Fig. 14b–d) may also be present.

Phase 4 or end stage is accompanied by secondary osteoarthritis, CE synovial proliferation (Fig. 13h), and cysts appearing in the necrotic bone (or fragments) (Fig. 15).

The evaluation on standard views alone may underestimate the extent end phase of AVN (Figs. 15 and 16). MRI is therefore recommended, as the evolution of AVN may be fast in between postponed consultations which state "normal findings" (Fig. 17).

Table 2 "Lichtman-like" MRI classification of AVN of carpal bones

STAGE ("Lichtman-like")	T1-WI	T2-WI FS	Other	CE	Standard views (Lichtman)
(Phase 0)	Normal or **Hypo-intense line (stress fracture)**	Normal	Normal bone contour	Uniform	Normal
Phase 1	**Low (first at the proximal convex side)**	**(Low with areas of) high SI**	Normal bone contour	Uniform	Normal
Phase 2	**Low**	**High SI**	**Abnormal contour (Lunate: radial-proximal)**	**Inhomogeneous or no CE**	**Osteosclerosis (necrotic segment or complete)**
Phase 3A	**Low (uniform)**	**Low**	**Collapse of the carpal bone**	**No CE**	**Collapse/ Fragmentation**
Phase 3B	**Low (uniform)**	**Low**	**(Scaphoid: rotatory instability)**	**No CE**	**(Scaphoid: + SL dissociation)**
Phase 4	**Low**	**Low**	**Cysts and fragmentation Radiocarpal degeneration**	**Synovial**	**Osteoarthritis (cartilage loss/joint space narrowing)**

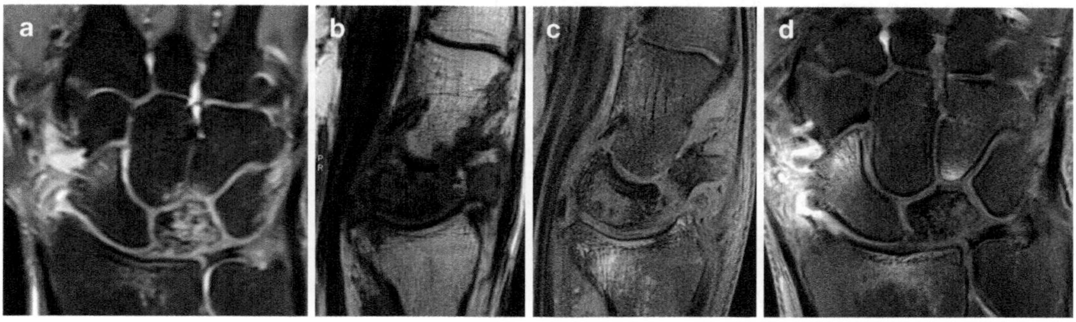

Fig. 2 Cor T2-WI FS (**a**); Sag T1-WI (**b**); Sag (**c**) and Cor (**d**) T1-WI FS with CE. Diffuse areas of high SI (**a**) and almost complete low SI (**b**) of the L. CE illustrates the still vital parts of the L (**c**, **d**)

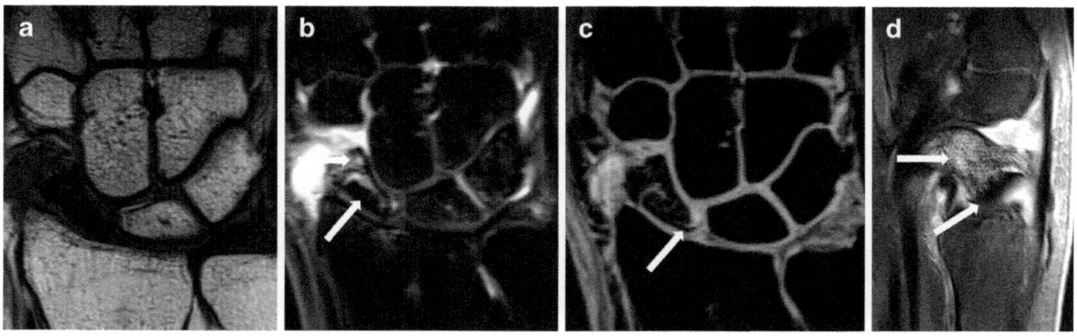

Fig. 3 Cor T1-WI (**a**); Cor T2-WI FS (**b**); and 3D GRE (**c**); Sag T1-WI FS with CE. Low signal (**a**, **b**) of the S with an oblique fracture line (**c**). The necrotic fragment is slightly displaced in the widened SL space (**c**). The proximal part of the S is necrotic (**b**, **d**) and the distal part shows hyperaemia, all clearly seen on the sagittal CE image (**d**)

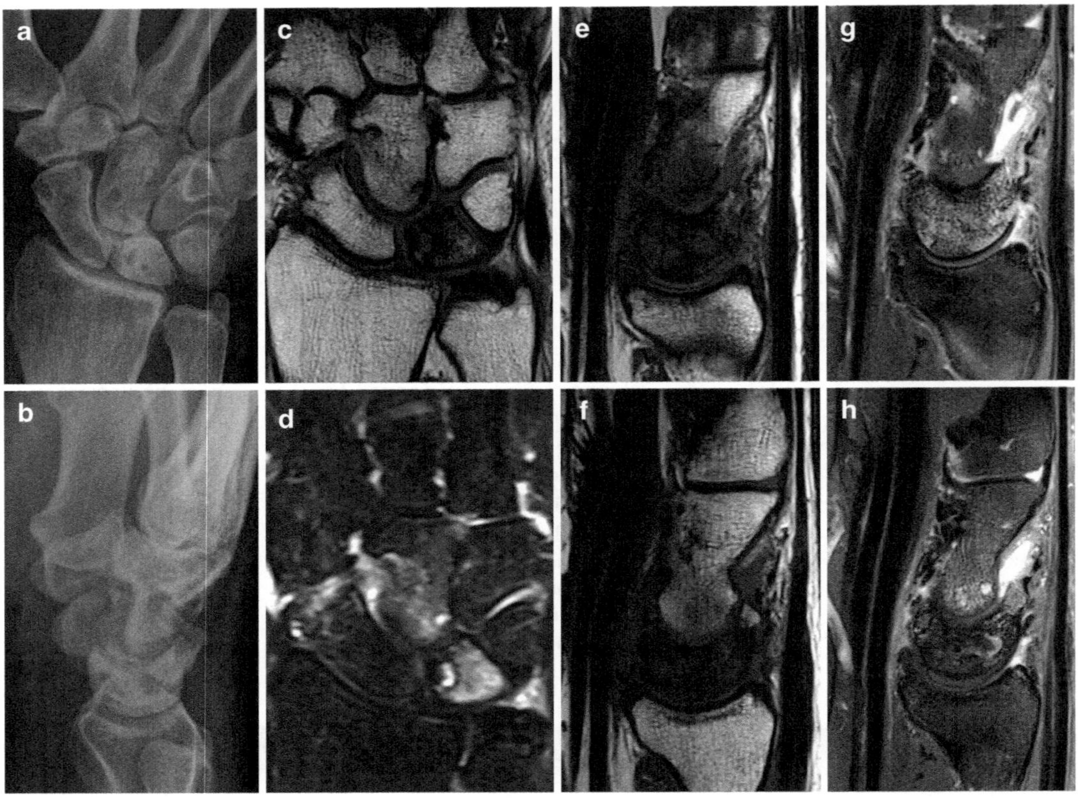

Fig. 4 Standard PA (**a**) and Lateral (**b**) views; Cor T1-WI (**c**); Cor T2-WI FS (**d**); Sag T1-WI (**e**, **f**) with FS CE (**g**, **h**). "Dense L" (**a**, **b**). Low T1-signal (**c**) combined with high T2-signal (**d**) reflect BMO. Low T1- and T2-signal (**e**, **f**) combined with CE reflect fibrosis (**g**) and without CE necrosis (**h**)

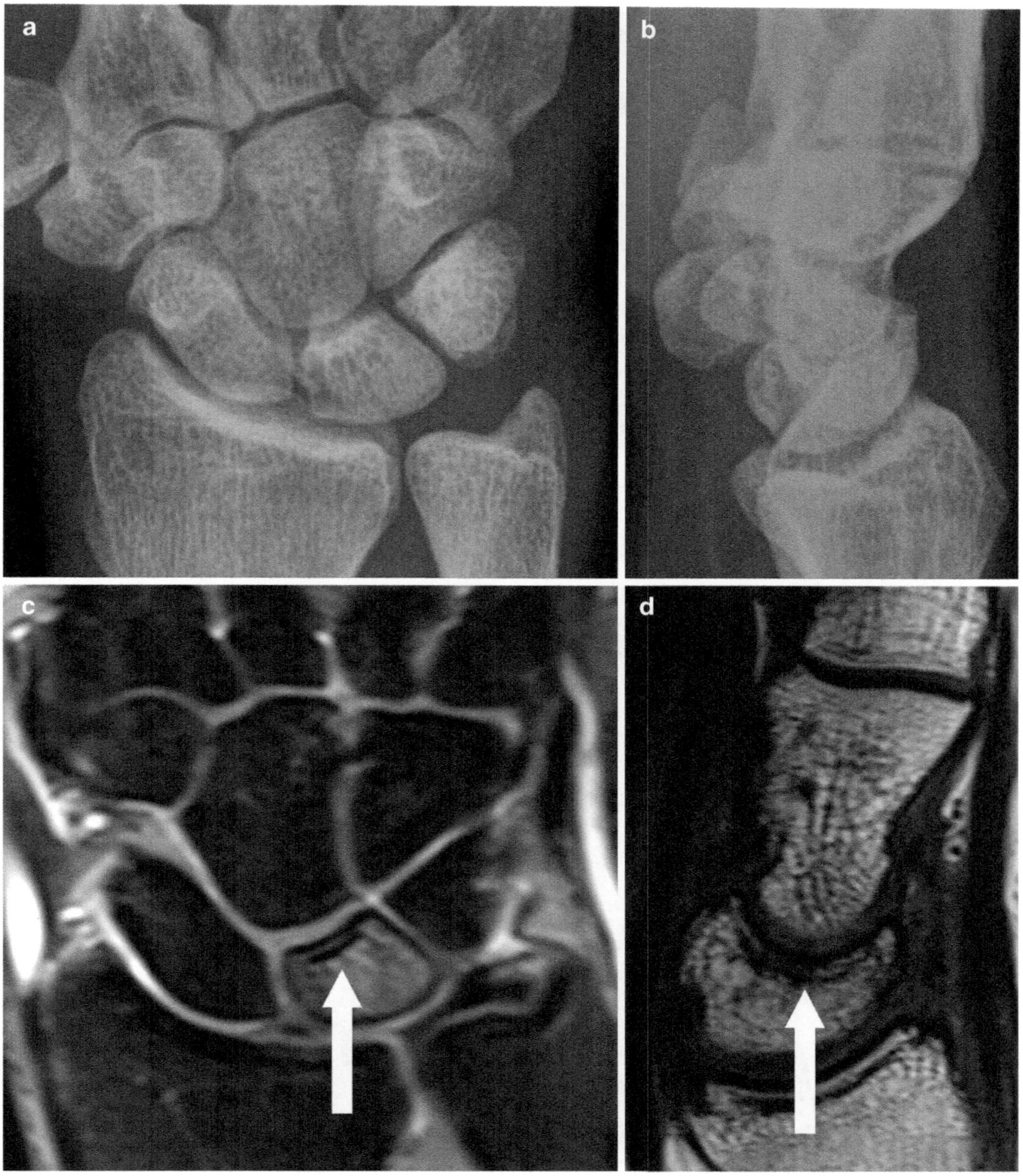

Fig. 5 Standard PA (**a**) and Lateral (**b**) views; Cor T2-WI FS (**c**); Sag T1-WI (**d**). Normal aspect (density and contour) of the L (**a**, **b**), subcortical stress fracture line (**c**, **d**) with starting BMO (**c**): considered between phase 1 and 2

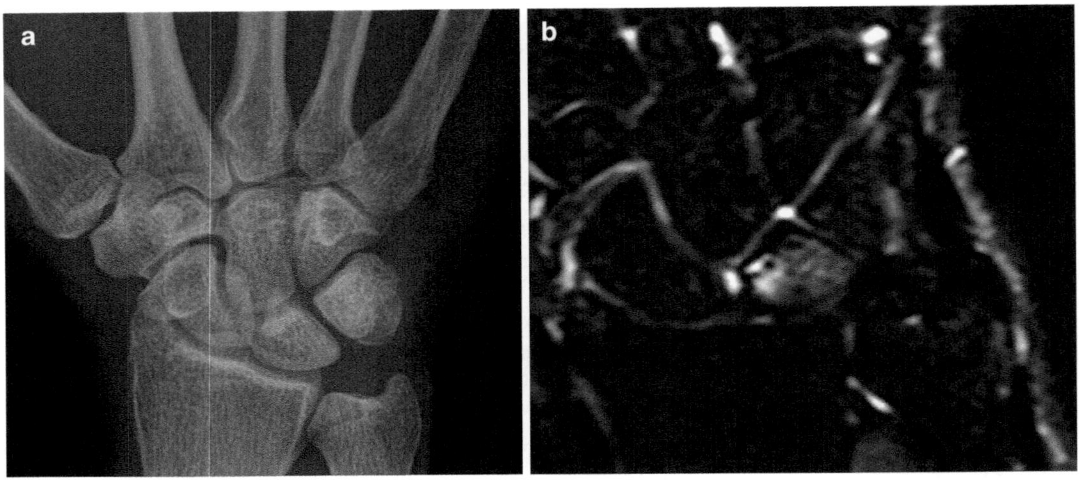

Fig. 6 Standard PA (**a**) view; Cor T2-WI FS (**b**). Normal aspect (density and contour) of the L (**a**) with areas of high SI on T2 of the L (**b**)

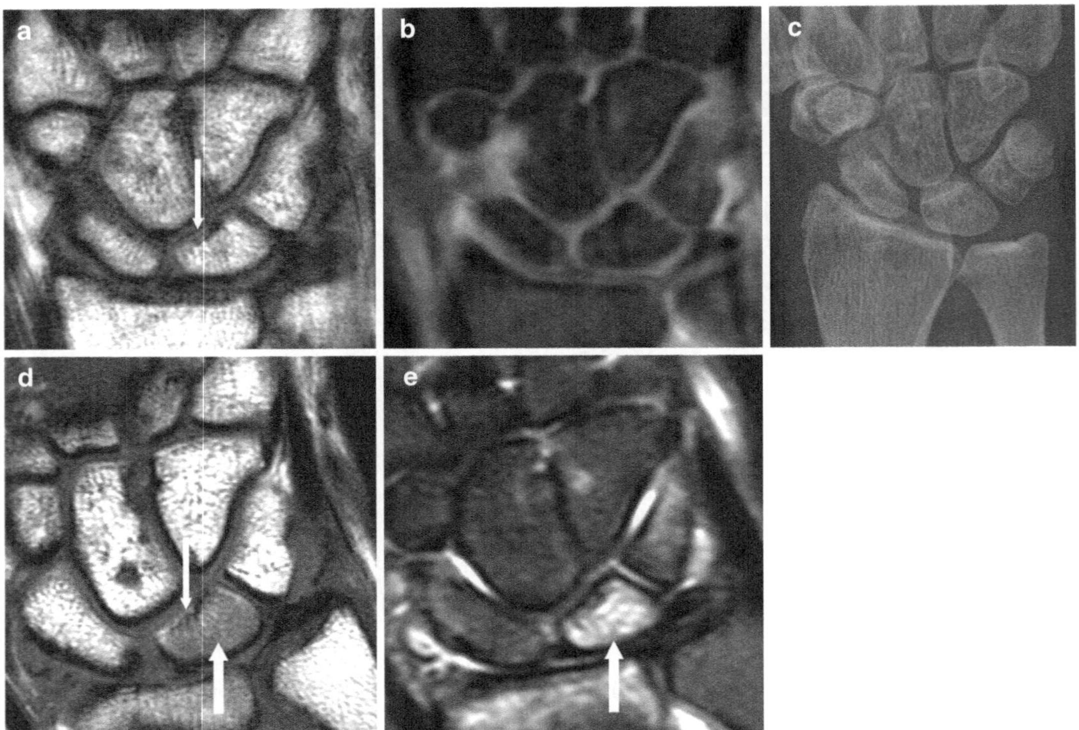

Fig. 7 Cor T1-WI (**a**) and T2-WI FS (**b**); Standard PA (**c**) view; Cor T1-WI (**d**); and T2-WI FS (**e**). Initially, only a subcortical fracture line (phase 0) is suspected (**a**, **b**; images distorted by motion artefacts). Control examinations 8 months later show a L with a normal density and contour (**c**) with oedema (**d**, **e**): AVN phase 1. The subcortical fracture line is confirmed (**d**)

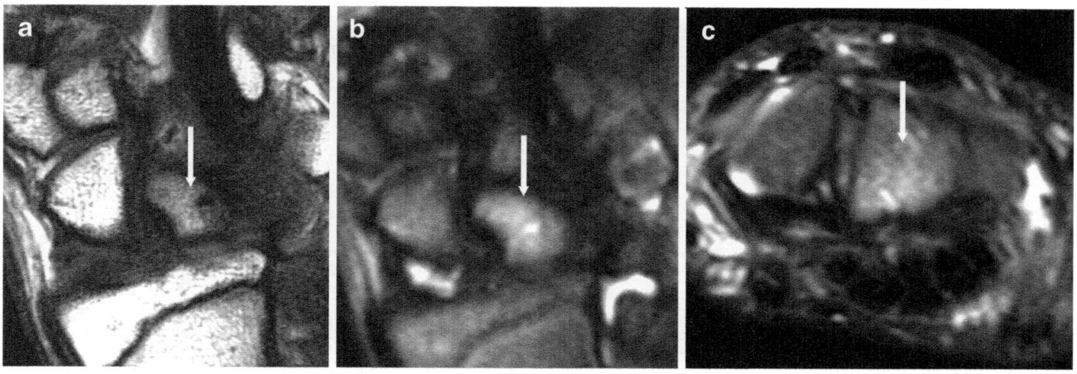

Fig. 8 Cor T1-WI (**a**) and T2-WI FS (**b**); Ax T2-WI FS (**c**). BMO of the L in an adolescent top athlete

Fig. 9 Cor T1-WI (**a**) and with FS CE (**b**). BMO of the S (**a**) with homogeneous CE (**b**)

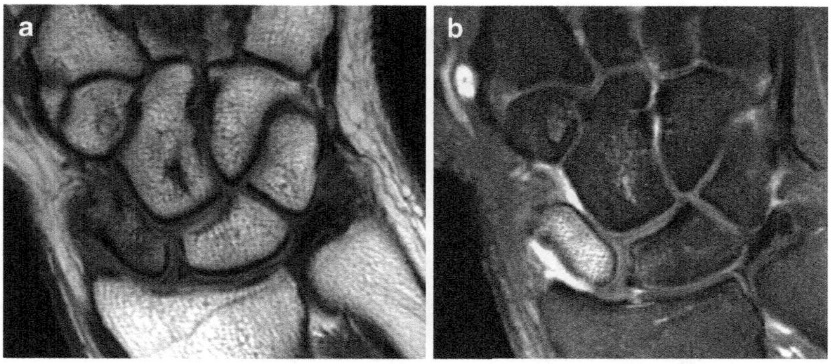

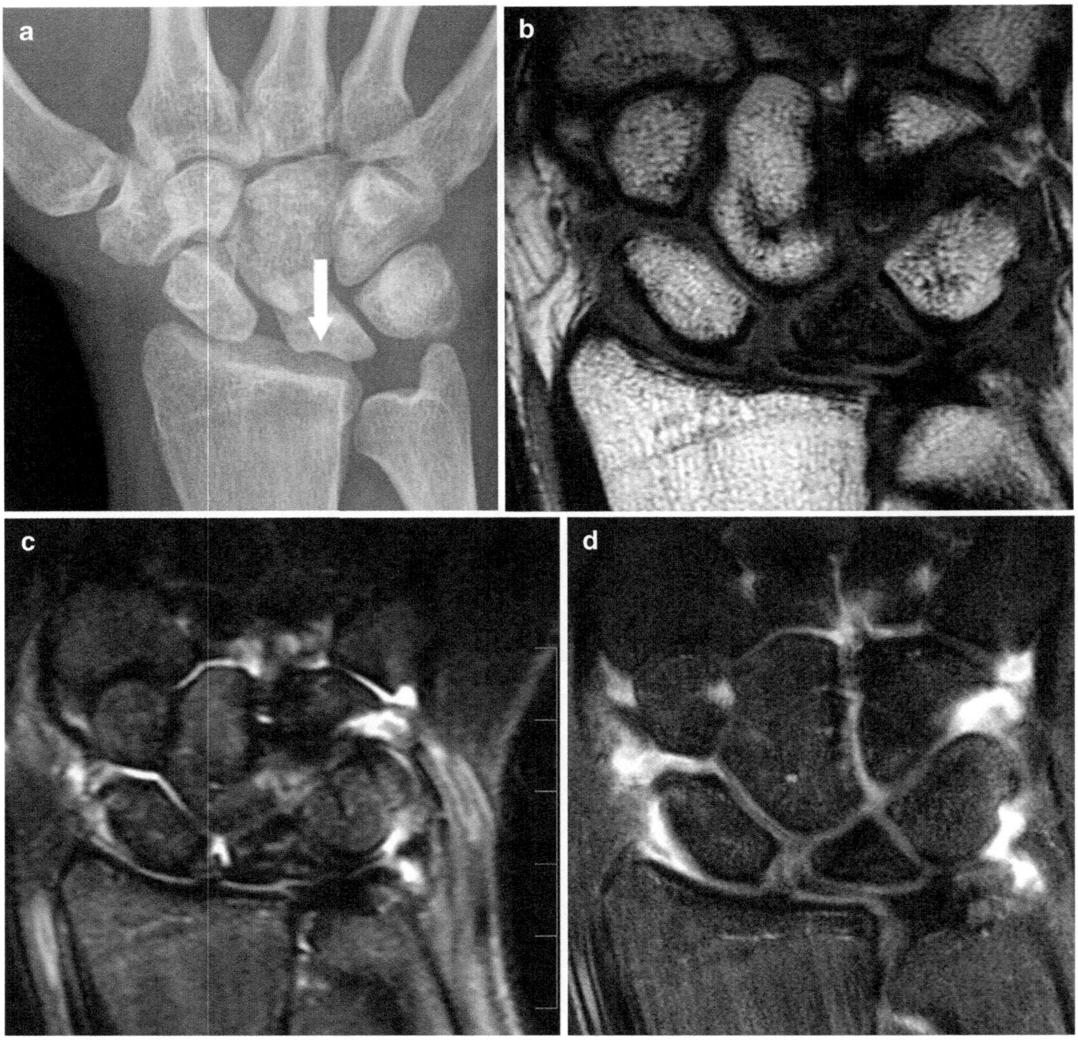

Fig. 10 Standard PA (**a**) view; Cor T1-WI (**b**), T2-WI FS (**c**), and T1-WI FS with CE. AVN of the L with cortical deformation at the proximal-radial side (**a**) graded as phase 2. Low signal on T1-WI (**b**) and T2-WI FS (**c**). No CE present (**d**). Note: SL tear with widening of SL joint and rotatory subluxation of the S

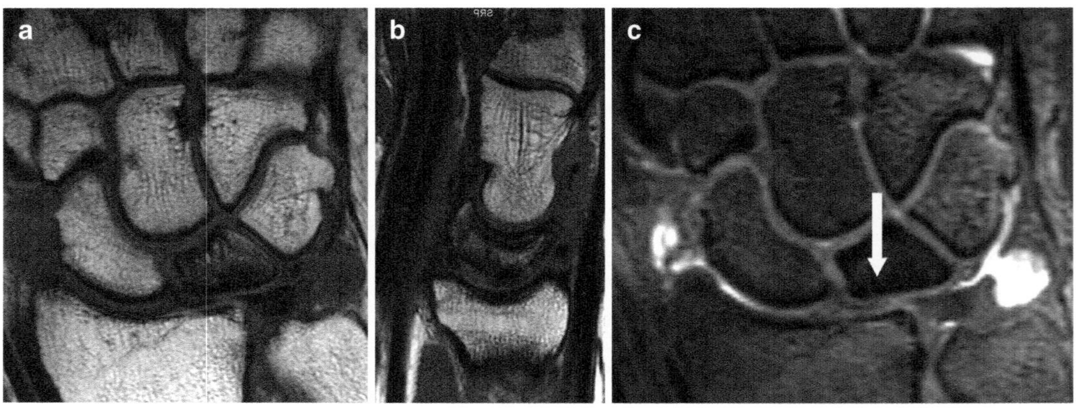

Fig. 11 Cor (**a**) and Sag (**b**) T1-WI; 3D GRE (**c**). AVN of the L with low SI (**a**, **b**). The deformation of the proximal-radial side (**a**) may be subtle in phase 2 (**c**)

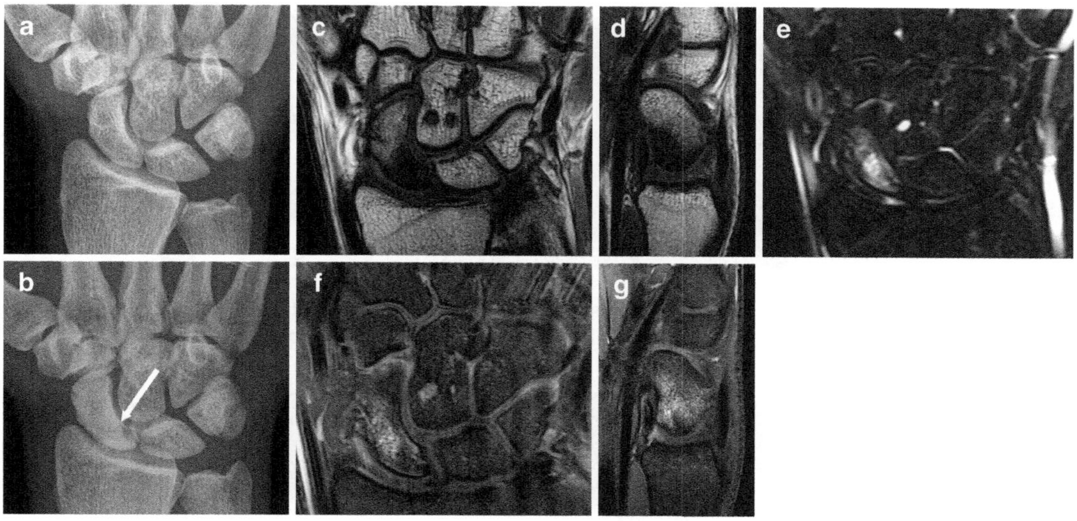

Fig. 12 Standard PA (**a**) views from 2006 (**a**) and 2011 (**b**); Cor (**c**) and Sag (**d**) T1-WI; Cor T2-WI FS (**e**); Cor (**f**) and Sag (**g**) T1-WI FS with CE. The negative standard view after trauma (**a**) changed 5 years later. The proximal pole of the S is obviously denser (**b**). The SI of the S was low on T1-WI (**c**, **d**) and high on T2-WI FS (**e**) with inhomogeneous CE (**f**, **g**). AVN phase 2 of the S

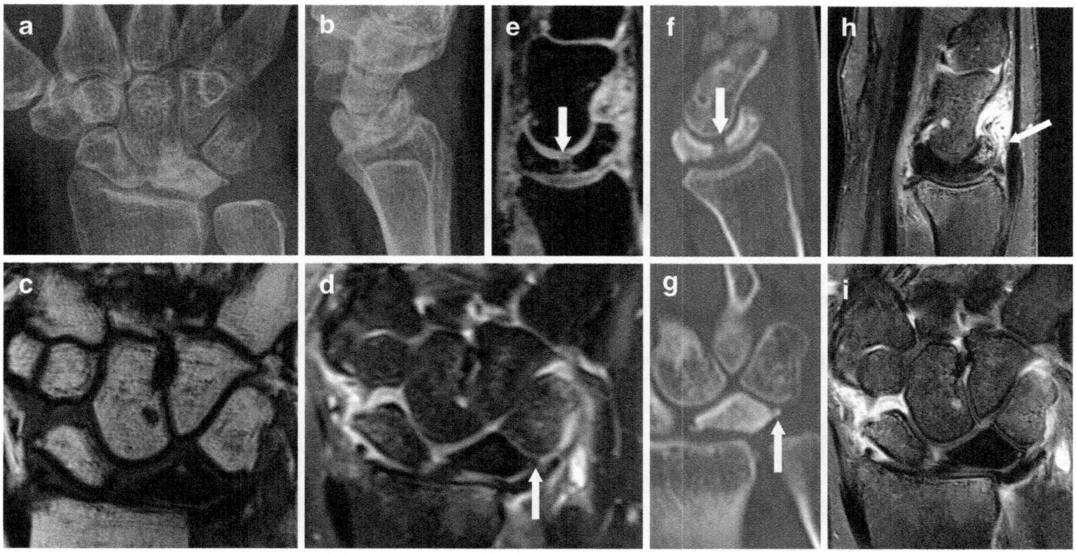

Fig. 13 Standard PA (**a**) and lateral (**b**) views; Cor T1-WI (**c**); Cor T2-WI FS (**d**); Sag 3D GRE (**e**); Sag (**f**) and Cor (**g**) reconstructed CT-image; Sag (**h**) and Cor (**i**) T1-WI FS with CE. The dens L has collapsed (**a**, **b**). SI on both T1-WI (**c**) and T2-WI FS (**d**) is low. 3D GRE (**e**) shows the fragmentation of the L in two parts, confirmed by CT (**f**). Small fragment at the LT-joint (**g**) on CT and, in retrospect, also on MR (**d**). CE is absent in the L (**h**, **i**). Phase 3A, although there is already synovial CE (**h**) and starting radiocarpal OA (**d**, **i**), initiating phase 4

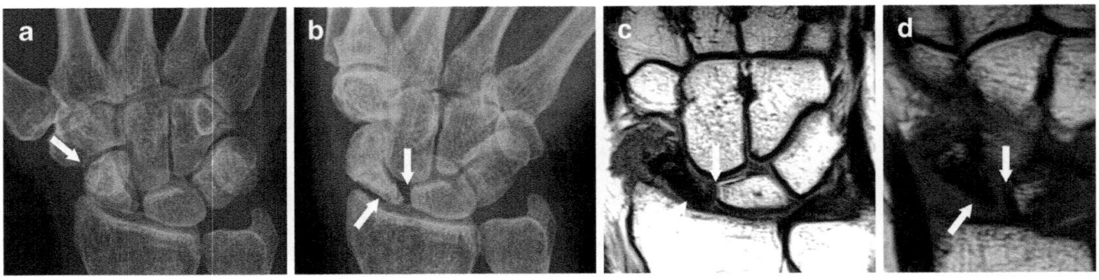

Fig. 14 Standard PA (**a**) with clenched fist (**b**) views; Cor T1-WI (**c**, **d**). Rotatory subluxation of the S with signet ring sign (**a**), collapse (**b–d**) of the dense (**b**) proximal pole and widening of the SL joint (**b–d**). Phase 3 AVN of the S

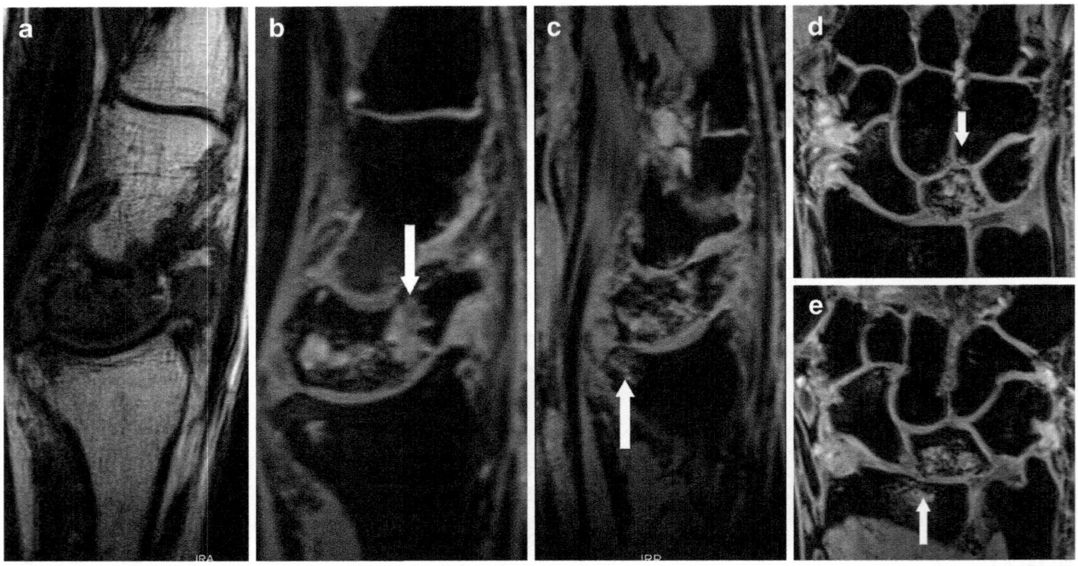

Fig. 15 Sag T1-WI (**a**); Sag (**b**, **c**) and Cor (**d**, **e**) 3D GRE. Fragmentation of the L (**a**, **b**) with cyst formation in the L (**a–c**) and radiocarpal and midcarpal OA (**c–e**): AVN phase 4 of the L

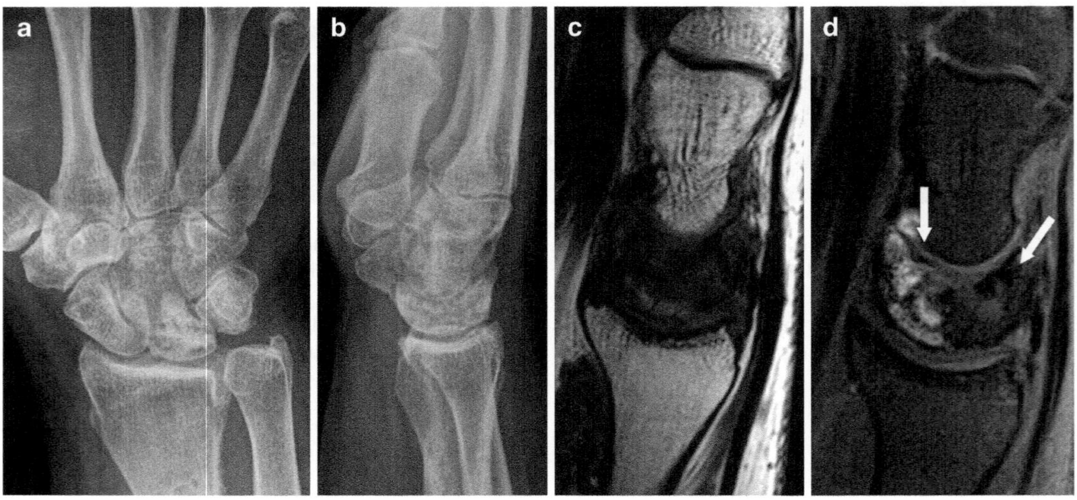

Fig. 16 Standard PA (**a**) and Lateral (**b**) views; Sag T1-WI (**c**) FS with CE (**d**). Same patient as 15 A. Inhomogeneous denser L (**a**, **b**), considered as phase 2. Some flattening of the dorsal L with necrosis (**c**, **d**), considered as phase 3A

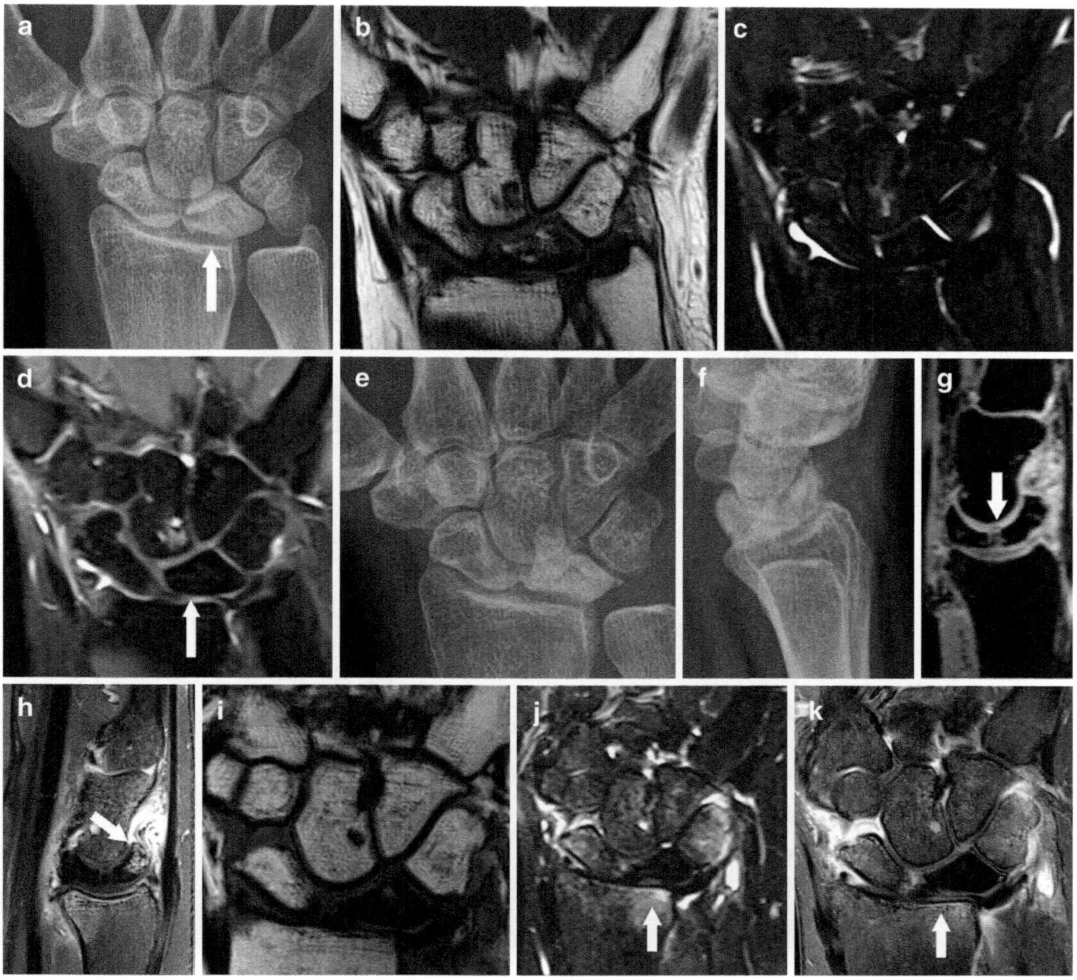

Fig. 17 Standard PA (**a**) view; Cor T1-WI (**b**), T2-WI FS (**c**), and 3D GRE (**d**) in September 2009. Standard PA (**e**) and Lateral (**f**) views; Sag 3D GRE (**g**) and T1-WI FS with CE (**h**); Cor T1-WI (**i**), T2-WI FS (**j**), and T1-WI FS with CE (**k**) in June 2010. Flattening of the radial side of the L with low signal on T1-WI and T2-WI FS (**a**–**d**), phase 2. Collapse (**e**–**k**) and fragmentation (**i**) of the L with synovial CE (**h**, **k**) and starting radiocarpal OA (**j**, **k**), phase 3–4

3 Association with Negative Ulnar Variance and Other

This association is still up for debate (van Leeuwen et al. 2016). The negative ulnar variance (Hulten 1928) is associated with AVN (Fig. 18) of the L (Zapico 1984). However, De Smet (De Smet 1994) found no association. Remarkably, 75% of the AVN of the L is present in a wrist with negative ulnar variance (Goldfarb et al. 2011; Nakamura et al. 1991; van Der Heijden et al. 2005), but a neutral or positive ulnar variance does not exclude AVN of the L (Figs. 19 and 20).

The mobility of the wrist normally diminishes as AVN is progressing (Fig. 21).

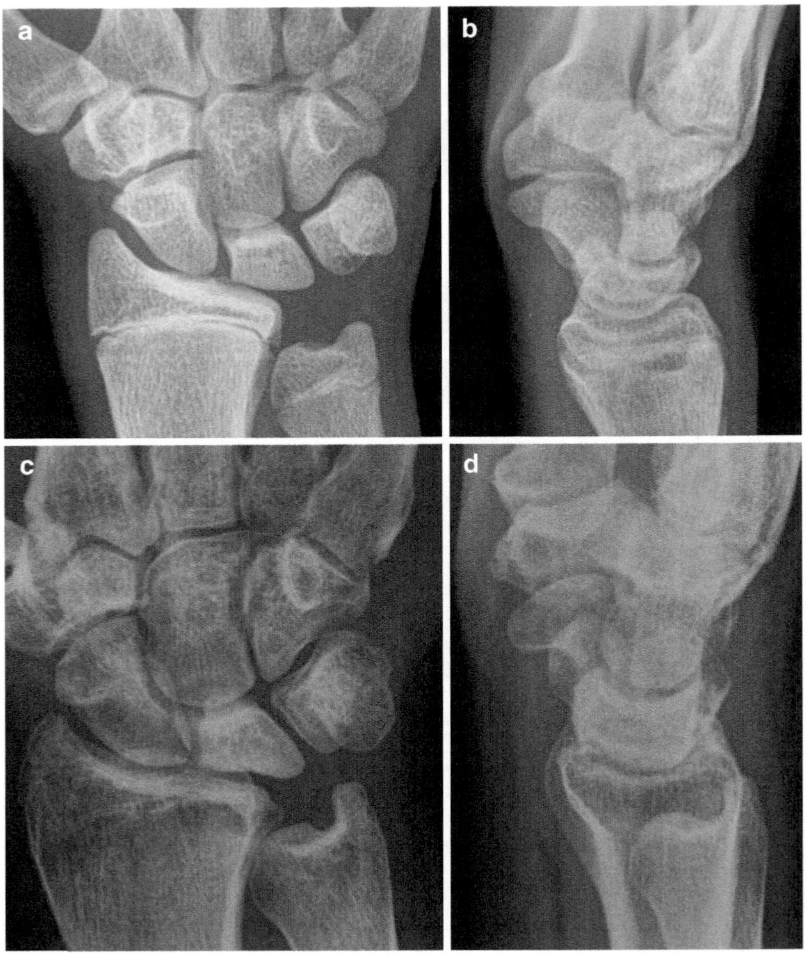

Fig. 18 Standard PA (**a**, **c**) and Lateral (**b**, **d**) views. Negative ulnar variance and elective wrist pain in an adolescent (**a**, **b**) and an adult (**c**, **d**), respectively AVN of the L phase 1 and 2

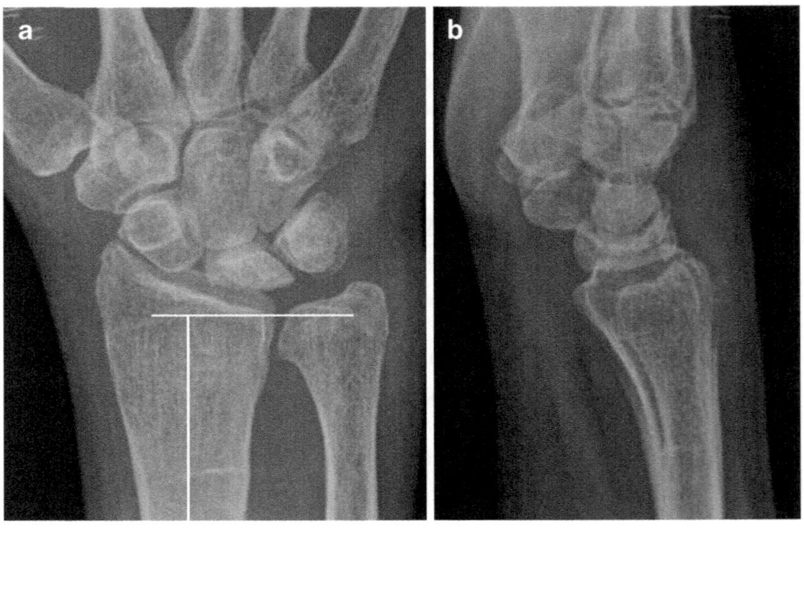

Fig. 19 Standard PA (**a**) and Lateral (**b**) views. Positive ulnar variance and AVN of the L phase 3

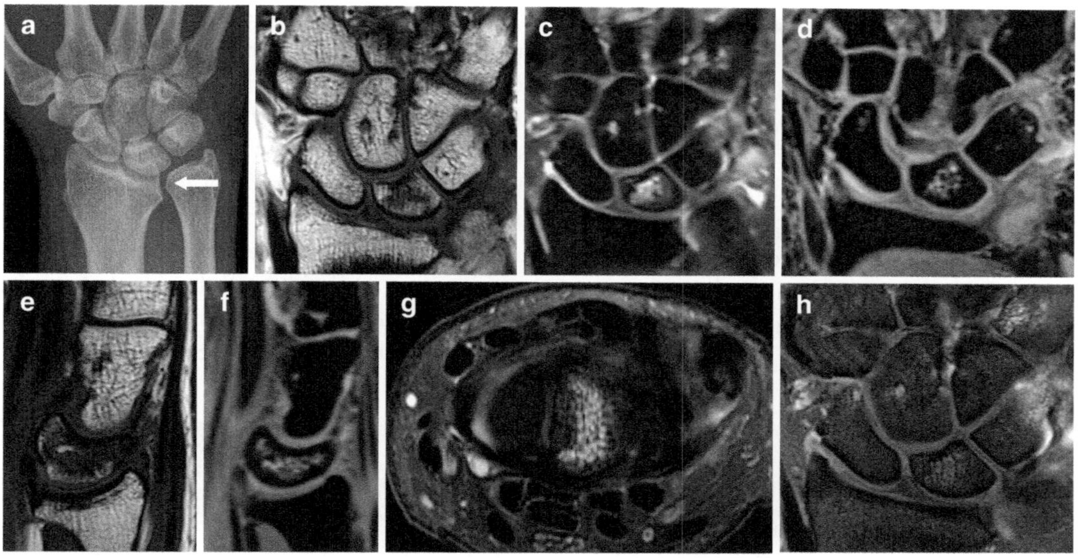

Fig. 20 Standard PA (**a**) view; Cor T1-WI (**b**), T2-WI FS (**c**) and 3D GRE (**d**); Sag T1-WI (**e**) and 3D GRE (**f**); Ax T2-WI FS (**g**), Cor T1-WI FS with CE (**h**). Positive ulnar variance (**a**) and AVN of the L phase 1 with normal contour (**b**–**h**), low signal on T1-WI (**b**, **e**) and high on T2-WI (**c**, **g**), and CE (**h**). Note the intact cartilage at the ulnar corner of the L (**b**, **d**, and **h**) in this positive ulnar variance

Fig. 21 Standard PA view in radial (**a**, **c**) and ulnar (**b**, **d**) deviation. AVN of the L progresses and mobility reduces

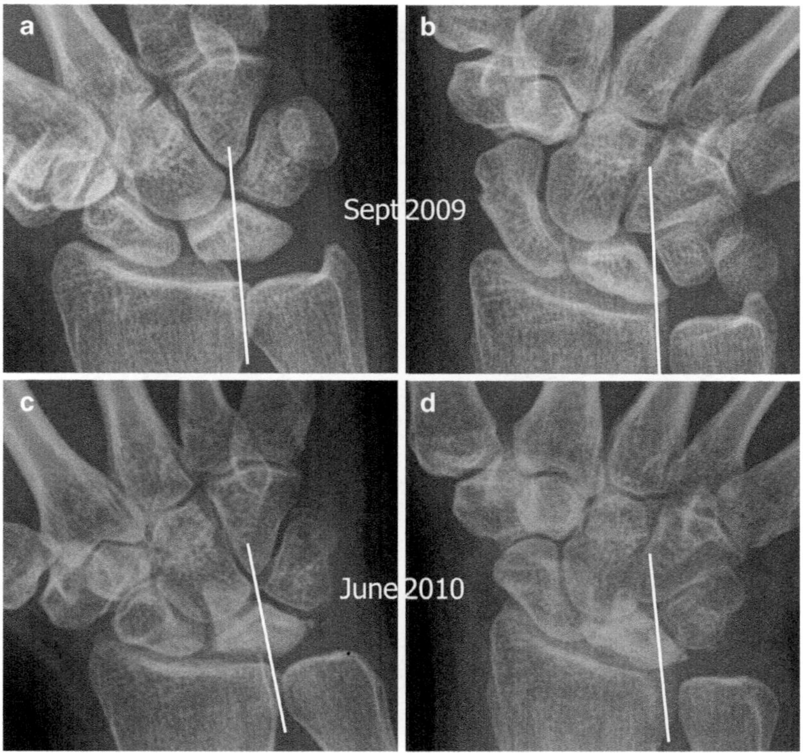

4 Differential Diagnosis

A coronal fracture of the L on coronal images (T1-WI) may resemble an AVN (Fig. 22).

Sagittal fractures of the L may also be confusing (Fig. 23). In that case, the central oedema (Eriksen and Ringe 2012; Margo and Seely 1963; Shabshin and Schweitzer 2009; Suh et al. 2018) pattern in anteroposterior direction on the axial image usually provides the solution.

Clinical and patient information may completely change the diagnosis. In the presented case, the clinician's question was "AVN?", which is obvious (Fig. 24a, b). However, the patient mainly complained about more recent ulnar sided pain and a recent resection of the pisiform bone was only mentioned afterwards (Fig. 24c–e).

The oedema pattern may also be confusing in a combination of lesions of the SL and TFCC (Fig. 25). Meticulous analysis may even lead towards a totally different imaging result (Fig. 26).

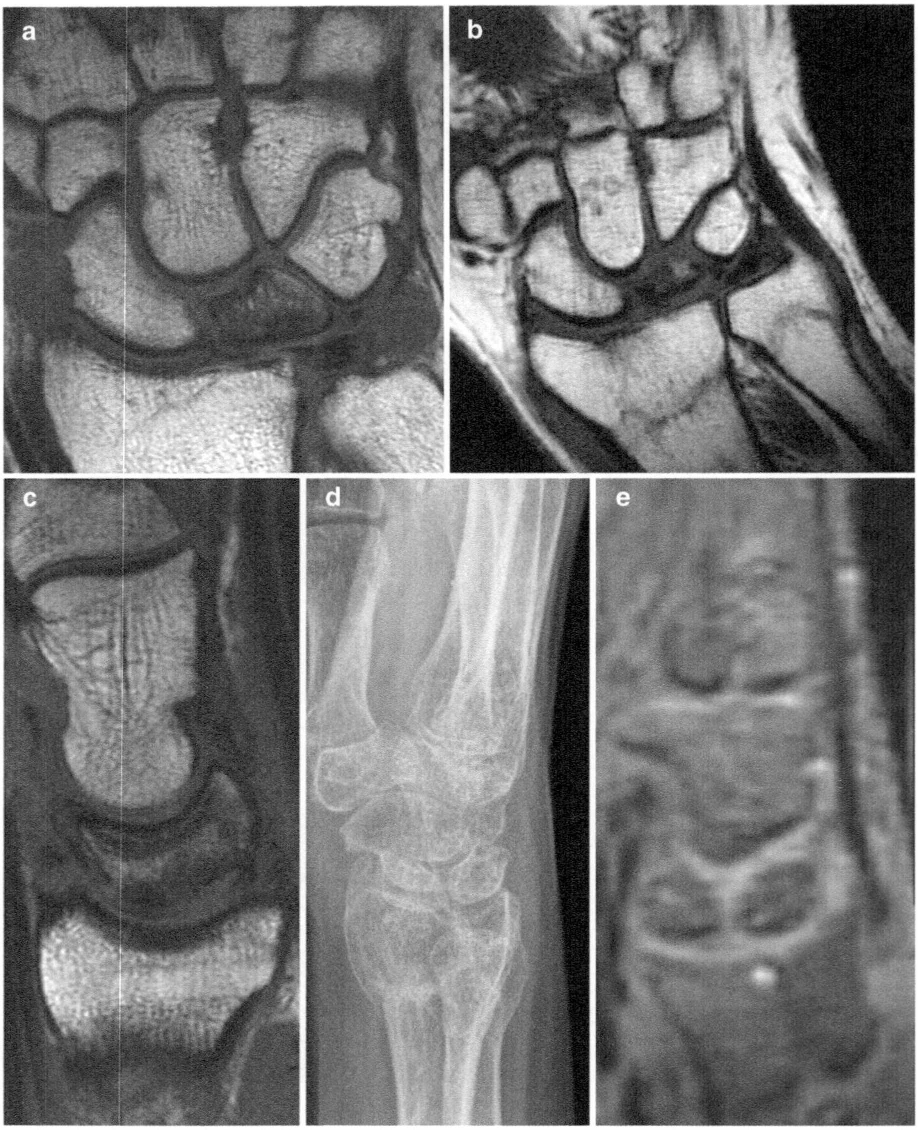

Fig. 22 Cor T1-WI (**a**, **b**); Sag T1-WI (**c**); Standard Lateral (**d**) views; Sag 3D GRE (**e**). An AVN of the L (**a**) and a sequel of a coronal fracture of the L (**b**) show both a low SI on coronal T1-WI. Sagittal imaging of the first patient shows an AVN of the L (**c**) and of the second patient sequelae of a coronal fracture of the L (**d**, **e**)

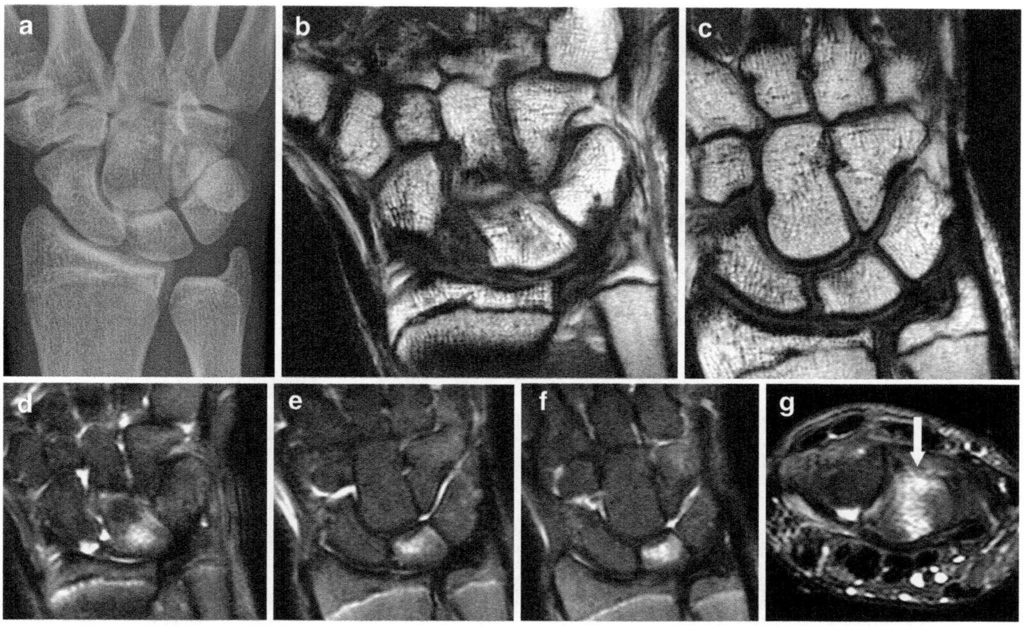

Fig. 23 Standard PA (**a**) view; Cor T1-WI (**b**, **c**); Cor T2-WI FS (**d**–**f**); Ax T2-WI FS (**g**). No abnormalities on the standard PA view (**a**) in an adolescent with vague pain. A hazy and limited oedema is noticed in the L (**b**–**f**). The oedema pattern in the axial image (**g**) from anterior to posterior is compatible with a sagittal L fracture

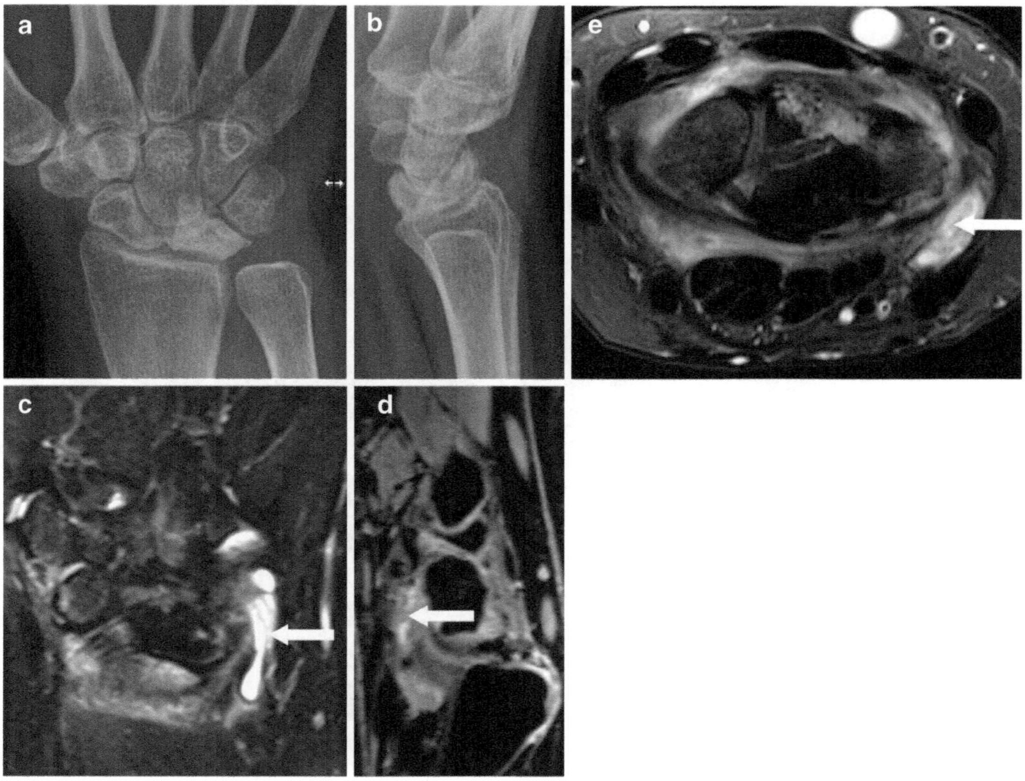

Fig. 24 Standard PA (**a**) and Lateral (**b**) view; Cor T2-WI FS (**c**); Sag 3D GRE (**d**); Ax T2-WI FS (**e**). Obvious AVN of the L (**a**, **b**). Fluid collection—liquefied hematoma after resection of the pisiform bone (**c**–**e**)

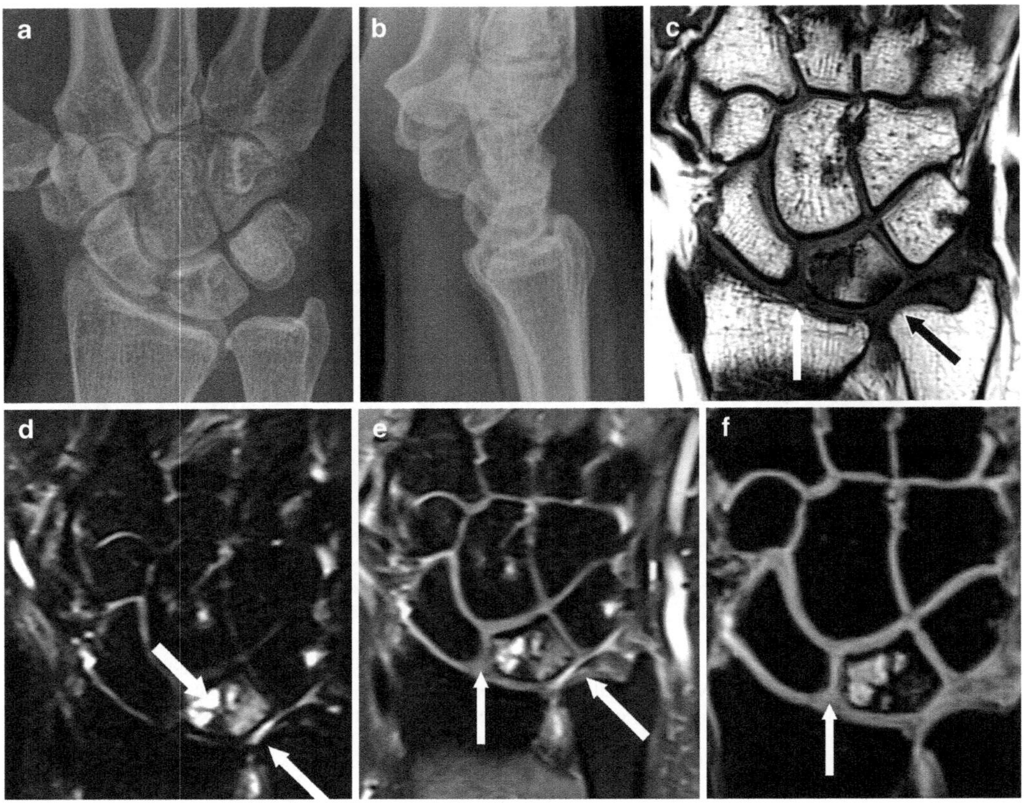

Fig. 25 Standard PA (**a**) and Lateral (**b**) view; Cor T1-WI (**c**), T2-WI FS (**d**), PD WI (**e**), and 3D GRE (**f**). Altered density (**a, b**) with bifocal oedema (**c–e**) at the radial and proximal-ulnar side of the L. Tear of the SL (**c, e, f**) and a Palmer lesion II E (**c–e**) with a positive ulnar variance (**a**)

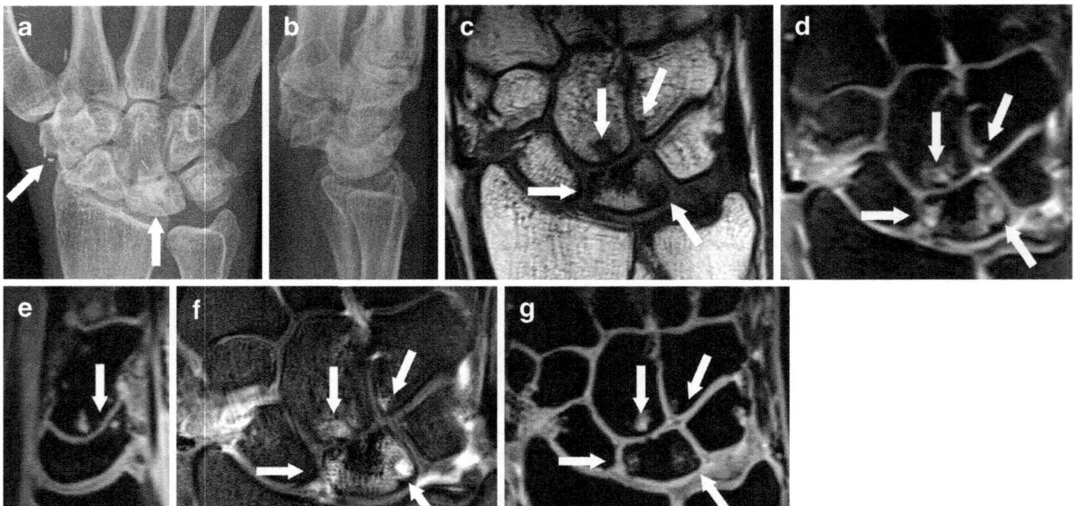

Fig. 26 Standard PA (**a**) and Lateral (**b**) view; Cor T1-WI (**c**), and T2-WI FS (**d**); Sag 3D GRE (**e**); Cor T1-WI FS with CE (**f**); Cor 3D GRE (**g**). Altered density of the L (**a, b**) and clips (**a**) after three operations for Kienbock and an STT-arthrodesis. Multifocal oedema in and around the L (**c, d**). Tear of the SL (**c, d, f, g**); dynamic UA (**c, d, f, g**) with a neutral ulnar variance (**a**); midcarpal OA (**c–g**); and incipient HLA (**c, d, f, g**)

5 Post-Operative Status

The evaluation of the post-operative status of the L (Fig. 27) or S (Fig. 28) remains a problem. The MRI marrow and soft tissue signals in general remain disturbed up to 6 months after surgery, CE may be present or absent, and remaining metal artefacts can disturb the images in an unpredictable way. However, the evolution to eventual collapse and/or fragmentation (Wilke and Kakar 2015) may be illustrated on MRI. Comparison with standard views and/or CT may be helpful in this difficult evaluation.

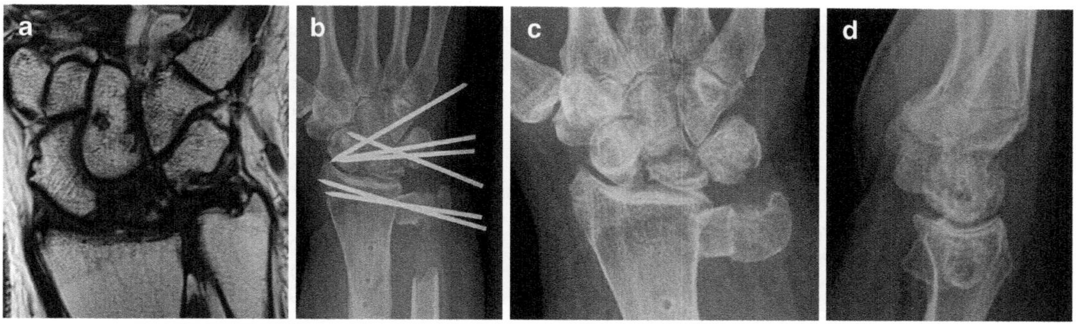

Fig. 27 Cor T1-WI (**a**); Standard PA (**b**, **c**) and Lateral (**d**) view. AVN of the L (**a**). Sauvé-Kapandji (SK) and carpal fixation procedure (**b**). Post-operative consolidation of SK (**c**, **d**). The status of the L is unclear

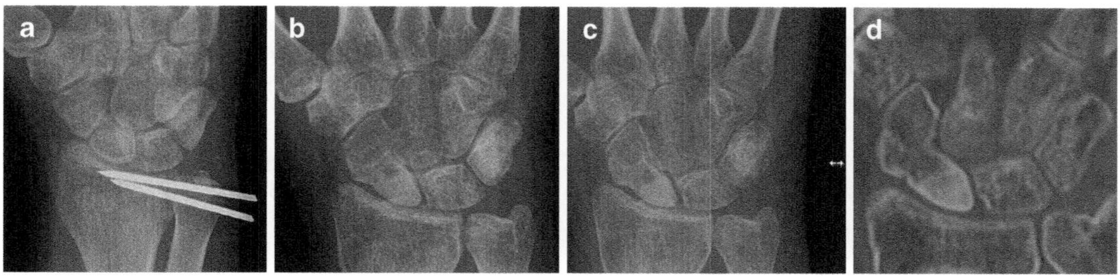

Fig. 28 Standard PA (**a–c**); Cor CT-image. Distal R-U fixation and scaphoid waist fracture on June 14th (**a**). AVN of the proximal pole of the S on August 4th (**b**) with increasing density on September 8th (**c**, **d**). No signs of fragmentation, nor collapse

References

Abascal F, Cerezal L, del Piñal F, García-Valtuille R, García-Valtuille A, Canga A, Torcida J (2001) Unilateral osteonecrosis in a patient with bilateral os centrale carpi: imaging findings. Skeletal Radiol 30(11):643–647. https://doi.org/10.1007/s002560100423. Epub 2001 Sep 14. PMID: 11810157

Arnaiz J, Piedra T, Cerezal L, Ward J, Thompson A, Vidal JA, Canga A (2014) Imaging of Kienböck disease. AJR Am J Roentgenol 203(1):131–139. https://doi.org/10.2214/AJR.13.11606. PMID: 24951206

De Smet L (1994) Ulnar variance: facts and fiction review article. Acta Orthop Belg 60(1):1–9. PMID: 8171975

Eriksen EF, Ringe JD (2012) Bone marrow lesions: a universal bone response to injury? Rheumatol Int 32(3):575–584. https://doi.org/10.1007/s00296-011-2141-2. Epub 2011 Sep 8. PMID: 21901347

Gelberman R, Richard H, Gross M (1986) The vascularity of the wrist: identification of arterial patterns at risk. Clin Orthop Relat Res 202:40–49

Goldfarb CA, Strauss NL, Wall LB, Calfee RP (2011) Defining ulnar variance in the adolescent wrist: measurement technique and interobserver reliability. J Hand Surg Am 36(2):272–277. https://doi.org/10.1016/j.jhsa.2010.11.008. PMID: 21276890

Hulten O (1928) Uber Anatomische Variationen der Handgelenkknochen. Acta Radiol 9(2):155–168. https://doi.org/10.3109/00016922809176658

Lichtman D, Lesley N, Simmons S (2010) The classification and treatment of Kienböck's disease: the state of the art and a look at the future. J Hand Surg Eur Vol 35(7):549–554

Margo MK, Seely JA (1963) A statistical review of 100 cases of fracture of the carpal navicular bone. Clin Orthop Relat Res 31:102–105. PMID: 5888847

Nakamura R, Tanaka Y, Imaeda T, Miura T (1991) The influence of age and sex on ulnar variance. J Hand Surg Br 16(1):84–88. https://doi.org/10.1016/0266-7681(91)90136-c. PMID: 2007823

Shabshin N, Schweitzer ME (2009) Age dependent T2 changes of bone marrow in pediatric wrist MRI. Skeletal Radiol 38(12):1163–1168. https://doi.org/10.1007/s00256-009-0752-4. Epub 2009 Aug 7. PMID: 19662404

Suh CH, Yun SJ, Jin W, Lee SH, Park SY, Ryu CW (2018) Diagnostic performance of dual-energy CT for the detection of bone marrow oedema: a systematic review and meta-analysis. Eur Radiol 28(10):4182–4194. https://doi.org/10.1007/s00330-018-5411-5. Epub 2018 Apr 20. PMID: 29679212

van Der Heijden B, Groot S, Schuurman AH (2005) Evaluation of ulnar styloid length. J Hand Surg Am 30(5):954–959. https://doi.org/10.1016/j.jhsa.2005.05.007. Erratum in: J Hand Surg [Am]. 2007 Jul-Aug;32(6):923. Groot, Sadra [corrected to Groot, Sandra]. PMID: 16182051

van Leeuwen WF, Oflazoglu K, Menendez ME, Ring D (2016) Negative ulnar variance and Kienböck disease. J Hand Surg Am 41(2):214–218. https://doi.org/10.1016/j.jhsa.2015.10.014. Epub 2015 Dec 11. PMID: 26686062

Wilke B, Kakar S (2015) Delayed avascular necrosis and fragmentation of the lunate following perilunate dislocation. Orthopedics 38(6):e539–e542. https://doi.org/10.3928/01477447-20150603-92. PMID: 26091230

Zapico A (1984) Enfermedad de Kienböck. Rev Ortop Trauma 28IB(3):353–355

TFCC Degeneration

Contents

1 Palmer Type II Lesions

TFC(C) (see also chapter "Ligament Injuries," Sect. 1) stands for triangular fibrocartilage (complex). The central degenerative tear at and around the TFC (Chong and Kandathil 2013; Anderson et al. 2008; Bille et al. 2007; Cerezal et al. 2005; Couzens et al. 2014; Davis and Blankenbaker 2010; De Filippo et al. 2010; Ekenstam and Hagert 1985; Girgis and Epstein 2000; Gornitzky and Carrigan 2016; Iordache et al. 2012; Lee et al. 2013; Luetkens et al. 2021; Mikić 1989; Nakamura 2012; Nakamura et al. 2001; Nevalainen et al. 2023; Oneson et al. 1997; Quinn et al. 1989; Ringler and Murthy 2015; Scheck et al. 1999; Spies et al. 2022; Theumann et al. 2001, 2006; Verhiel et al. 2022; Wang et al. 2023; Watanabe et al. 2010; Zanetti et al. 1997; Zlatkin and Rosner 2006) and its extent are evaluated on at least two perpendicular images. Degenerative tears are classified using the Palmer classification (Palmer 1989, 1990; Palmer and Werner 1981; Palmer et al. 1985; Goldfarb et al. 2011; Nakamura et al. 1991; Yaghoubian et al. 2001; Zhan et al. 2020) (Fig. 1).

Degenerative TFC(C) - lesions:

II A : wear / erosion of the central part (without perforation) of the TFC

II B = II A + lunar or ulnar chondromalacia*

II C : perforation of the TFC + *

II D = II C + LT ligament perforation

II E = II D + ulnocarpal osteoarthritis

Fig. 1 Palmer classification

The type II A tear (Fig. 2) with a central wear/erosion of the TFC may be very subtle. Thinning of the central zone of the TFC and a focal slightly higher T2/T1-signal are present. Fluid in the DRUJ should always be an alert sign (Fig. 2). Immediately, the ulnar length should be checked in the correct wrist position (Fig. 3b, c) to confirm or exclude an accompanying positive ulnar variance (Fig. 3b).

Chondromalacia of the lunate bone or ulna is added to a type II B lesion (Fig. 4).

M. Mespreuve, K. Waked, *MRI of the Wrist*, Medical Radiology,
https://doi.org/10.1007/978-3-031-63973-9_9

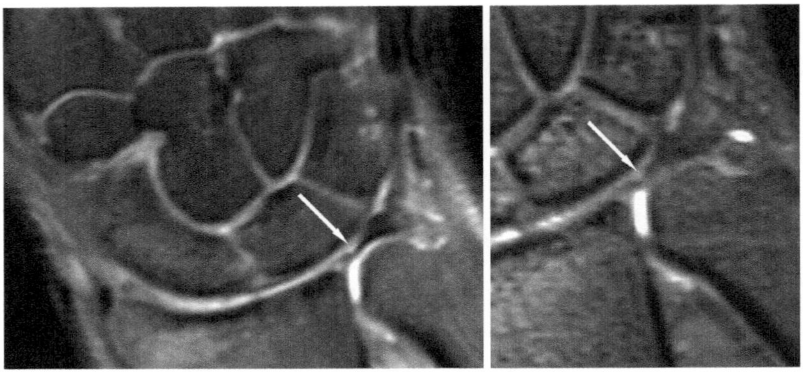

Fig. 2 Cor T2-WI FS. Palmer type II A wear/erosion of the central part of the TFC with hydrops at the DRUJ

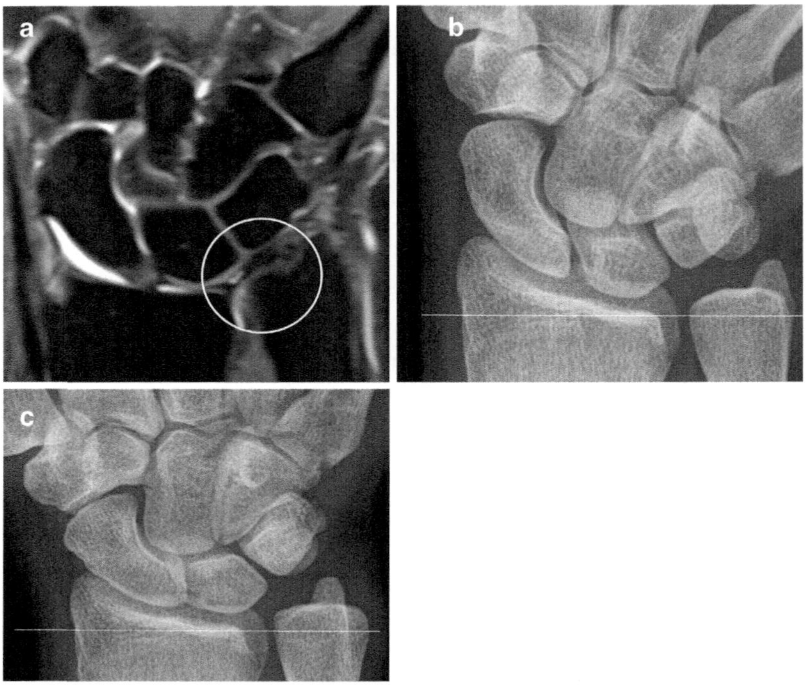

Fig. 3 Cor T2-WI FS (**a**); Standard PA correctly exposed ulnar styloid (**b**) versus the partially internally rotated styloid (**c**). Palmer type II A lesion (**a**) and a true positive ulnar variance (**b**) without pronation (**c**) of the ulna

The type II C has a central perforation of the TFC (Figs. 5 and 6), which needs to be quantified in size (Fig. 6). The difference between the II B and II C type may be a subject of discussion in case of small perforations. The absence of fluid in the defect may correlates to II B, whereas the presence of fluid defines a II C type.

When the LTL is also perforated (Fig. 7e), the lesion is upgraded to a II D type and, in case of ulnocarpal osteoarthritis (Fig. 7a, b), to a II E type.

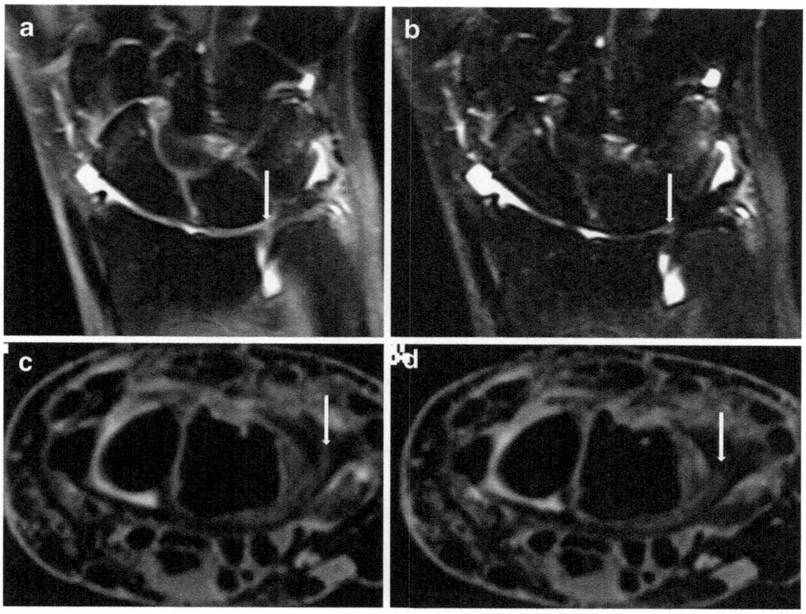

Fig. 4 Cor T2-WI FS (**a**, **b**); Ax 3D GRE (**c**, **d**). Palmer type II B lesion with a central wear and ulnar chondromalacia

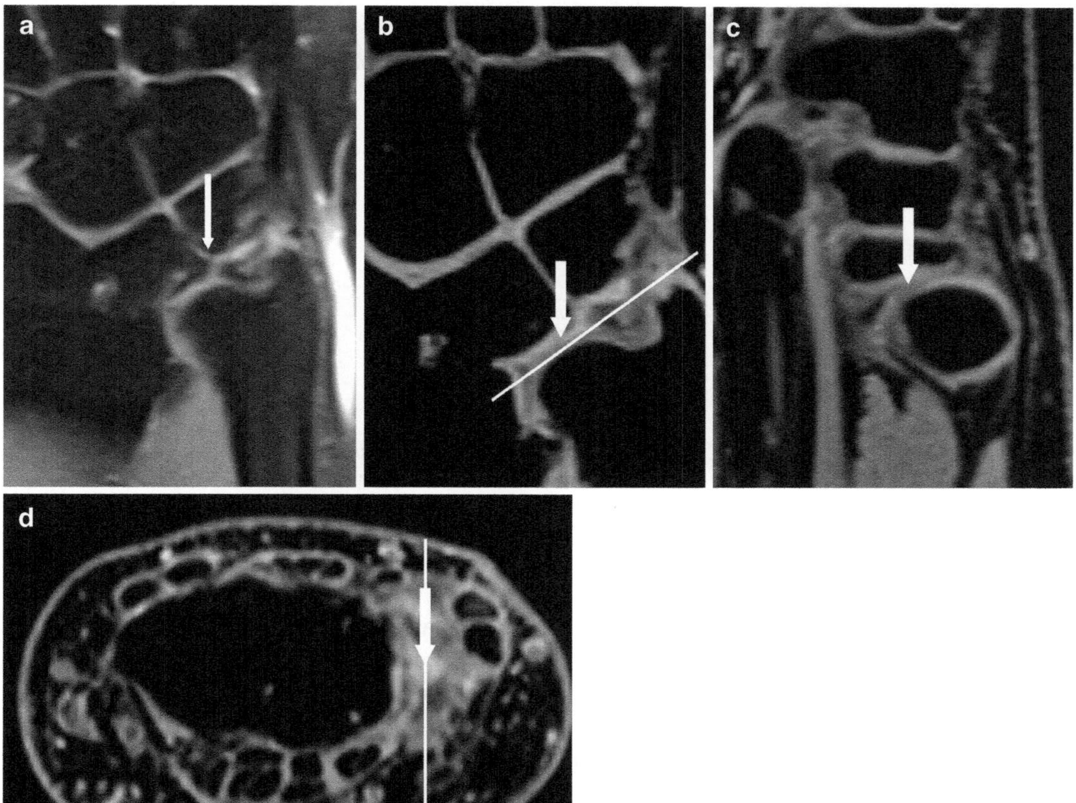

Fig. 5 Cor T2-WI FS (**a**) and 3D GRE (**b**); Sag (**c**) and Ax (**d**) 3D GRE. Palmer type II C lesion in 3D with a clear central defect in the TFC and blunt margins

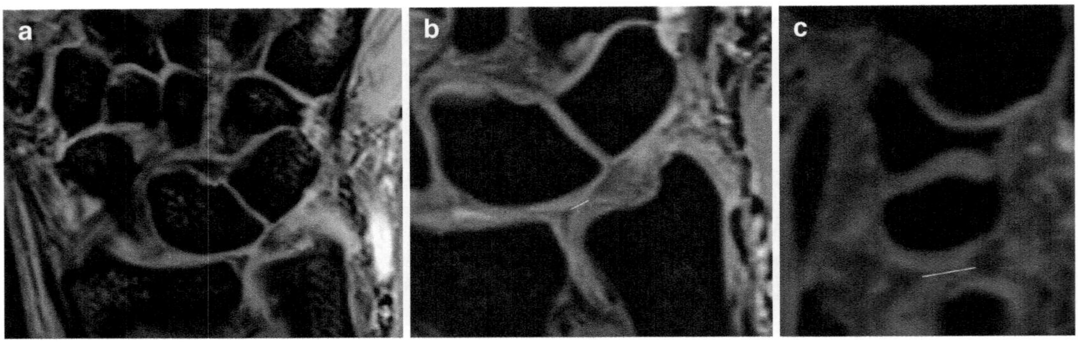

Fig. 6 Cor (**a**, **b**) and Sag (**c**) 3D GRE. Evaluation of the 2D-size of a Palmer type II C lesion

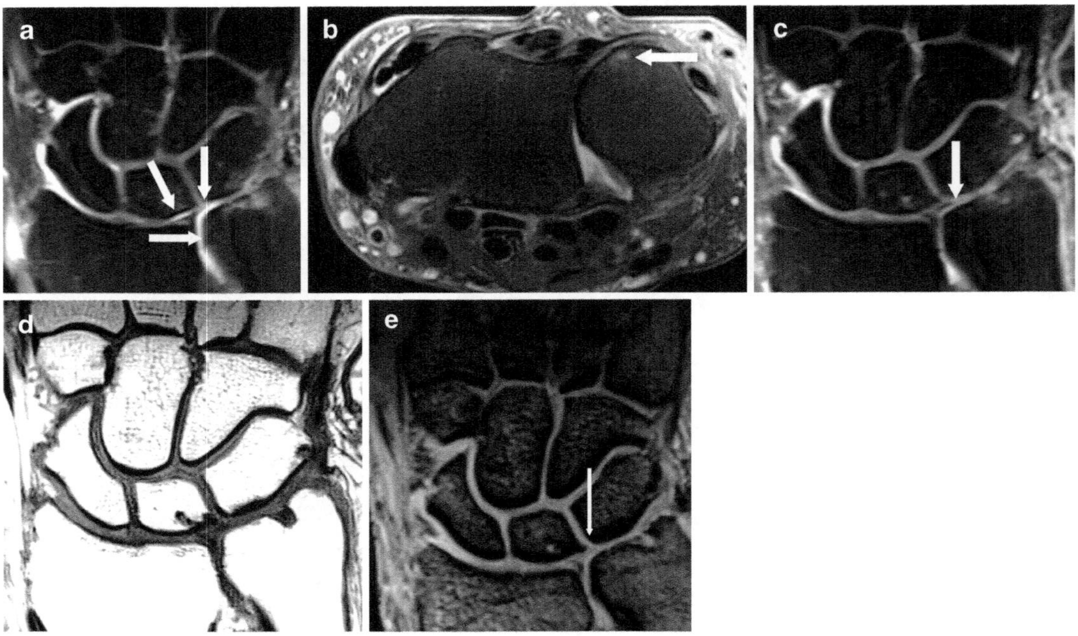

Fig. 7 Cor (**a**) and Ax (**b**) T2-WI FS; Cor T2-WI FS (**c**), T1-WI (**d**); and 2D GRE (**e**). Palmer type II E lesion with a clear central defect in the TFC (**a**, **b**), ulnar (**b**), and lunar (**c**) chondromalacia, LTL perforation (**d**, **e**), and ulnocarpal osteoarthritis (**a**, **b**)

2 Additional Lesions

Long-standing and substantial degenerative lesions may be accompanied (Gillis et al. 2019; Mannil et al. 2016; Reghunath et al. 2022; Yoshioka et al. 2007) by extensive hydrops and secondary osteochondromatosis (Adams and Berger 2002) (Fig. 8). A degenerative cyst may arise from the TFC (Fig. 9).

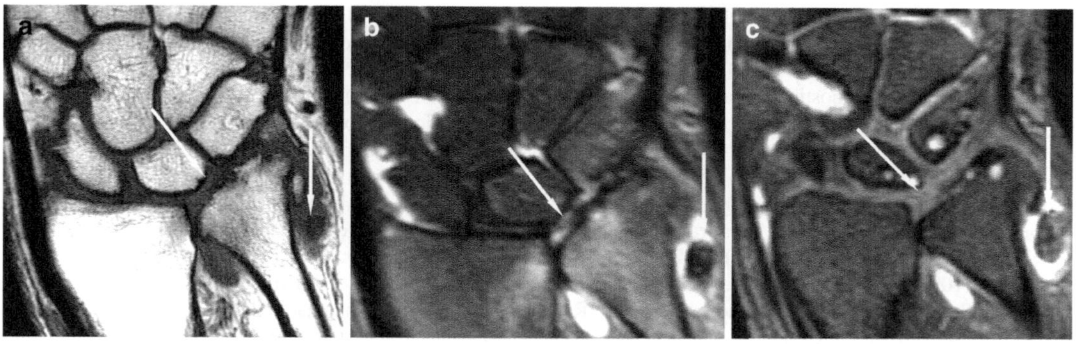

Fig. 8 Cor T1-WI (**a**), T2-WI FS (**b**), and 3D GRE (**c**). Palmer type II E lesion with secondary osteochondromatosis and hydrops in the distended DRUJ

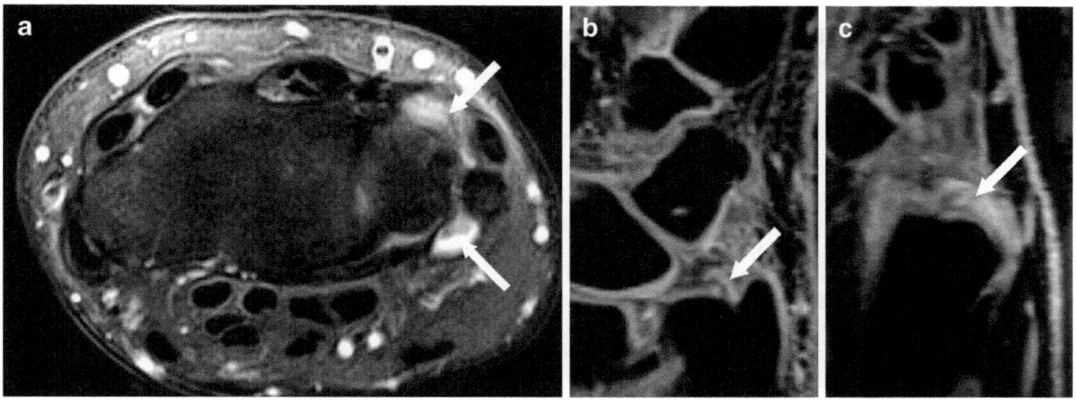

Fig. 9 Ax T2-WI FS (**a**); Cor (**b**) and Sag (**c**) 3D GRE. Degenerative cyst of TFC

References

Adams BD, Berger RA (2002) An anatomic reconstruction of the distal radioulnar ligaments for posttraumatic distal radioulnar joint instability. J Hand Surg Am 27(2):243–251. https://doi.org/10.1053/jhsu.2002.31731. PMID: 11901383

Anderson ML, Skinner JA, Felmlee JP, Berger RA, Amrami KK (2008) Diagnostic comparison of 1.5 Tesla and 3.0 Tesla preoperative MRI of the wrist in patients with ulnar-sided wrist pain. J Hand Surg Am 33(7):1153–1159. https://doi.org/10.1016/j.jhsa.2008.02.028. PMID: 18762112

Bille B, Harley B, Cohen H (2007) A comparison of CT arthrography of the wrist to findings during wrist arthroscopy. J Hand Surg Am 32(6):834–841. https://doi.org/10.1016/j.jhsa.2007.04.005. PMID: 17606063

Cerezal L, Abascal F, García-Valtuille R, Del Piñal F (2005) Wrist MR arthrography: how, why, when. Radiol Clin North Am 43(4):709–731. https://doi.org/10.1016/j.rcl.2005.02.004, viii. PMID: 15893533

Chong C, Kandathil JC (2013) MR imaging of TFCC, what every radiologist need to know. Eur Congress of Radiology:poster C-1841. https://doi.org/10.1594/ecr2013/C-1841

Couzens G, Daunt N, Crawford R, Ross M (2014) Positive magnetic resonance imaging findings in the asymptomatic wrist. ANZ J Surg 84(7–8):528–532. https://doi.org/10.1111/ans.12552. Epub 2014 Feb 26. PMID: 24612468

Davis KW, Blankenbaker DG (2010) Imaging the ligaments and tendons of the wrist. Semin Roentgenol 45(3):194–217. https://doi.org/10.1053/j.ro.2009.12.005. PMID: 20483115

De Filippo M, Pogliacomi F, Bertellini A, Araoz PA, Averna R, Sverzellati N, Ingegnoli A, Corradi M, Costantino C, Zompatori M (2010) MDCT arthrography of the wrist: diagnostic accuracy and indications. Eur J Radiol 74(1):221–225. https://doi.org/10.1016/j.ejrad.2009.01.023. Epub 2009 Feb 23. PMID: 19233582

Ekenstam F, Hagert CG (1985) Anatomical studies on the geometry and stability of the distal radio ulnar joint. Scand J Plast Reconstr Surg 19(1):17–25. https://doi.org/10.3109/02844318509052861. PMID: 4023639

Gillis JA, Soreide E, Khouri JS, Kadar A, Berger RA, Moran SL (2019) Outcomes of the Adams-Berger ligament reconstruction for the distal radioulnar joint instability in 95 consecutive cases. J Wrist Surg 8(4):268–275. https://doi.org/10.1055/s--0039-1685235. Epub 2019 Apr 22. PMID: 31404256; PMCID: PMC6685731

Girgis WS, Epstein RE (2000) Magnetic resonance imaging of the hand and wrist. Semin Roentgenol 35(3):286–296. https://doi.org/10.1053/sroe.2000.7339. PMID: 10939130

Goldfarb CA, Strauss NL, Wall LB, Calfee RP (2011) Defining ulnar variance in the adolescent wrist: measurement technique and interobserver reliability. J Hand Surg Am 36(2):272–277. https://doi.org/10.1016/j.jhsa.2010.11.008. PMID: 21276890

Gornitzky AL, Carrigan RB (2016) The diagnostic utility of MRI in the painful wrist: when to reconsider advanced imaging in the pediatric patient. Pediatrics (Evanston) 137(Suppl 3):596–596A. https://doi.org/10.1542/peds.137.Supplement_3.596A

Iordache SD, Rowan R, Garvin GJ, Osman S, Grewal R, Faber KJ (2012) Prevalence of triangular fibrocartilage complex abnormalities on MRI scans of asymptomatic wrists. J Hand Surg Am 37(1):98–103. https://doi.org/10.1016/j.jhsa.2011.10.006. Epub 2011 Nov 30. PMID: 22129657

Lee YH, Choi YR, Kim S, Song HT, Suh JS (2013) Intrinsic ligament and triangular fibrocartilage complex (TFCC) tears of the wrist: comparison of isovolumetric 3D-THRIVE sequence MR arthrography and conventional MR image at 3 T. Magn Reson Imaging 31(2):221–226. https://doi.org/10.1016/j.mri.2012.06.024. Epub 2012 Sep 7. PMID: 22959873

Luetkens KS, Laas SF, Haßler S, Gassenmaier T, Gietzen CH, Christopoulos G, Huflage H, Kunz AS, Bley TA, Schmitt R, Grunz JP (2021) Contrast-enhanced MRI of the wrist: intravenous application of gadolinium improves diagnosis in ulnar-sided injuries of the TFCC. Eur J Radiol 143:109901. https://doi.org/10.1016/j.ejrad.2021.109901. Epub 2021 Aug 10. PMID: 34392004

Mannil L, Martin W, Dahmen J, Witte T, Juten PG, Deneken F, Räder M, Homann HH (2016) Arthroscopic treatment for ulnar-sided TFCC-tears. Eur J Trauma Emerg Surg 42(1):29–35. https://doi.org/10.1007/s00068-015-0593-x. Epub 2015 Nov 13. PMID: 26566794

Mikić ZD (1989) Detailed anatomy of the articular disc of the distal radioulnar joint. Clin Orthop Relat Res 245:123–132. PMID: 2752612

Nakamura T (2012) Anatomy and biomechanics of the distal radioulnar joint (DRUJ). In: Arthroscopic management of ulnar pain. Springer, Heidelberg, pp 15–23. https://doi.org/10.1007/978-3-642-30544-3_2

Nakamura R, Tanaka Y, Imaeda T, Miura T (1991) The influence of age and sex on ulnar variance. J Hand Surg Br 16(1):84–88. https://doi.org/10.1016/0266-7681(91)90136-c. PMID: 2007823

Nakamura T, Takayama S, Horiuchi Y, Yabe Y (2001) Origins and insertions of the triangular fibrocartilage complex: a histological study. J Hand Surg Br 26(5):446–454. https://doi.org/10.1054/jhsb.2001.0562. PMID: 11560427

Nevalainen MT, Zoga AC, Rivlin M, Morrison WB, Roedl JB (2023) Extensor carpi ulnaris tendon pathology and ulnar styloid bone marrow edema as diagnostic markers of peripheral triangular fibrocartilage complex tears on wrist MRI: a case-control study. Eur Radiol 33(5):3172–3177. https://doi.org/10.1007/s00330-023-09446-x. Epub 2023 Feb 21. PMID: 36809434; PMCID: PMC10121535

Oneson SR, Timins ME, Scales LM, Erickson SJ, Chamoy L (1997) MR imaging diagnosis of triangular fibrocartilage pathology with arthroscopic correlation. AJR Am J Roentgenol 168(6):1513–1518. https://doi.org/10.2214/ajr.168.6.9168716. PMID: 9168716

Palmer AK (1989) Triangular fibrocartilage complex lesions: a classification. J Hand Surg Am 14(4):594–606. https://doi.org/10.1016/0363-5023(89)90174-3. PMID: 2666492

Palmer AK (1990) Triangular fibrocartilage disorders: injury patterns and treatment. Arthroscopy 6(2):125–132. https://doi.org/10.1016/0749-8063(90)90013-4. PMID: 2363780

Palmer AK, Werner FW (1981) The triangular fibrocartilage complex of the wrist – anatomy and function. J Hand Surg Am 6(2):153–162. https://doi.org/10.1016/s0363-5023(81)80170-0. PMID: 7229292

Palmer AK, Werner FW, Murphy D, Glisson R (1985) Functional wrist motion: a biomechanical study. J Hand Surg Am 10(1):39–46. https://doi.org/10.1016/s0363-5023(85)80246-x. PMID: 3968403

Quinn SF, Belsole RJ, Greene TL, Rayhack JM (1989) Advanced imaging of the wrist. Radiographics 9(2):229–246. https://doi.org/10.1148/radiographics.9.2.2928572. PMID: 2928572

Reghunath A, Singh DK, Aggarwal A, Babbar N, Choudhary R, Surya S (2022) MRI and MR arthrography imaging of the pathologies of the wrist: a pictorial essay. J Clin Diagn Res 16(12):TE01–TE07. https://doi.org/10.7860/JCDR/2022/59277.17323

Ringler MD, Murthy NS (2015) MR imaging of wrist ligaments. Magn Reson Imaging Clin N Am 23(3):367–391. https://doi.org/10.1016/j.mric.2015.04.007. PMID: 26216769

Scheck RJ, Romagnolo A, Hierner R, Pfluger T, Wilhelm K, Hahn K (1999) The carpal ligaments in MR arthrography of the wrist: correlation with standard MRI and wrist arthroscopy. J Magn Reson Imaging 9(3):468–474. https://doi.org/10.1002/(sici)1522-2586(199903)9:3<468::aid-jmri16>3.0.co;2-t. PMID: 10194719

Spies CK, Unglaub F, Bruckner T, Müller L, Eysel P, Rau J (2022) Diagnostic accuracy of wrist MRI in comparison to wrist arthroscopy regarding TFCC lesions in clinical practice. Arch Orthop Trauma Surg 142(5):879–885. https://doi.org/10.1007/s00402-021-04329-6. Epub 2022 Jan 10. PMID: 35006371

Theumann N, Favarger N, Schnyder P, Meuli R (2001) Wrist ligament injuries: value of post-arthrography computed tomography. Skeletal Radiol 30(2):88–93. https://doi.org/10.1007/s002560000302. PMID: 11310205

Theumann NH, Etechami G, Duvoisin B, Wintermark M, Schnyder P, Favarger N, Gilula LA (2006) Association between extrinsic and intrinsic carpal ligament injuries at MR arthrography and carpal instability at radiography: initial observations. Radiology 238(3):950–957. https://doi.org/10.1148/radiol.2383050013. Epub 2006 Jan 19. PMID: 16424247

Verhiel SHWL, Blackburn J, Ritt MJPF, Simeone FJ, Chen NC (2022) MRI findings in patients undergoing triangular fibrocartilage complex repairs versus patients without ulnar-sided wrist pain. Hand (N Y) 17(3):483–490. https://doi.org/10.1177/1558944720937369. Epub 2020 Jul 19. PMID: 32686539; PMCID: PMC9112747

Wang Z, Chen S, Liu B, Qian Z, Zhu J, Wang Q (2023) Abnormal MRI signal intensity of the triangular fibrocartilage complex in asymptomatic wrists. J Hand Surg Eur Vol 48(4):326–332. https://doi.org/10.1177/17531934221141986. Epub 2022 Dec 8. PMID: 36482744

Watanabe A, Souza F, Vezeridis PS, Blazar P, Yoshioka H (2010) Ulnar-sided wrist pain. II. Clinical imaging and treatment. Skeletal Radiol 39(9):837–857. https://doi.org/10.1007/s00256-009-0842-3. Epub 2009 Dec 10. PMID: 20012039; PMCID: PMC2904904

Yaghoubian R, Goebel F, Musgrave DS, Sotereanos DG (2001) Diagnosis and management of acute fracture-dislocation of the carpus. Orthop Clin North Am 32(2):295–305. https://doi.org/10.1016/s0030-5898(05)70250-9, viii. PMID: 11331542

Yoshioka H, Tanaka T, Ueno T, Carrino JA, Winalski CS, Aliabadi P, Lang P, Weissman BN (2007) Study of ulnar variance with high-resolution MRI: correlation with triangular fibrocartilage complex and cartilage of ulnar side of wrist. J Magn Reson Imaging 26(3):714–719. https://doi.org/10.1002/jmri.21084. PMID: 17729368

Zanetti M, Bräm J, Hodler J (1997) Triangular fibrocartilage and intercarpal ligaments of the wrist: does MR arthrography improve standard MRI? J Magn Reson Imaging 7(3):590–594. https://doi.org/10.1002/jmri.1880070322. PMID: 9170047

Zhan H, Bai R, Qian Z, Yang Y, Zhang H, Yin Y (2020) Traumatic injury of the triangular fibrocartilage complex (TFCC)-a refinement to the Palmer classification by using high-resolution 3-T MRI. Skeletal Radiol 49(10):1567–1579. https://doi.org/10.1007/s00256-020-03438-4. Epub 2020 May 5. PMID: 32372253

Zlatkin MB, Rosner J (2006) MR imaging of ligaments and triangular fibrocartilage complex of the wrist. Radiol Clin North Am 44(4):595–623. https://doi.org/10.1016/j.rcl.2006.04.010, ix. PMID: 16829252

Cartilage

Contents

Indirect, abnormal (restricted) motion signs, such as degenerative sclerotic lining, marginal osteophytes, subchondral cysts, and thinning of the joint space at the radiocarpal joint are obvious (Bhat et al. 2011; Loredo et al. 2005) (Fig. 1a). On standard views, suspected (Fig. 1a, b), or unsuspected (Fig. 2a, b) degenerative changes become clear on MRI—especially the extent—at unusual carpal locations (Arora et al. 2010; Balci et al. 2015; Bell et al. 1985; Cerezal et al. 2005; Eriksen and Ringe 2012; Gondim Teixeira et al. 2016; Gornitzky and Carrigan 2016; Hunt 2006; Lee et al. 2021; Lok et al. 2014; Mutimer et al. 2008; Ochman et al. 2017; Ramdhian-Wihlm et al. 2012; Reghunath et al. 2022; Ruston et al. 2013; Schmitt et al. 2003; Zheng et al. 2010) (Figs. 1c, d and 2c–f).

In general, too little attention is paid the TP joint. (Isolated) degenerative changes are frequently discovered as such (Anderson et al. 2008; Kofman et al. 2014) (Fig. 3), eventually with secondary degenerative (osteo)chondromatosis. Differentiation of primary synovial (osteo)chondromatosis (Fig. 4) with more fragments (usually of the same size) in the joint of a younger patient without degenerative associated abnormalities is not always possible in the earlier phase. Moreover, the visibility of the IA fragments depends on the low(er) T1/T2 signal related to the degree of calcification.

M. Mespreuve, K. Waked, *MRI of the Wrist*, Medical Radiology,
https://doi.org/10.1007/978-3-031-63973-9_10

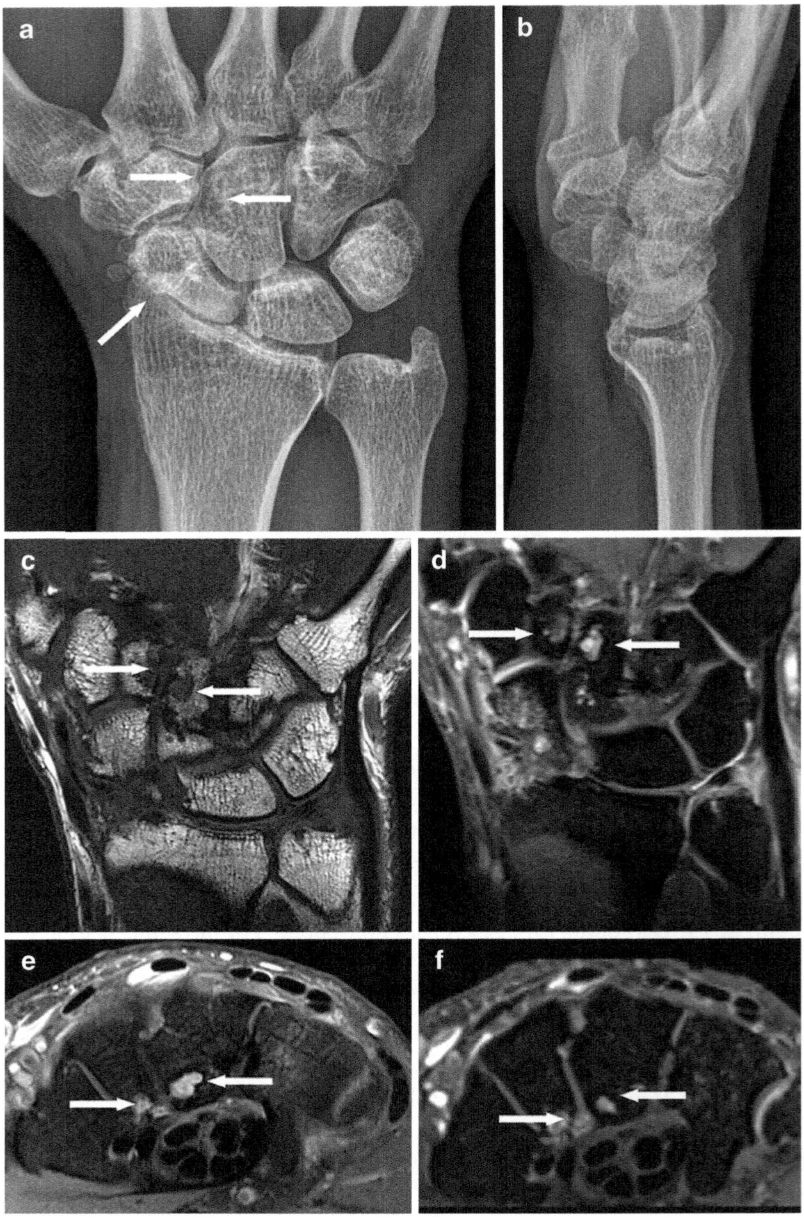

Fig. 1 Standard PA (**a**) and Lateral (**b**) views; Cor T1-WI (**c**) and T2-WI FS (**d**); Ax T2-WI FS (**e**) and 3D GRE (**f**). Degenerative cartilage thinning radiocarpal (**a**). Subchondral juxta-articular cysts tra-C (**a**, **c**–**f**)

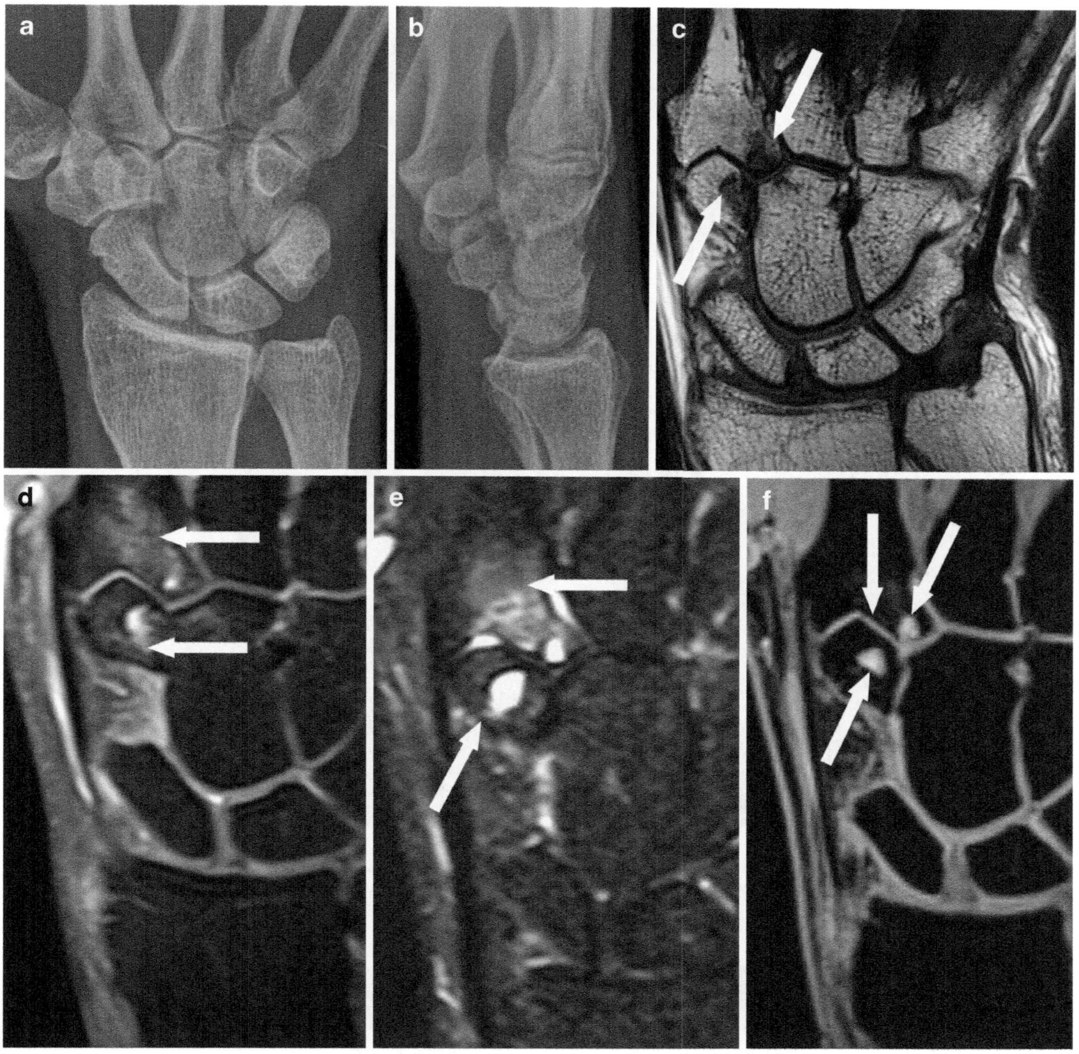

Fig. 2 Standard PA (**a**) and lateral (**b**) views; Cor T1-WI (**c**), T2-WI FS (**e**); and 3D GRE (**d**, **f**). Degenerative cartilage thinning CMC II (**a**) with subchondral juxta-articular cysts of the tra (**c**, **e**) and surrounding BMO (**d**, **e**)

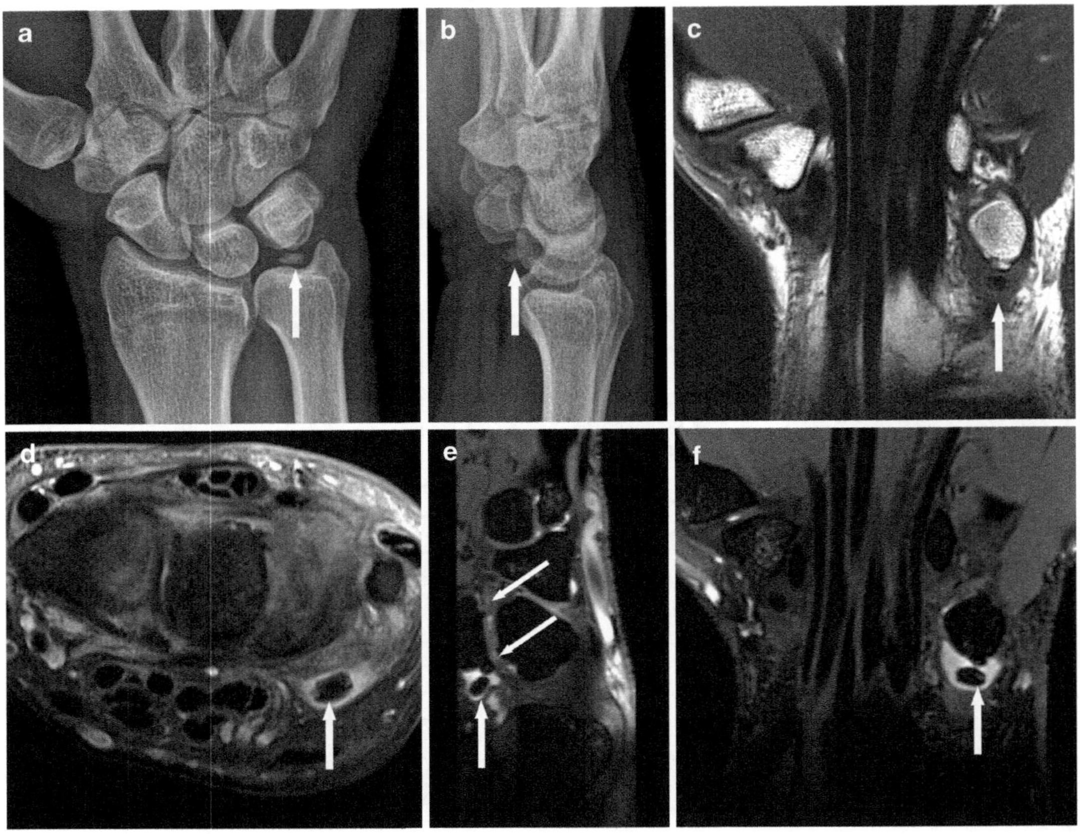

Fig. 3 Standard PA (**a**) and lateral (**b**) views; Cor T1-WI (**c**) and T2-WI FS (**d**); Sag (**e**) and Cor (**f**) 3D GRE. Loose bone fragment proximal from the TP joint (**a–f**) with capsular distension and hydrops (**c–f**) and marginal osteophytes (**e**)

Fig. 4 Standard PA (**a**) and lateral (**b**) views; Cor T1-WI (**c**) and T2-WI FS (**d**). Loose bone fragments (**a**, **b**) in the RC joint and its prestyloid capsule recessus (**c**, **d**) without obvious degenerative changes

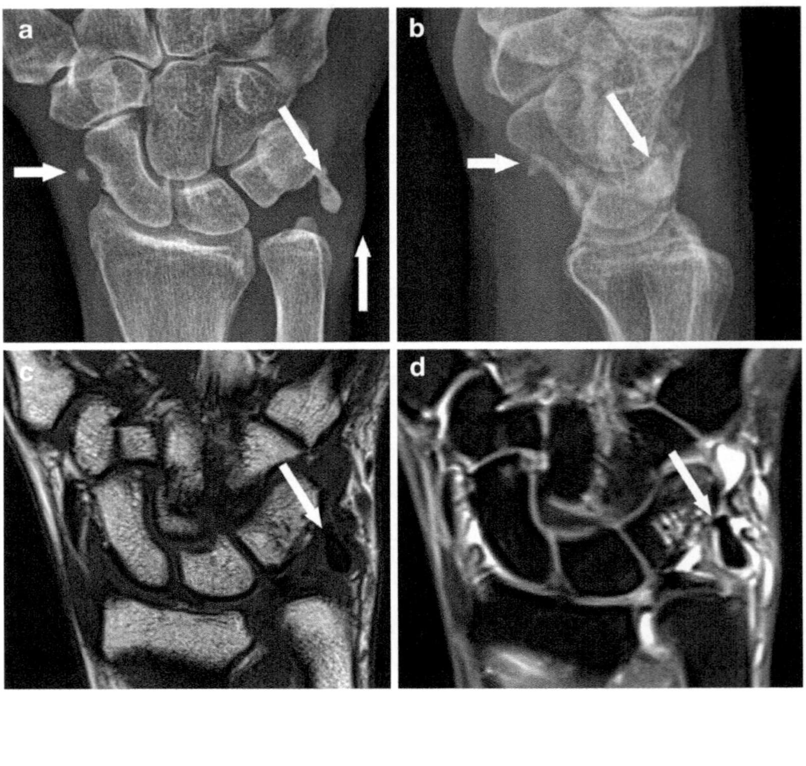

References

Anderson ML, Skinner JA, Felmlee JP, Berger RA, Amrami KK (2008) Diagnostic comparison of 1.5 Tesla and 3.0 Tesla preoperative MRI of the wrist in patients with ulnar-sided wrist pain. J Hand Surg Am 33(7):1153–1159. https://doi.org/10.1016/j.jhsa.2008.02.028. PMID: 18762112

Arora S, Grover SB, Batra S, Sharma VK (2010) Comparative evaluation of postreduction intra-articular distal radial fractures by radiographs and multidetector computed tomography. J Bone Joint Surg Am 92(15):2523–2532. https://doi.org/10.2106/JBJS.I.01617. PMID: 21048172

Balci A, Basara I, Çekdemir EY, Tetik F, Aktaş G, Acarer A, Özaksoy D (2015) Wrist fractures: sensitivity of radiography, prevalence, and patterns in MDCT. Emerg Radiol 22(3):251–256. https://doi.org/10.1007/s10140-014-1278-1. Epub 2014 Oct 18. PMID: 25325932

Bell MJ, Hill RJ, McMurtry RY (1985) Ulnar impingement syndrome. J Bone Joint Surg Br 67(1):126–129. https://doi.org/10.1302/0301-620X.67B1.3968131. PMID: 3968131

Bhat AK, Kumar B, Acharya A (2011) Radiographic imaging of the wrist. Indian J Plast Surg 44(2):186–196. https://doi.org/10.4103/0970-0358.85339. PMID: 22022028; PMCID: PMC3193630

Cerezal L, Abascal F, García-Valtuille R, Del Piñal F (2005) Wrist MR arthrography: how, why, when. Radiol Clin North Am 43(4):709–731. https://doi.org/10.1016/j.rcl.2005.02.004, viii. PMID: 15893533

Eriksen EF, Ringe JD (2012) Bone marrow lesions: a universal bone response to injury? Rheumatol Int 32(3):575–584. https://doi.org/10.1007/s00296-011-2141-2. Epub 2011 Sep 8. PMID: 21901347

Gondim Teixeira PA, De Verbizier J, Aptel S, Wack M, Dap F, Dautel G, Blum A (2016) Posterior radioscaphoid angle as a predictor of wrist degenerative joint disease in patients with scapholunate ligament tears. AJR Am J Roentgenol 206(1):144–150. https://doi.org/10.2214/AJR.15.14606. PMID: 26700346

Gornitzky AL, Carrigan RB (2016) The diagnostic utility of MRI in the painful wrist: when to reconsider advanced imaging in the pediatric patient. Pediatrics (Evanston) 137(Suppl 3):596–596A. https://doi.org/10.1542/peds.137.Supplement_3.596A

Hunt TR 3rd (2006) Degenerative and post-traumatic arthritis affecting the carpometacarpal joints of the fingers. Hand Clin 22(2):221–228. https://doi.org/10.1016/j.hcl.2006.02.004. PMID: 16701136

Kofman KE, Schuurman AH, Mulder MC, Verlinde SA, Gierman LM, van Diest PJ, Bleys RL (2014) The pisotriquetral joint: osteoarthritis and enthesopathy. J Hand Microsurg 6(1):18–25. https://doi.org/10.1007/s12593-014-0129-3. Epub 2014 Apr 18. PMID: 24876685; PMCID: PMC4037443

Lee GE, Forster GL, Freilich AM, DeGeorge BR Jr (2021) Magnetic resonance arthrography of the wrist: the impact on operative management of wrist injuries. J Wrist Surg 11(2):120–126. https://doi.org/10.1055/s-0041-1735305. PMID: 35478944; PMCID: PMC9038300

Lok RL, Griffith JF, Ng AW, Wong CW (2014) Imaging of radial wrist pain. Part II: pathology. Skeletal Radiol 43(6):725–743. https://doi.org/10.1007/s00256-014-1826-5. Epub 2014 Feb 14. PMID: 24522772

Loredo RA, Sorge DG, Garcia G (2005) Radiographic evaluation of the wrist: a vanishing art. Semin Roentgenol 40(3):248–289. https://doi.org/10.1053/j.ro.2005.01.014. PMID: 16060116

Mutimer J, Green J, Field J (2008) Comparison of MRI and wrist arthroscopy for assessment of wrist cartilage. J Hand Surg Eur Vol 33(3):380–382. https://doi.org/10.1177/1753193408090395. PMID: 18562375

Ochman S, Wieskötter B, Langer M, Vieth V, Raschke MJ, Stehling C (2017) High-resolution MRI (3T-MRI) in diagnosis of wrist pain: is diagnostic arthroscopy still necessary? Arch Orthop Trauma Surg 137(10):1443–1450. https://doi.org/10.1007/s00402-017-2747-2. Epub 2017 Aug 14. PMID: 2880876

Ramdhian-Wihlm R, Le Minor JM, Schmittbuhl M, Jeantroux J, Mahon PM, Veillon F, Dosch JC, Dietemann JL, Bierry G (2012) Cone-beam computed tomography arthrography: an innovative modality for the evaluation of wrist ligament and cartilage injuries. Skeletal Radiol 41(8):963–969. https://doi.org/10.1007/s00256-011-1305-1. Epub 2011 Nov 8. PMID: 22064983

Reghunath A, Singh DK, Aggarwal A, Babbar N, Choudhary R, Surya S (2022) MRI and MR arthrography imaging of the pathologies of the wrist: a pictorial essay. J Clin Diagn Res 16(12):TE01–TE07. https://doi.org/10.7860/JCDR/2022/59277.17323

Ruston J, Konan S, Rubinraut E, Sorene E (2013) Diagnostic accuracy of clinical examination and magnetic resonance imaging for common articular wrist pathology. Acta Orthop Belg 79(4):375–380. PMID: 24205765

Schmitt R, Christopoulos G, Meier R, Coblenz G, Fröhner S, Lanz U, Krimmer H (2003) Direkte MR-Arthrographie des Handgelenks im Vergleich zur Arthroskopie: Eine prospektive Studie an 125 Patienten [Direct MR arthrography of the wrist in comparison with arthroscopy: a prospective study on 125 patients]. Rofo 175(7):911–919. https://doi.org/10.1055/s-2003-40434. German. PMID: 12847645

Zheng ZZ, Shan H, Li X (2010) Fat-suppressed 3D T1-weighted gradient-echo imaging of the cartilage with a volumetric interpolated breath-hold examination. AJR Am J Roentgenol 194(5):W414–W419. https://doi.org/10.2214/AJR.09.2423. PMID: 20410387

Abutment Syndromes (AS)

Contents

The location at which two or more bones border and abut another may suffer from bone impaction. The bone marrow oedema and resulting spongiosa inflammation causes a local high signal on a T2-WI FS (Fig. 1a) and a low signal on T1-WI (Fig. 1b).

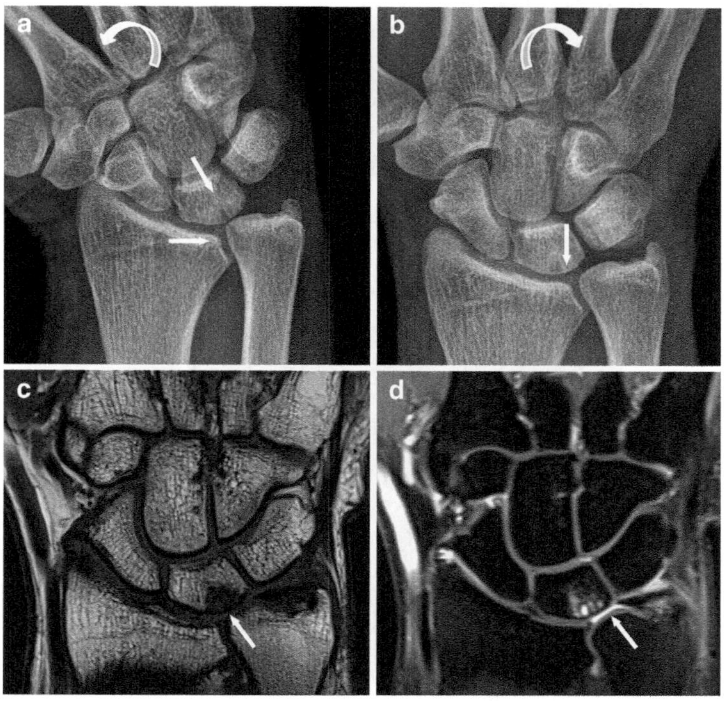

Fig. 1 Standard PA view in radial (**a**) and ulnar (**b**) deviation; Cor T1-WI (**c**); Cor T2-WI FS (**d**). Bone marrow oedema at the ulnar side of the lunate bone

M. Mespreuve, K. Waked, *MRI of the Wrist*, Medical Radiology,
https://doi.org/10.1007/978-3-031-63973-9_11

A primary AS is a consequence of the anatomical status, while a secondary AS results from deformed anatomical bony elements and/or disturbed interosseus relations.

1 Primary Abutment Syndromes

1. **Ulnar abutment syndrome** is the most common primary AS and is due to the abutment of the distal ulna on the ulnar side of the proximal part of the lunate bone (Bhat et al. 2011; Cerezal et al. 2004; Couzens et al. 2014; Eriksen and Ringe 2012) (Fig. 1, 4a).

   Initially, changes may be limited to oedema of the thickened cartilage at the ulnar side of the L (Fig. 2) with an intact triangular fibrocartilage. Progression of this ulnar abutment will lead to chondromalacia with subchondral degenerative cysts, thinning of the cartilage at the ulnar side of the lunate, central perforation of the TFC, and lunotriquetral ligament perforation (Fig. 3).

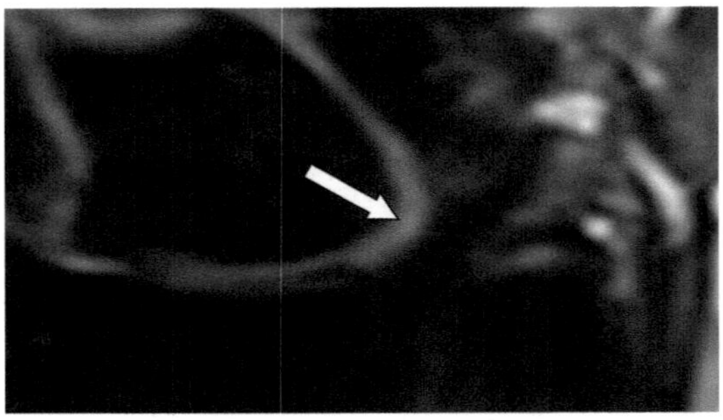

Fig. 2 Cor T2-WI FS. Oedema of the cartilage at the ulnar side of the lunate bone

   The ulnar impacted side of the L will enhance in most cases of UA (Fig. 4b, c), but CE is not needed for the diagnosis. Note that avascular necrosis, sometimes considered in the clinical differential diagnosis, starts at the radial side of the L (Fig. 17).

   Classically, a positive ulnar variance (Goldfarb et al. 2011; Hulten 1928) is found in UA (Fig. 4d). The evaluation of the ulnar variance should always be made on standard PA view in a neutral position, using the Hulten criteria (Hulten 1928; Lawson 1985; Nakamura et al. 1991). A neutral (Fig. 5a), and even a negative (Fig. 6a), ulnar variance, however, do not exclude UA and is referred to as "dynamic ulnar abutment". The "length" of the ulna varies relative to the distal radius and is most pronounced in pronation.

   UA may also be a relatively rapid progressive phenomenon developing over months (Fig. 7). The impaction component may extend also to the triquetral bone (Tri) (Fig. 6b).
2. **Ulnotriquetral abutment** is considered if the ulnar abutment is exclusively centred on the triquetral bone (Cerezal et al. 2004; Eriksen and Ringe 2012) (Fig. 8).
3. **Stylotriquetral abutment** (Figs. 9 and 10) is related to the length of the ulnar styloid pro-

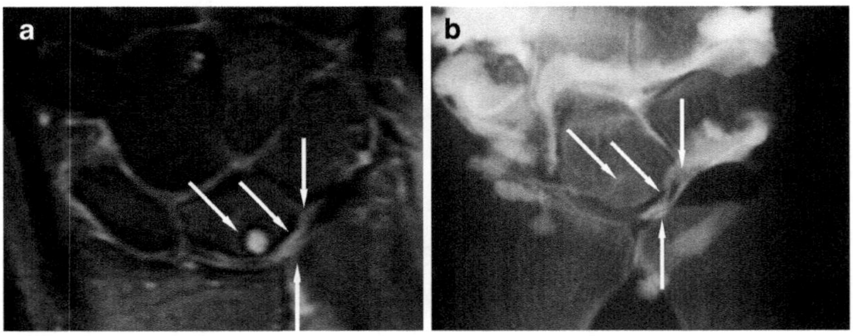

Fig. 3 Cor T2-WI FS (**a**); Corresponding arthrography (**b**). Chondromalacia with subchondral degenerative cyst and thinning of the cartilage at the ulnar side of the lunate (oblique arrows), central perforation of the TFC (ascending arrow) and LTL perforation (descending arrow)

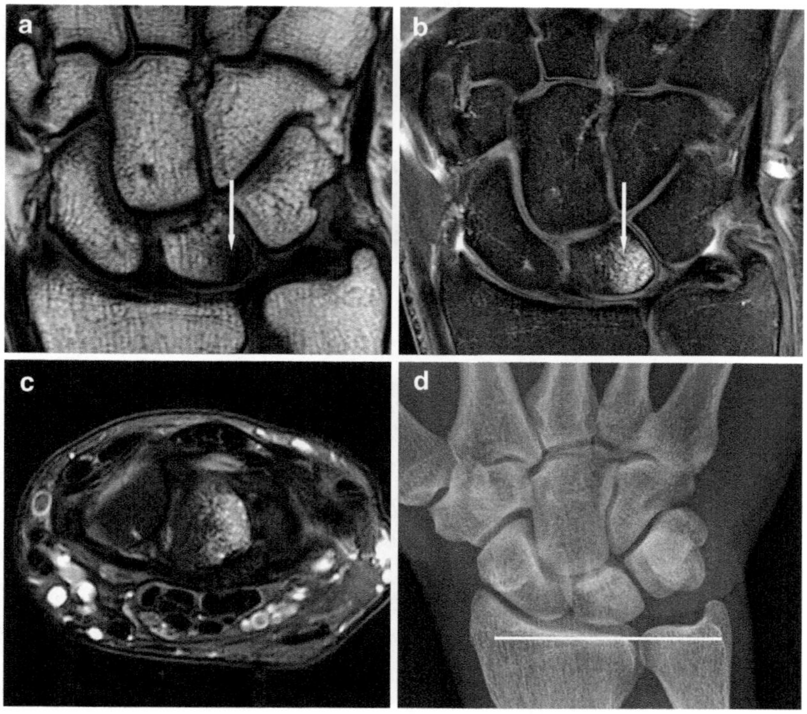

Fig. 4 Cor T1-WI (**a**), and T1-WI FS + CE (**b**); Ax T2-WI FS (**c**); Standard PA view (**d**). UA with CE at the ulnar side of the L (**a–c**). Positive ulnar variance (Hulten criteria) (**d**)

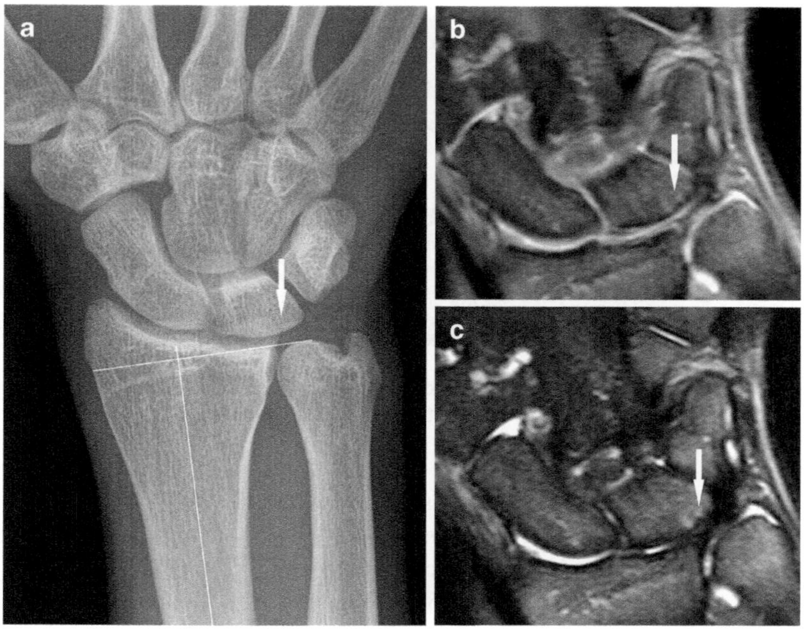

Fig. 5 Standard PA view (**a**); Cor PD (**b**), and T2-WI FS (**c**). Neutral ulnar variance (Hulten criteria) (**a**). Subchondral cysts, cartilage thinning, and weak oedema at the ulnar side of the L (**b**, **c**)

cess (Cerezal et al. 2004; Anderson et al. 2008; D'Agostino et al. 2011) (USPI or Garcia-Elias index). The styloid abuts the triquetral bone in ulnar deviation (Fig. 9b). It is often called prestyloid recess synovitis, due to the frequent local synovial proliferation (Fig. 10f). Surgical correction may involve the resection of the ulnar styloid and the local synovial proliferation (Fig. 10c).

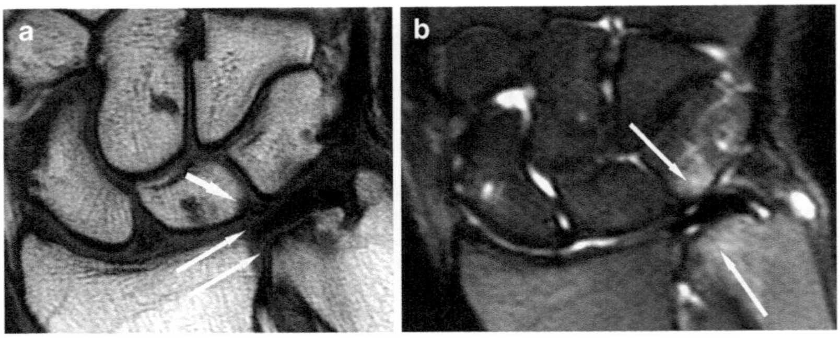

Fig. 6 Cor T1-WI (**a**), and T2-WI FS (**b**). Negative ulnar variance with UA (**a**). UA with mainly ulnotriquetral impaction (**b**)

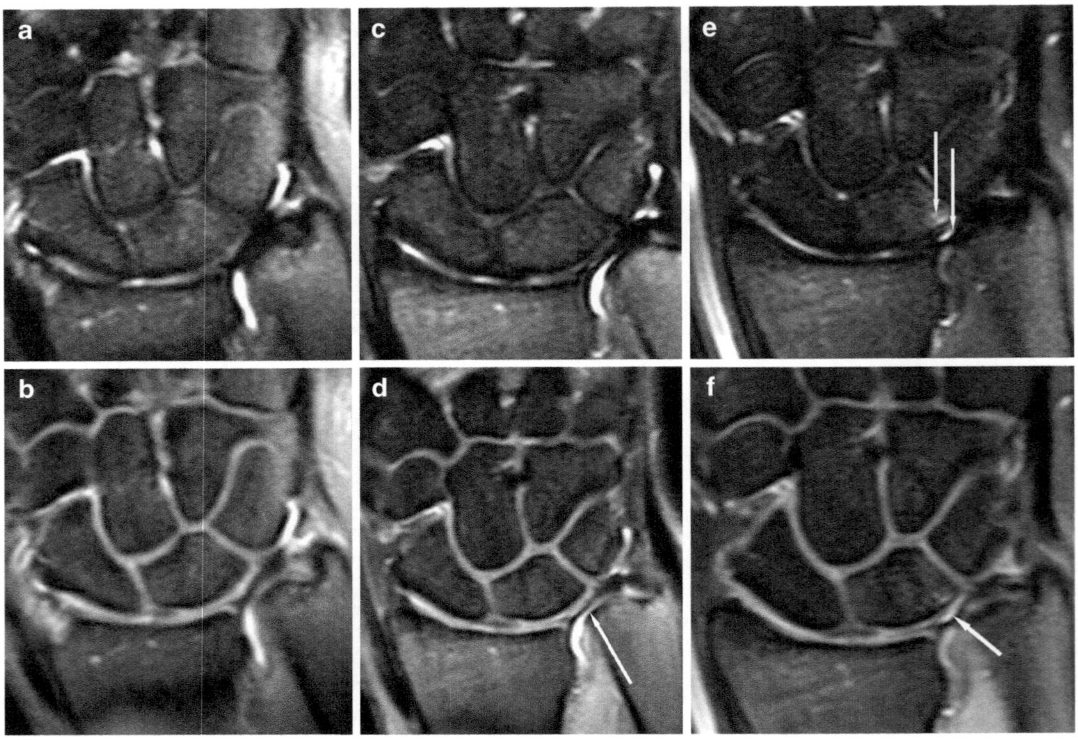

Fig. 7 Cor T2-WI FS. July: no obvious signs of UA (**a, b**). October: thinning of the TFC (**c, d**). November: subchondral degenerative cysts and weak BMO start to develop at the ulnar side of the lunate bone (**e, f**)

4. **Hamatolunate abutment** is associated with lunate bone Vegas type II (Lawson 1985) with an additional distal articular facet at the ulnar side of the L for the hamate bone (Fig. 11). The BMO starts at the proximal pole of the H (Fig. 11), evolving to kissing bone marrow oedema around the hamatolunate joint (Fig. 12).
5. **Quadrangular joint abutment** related to an accessory os styloideum (Eriksen and Ringe 2012; Apple et al. 1984; Capo et al. 2009; Conway et al. 1985; Cuono and Watson 1979; Fiolle 1967; Fusi et al. 1995; Geutjens 1994; Gomes et al. 2010; Gunther 1984; Hultgren and Lugnegård 1986; Keats 1981; Kootstra et al. 1974; Lenoble and Foucher 1992; Park et al. 2008; Timins 1999; Vermeulen et al. 2009) causes abutment, with the base of the third metacarpal as the most common presentation (Fig. 13), resulting in (kissing)

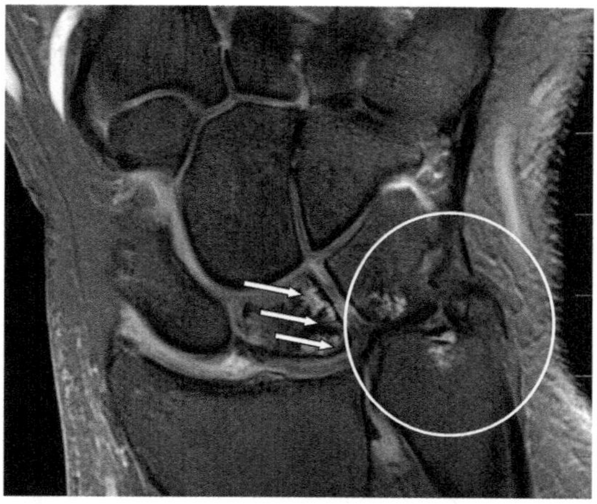

Fig. 8 T2-WI FS. Ulnotriquetral abutment (circle). A secondary lunotriquetral abutment (arrows) developed as well following a LTL rupture

BMO. The base of the second metacarpal is only rarely involved. The elective focal pain during hyperextension of the wrist of this professional pianoplayer disappeared after surgical resection of the os styloideum (Gomes et al. 2010; Hauck et al. 1996; Kalantari et al. 2007; Mespreuve et al. 2017).

6. **Ulnar impingement** is considered in this group as well. A too short ulna (Bell et al. 1985; Ekenstam and Hagert 1985; Stein et al. 2011) may cause a incongruent contact between the articular faces of the distal radio-ulnar joint. Degenerative alterations usually follow.

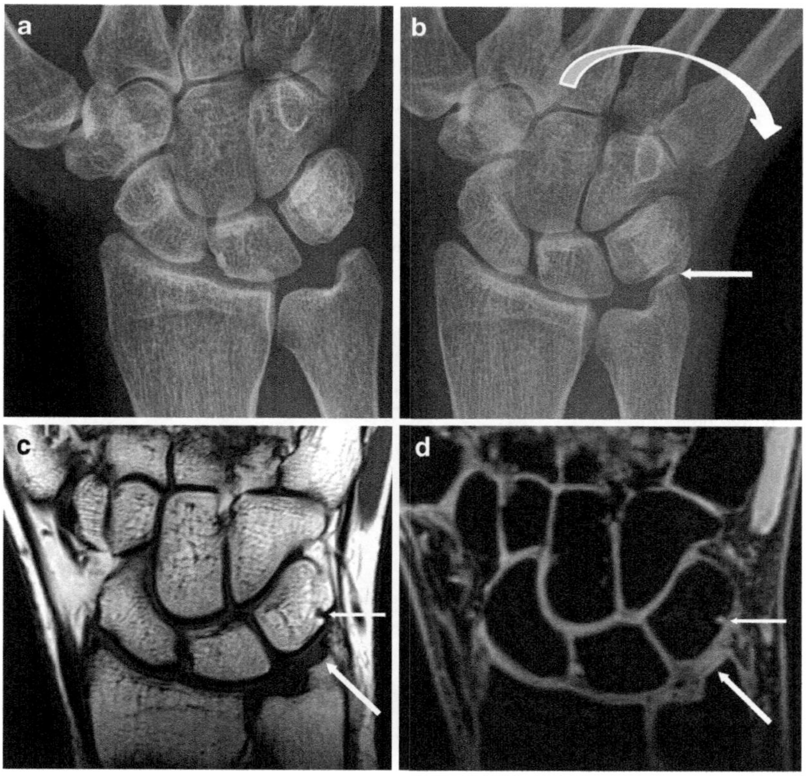

Fig. 9 Standard PA view (**a**) in ulnar deviation (**b**); Cor T1-WI (**c**), and 3D GRE (**d**). Slightly sclerotic tip of the ulnar styloid process (**a**) in contact with the triquetral bone (**b**). Flattening of the tip of the styloid process (**c**, **d**). A small subchondral cyst developed at the Tri contact site (**c**, **d**)

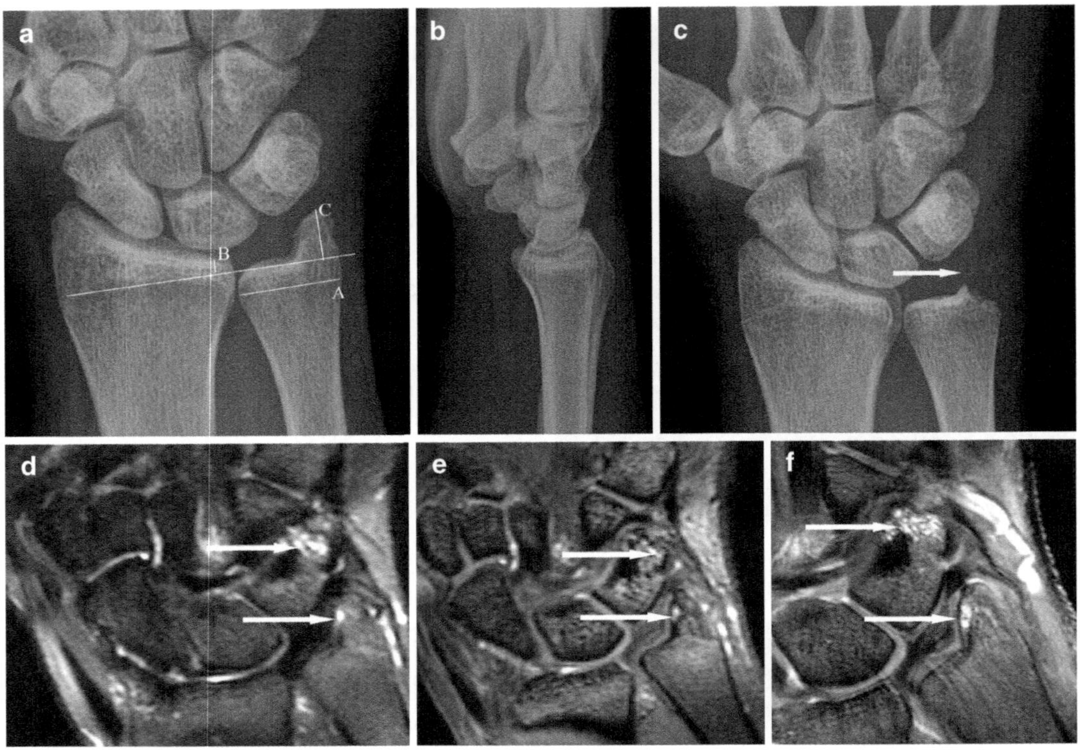

Fig. 10 Standard PA (**a**) and lateral (**b**) views; Standard PA view after surgery (**c**); Cor T2-WI FS (**d**), 3D GRE (**e**), and T1-WI FS + CE (**f**). Enlarged ulnar styloid process (**a**) with USPI (C-B/A > 0,21 +/− 0.07). Stylotriquetral abutment (**a**, **d**–**f**) with oedema (**d**), subcortical cysts (**e**), and CE synovial proliferation (**f**) treated with ulnar styloid and synovial resection (**c**)

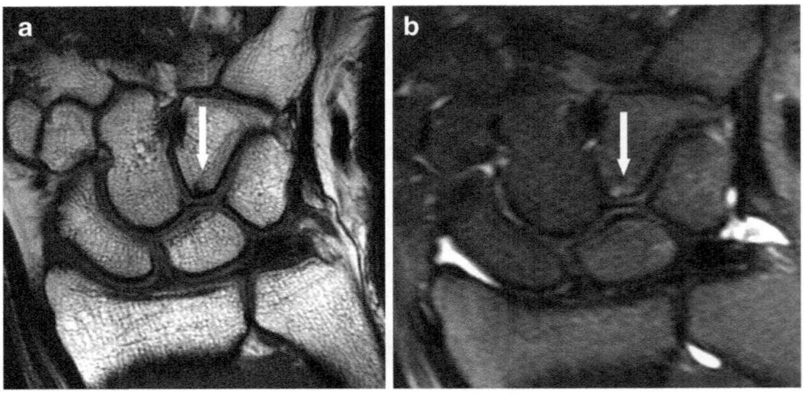

Fig. 11 Cor T1-WI (**a**), and T2-WI FS (**b**). Starting oedema at the proximal pole of the hamate in front of the additional distal articular facet for the hamate at the lunate bone (Vegas type II)

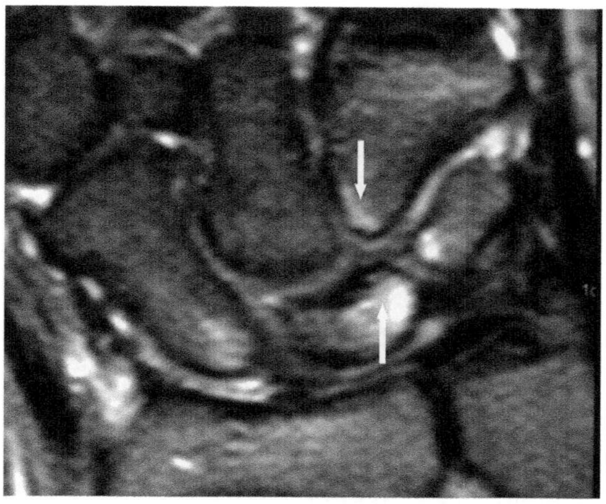

Fig. 12 Cor T2-WI FS. Kissing BMO at the proximal pole of the hamate in front of the additional distal articular facet at the lunate bone (Vegas type II)

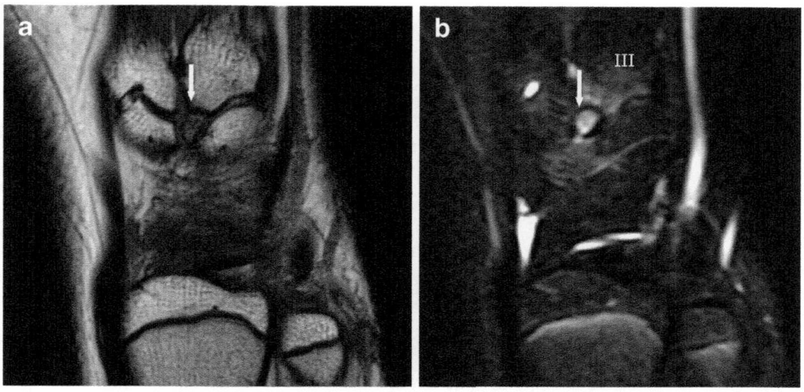

Fig. 13 Cor T1-WI (**a**), and. T2-WI FS (**b**). Presence of an accessory os styloideum with focal bone marrow oedema due to abutment with the base of the third metacarpal

2 Secondary Abutment Syndromes

1. **Scapholunate abutment** appears after laceration of the SL ligament (Metz et al. 1993) with secondary increased mobility at the joint during radio-ulnar deviation. Juxta-articular BMO parallel to the SL joint with small subchondral cysts appear (Fig. 14).
2. **Lunotriquetral abutment** appears after laceration of the LT ligament with secondary increased mobility at the joint during radio-ulnar deviation. Juxta-articular BMO parallel to the LT joint with small subchondral cysts appear (Fig. 15). Differential diagnosis with fibro-cartilaginous L-T coalition Minnaar type 1 (Metz et al. 1993; Defazio et al. 2013; Devilliers Minnaar 1952; Lotter et al. 2010; Mertens et al. 2023; Ritt et al. 2001; van Schoonhoven et al. 2001) (Fig. 16) usually is made on the standard PA view. The margins of the LTJ are irregular and sclerotic (Fig. 16a).
3. **Ulnar abutment syndrome** as a secondary AS is due to abutment of the distal ulna on the ulnar side of the proximal part of the lunate bone (Fig. 17). The height of the L has diminished at the radial side because of an old AVN. A neo-articulation developed between the distal ulna and the L (Fig. 1) with secondary abutment (Fig. 17b, c).

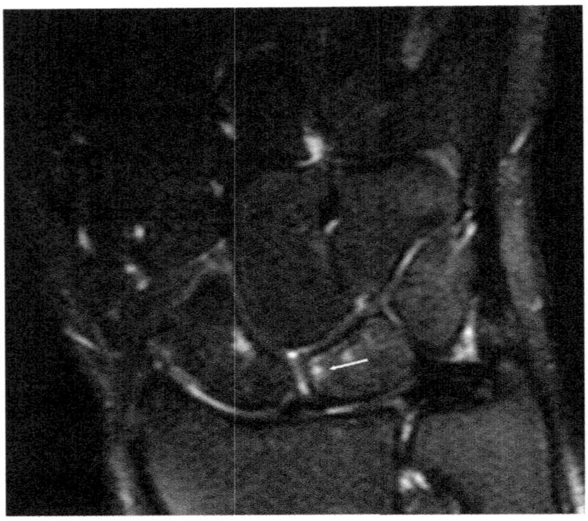

Fig. 14 Cor T2-WI FS. Presence of juxta-articular BMO and a small subchondral cyst due to increased mobility at the SL joint

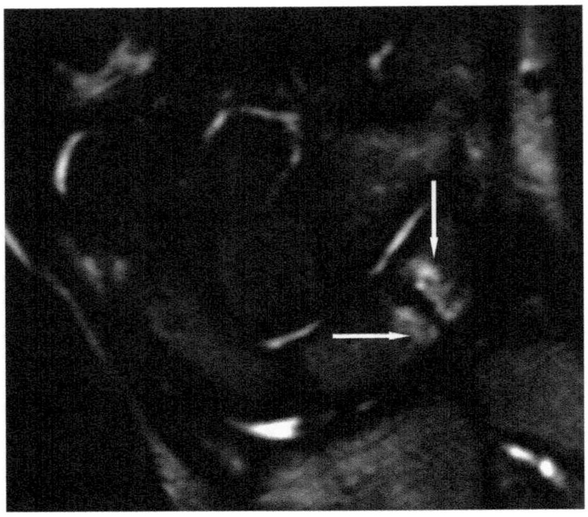

Fig. 15 Cor T2-WI FS. Presence of juxta-articular BMO due to increased mobility at the LT joint

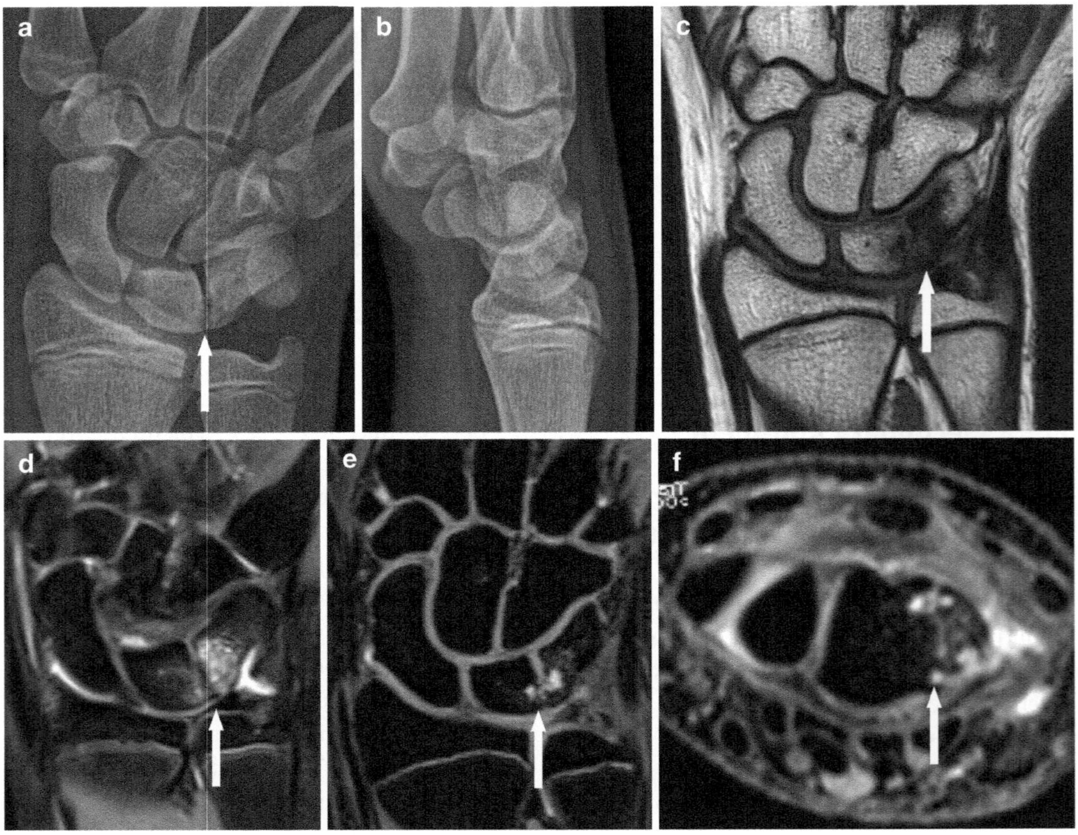

Fig. 16 Standard PA (**a**) and lateral (**b**) views; Cor T1-WI (**c**), T2-WI FS (**d**), and 3D GRE (**e**); Ax T2-WI (**f**). Symptomatic fibro-cartilaginous coalition

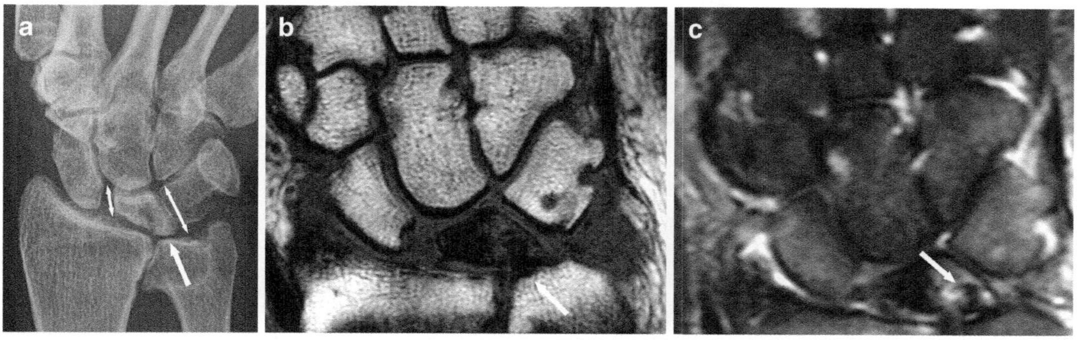

Fig. 17 Standard PA view (**a**); Cor T1-WI (**b**), and T2-WI FS (**c**). Old AVN of the deformed L with diminished height of the radial side (**a**). A neo-articulation developed between the distal ulna and the L (**a**, **b**) with secondary abutment (**c**)

4. **Ulnotriquetral abutment** may appear after a post-traumatic deformation of the R and/or U with a relative length increase (Topper et al. 1997; van Der Heijden et al. 2005; Watanabe et al. 2010) of the U causing secondary ulnotriquetral abutment (Fig. 18).
5. **Stylotriquetral abutment** (Fig. 19) after collapse of the L prosthesis at the radial side (Fig. 19a, c, e) and step off at the LTJ (Fig. 19c, e, f).
6. **Hamatolunate abutment** (Fig. 20) presents as a secondary AS in ulnar deviation after an old LT rupture and midcarpal degeneration.
7. **Capitatolunar abutment** arising with midcarpal degeneration (Garcia-Elias 2008) (Fig. 21).
8. **Scaphoradial abutment** occurs after a traumatic depression of the radial fossa (Gornitzky and Carrigan 2016) for the scaphoid bone. The radial deviation may be restricted and the repetitive impaction of the scaphoid bone on the step up of the articular fossa will give rise to an abutment syndrome (Fig. 22). This step up—if present in a central location (Fig. 23)—may be masked by an intact anterior and posterior rim on radiographs.

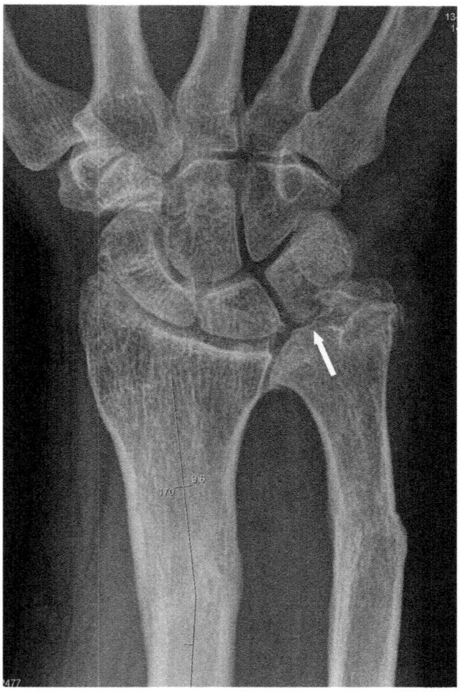

Fig. 18 Standard PA view. Post-traumatic deformation of R and U with a relative length increase of the U causing ulnotriquetral abutment

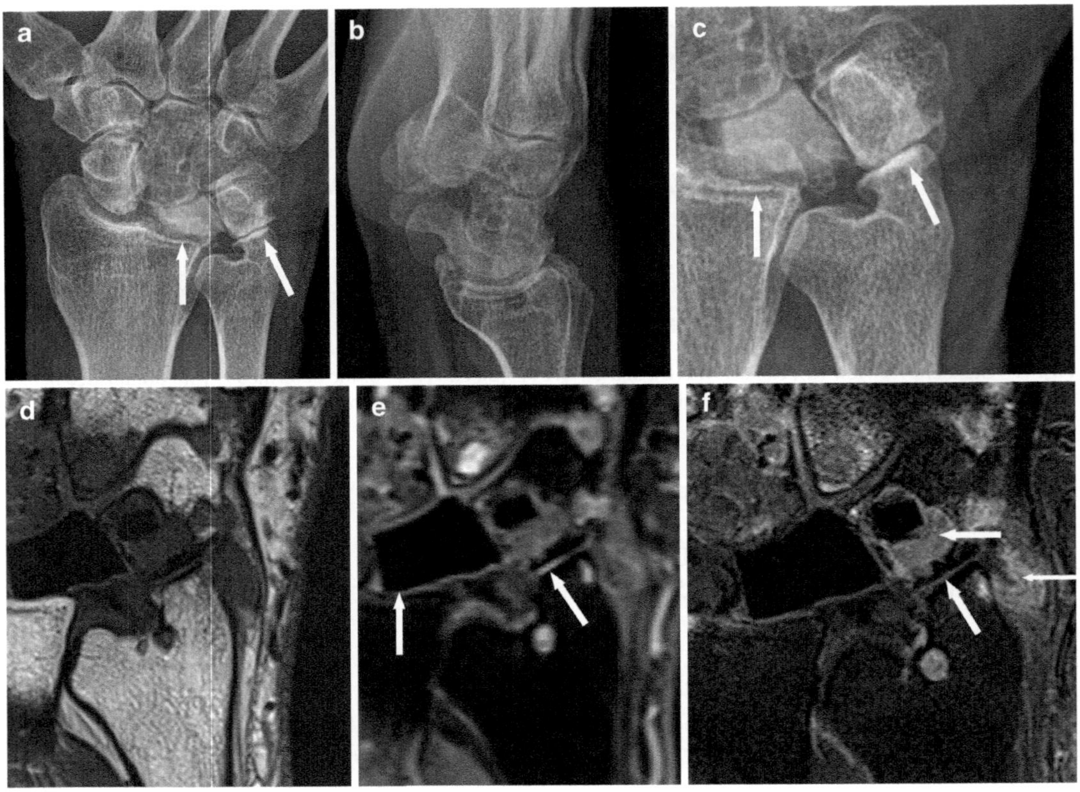

Fig. 19 Standard PA (**a**), lateral (**b**), and enlarged PA (**c**) views; Cor T1-WI (**d**), T2-WI FS (**e**), and T1-WI FS with CE (**f**). SLAC wrist with stylotriquetral abutment (**a**, **c**, **e**, and **f**) after collapse of the L prosthesis at the radial side (**a**, **c**, **e**) and step off at the LTJ (**c**, **e**, **f**). CE synovitis (**d**, **f**)

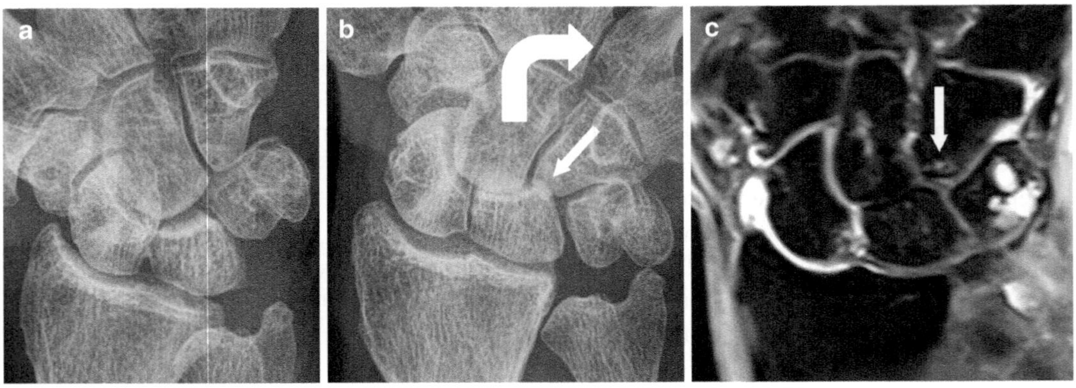

Fig. 20 Standard PA view in radial (**a**) and in ulnar (**b**) deviation; Cor T2-WI FS (**c**). The first and second line of Gilula show a step off sign at LT joint (**a**, **b**). Hamatolunate abutment (straight arrows) in ulnar deviation (**b**, **c**) after LT laceration. Midcarpal degeneration (**b**, **c**)

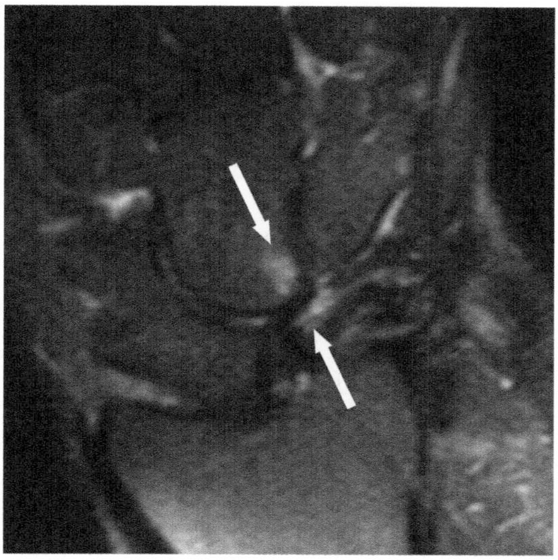

Fig. 21 Cor T2-WI FS. Capitatolunate abutment in ulnar deviation with midcarpal degeneration

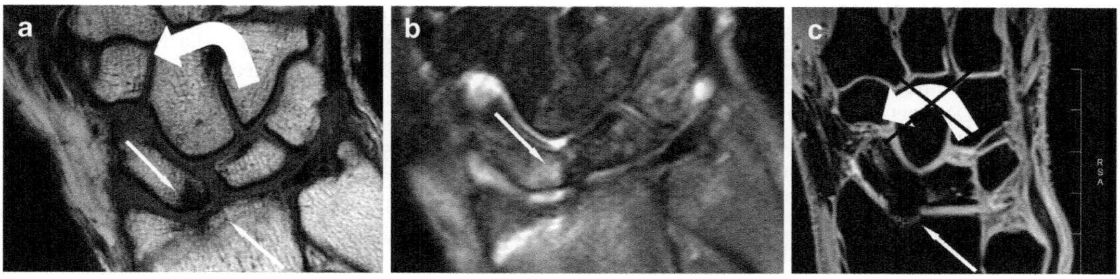

Fig. 22 Cor T1-WI (**a**), T2-WI FS (**b**), and 3D GRE (**c**). Scaphoradial abutment (straight arrows) in (restricted) radial deviation (curved arrows) after traumatic depression of the corresponding radial articular area

Fig. 23 Ax 3D GRE (**a**), and T2-WI FS (**b**). Central depression of the radial epiphysis with BMO

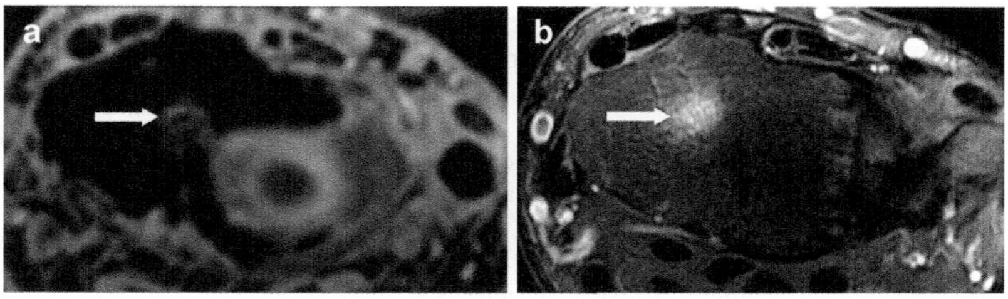

References

Anderson ML, Skinner JA, Felmlee JP, Berger RA, Amrami KK (2008) Diagnostic comparison of 1.5 Tesla and 3.0 Tesla preoperative MRI of the wrist in patients with ulnar-sided wrist pain. J Hand Surg Am 33(7):1153–1159. https://doi.org/10.1016/j.jhsa.2008.02.028. PMID: 18762112

Apple JS, Martinez S, Nunley JA (1984) Painful os styloideum: bone scintigraphy in carpe bossu disease. AJR Am J Roentgenol 142(1):181–182. https://doi.org/10.2214/ajr.142.1.181. PMID: 6229168

Bell MJ, Hill RJ, McMurtry RY (1985) Ulnar impingement syndrome. J Bone Joint Surg Br 67(1):126–129. https://doi.org/10.1302/0301-620X.67B1.3968131. PMID: 3968131

Bhat AK, Kumar B, Acharya A (2011) Radiographic imaging of the wrist. Indian J Plast Surg 44(2):186–196. https://doi.org/10.4103/0970-0358.85339. PMID: 22022028; PMCID: PMC3193630

Capo JT, Orillaza NS, Lim PK (2009) Carpal boss in an adolescent: case report. J Hand Surg Am 34(10):1808–1810. https://doi.org/10.1016/j.jhsa.2009.07.022. Epub 2009 Nov 7. PMID: 19897321

Cerezal L, del Piñal F, Abascal F (2004) MR imaging findings in ulnar-sided wrist impaction syndromes. Magn Reson Imaging Clin N Am 12(2):281–299. https://doi.org/10.1016/j.mric.2004.02.005, vi. PMID: 15172387

Conway WF, Destouet JM, Gilula LA, Bellinghausen HW, Weeks PM (1985) The carpal boss: an overview of radiographic evaluation. Radiology 156(1):29–31. https://doi.org/10.1148/radiology.156.1.3923555. PMID: 3923555

Couzens G, Daunt N, Crawford R, Ross M (2014) Positive magnetic resonance imaging findings in the asymptomatic wrist. ANZ J Surg 84(7–8):528–532. https://doi.org/10.1111/ans.12552. Epub 2014 Feb 26. PMID: 24612468

Cuono CB, Watson HK (1979) The carpal boss: surgical treatment and etiological considerations. Plast Reconstr Surg 63(1):88–93. PMID: 432327

D'Agostino P, Townley WA, Le Viet D, Roulot E (2011) Oblique ulnar styloid osteotomy – a treatment for ulnar styloid impaction syndrome. J Hand Surg Am 36(11):1785–1789. https://doi.org/10.1016/j.jhsa.2011.07.023. Epub 2011 Oct 5. PMID: 21975097

Defazio MV, Cousins BJ, Miversuski RA Jr, Cardoso R (2013) Carpal coalition: a review of current knowledge and report of a single institution's experience with asymptomatic intercarpal fusion. Hand (N Y) 8(2):157–163. https://doi.org/10.1007/s11552-013-9498-5. Erratum in: Hand (N Y). 2013;8(2):245. PMID: 24426912; PMCID: PMC3653005

Devilliers Minnaar AB (1952) Congenital fusion of the lunate and triquetral bones in the South African Bantu. J Bone Joint Surg Br 34-B(1):45–48. https://doi.org/10.1302/0301-620X.34B1.45. PMID: 12999869

Ekenstam F, Hagert CG (1985) Anatomical studies on the geometry and stability of the distal radio ulnar joint. Scand J Plast Reconstr Surg 19(1):17–25. https://doi.org/10.3109/02844318509052861. PMID: 4023639

Eriksen EF, Ringe JD (2012) Bone marrow lesions: a universal bone response to injury? Rheumatol Int 32(3):575–584. https://doi.org/10.1007/s00296-011-2141-2. Epub 2011 Sep 8. PMID: 21901347

Fiolle J (1967) Le "carpe bossu". Bull Mkm SocNat Chir 1687–1690

Fusi S, Watson HK, Cuono CB (1995) The carpal boss. A 20-year review of operative management. J Hand Surg Br 20(3):405–408. https://doi.org/10.1016/s0266-7681(05)80104-4. PMID: 7561423

Garcia-Elias M (2008) The non-dissociative clunking wrist: a personal view. J Hand Surg Eur Vol 33(6):698–711. https://doi.org/10.1177/1753193408090148. Epub 2008 Oct 20. PMID: 18936125

Geutjens G (1994) Carpal bossing with capitate-trapezoid fusion. A case report. Acta Orthop Scand 65(1):97–98. https://doi.org/10.3109/17453679408993728. PMID: 8154295

Goldfarb CA, Strauss NL, Wall LB, Calfee RP (2011) Defining ulnar variance in the adolescent wrist: measurement technique and interobserver reliability. J Hand Surg Am 36(2):272–277. https://doi.org/10.1016/j.jhsa.2010.11.008. PMID: 21276890

Gomes AF, Paganella VC, Paganella MC, Henkin CS, Giostri G (2010) Computed tomography and magnetic resonance imaging findings of os styloideum in a symptomatic athlete. Radiol Bras 43:207–209. https://doi.org/10.1590/S0100-39842010000300014

Gornitzky AL, Carrigan RB (2016) The diagnostic utility of MRI in the painful wrist: when to reconsider advanced imaging in the pediatric patient. Pediatrics (Evanston) 137(Suppl 3):596–596A. https://doi.org/10.1542/peds.137.Supplement_3.596A

Gunther SF (1984) The carpometacarpal joints. Orthop Clin North Am 15(2):259–277. PMID: 6728445

Hauck RM, Skahen J 3rd, Palmer AK (1996) Classification and treatment of ulnar styloid nonunion. J Hand Surg Am 21(3):418–422. https://doi.org/10.1016/S0363-5023(96)80355-8. PMID: 8724472

Hulten O (1928) Uber Anatomische Variationen der Handgelenkknochen. Acta Radiol 9(2):155–168. https://doi.org/10.3109/00016922809176658

Hultgren T, Lugnegård H (1986) Carpal boss. Acta Orthop Scand 57(6):547–550. https://doi.org/10.3109/17453678609014791. PMID: 3577728

Kalantari BN, Seeger L, Motamedi K et al (2007) Accessory ossicles and sesamoid bones: spectrum of pathology and imaging evaluation. Appl Radiol 10:28–37

Keats TE (1981) Some new normal roentgen variants that may simulate disease. Curr Probl Diagn Radiol 10(3):1–52. https://doi.org/10.1016/0363-0188(81)90006-2. PMID: 6791877

Kootstra G, Huffstadt JC, Kauer JM (1974) The styloid bone. A clinical and embryological study. Hand 6(2):185–189. https://doi.org/10.1016/0072-968x(74)90088-6. PMID: 4846215

Lawson JP (1985) Symptomatic radiographic variants in extremities. Radiology 157(3):625–631. https://

doi.org/10.1148/radiology.157.3.4059550. PMID: 4059550
Lenoble E, Foucher G (1992) Le carpe bossu [The carpal bump]. Ann Chir Main Memb Super 11(1):46–50. https://doi.org/10.1016/s0753-9053(05)80052-3. French. PMID: 1375493
Lotter O, Stahl S, Luz O, Pfau M, Schaller HE (2010) CASE REPORT bilateral paradoxically symptomatic luno-triquetral coalition: a case report. Eplasty 10:e47. PMID: 20596547; PMCID: PMC2893531
Mertens K, Mespreuve M, Vanhoenacker FM (2023) Lunotriquetral coalition. Semin Musculoskelet Radiol 27(3):378–380. https://doi.org/10.1055/s--0043-1766108. Epub 2023 May 25. PMID: 37230136
Mespreuve M, De Smet L, De Cuyper K, Waked K, Vanhoenacker F (2017) MRI diagnosis of carpal boss and comparison with radiography. Acta Radiol 58(10):1245–1251. https://doi.org/10.1177/0284185116685925. Epub 2017 Jan 13. PMID: 28084813
Metz VM, Schimmerl SM, Gilula LA, Viegas SF, Saffar P (1993) Wide scapholunate joint space in lunotriquetral coalition: a normal variant? Radiology 188(2):557–559. https://doi.org/10.1148/radiology.188.2.8327715. PMID: 8327715
Nakamura R, Tanaka Y, Imaeda T, Miura T (1991) The influence of age and sex on ulnar variance. J Hand Surg Br 16(1):84–88. https://doi.org/10.1016/0266-7681(91)90136-c. PMID: 2007823
Park MJ, Namdari S, Weiss AP (2008) The carpal boss: review of diagnosis and treatment. J Hand Surg Am 33(3):446–449. https://doi.org/10.1016/j.jhsa.2007.11.029. PMID: 18343306
Ritt MJ, Maas M, Bos KE (2001) Minnaar type 1 symptomatic lunotriquetral coalition: a report of nine patients. J Hand Surg Am 26(2):261–270. https://doi.org/10.1053/jhsu.2001.21520. PMID: 11279572
Stein JM, Cook TS, Simonson S, Kim W (2011) Normal and variant anatomy of the wrist and hand on MR imaging. Magn Reson Imaging Clin N Am 19(3):595–608. https://doi.org/10.1016/j.mric.2011.05.007, ix. PMID: 21816333
Timins ME (1999) Osseous anatomic variants of the wrist: findings on MR imaging. AJR Am J Roentgenol 173(2):339–344. https://doi.org/10.2214/ajr.173.2.10430131. PMID: 10430131
Topper SM, Wood MB, Ruby LK (1997) Ulnar styloid impaction syndrome. J Hand Surg Am 22(4):699–704. https://doi.org/10.1016/S0363-5023(97)80131-1. PMID: 9260629
van Der Heijden B, Groot S, Schuurman AH (2005) Evaluation of ulnar styloid length. J Hand Surg Am 30(5):954–959. https://doi.org/10.1016/j.jhsa.2005.05.007. Erratum in: J Hand Surg [Am]. 2007 Jul–Aug;32(6):923. Groot, Sadra [corrected to Groot, Sandra]. PMID: 16182051
van Schoonhoven J, Prommersberger KJ, Schmitt R (2001) Traumatic disruption of a fibrocartilage lunate-triquetral coalition – a case report and review of the literature. Hand Surg 6(1):103–108. https://doi.org/10.1142/s0218810401000497. PMID: 11677672
Vermeulen GM, de With MC, Bleys RL, Schuurman AH (2009) Carpal boss: effect of wedge excision depth on third carpometacarpal joint stability. J Hand Surg Am 34(1):7–13. https://doi.org/10.1016/j.jhsa.2008.09.010. PMID: 19121724
Watanabe A, Souza F, Vezeridis PS, Blazar P, Yoshioka H (2010) Ulnar-sided wrist pain. II. Clinical imaging and treatment. Skeletal Radiol 39(9):837–857. https://doi.org/10.1007/s00256-009-0842-3. Epub 2009 Dec 10. PMID: 20012039; PMCID: PMC2904904

Tendons

Contents

1 General

The theoretical terms used for tendon pathology are summarised in Table 1. Although evaluation by US of the superficial tendons is usually the first choice, the combination of 3D imaging and T2-sequences very sensitive to fluid imply that MRI is a very good technique to illustrate tendon pathology discovered in a more general context. Especially in a complex structure such as the wrist, all dorsal and palmar as well as the superficial and deep tendons (Fig. 1) and eventual symptomatic variants are illustrated at once (Albright and Linburg 1978; Bruno et al. 2019; Davis and Blankenbaker 2010; Gornitzky and Carrigan 2016; Martinoli et al. 2010; Meraj et al. 2017; Mespreuve et al. 2005; Nayak et al. 2008; Rixey et al. 2021; Rodríguez-Niedenführ et al. 2002; Sookur et al. 2008; Theumann et al. 2002; Zeiss and Guilliam-Haidet 1996). The aetiology is very variable. Trauma; chronic overload; RA; Gout; PVNS; Sarcoidosis; Amyloidosis; and Fungal infection are the most frequent ones. A specific aetiology is related to many compartments.

Table 1 Terms used for tendon pathology

	Tendon PD-WI	Tendon T2-WI	Tendon
Tendinosis	Intermediary	Intermediary	Thickened
Tendinitis	Intermediary	High	Thickened
Tenosynovitis		Fluid around	Normal
Partial tear		Increased	Thickened
Complete tear		Increased	Defect Retraction Serpiginous

M. Mespreuve, K. Waked, *MRI of the Wrist*, Medical Radiology,
https://doi.org/10.1007/978-3-031-63973-9_12

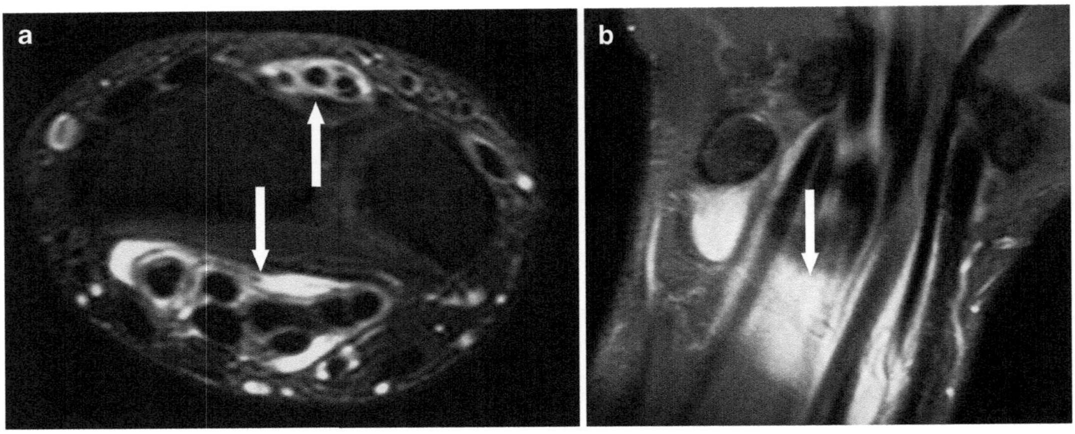

Fig. 1 Ax (**a**) and Coronal (**b**) T2-WI FS. Tenosynovitis with fluid in the tendon sheaths around the palmar flexor tendons and the dorsal extensor IV compartment

2 Extensor compartments

The tendon pathology of the first extensor compartment (abductor pollicis longus and extensor pollicis brevis) (Chang et al. 2017) is very frequent. A (firm) localised radial swelling (Fig. 2a) is provoked by a (De Quervain's) tenosynovitis of these tendons (Fig. 2b–d) with surrounding subcutaneous oedema. The CMC-I joint should be evaluated reflexively for frequently underlying osteoarthritis (Fig. 3). After surgical release, the position of the tendons may change to a more superficial and radiopalmar position, sometimes with a (residual) fluid collection adjacent to the radius (Fig. 4).

The proximal crossover from compartment I (abductor pollicis longus and extensor pollicis brevis) over II (extensor carpi radialis longus and brevis) (Gümüşalan et al. 1997) (Fig. 5) may give rise to tenosynovitis in both compartments (Fig. 6) known as the (more classical) proximal intersection syndrome. In contrast to US (Fig. 7), the mobility and/or friction of the tendons cannot be illustrated dynamically and comparison with the other side is not routinely performed.

The distal intersection syndrome occurs less frequent (Fig. 8). The extensor pollicis longus (compartment III) crosses over the tendons of the extensor carpi radialis longus and brevis (compartment II). A congenital or post-traumatic hypertrophic and deformed Lister tubercle may clamp the extensor pollicis longus tendon (Fig. 9). Drummer's tendonitis specifically affects the tendon of the extensor pollicis longus. Ultimately, all may be at the origin of a rupture of the extensor pollicis longus (Figs. 10 and 11).

The tendons of compartment IV are almost always part of an overuse multicompartmental tenosynovitis (Fig. 12). Synovial proliferation between the tendons of compartment IV may result in clumping of the tendons, presenting as an undifferentiated cluster (Fig. 13).

In compartment VI, the extensor carpi ulnaris tendon is prone to (sub)luxation (Anderson et al. 2008; Kaiser et al. 2018; Luijkx et al. 2019). The luxated tendon results in an empty sulcus sign at the ulna (Paley et al. 1987) (Fig. 14). Longitudinal cleavage of the ecu is a relatively frequent finding around the ulnar styloid process (Fig. 15). This may eventually lead to a rupture (Fig. 16). The proximal (Fig. 16a–c) and distal part (Fig. 16a, f) of the ecu should be looked for in order to inform the surgeon about the tendinous gap. After repair (Fig. 17), metal artefacts may disturb the image focally (Fig. 17a), but the continuity is proven (Fig. 17b). An adjacent "tendinous" structure appears in compartment VI (Fig. 17b–f) due to a supporting transfer from the extensor digiti minimi of compartment V (Fig. 17d).

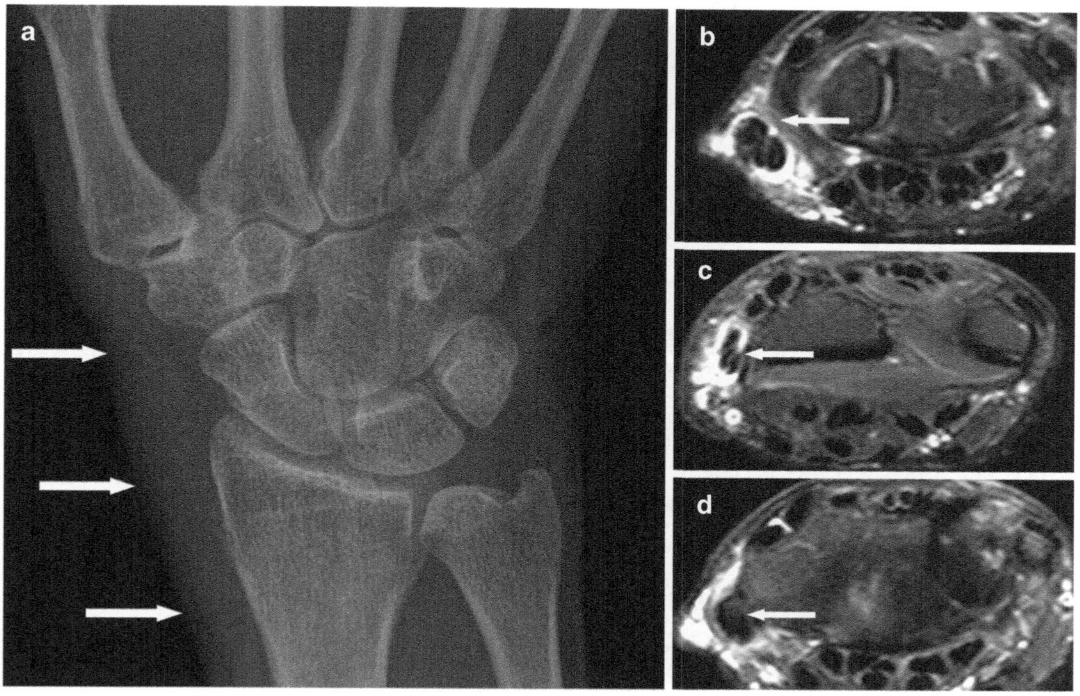

Fig. 2 Standard PA view (**a**); Ax T2-WI FS (**b–d**). Swelling of the soft tissues at the radial side of the wrist (**a**). Tenosynovitis at the extensor compartment I (apl and epb) with surrounding subcutaneous oedema (**b–d**)

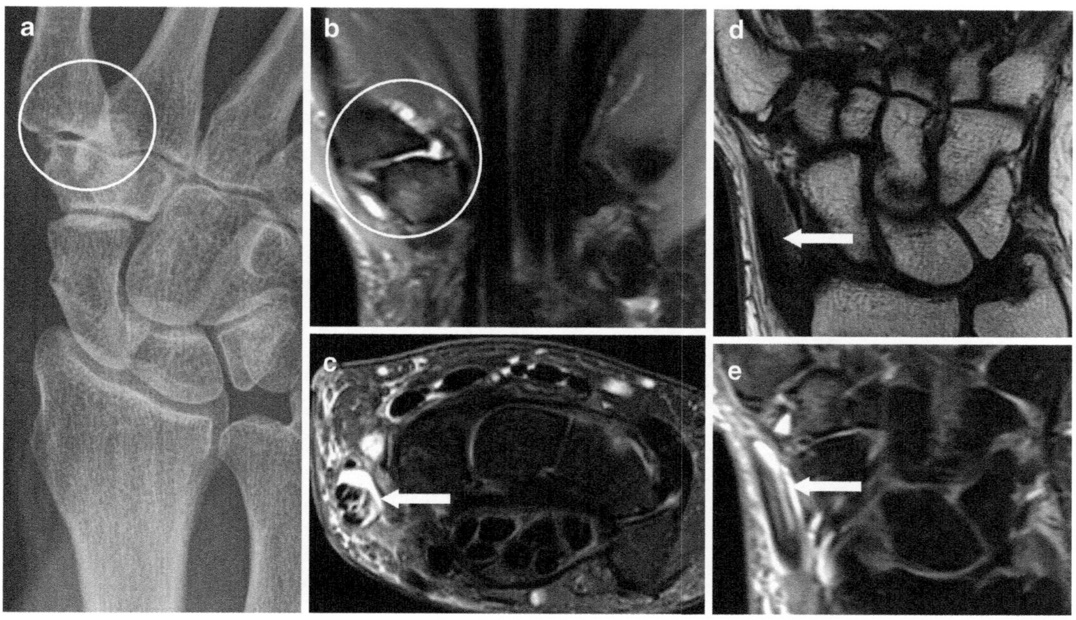

Fig. 3 Standard PA view (**a**); Cor (**b**) and Ax T2-WI FS (**c**); Cor T1-WI (**d**); and T2-WI FS (**e**). Osteoarthritis at the CMC-I joint (**a**, **b**) with hydrops (**b**). Tenosynovitis of the apl and epb (**c–e**)

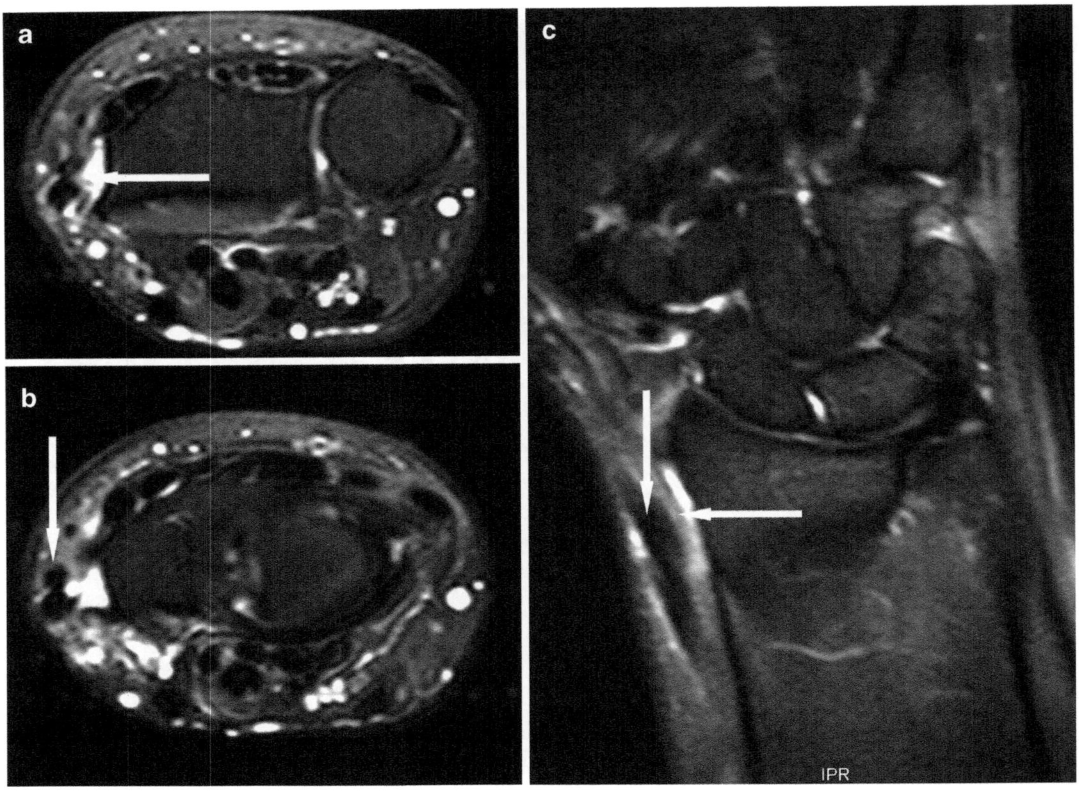

Fig. 4 Ax (**a**, **b**) and Cor (**c**) T2-WI FS. Status after surgical release with a more superficial and radiopalmar position of the tendons (apl, epb), sometimes with a (residual) fluid collection adjacent to the radius

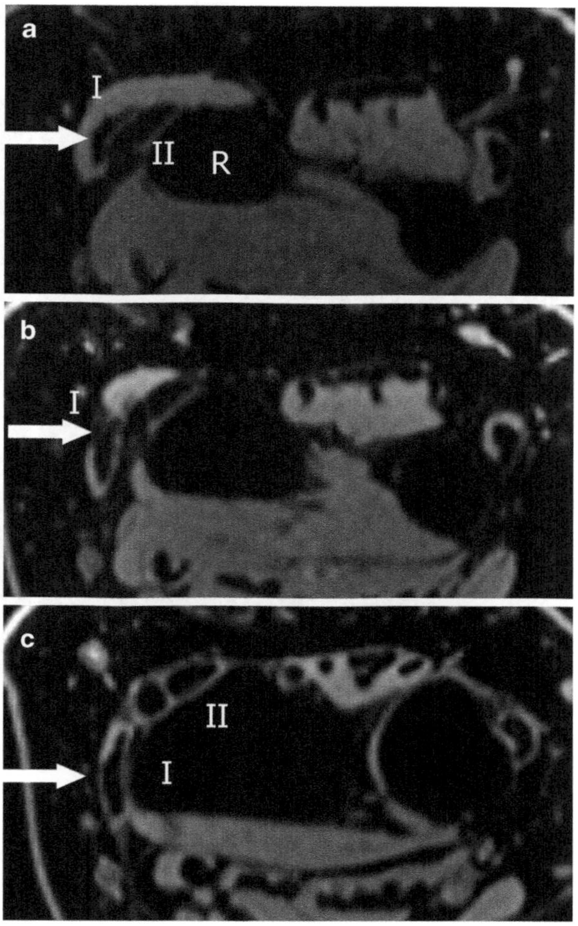

Fig. 5 Cor 3D GRE (**a–c**). The distal crossover from compartment I (apl and epb) over compartment II (ecrl and ecrb)

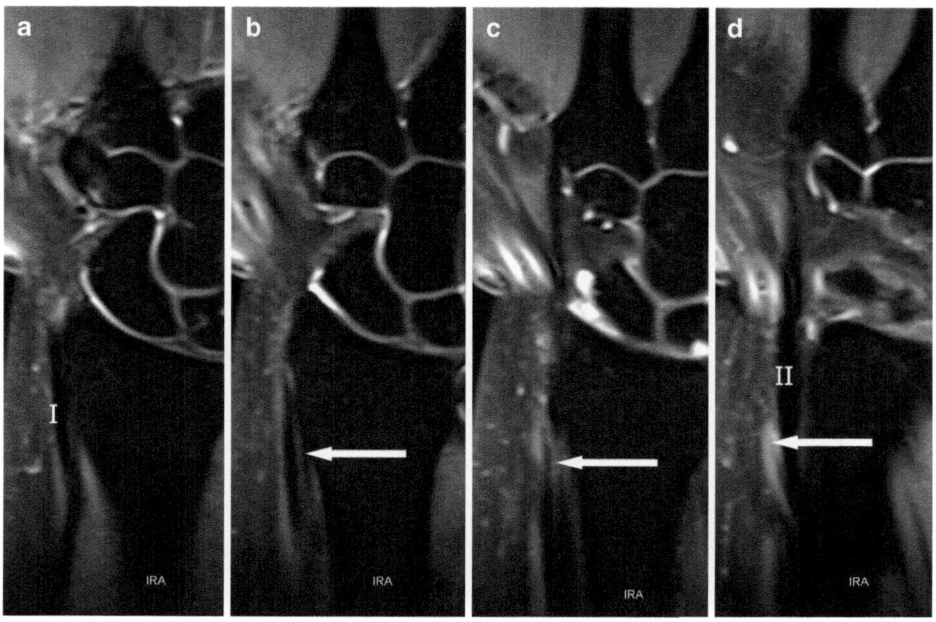

Fig. 6 Cor T2-WI FS (**a–d**). The proximal crossover from compartment I (apl and epb) over compartment II (ecrl and ecrb) with fluid along the tendons

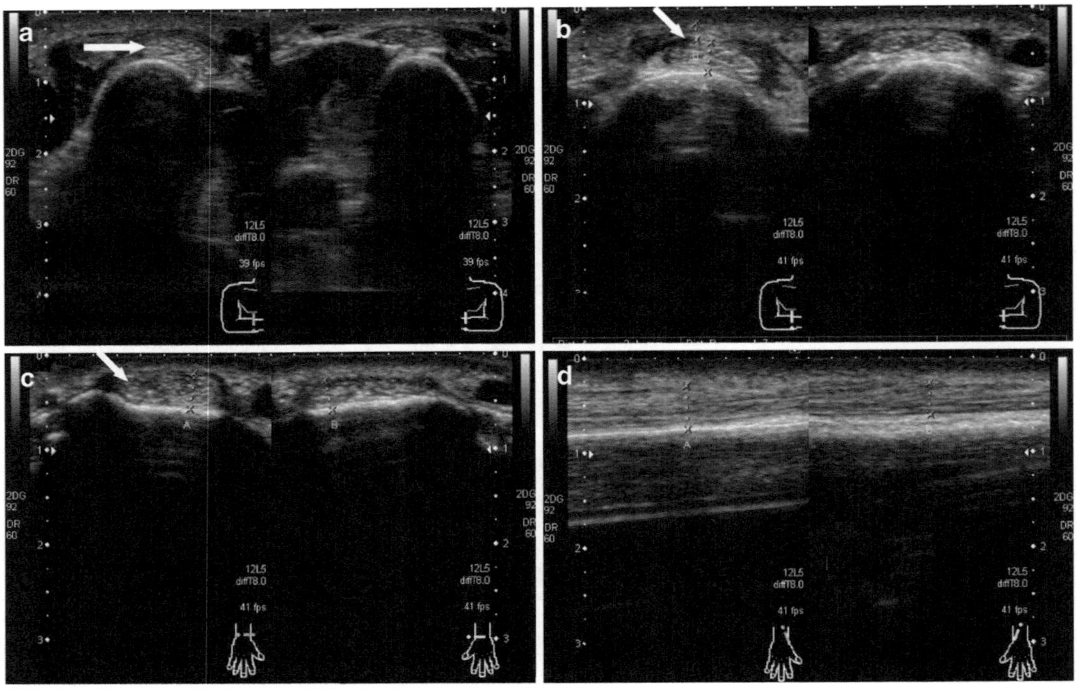

Fig. 7 US of the right-side axial (**a**–**c**) and longitudinal (**d**) compared to the normal left side. The distal crossover from compartment I (apl and epb) over compartment II (ecrl and ecrb) with fluid along the swollen tendons

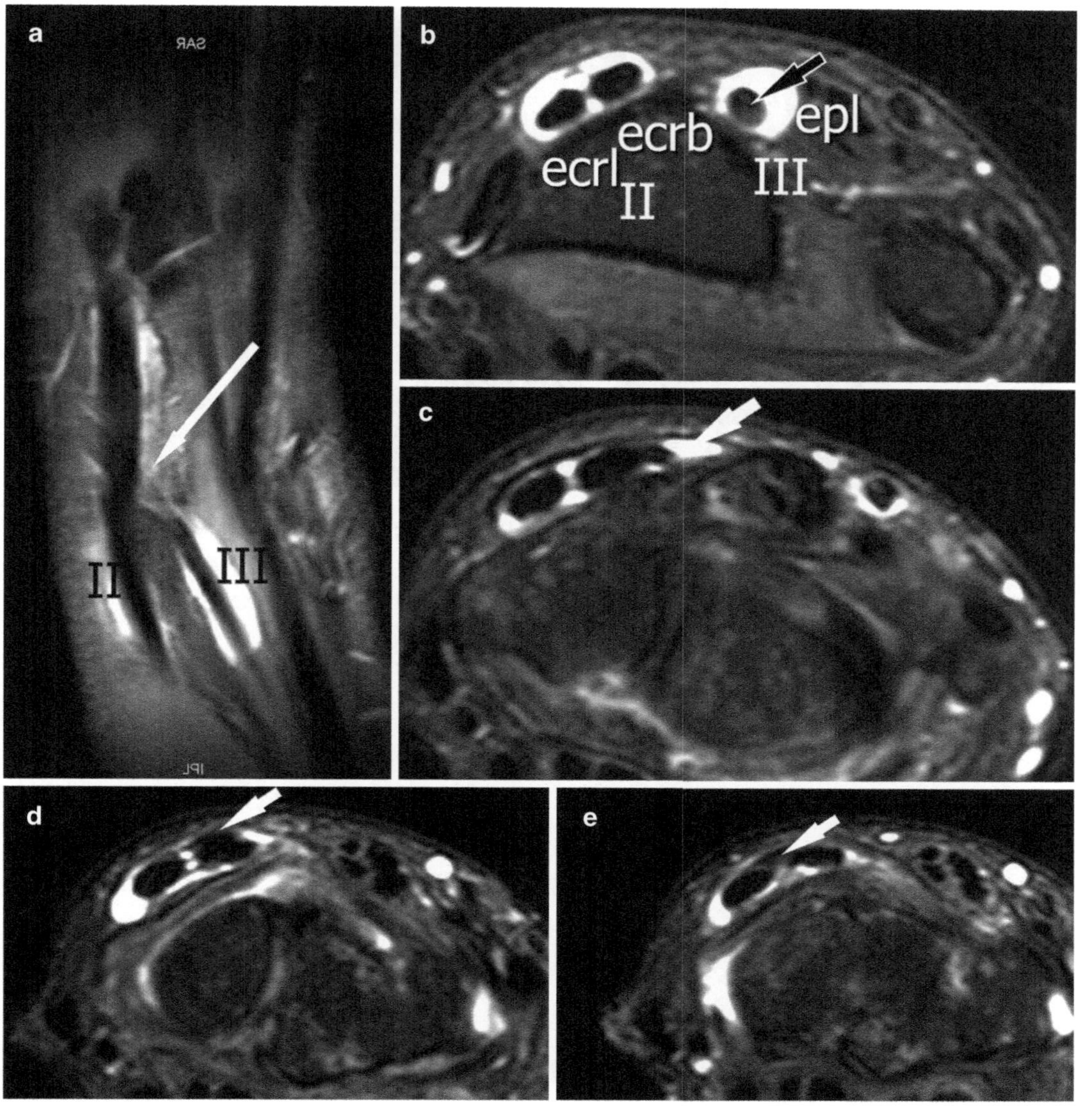

Fig. 8 Cor (**a**) and Axial (**b–e**) T2-WI FS. The distal crossover from compartment III (epl) over compartment II (ecrl and ecrb) with fluid along the tendons

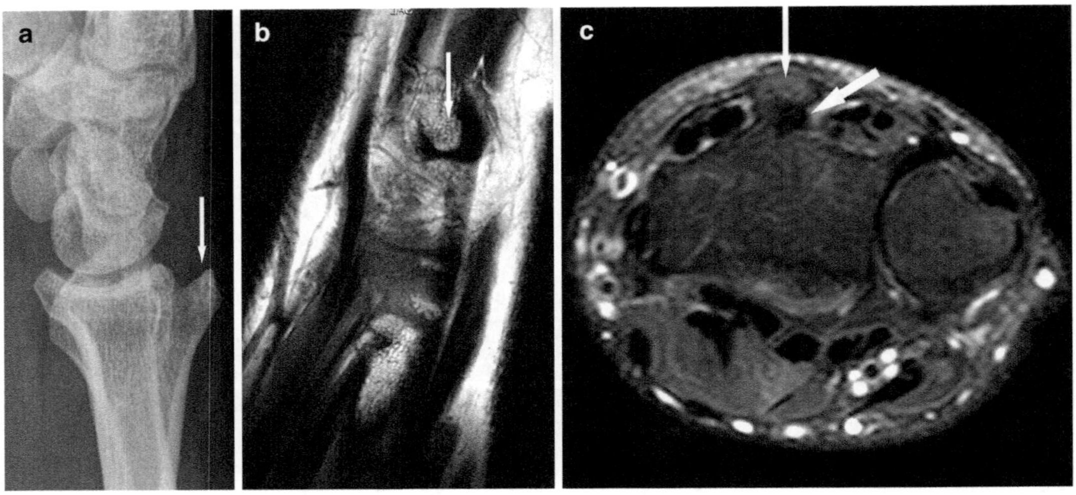

Fig. 9 Standard lateral view (**a**); Cor T1-WI (**b**); and Ax T2-WI FS (**c**). The Lister tubercle is hypertrophic and deformed, clamping the epl tendon

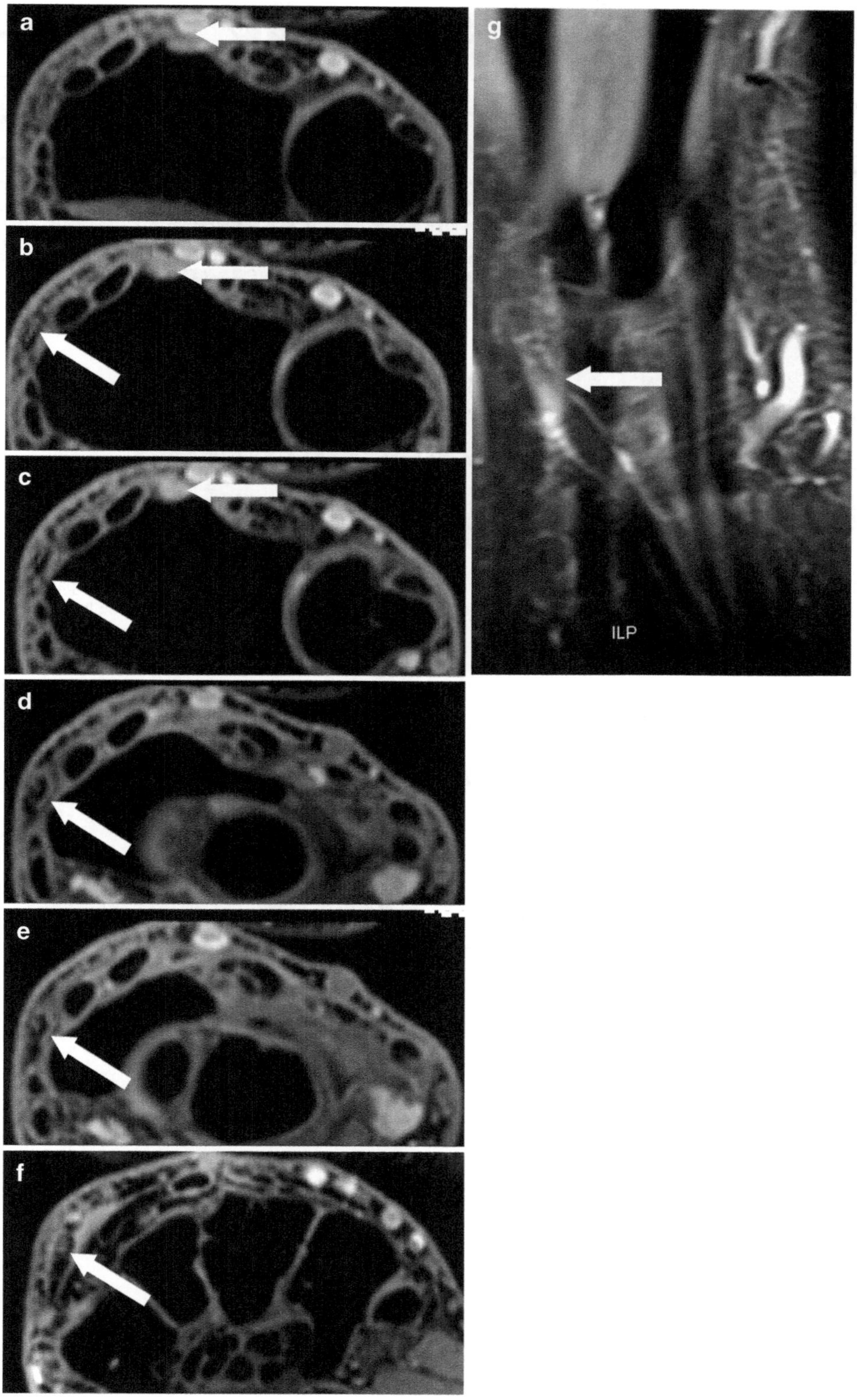

Fig. 10 Ax (**a–f**) and Cor 3D GRE. In chronic drummer's tendonitis, the epl tendon may rupture. The compartment III is empty (**a–c**, **g**) with visualisation of the distal fragment (**b–f**)

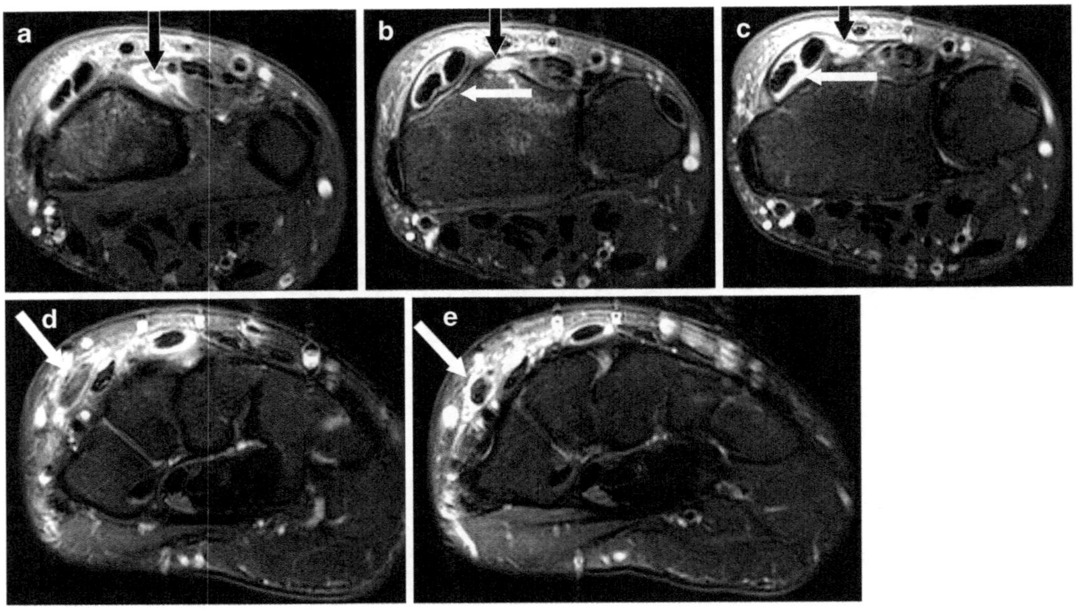

Fig. 11 Ax T2-WI FS (**a**–**e**). Chronic distal intersection syndrome with tenosynovitis at compartment II and III. Secondary rupture of the epl with an empty compartment III (**a**–**c**) and a loose distal part of the tendon (**d**, **e**)

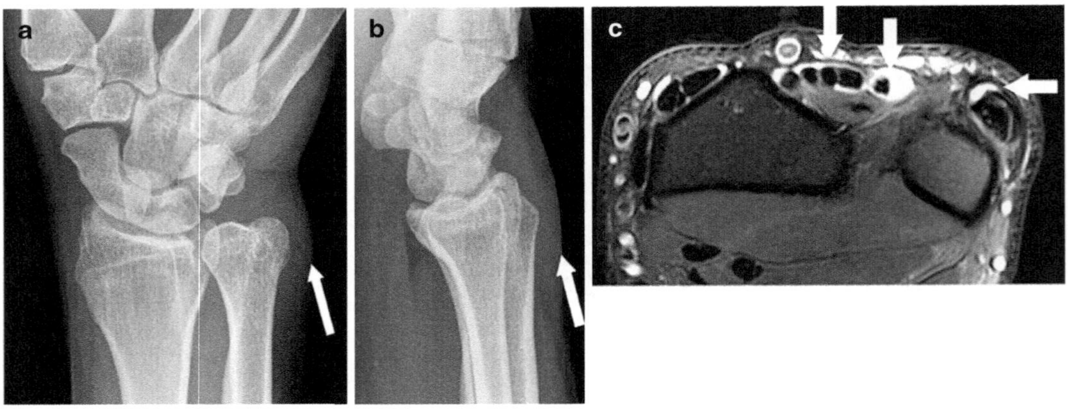

Fig. 12 Standard oblique (**a**) and Lateral (**b**) view; Ax T2-WI FS (**c**). Swelling at the ulnar (**a**) and dorsal (**b**) side of the wrist. Tenosynovitis of the extensor compartment (II); III; IV; V; and VI

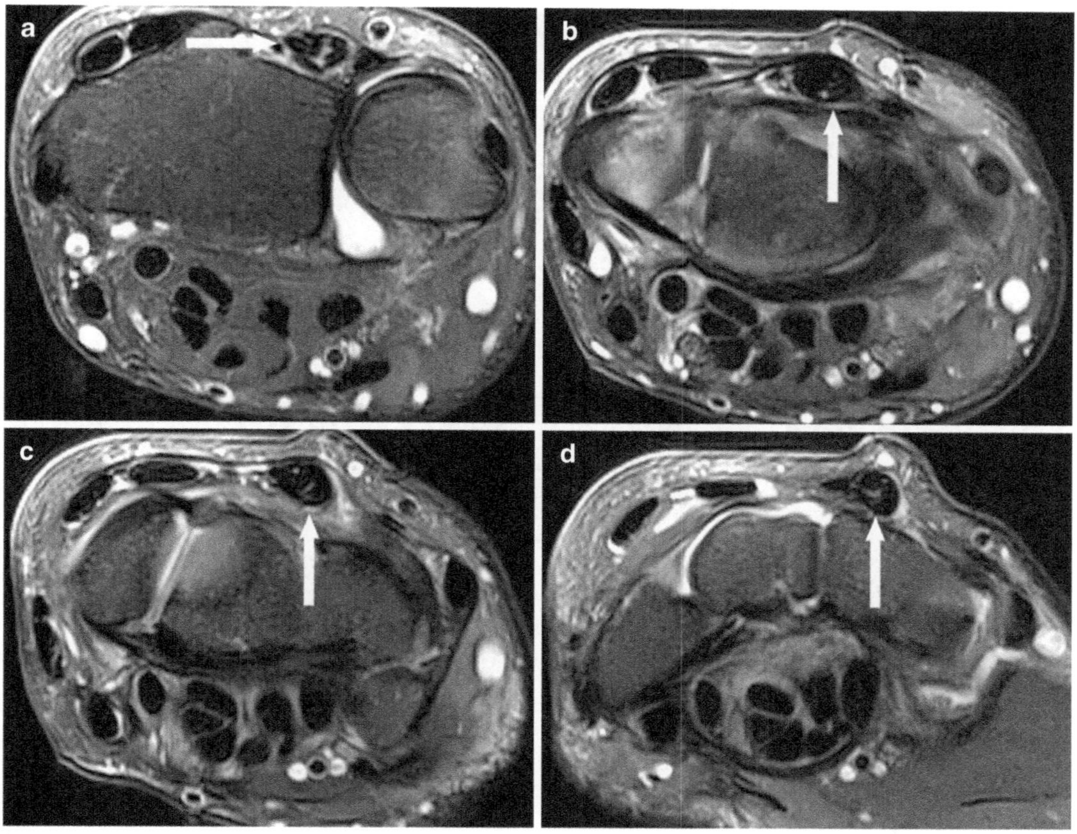

Fig. 13 Ax T2-WI FS (**a–d**). Clumping of the tendons (ed) of compartment IV

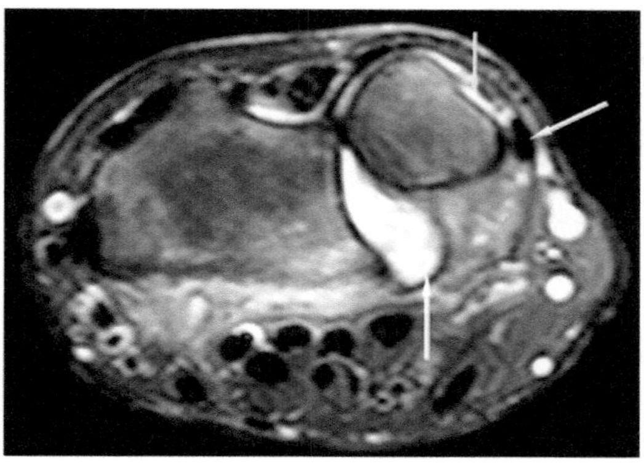

Fig. 14 Ax T2-WI FS. Luxation of the ecu with an empty sulcus. Accompanying dorsal U subluxation and DRUJ hydrops

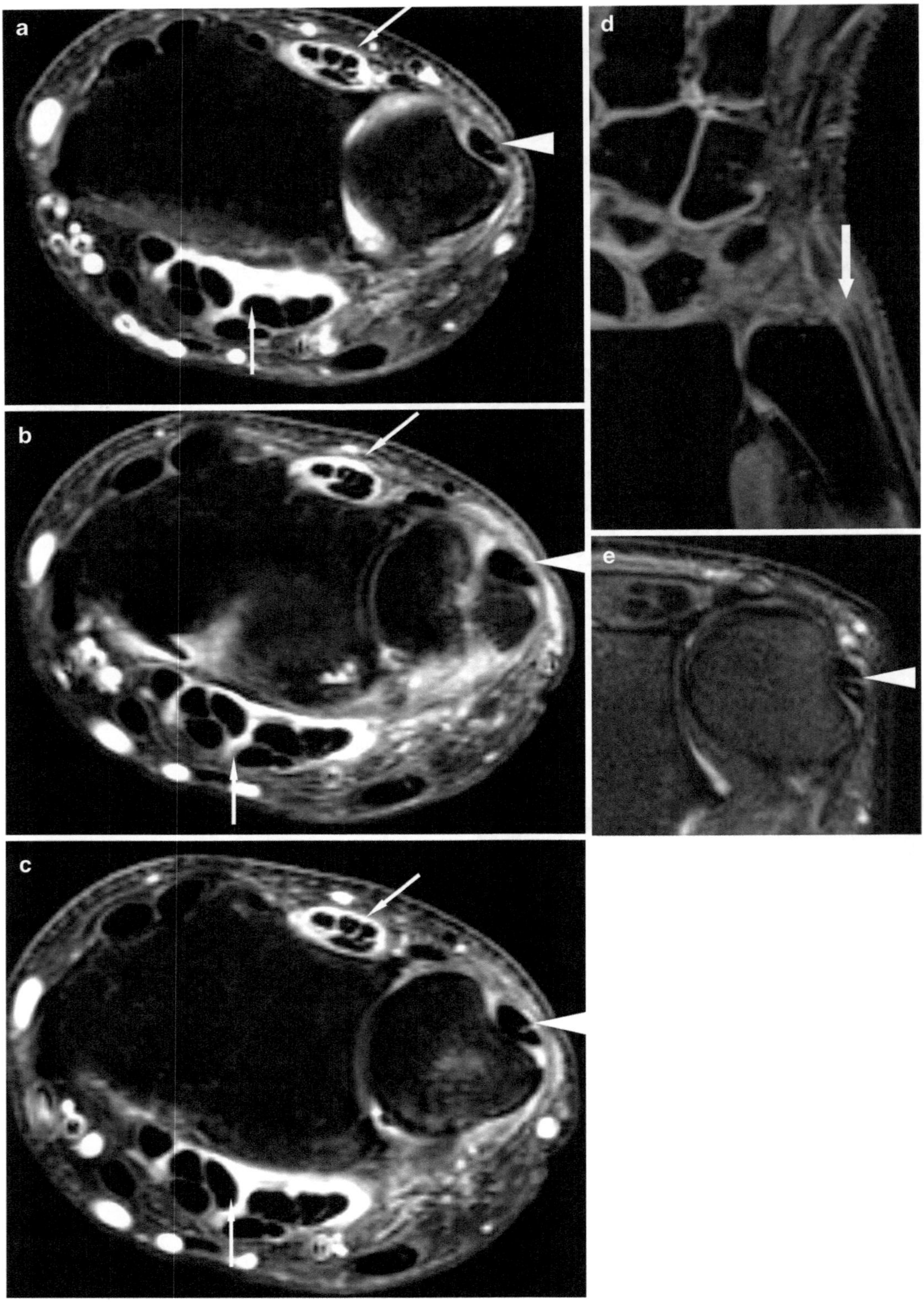

Fig. 15 Ax T2-WI FS (**a–c**), Cor 3D GRE (**d**); and T1-WI FS with CE. Longitudinal cleavage of the ecu (**a–e**) with multiple compartment (IV and flexors) tenosynovitis (**a–c**)

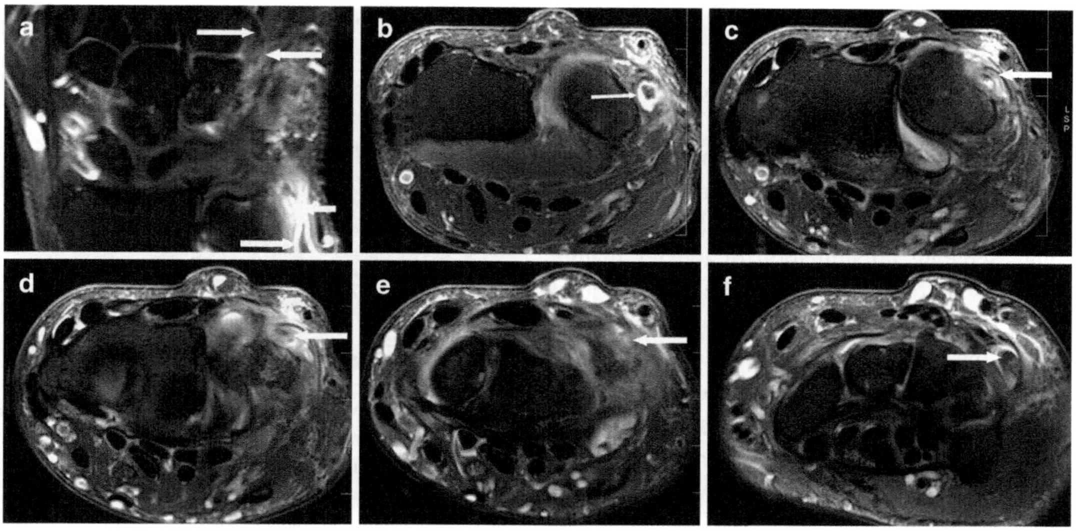

Fig. 16 Cor (**a**) and Ax (**b–f**) T2-WI FS. Rupture of the ecu with large diastasis (**a–f**). Signs of underlying tenosynovitis and tendinitis (**b, f**)

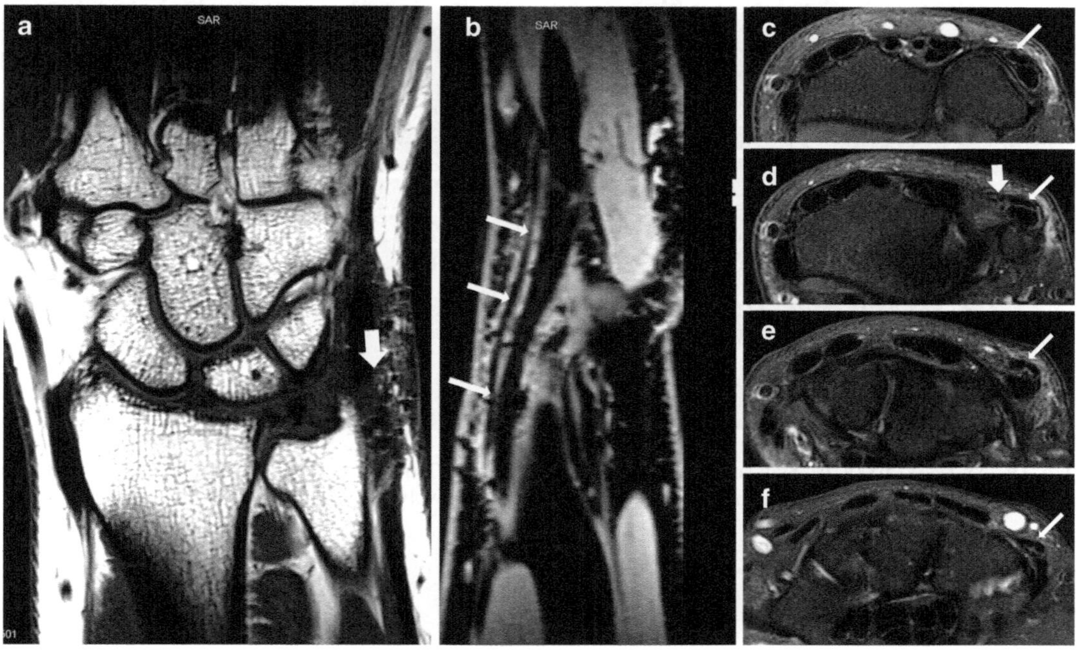

Fig. 17 Cor (**a**) T1-WI (**a**); Sag 3D GRE (**b**); Ax T2-WI FS (**c–f**). Rupture of the ecu with repair. Transfer of the edm (compartment V) to compartment VI

3 Flexor tendons

In the group of the palmar flexor tendons, the flexor carpi radialis is a separate entity. It runs close to the tubercle of the trapezium. Tenosynovitis of the fcr (Figs. 18 and 19) should immediately draw the attention to the CMC-I joint. Separate inflammation of the fcr mainly occurs with osteoarthritis of the CMC-I joint (Figs. 18 and 19c). On the other hand, tenosynovitis of the fcr (Fig. 19a, b) without degenerative anomalies (Fig. 19d) and/or with other compartments involved (Fig. 19e) is suggestive for inflammatory pathology, in particular RA (Eshed et al. 2009).

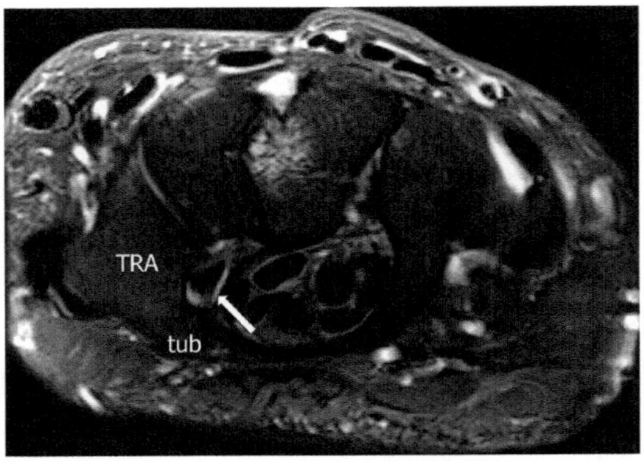

Fig. 18 Ax T2-WI FS. Tenosynovitis of the fcr, which runs separately in the bony carpal tunnel close to the tubercle of the Tra

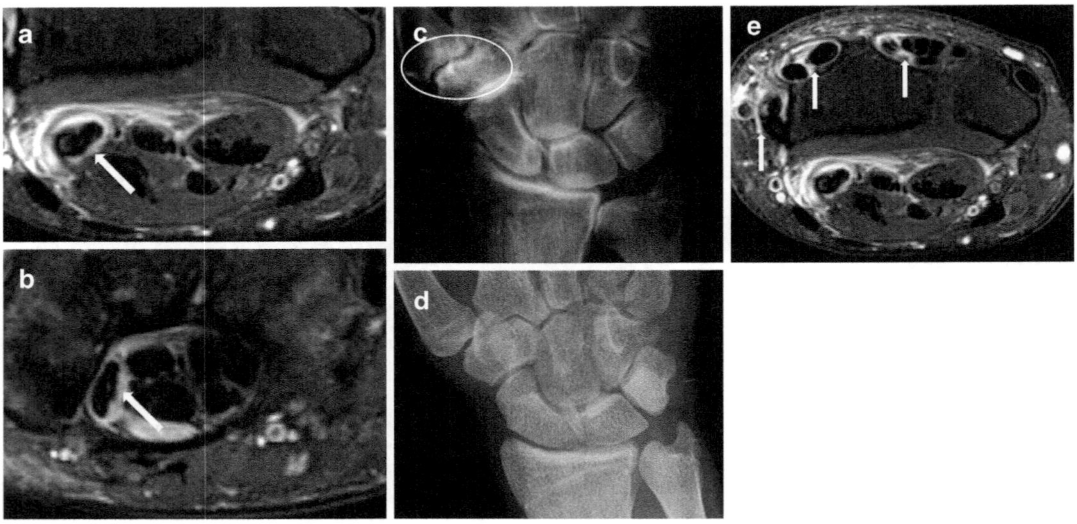

Fig. 19 Ax T2-WI FS (**a**, **b**); Standard PA (**c**, **d**); Ax T1-WI with CE. Tenosynovitis of the fcr (**a**, **b**). CMC-I joint with (**c**) and without degenerative anomalies (**d**). Multiple compartments involved (**e**)

In tenosynovitis of the flexor digitorum tendons (Elias and Schulter-Ellis 1985; Jones et al. 1997), the fluid tends to collect mainly deep in the carpal tunnel (Figs. 1 and 20). An anteriorly displaced irregular pronator fat pad, however, may indicate an underlying occult fracture of the radius (Fig. 21a). A fluid collection of any kind in the Parona space (Fig. 21b, c) should also be differentiated. Standard views may be of help (Fig. 22a, b), but MRI gives an entire picture of the wrist bones and soft tissues (Fig. 22c–e) and allows to suggest the diagnosis of RA.

However, tendon calcifications as typically in the fcu in hairdressers may be missed on MRI. The essential principle of analysing an MRI together with standard views (Fig. 23a, b) and the primary importance of US (Fig. 23c–e) in tendinopathy cannot be emphasised enough.

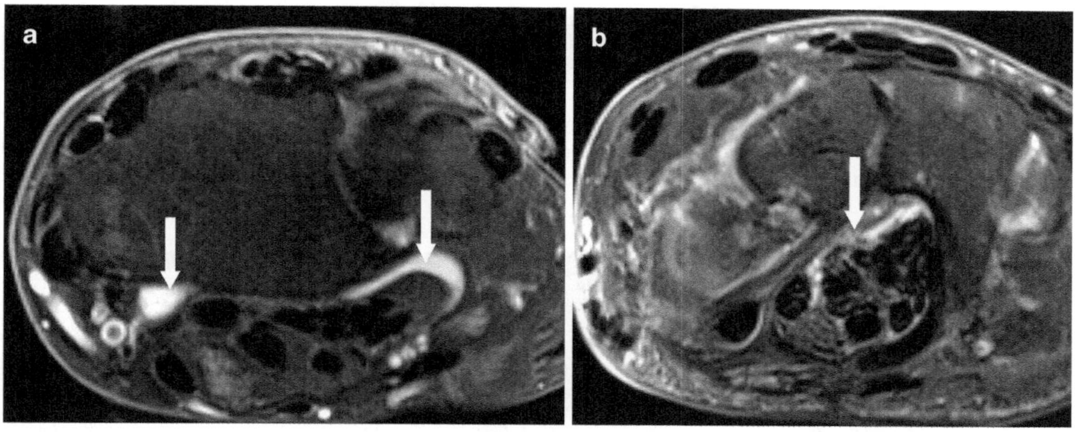

Fig. 20 Ax T2-WI FS (**a**); Standard PA (**b**); Ax T1-WI with CE. Tenosynovitis of the flexor digitorum

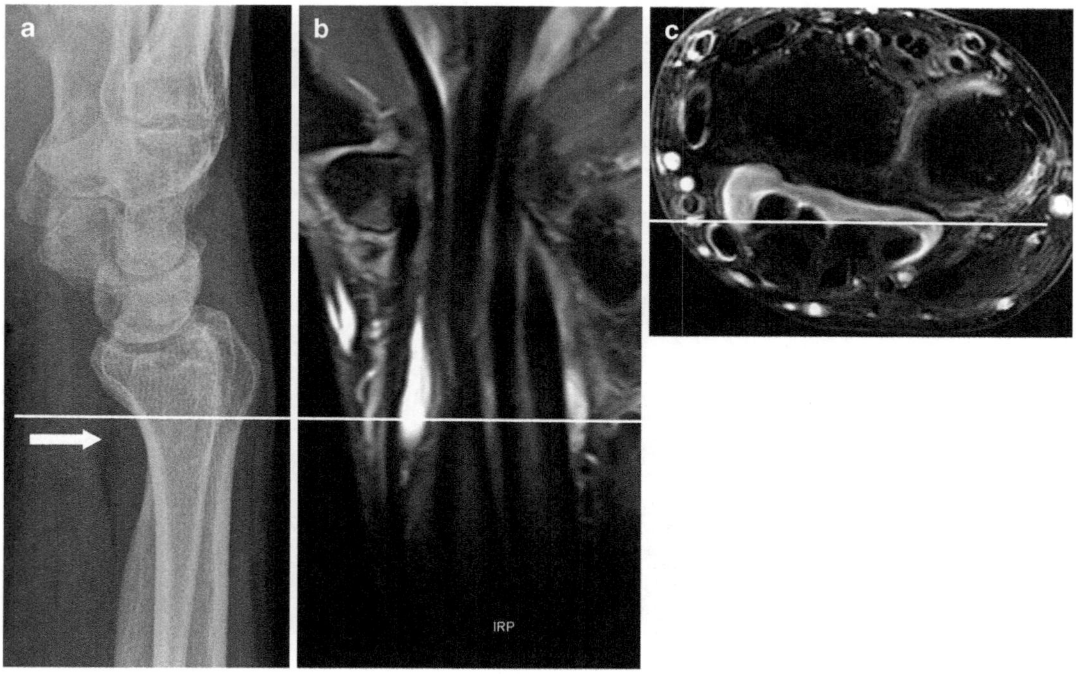

Fig. 21 Standard Lateral view (**a**); Cor (**b**) and Ax (**c**) T2-WI FS. Displaced and irregular pronator fat pad (**a**). Extensive fluid collection in Parona space

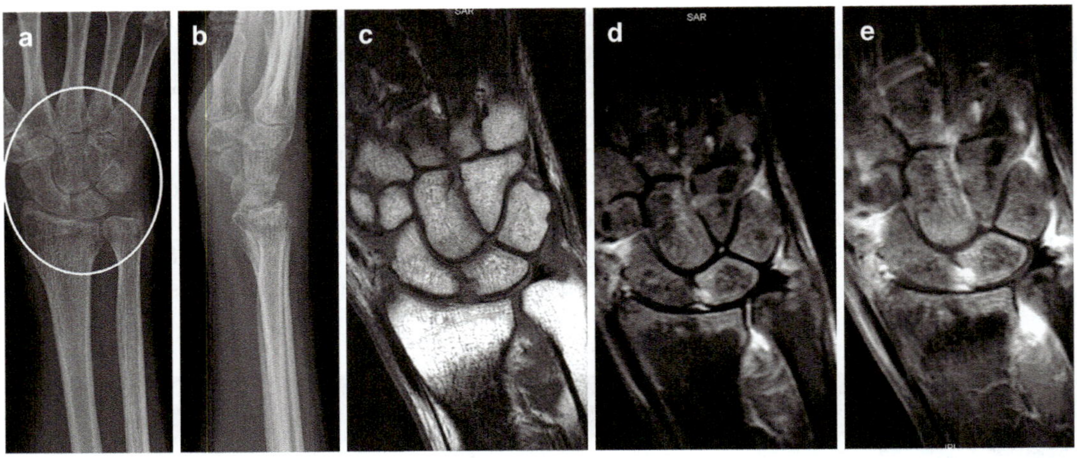

Fig. 22 Standard PA (**a**) and Lateral (**b**) view; Cor T1-WI (**c**), T2-WI FS (**d**), and T1-WI FS with CE (**e**). Diffuse osteoporosis at the wrist (**a**, **b**). Diffuse BMO, infiltration of the SL with small L bony erosion, hydrops at the DRUJ and small synovial proliferations (**c**, **d**) with CE (**e**), all pointing to RA

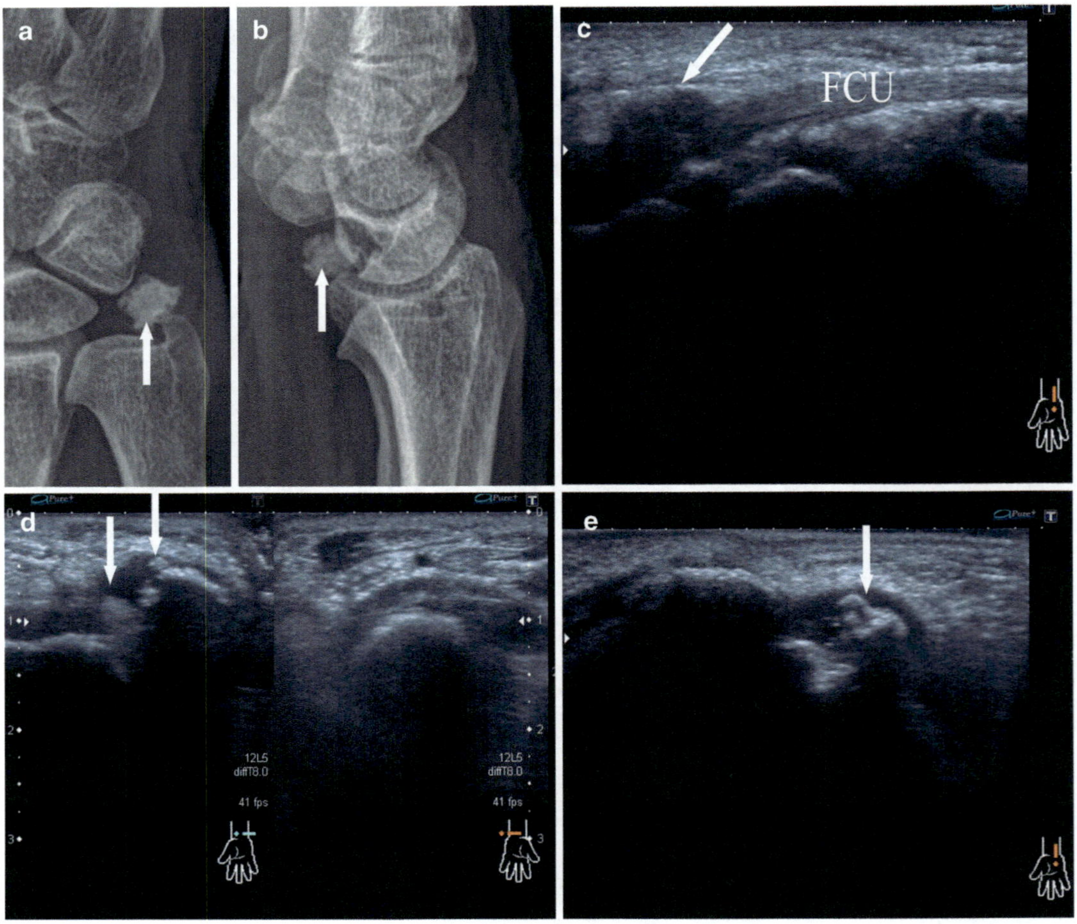

Fig. 23 Standard PA (**a**) and Lateral (**b**) view; longitudinal (**c**, **e**) and comparative transversal (**d**) US. Coarse calcification proximal of the P (**a**, **b**) within a swollen fcu proximal to the insertion on the P (**c–e**)

References

Albright JA, Linburg RM (1978) Common variations of the radial wrist extensors. J Hand Surg Am 3(2):134–138. https://doi.org/10.1016/s0363-5023(78)80060-4. PMID: 632542

Anderson ML, Skinner JA, Felmlee JP, Berger RA, Amrami KK (2008) Diagnostic comparison of 1.5 Tesla and 3.0 Tesla preoperative MRI of the wrist in patients with ulnar-sided wrist pain. J Hand Surg Am 33(7):1153–1159. https://doi.org/10.1016/j.jhsa.2008.02.028. PMID: 18762112

Bruno F, Arrigoni F, Palumbo P, Natella R, Maggialetti N, Reginelli A, Splendiani A, Di Cesare E, Bazzocchi A, Guglielmi G, Masciocchi C, Barile A (2019) The acutely injured wrist. Radiol Clin North Am 57(5):943–955. https://doi.org/10.1016/j.rcl.2019.05.003. Epub 2019 Jun 26. PMID: 31351543

Chang CY, Kheterpal AB, Vicentini JRT, Huang AJ (2017) Variations of anatomy on MRI of the first extensor compartment of the wrist and association with DeQuervain tenosynovitis. Skeletal Radiol 46(8):1047–1056. https://doi.org/10.1007/s00256-017-2639-0. Epub 2017 Apr 7. PMID: 28389821

Davis KW, Blankenbaker DG (2010) Imaging the ligaments and tendons of the wrist. Semin Roentgenol 45(3):194–217. https://doi.org/10.1053/j.ro.2009.12.005. PMID: 20483115

Elias LS, Schulter-Ellis FP (1985) Anomalous flexor superficialis indicis: two case reports and literature review. J Hand Surg Am 10(2):296–299. https://doi.org/10.1016/s0363-5023(85)80128-3. PMID: 3980950

Eshed I, Feist E, Althoff CE, Hamm B, Konen E, Burmester GR, Backhaus M, Hermann KG (2009) Tenosynovitis of the flexor tendons of the hand detected by MRI: an early indicator of rheumatoid arthritis. Rheumatology (Oxford) 48(8):887–891. https://doi.org/10.1093/rheumatology/kep136. Epub 2009 May 27. PMID: 19474128

Gornitzky AL, Carrigan RB (2016) The diagnostic utility of MRI in the painful wrist: when to reconsider advanced imaging in the pediatric patient. Pediatrics (Evanston) 137(Suppl 3):596–596A. https://doi.org/10.1542/peds.137.Supplement_3.596A

Gümüşalan Y, Kalaycioğlu A, Yazar F, Arifoğlu Y, Sinav A (1997) Accessory extensor carpi radialis muscle and interconnecting muscular bundle. Acta Anat (Basel) 159(1):57–60. PMID: 9522898

Jones M, Abrahams PH, Sañudo JR, Campillo M (1997) Incidence and morphology of accessory heads of flexor pollicis longus and flexor digitorum profundus (Gantzer's muscles). J Anat 191(Pt 3):451–455. https://doi.org/10.1046/j.1469-7580.1997.19130451.x. PMID: 9419002; PMCID: PMC1467702

Kaiser P, Kellermann F, Arora R, Henninger B, Rudisch A (2018) Diagnosing extensor carpi ulnaris tendon dislocation with dynamic rotation MRI of the wrist. Clin Imaging 51:323–326. https://doi.org/10.1016/j.clinimag.2018.06.015. Epub 2018 Jun 23. PMID: 29958158

Luijkx T, Buckens CF, van Seeters T, Pegge SA, Maas M (2019) ECU tendon subluxation: a nonspecific MRI finding occurring in all wrist positions irrespective of ulnar-sided symptoms? Eur J Radiol 116:192–197. https://doi.org/10.1016/j.ejrad.2019.05.011. Epub 2019 May 10. PMID: 31153564

Martinoli C, Perez MM, Padua L, Valle M, Capaccio E, Altafini L, Michaud J, Tagliafico A (2010) Muscle variants of the upper and lower limb (with anatomical correlation). Semin Musculoskelet Radiol 14(2):106–121. https://doi.org/10.1055/s-0030-1253155. Epub 2010 May 18. PMID: 20486022

Meraj S, Gyftopoulos S, Nellans K, Walz D, Brown MS (2017) MRI of the extensor tendons of the wrist. AJR Am J Roentgenol 209(5):1093–1102. https://doi.org/10.2214/AJR.17.17791. Epub 2017 Aug 31. PMID: 28858545

Mespreuve M, Vanhoenacker F, Malfait F, Mortier D, Mertens G (2005) Postaxial polydactyly type A in a patient with Ellis – van Creveld syndrome: additional value of MR-imaging. Eurorad:case12665. http://www.eurorad.org/case.php?id=12665

Nayak SR, Krishnamurthy A, Prabhu LV, Rai R, Ranade AV, Madhyastha S (2008) Anatomical variation of radial wrist extensor muscles: a study in cadavers. Clinics (Sao Paulo) 63(1):85–90. https://doi.org/10.1590/s1807-59322008000100015. PMID: 18297212; PMCID: PMC2664178

Paley D, McMurtry RY, Murray JF (1987) Dorsal dislocation of the ulnar styloid and extensor carpi ulnaris tendon into the distal radioulnar joint: the empty sulcus sign. J Hand Surg Am 12(6):1029–1032. https://doi.org/10.1016/s0363-5023(87)80104-1. PMID: 3693829

Rixey A, Wenger D, Baffour F, Kakar S, McKenzie G (2021) Accessory abductor digiti minimi muscle, less muscular than thought: an update on prevalence, morphology, and review of the literature. Skeletal Radiol 50(8):1687–1695. https://doi.org/10.1007/s00256-021-03728-5. Epub 2021 Feb 3 PMID: 33533963

Rodríguez-Niedenführ M, Vázquez T, Golanó P, Parkin I, Sañudo JR (2002) Extensor digitorum brevis manus: anatomical, radiological and clinical relevance. A review. Clin Anat 15(4):286–292. https://doi.org/10.1002/ca.10027. PMID: 12112357

Sookur PA, Naraghi AM, Bleakney RR, Jalan R, Chan O, White LM (2008) Accessory muscles: anatomy, symptoms, and radiologic evaluation. Radiographics 28(2):481–499. https://doi.org/10.1148/rg.282075064. PMID: 18349452

Theumann NH, Pfirrmann CW, Chung CB, Antonio GE, Trudell DJ, Resnick D (2002) Ligamentous and tendinous anatomy of the intermetacarpal and common carpometacarpal joints: evaluation with MR imaging and MR arthrography. J Comput Assist Tomogr 26(1):145–152. https://doi.org/10.1097/00004728-200201000-00026. PMID: 11801922

Zeiss J, Guilliam-Haidet L (1996) MR demonstration of anomalous muscles about the volar aspect of the wrist and forearm. Clin Imaging 20(3):219–221. https://doi.org/10.1016/0899-7071(95)00013-5. PMID: 8877177

Arthritis

Contents

1 General

More localised infectious or (in a later stage) more generalised inflammatory arthritis are initially sometimes difficult to diagnose and to differentiate. The 3D imaging of MRI eliminates the bony superposition, gives an objective idea of the width of the joint spaces, and visualises directly in high contrast the soft tissues and bone marrow. It therefore substantially contributes to the (differential) diagnosis (Aizenberg et al. 2018; Boeren et al. 2023; Eriksen and Ringe 2012; Jans and Chen 2021).

In RA, the wrist is frequently affected and is also a good marker for the general joint involvement. Standard views will only show irreversible destructive bony erosions and soft tissue swelling. MRI on the other hand may show BMO as a precursor of erosions, IA fluid, synovial proliferation with bone and cartilage destruction, active zones of osteitis, tenosynovitis, tendon laceration or rupture, and ligament lesions. Nowadays, the evolution to final ankylosis is rare. Peri-articular CE on MRI has a sensitivity of about 100% and a specificity of about 89% for RA (Ejbjerg et al. 2005).

2 Infectious Arthritis

After hematogenous spread of a germ, further extension to the joint will be age-dependent (Fig. 1). Within the first year of a newborn, the arteries cross the growth plate and infection may thus spread from the bone directly into the joint. During the following growing phase (approximately from 1 to 18 years), the arteries do not cross the growth plate anymore and the infectious

M. Mespreuve, K. Waked, *MRI of the Wrist*, Medical Radiology,
https://doi.org/10.1007/978-3-031-63973-9_13

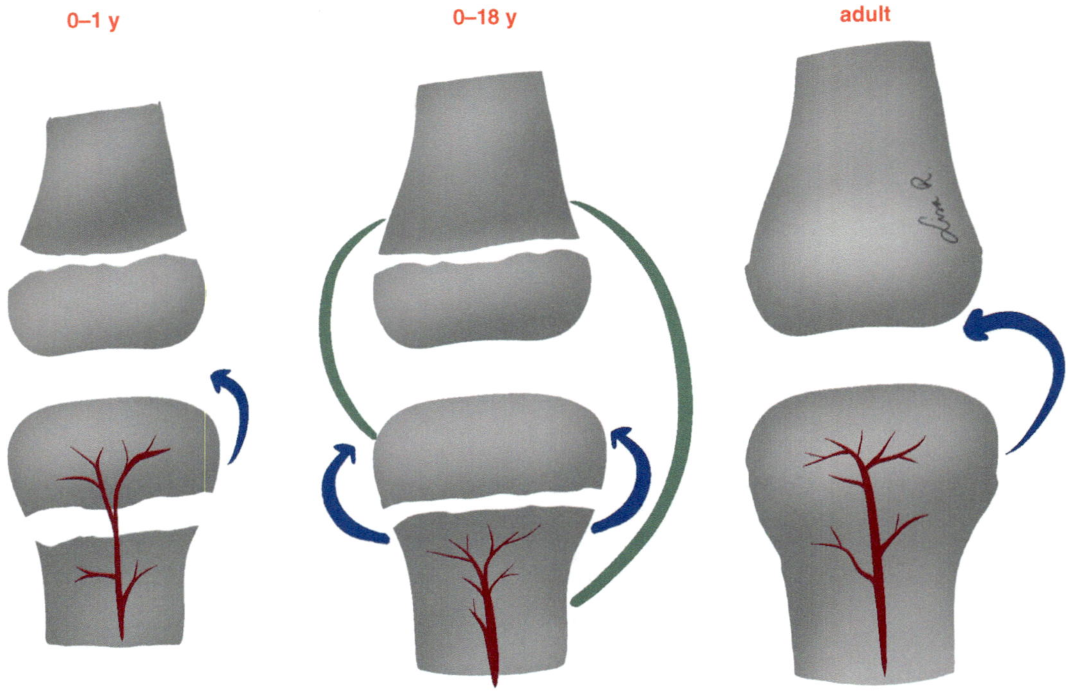

Fig. 1 After hematogenous spread of a germ, further extension depends on the growth phase related to bone development. (Illustrated by Lisa Ramaut, MD)

spread depends solely on the type of the proximal capsule insertion, resulting in a para-articular or an intra-articular spread. After closure of the growth plate, the germ spread returns to the initial phase, i.e., directly into the joint. A mostly obvious direct penetration in the joint may also cause infectious arthritis.

Standard views will remain the first approach in the routine diagnostic process (Fig. 2a) and CT may illustrate in a clear way the destruction of the trabeculae and cortex (Fig. 2b–d). MRI has the same 3D diagnostic power as CT, but the superior natural soft tissue contrast and the contrast enhancement remain powerful diagnostic tools in this imaging process (Couzens et al. 2014) (Fig. 2e–h).

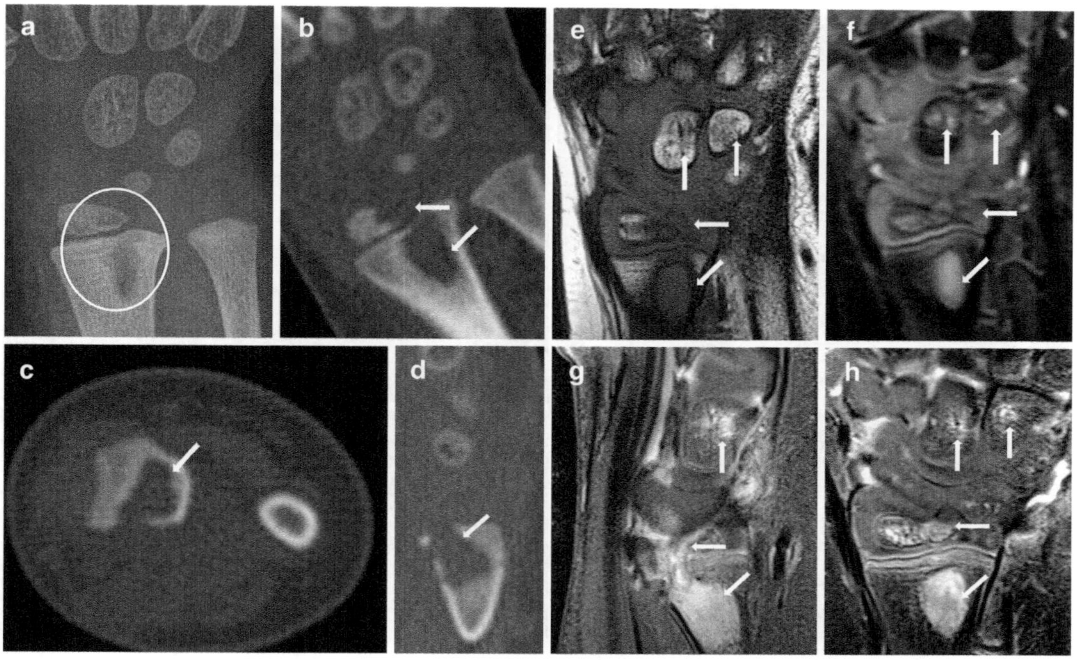

Fig. 2 Standard PA view (**a**); Cor (**b**), Ax (**c**), and Sag (**d**) CT; Cor T1-WI (**e**), T2-WI FS (**f**); Sag (**g**), and Cor (**h**) T1-WI FS with CE. Translucent area with trabecular destruction in the distal R on both sides of the growth plate- metaphysis (**a**). CT (**b–d**) shows a lytic zone with cortical destruction of the R epi- and diaphysis. Apart from the lytic (**e, f**) and CE (**g, h**) areas in the R a similar small lesion of the C and H is shown (**e–h**). The additional lesion of the H is probably visible on the CT (**b**)

3 Rheumatoid Arthritis

In RA, the risk of developing an erosion within 1 year is six times higher at the early detected location of fuzzy bounded BMO (Boeren et al. 2023; Xiao et al. 2021; Yang et al. 2015) with intact trabecular pattern (Fig. 3). Using MRI, erosions will be seen up to 1 year earlier than on standard views. These primary destructions due to synovial proliferation and granulation (pannus) are located at the cartilage border and the insertion of the capsule and the ligaments. It causes round, well circumscribed erosions with internal synovial fluid or proliferation (Figs. 4 and 5). The cartilage damage and ligament destruction are directly shown by MRI, as are tendinitis, tenosynovitis, and tendon rupture (Fujimori et al. 2017; Gandjbakhch et al. 2011).

Some solitary abnormalities need further diagnostic attention when discovered. Peritendinous CE (Eshed et al. 2009; Valeri et al. 2001) at multiple compartments (Fig. 6) may indicate RA and should at least be followed-up. A small erosion (Fig. 7a) and/or synovial proliferation (Fig. 7b, c), which may be mixed with coincident degenerative alterations may reveal after CE (Fig. 7e, f) a RA pattern (Fig. 7). Even an isolated lesion with a typical aspect and location needs to be evaluated further to confirm (or exclude) RA (Fig. 8). Follow-up may reveal a new appearing BMO (Hetland et al. 2009; Kamp et al. 2013; Palosaari et al. 2006; Shabshin and Schweitzer 2009) (Fig. 9), which is frequently a

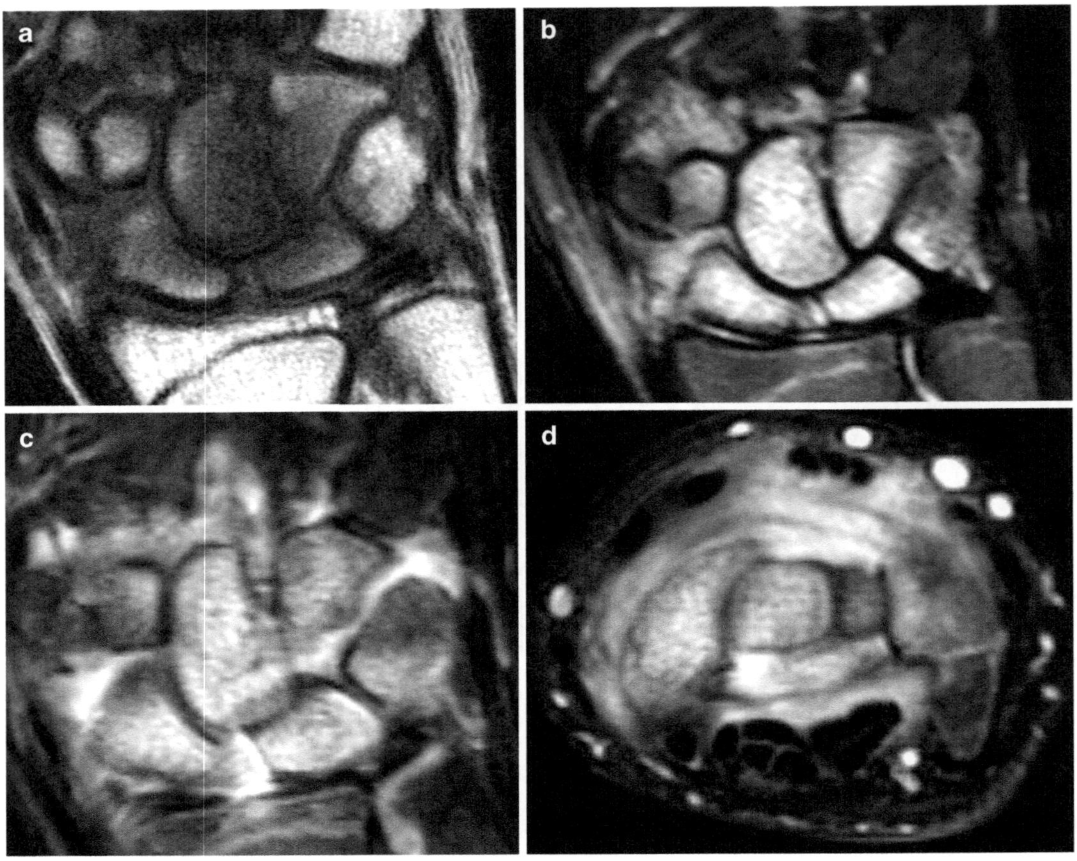

Fig. 3 Cor T1-WI (**a**) and T2-WI FS (**b**); Cor (**c**) and AX (**d**) T1-WI FS with CE. Accidentally early detected diffuse carpal locations of fuzzy bounded BMO with an intact trabecular pattern and hydrops (**a**, **b**). Diffuse CE of synovia and bone marrow (**c**, **d**)

precursor of an erosion. The intrinsic ligaments and the TFCC are also prone to infiltration by synovial proliferation (Fig. 10) as are the extrinsic ligaments (Fig. 11). Multiple small synovial cysts (Fig. 12) are striking attention-getters (Mysling et al. 2013; Rubin 2019).

A combination of tiny erosions, ligament infiltration, and (multi-compartment) hydrops (especially at the DRUJ) are very alarming and suggestive for a deterioration towards RA (Fig. 13). The visualisation of diffuse BMO and hydrops (Gornitzky and Carrigan 2016) (Fig. 14a) should also prompt for CE (Fig. 14b). These zones are prone to the development of erosions.

Diffuse and persisting tenosynovitis (Eshed et al. 2009; Nieuwenhuis et al. 2015) of the extensor and/or flexor tendons should be an alarm sign (Fig. 15), especially in the juvenile form (Nusman et al. 2016; Ording Muller et al. 2013). The joint is frequently spared in this form of RA. Epiphysial overgrowth, early closure of the growth plate, underdevelopment or partial resorption of carpal bones, and periostitis are late and to be avoided complications of juvenile RA. In adults, a persist-

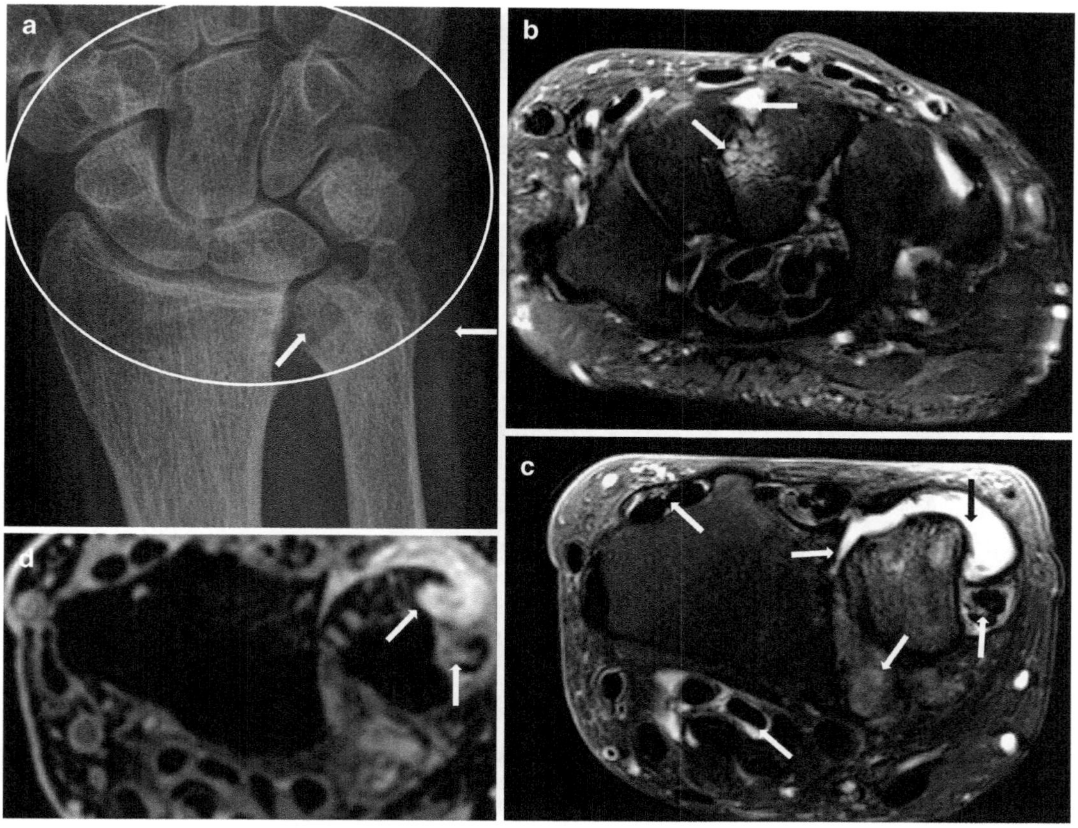

Fig. 4 Standard PA view (**a**); Ax T1-WI FS with CE (**b**, **c**); 3D GRE (**d**). Accidentally detected translucency at the U head with soft tissue swelling and minimal (peri)carpal osteoporosis (**a**). Fuzzy bounded BMO with intact trabecular pattern and CE, also at an intrinsic distal carpal ligament (**b**). Ecu cleavage (**c**, **d**) and mild tenosynovitis of compartment II, VI and the flexor tendons (**c**). Destruction of the palmar rul (**c**) and DRUJ hydrops (**c**). Erosion at the ulnar head (**d**) due to synovial proliferation

ing tenosynovitis eventually combined with CTS may be the first manifestation of RA (Fig. 16).

The retraction of the capsule is difficult to evaluate as is the fast lymphogenic drainage (Fig. 17) due to the inflammation. Classical arthrography may show the extent of the fibrotic retraction and eventual IA adhesions.

CE MRI sequences can show synovial hyperplasia before the erosive lesions develop. Consequently, the (anti-TNF) therapy will—due to an earlier start—prevent destruction of bone, cartilage, and soft tissues. Grading may be done among others by the RAMRIS protocol (Aizenberg et al. 2018; Fujimori et al. 2017; Barbieri et al. 2013; Dakkak et al. 2020). Follow-up during the therapy may show reduced BMO and CE at the synovial proliferations and absence of newly developed erosions.

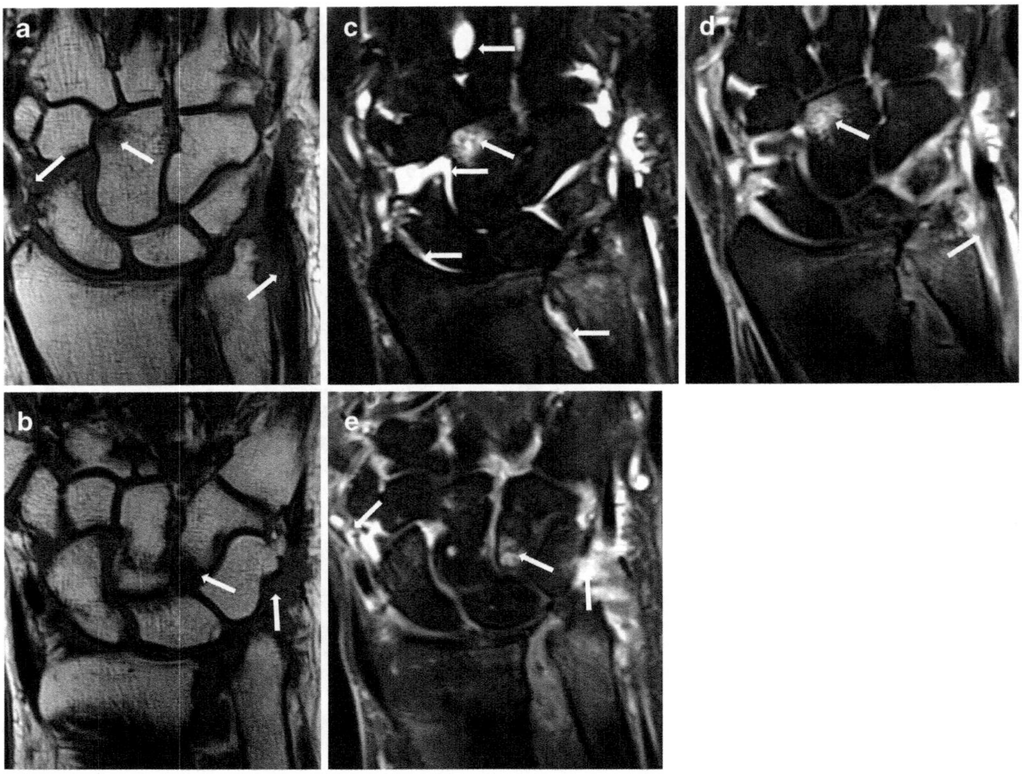

Fig. 5 Cor T1-WI (**a**, **b**), T2-WI FS (**c**), and T1-WI FS with CE (**d**, **e**). BMO with CE at the C and H (**a**–**e**). Destruction of the S-Tra ligament (**a**). CMC, midcarpal, radiocarpal, and DRUJ hydrops (**c**). CE synovial proliferation around the ecu and meniscus homologue (**b**, **d**, and **e**) with small erosion at the U styloid and Tri (**a**, **b**)

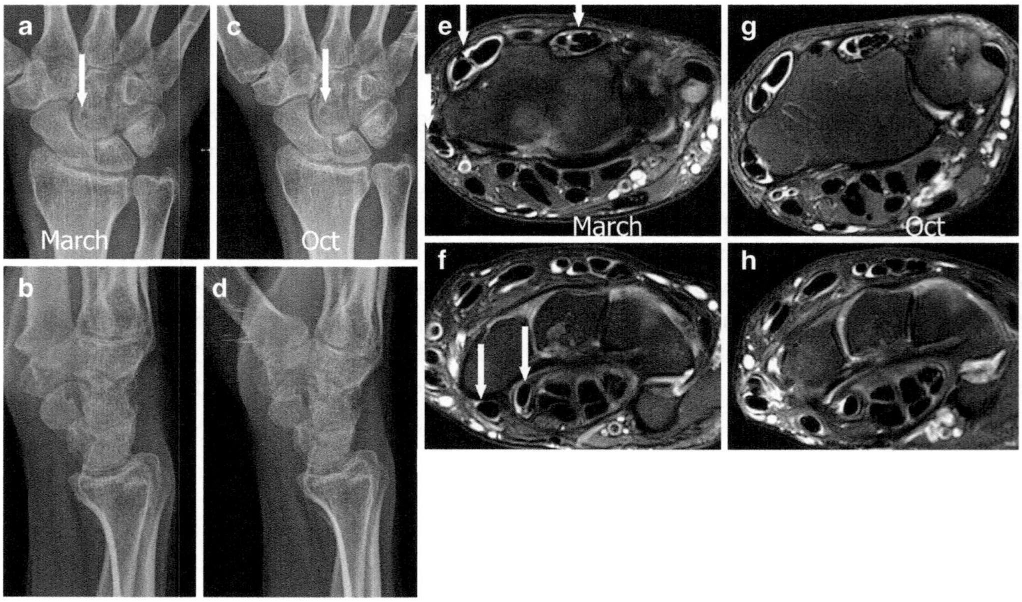

Fig. 6 Standard PA (**a**, **c**) and Lat (**b**, **d**) views; Ax T1-WI FS with CE (**e**, **f**) and follow-up (**g**, **h**). A small erosion at the C (**a**) without evolution over 6 months (**c**) on standard views. Clear CE around the tendons of compartments I, II, (III), and IV, the fcr and fpl (**e**, **f**), slightly increasing at compartment I (**g**, **h**) due to RA

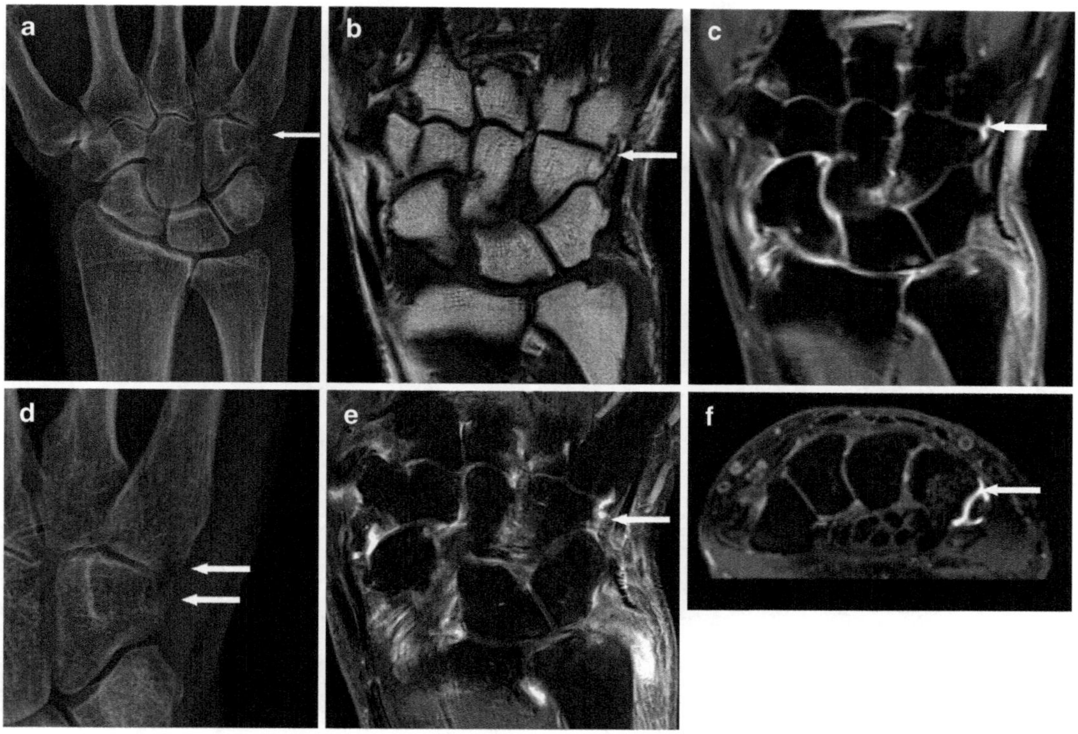

Fig. 7 Standard PA (**a**, **d**) views; Cor T1-WI (**b**) and T2-WI FS (**c**); Cor (**e**) and Ax (**f**) T1-WI FS with CE. A small erosion at the CMC-V joint (**a**, **d**) due to a small peri-ligamentous synovial proliferation (**b**, **c**–**f**). Also note CE at DRUJ, the proximal pole of the H and the SLC/SLT ligament and a diffuse small amount of hydrops (**e**). Signs of UA with TFCC lesion Palmer II E

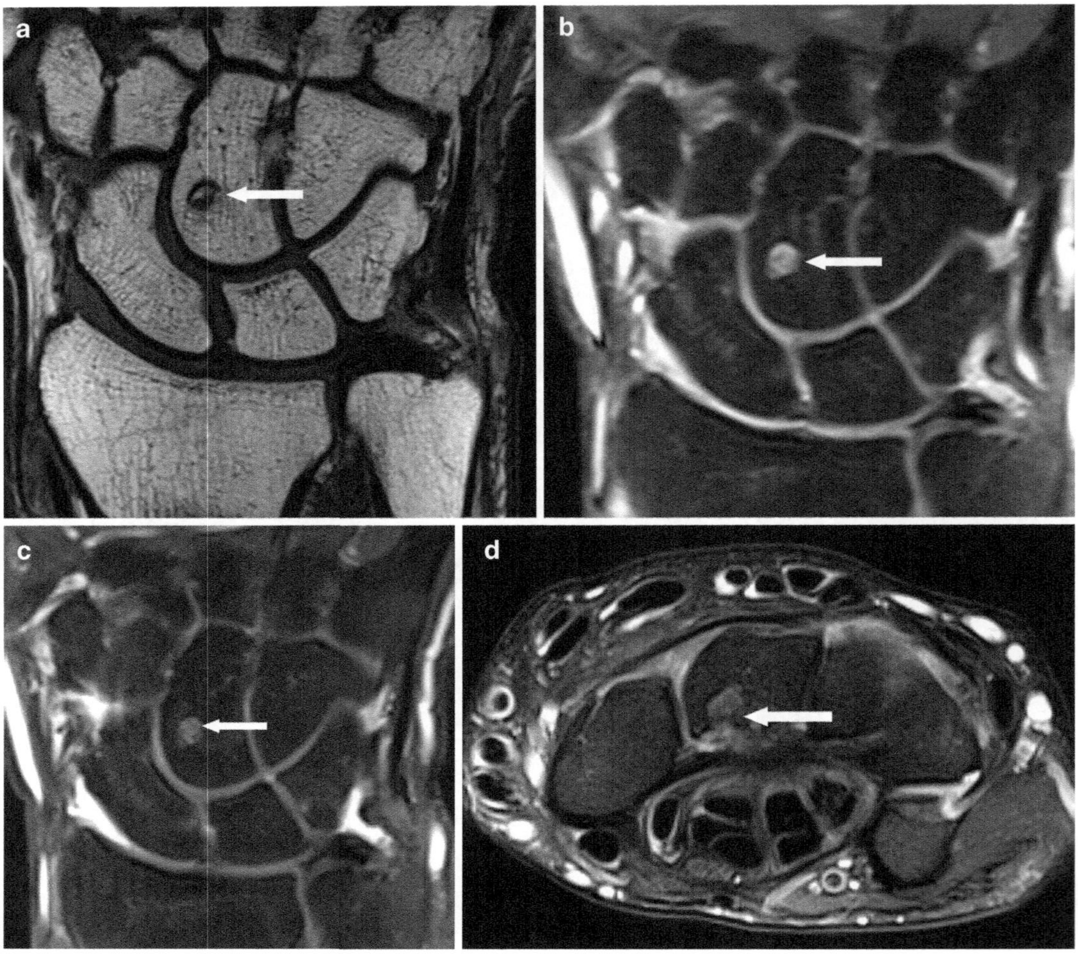

Fig. 8 Cor T1-WI (**a**), T2-WI FS (**b**); Cor (**c**) and Ax (**d**) T1-WI with CE. Synovial proliferation with small CE erosion of the C at the distal insertion of the palmar RSC extrinsic ligament

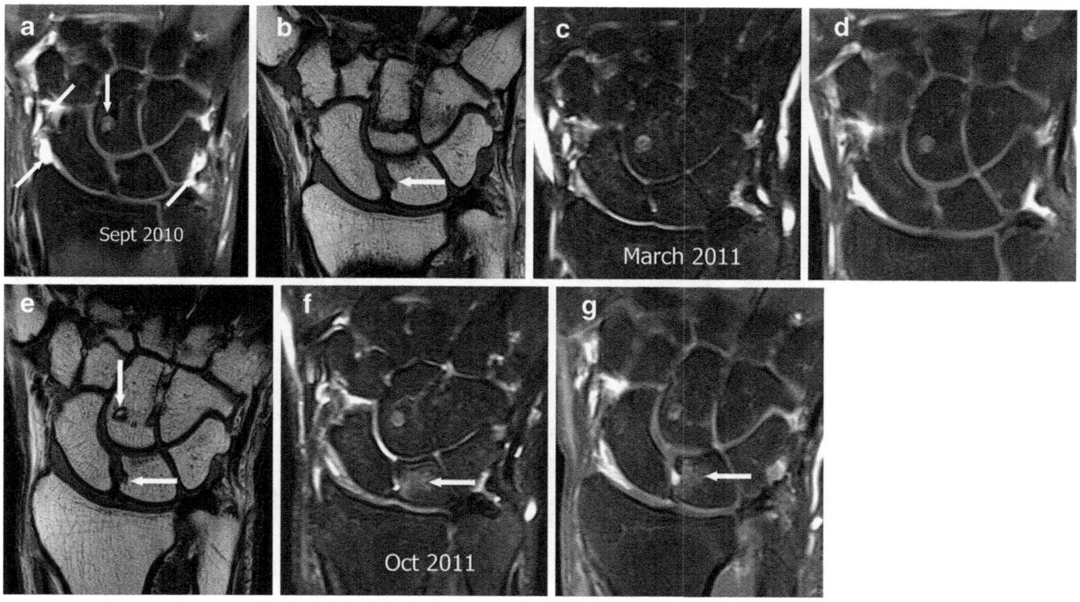

Fig. 9 Cor T1-WI FS with CE (**a**); Cor T1-WI (**b**, **e**), T2-WI FS (**c**, **f**), and T1-WI FS with CE (**e**, **g**). Synovial proliferations and a small erosion of the C (**a**). During follow-up, a small erosion of the L (**b–d**; **March 2011**) becomes more prominent (**e–g**; **Oct 2011**) and BMO of the L appears (**f**, **g**)

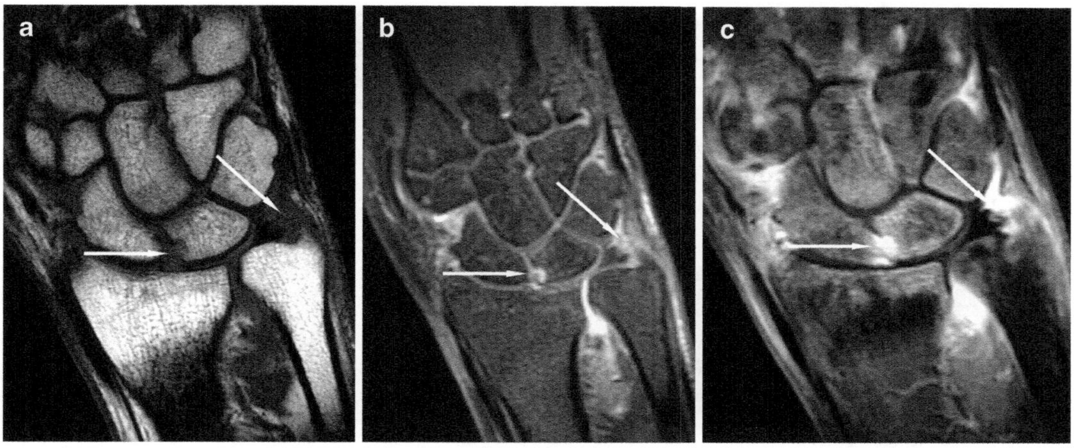

Fig. 10 Cor T1-WI (**a**), T2-WI FS (**b**), and T1-WI FS with CE (**c**). Synovial proliferations with also infiltration of the SLL at the L side, around the meniscus homologue and the ulnar insertion of the TFCC

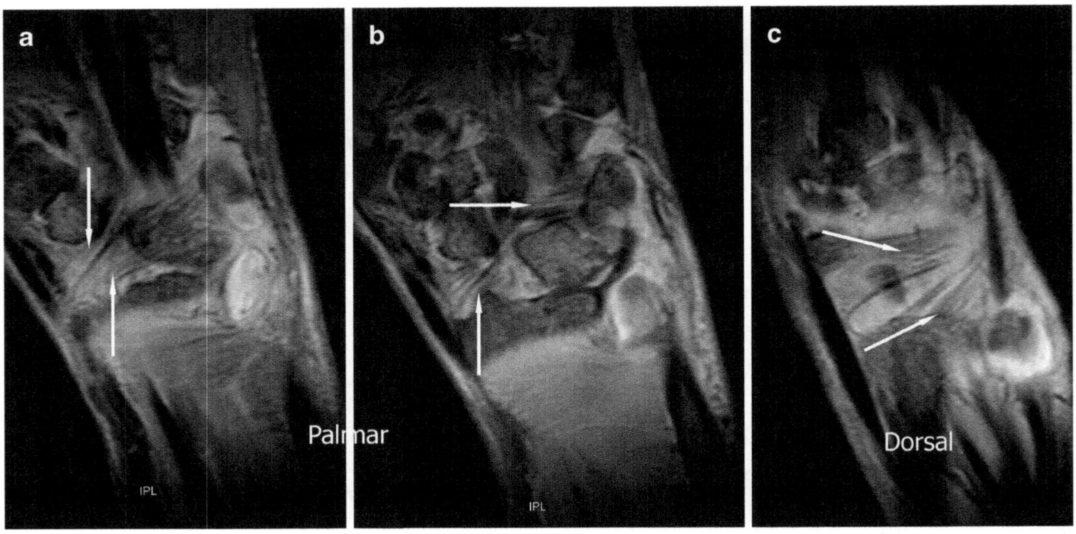

Fig. 11 Cor T2-WI FS (**a**–**c**). Synovial proliferations with oedema and infiltration of the palmar and dorsal extrinsic ligaments

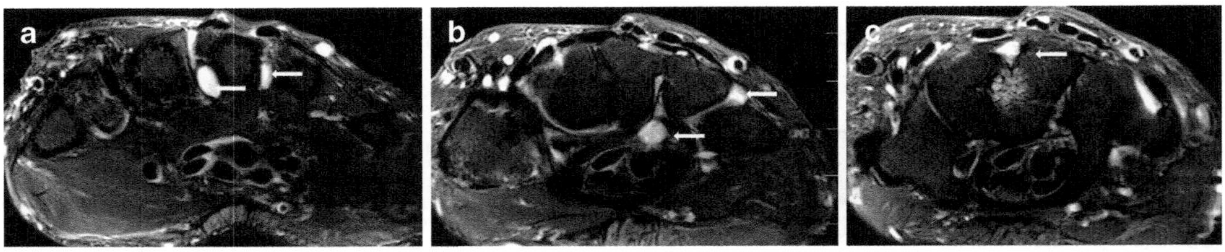

Fig. 12 Ax T2-WI FS (**a**–**c**); Standard PA view (**d**). Multiple small synovial cysts (**a**–**c**) and a small zone of BMO in the C

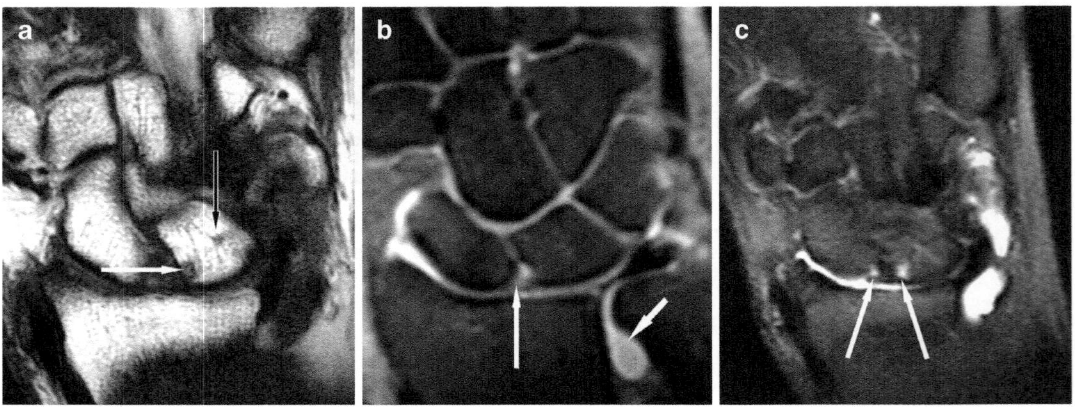

Fig. 13 Cor T1-WI (**a**), T2-WI FS (**b**), and T1-WI FS with CE. Tiny erosions (**a**) with multi-compartmental hydrops, especially prominent at the DRUJ (**b**), and a tiny CE infiltration at the insertion site of the SLL (**b**, **c**)

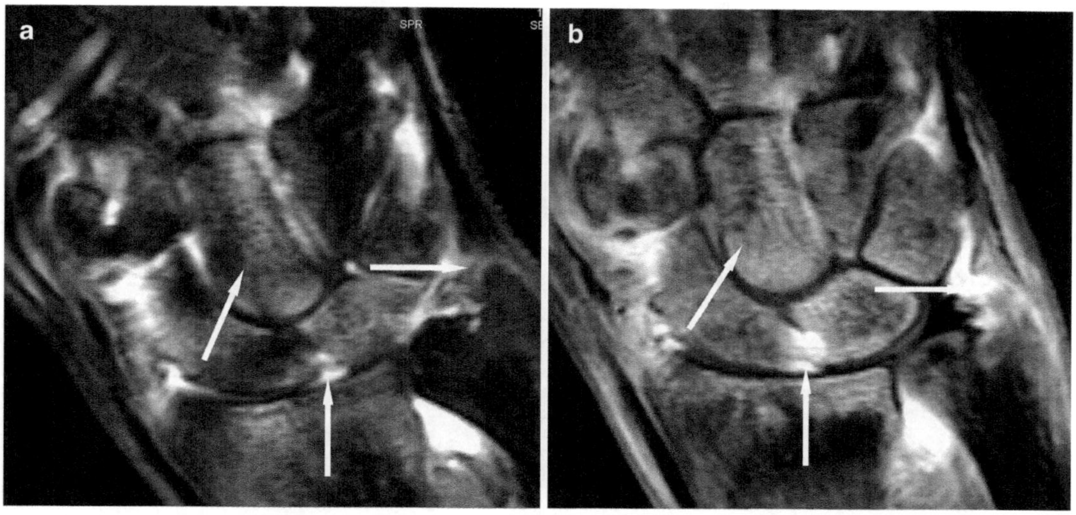

Fig. 14 Cor T2-WI FS (**a**) and T1-WI FS with CE. Diffuse BMO with multi-compartmental hydrops (**a**) and diffuse CE (**b**). Note the small infiltration of the SLL (**a, b**) and CE around the meniscus homologue and the TFCC base (**a, b**)

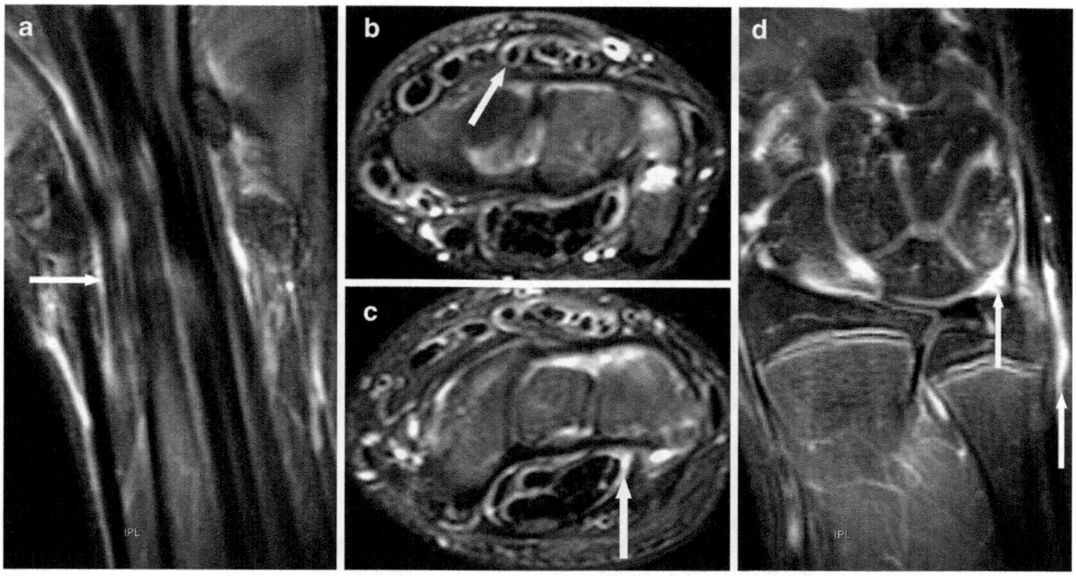

Fig. 15 Cor (**a**) and Ax (**b, c**) T2-WI FS; T1-WI FS with CE. Diffuse tenosynovitis with target sign of extensor and flexor tendons (**a–c**) with CE, pronounced around the ecu and the meniscus homologue in a 14-year-old child (**d**)

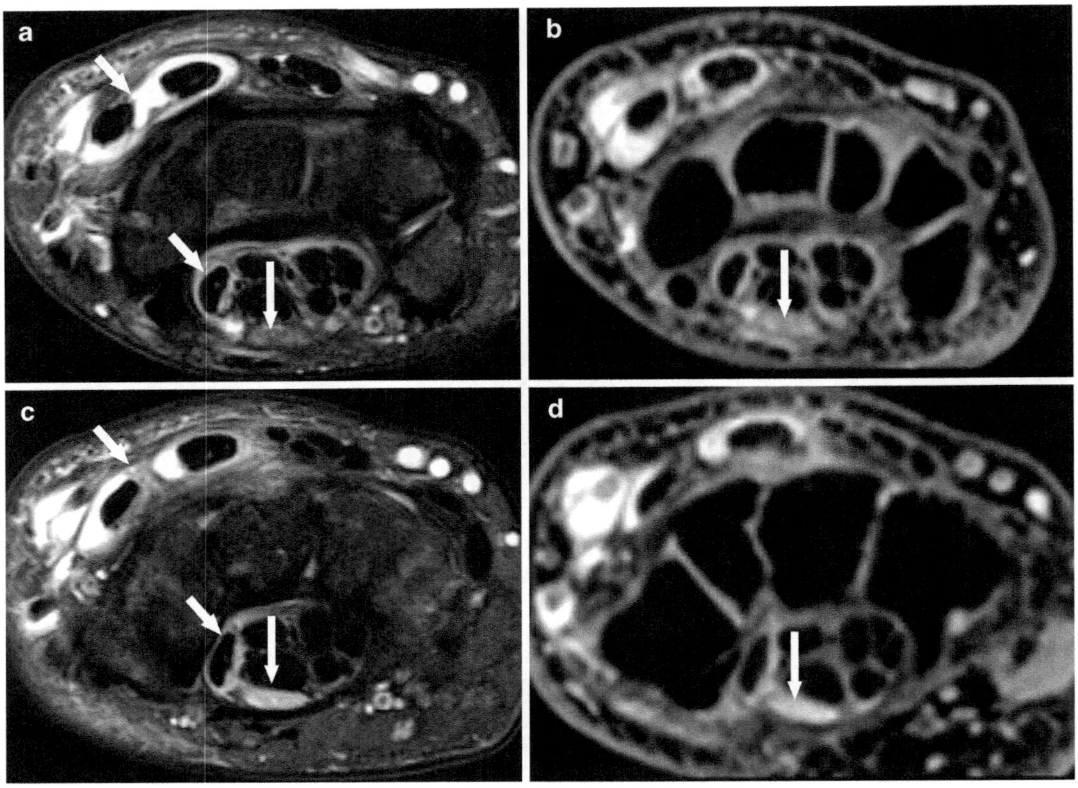

Fig. 16 Ax T2-WI FS (**a**, **c**) and 3D GRE (**b**, **d**). Fasciculation proximal (**a**) and high signal distal (**c**) in the carpal tunnel of the swollen median nerve with convex flexor retinaculum (**a**–D). Tenosynovitis with target sign of extensor (II) (**a**) and flexor (fcr) (**c**) tendons

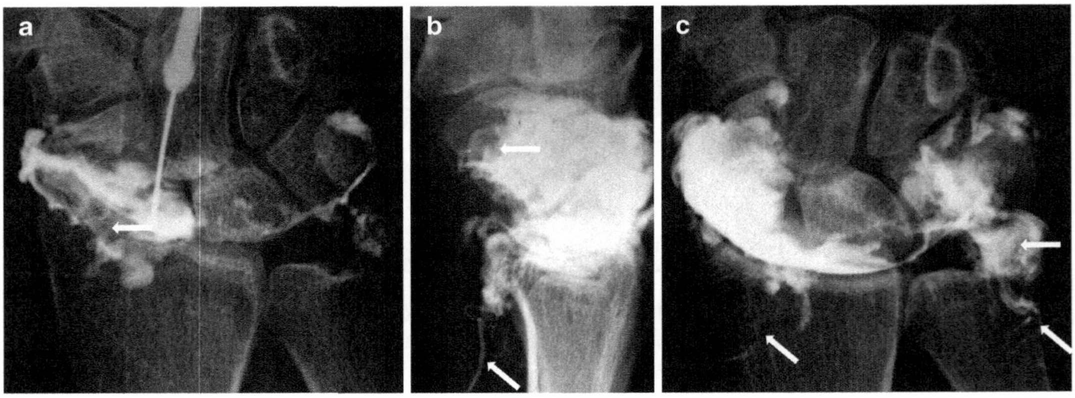

Fig. 17 RC arthrography. RA with diffuse capsular retraction (**a**–**c**) and fast lymphogenic drainage (**b**, **c**). Irregular lining and inhomogeneous contrast density due to internal synovial proliferations, especially at the pre-styloid recess (**c**)

4 Differential Diagnosis

The illustration (Fig. 18) of areas of carpal BMO, hydrops in multiple compartments, and (extensor and flexor) tenosynovitis may be misleading and due to other inflammatory pathology (Bennett and O'Connell 1978; Corzo et al. 2020; Hsu et al. 2004; Matthews et al. 2019; Nusman et al. 2019; Savnik et al. 2002). The main involvement of the typical STT-location and the elective destruction of the Tra-S ligament should raise the suspicion of CPPD (Calcium Pyrophosphate Deposition Disease). The standard views are important. Faintly opaque calcifications at the hyaline (and as well at the less specific fibro) cartilage, elective and pronounced narrowing with sclerotic borders of the Tra-tra-S joint, and widening of this joint in ulnar deviation (Fig. 19) are highly compatible with CPPD. Typical arthrosynovial cysts at the radial side of the STT joint (Fig. 20) also point to the diagnosis of CPPD. A "degenerative image of an in height collapsing wrist" (Fig. 21) may hide a CPPD. Even extensive and diffuse deposits of CPPD (Fig. 22) may be missed on MRI (Fig. 21).

A RA-like psoriatic arthritis (Tehranzadeh et al. 2008; Yuen et al. 1992) may also give a similar inflammatory pattern (Fig. 23a, b, 25, and 26). The follow-up MRI typically shows regressions through therapy (Fig. 23c, d). Typical osteoperiostitis indicates PsA (Figs. 24a, b and 26a, b). CE also correlates well with the activity in erosions (Figs. 24c–f and 25).

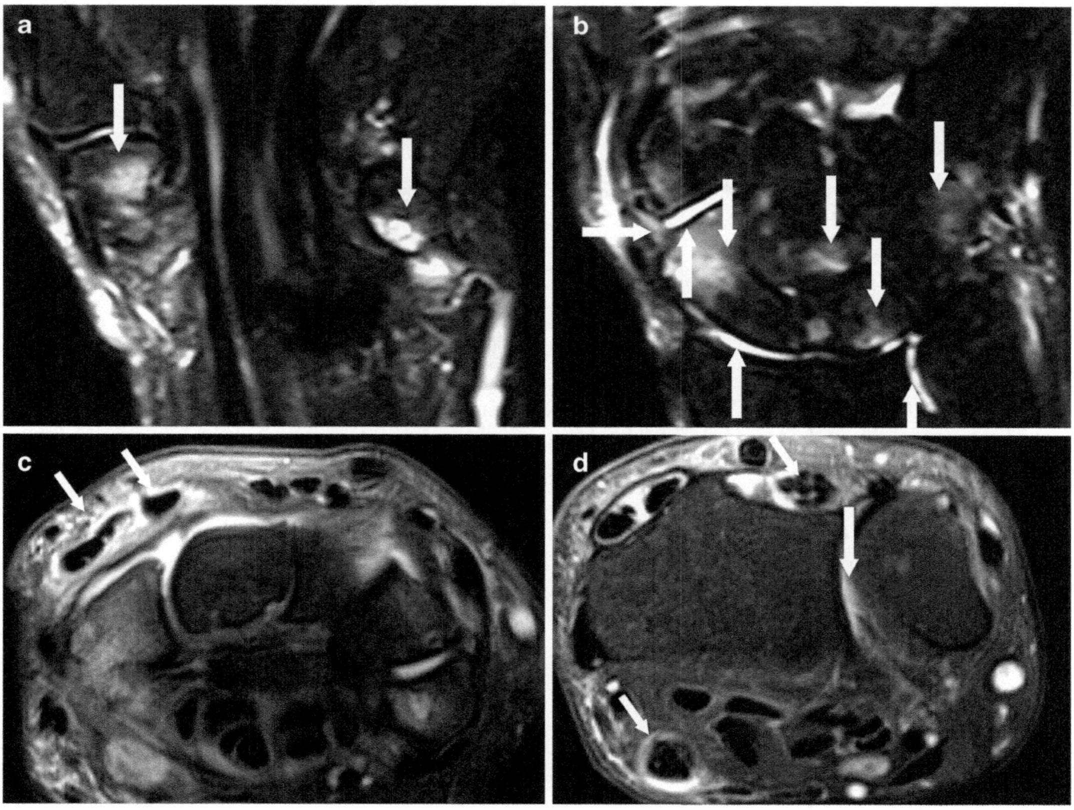

Fig. 18 Cor (**a**, **b**) and Ax (C-D) T2-WI. Diffuse areas of carpal BMO (**a**, **b**), hydrops RC, DRU and at the wide Tra-S joint (**b**, **d**), tenosynovitis II, III, and IV and flexor (fpl) (**c**, **d**)

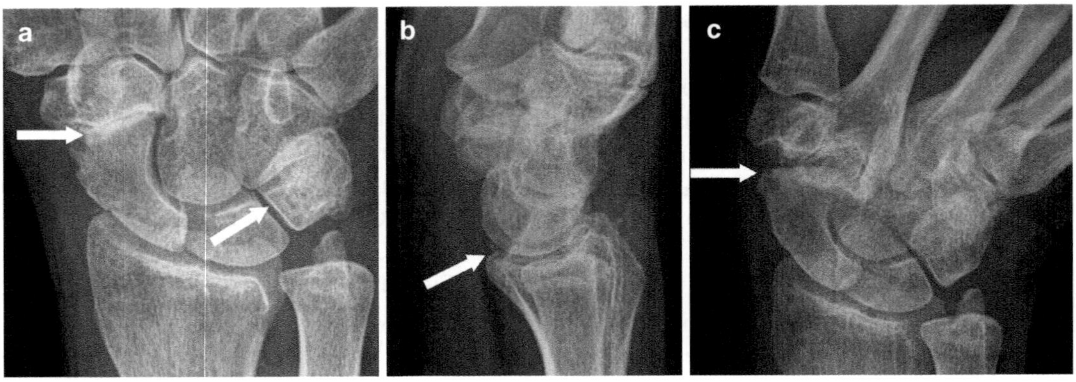

Fig. 19 Standard PA (**a**), Lateral (**b**), and oblique UD (**c**) views. Elective and pronounced narrowing with sclerotic borders of the Tra-tra-S joint (**a**). Faintly opaque calcifications at the hyaline cartilage of the LT (**a**) and RC (**b**) joint. Widening of the Tra-S joint in ulnar deviation (**c**)

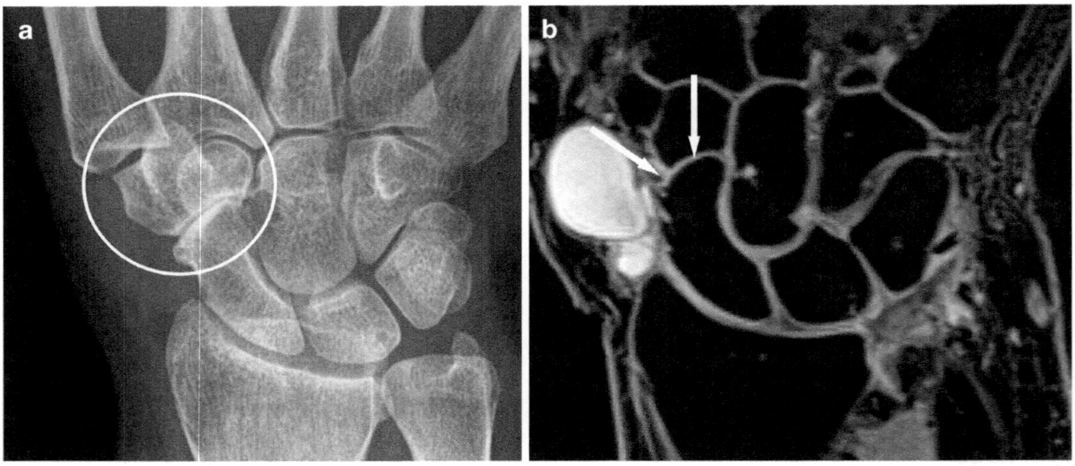

Fig. 20 Standard PA view (**a**); Cor 3D GRE (**b**). Even STT narrowing with sclerotic borders (**a**). Multilocular cyst centred at the radial side of the narrowed STT joint (**b**)

Concurrent with a fracture of the trapezoid bone after an acute trauma (Fig. 27a, b), signs of inflammation are detected (Fig. 27). A few months later, in response to an acute inflammatory pain surge (Fig. 28), a severe hyperuricemia is discovered and the diagnosis of gout (McQueen et al. 2014) is made.

Prosthesis may induce arthritis with surrounding CE, synovial proliferation, erosions, and extensive destruction (Fig. 29).

A long-lasting painful demineralisation after (unmentioned) immobilisation may mislead the interpretation of the standard views (Fig. 30a, b) and incidental normal findings will exclude inflammatory pathology (Fig. 30c, d).

A painful non inflammatory demineralisation on standard views (Fig. 31a, b) is sometimes due to an accidental finding of carpal fracture(s) (Fig. 30c–f).

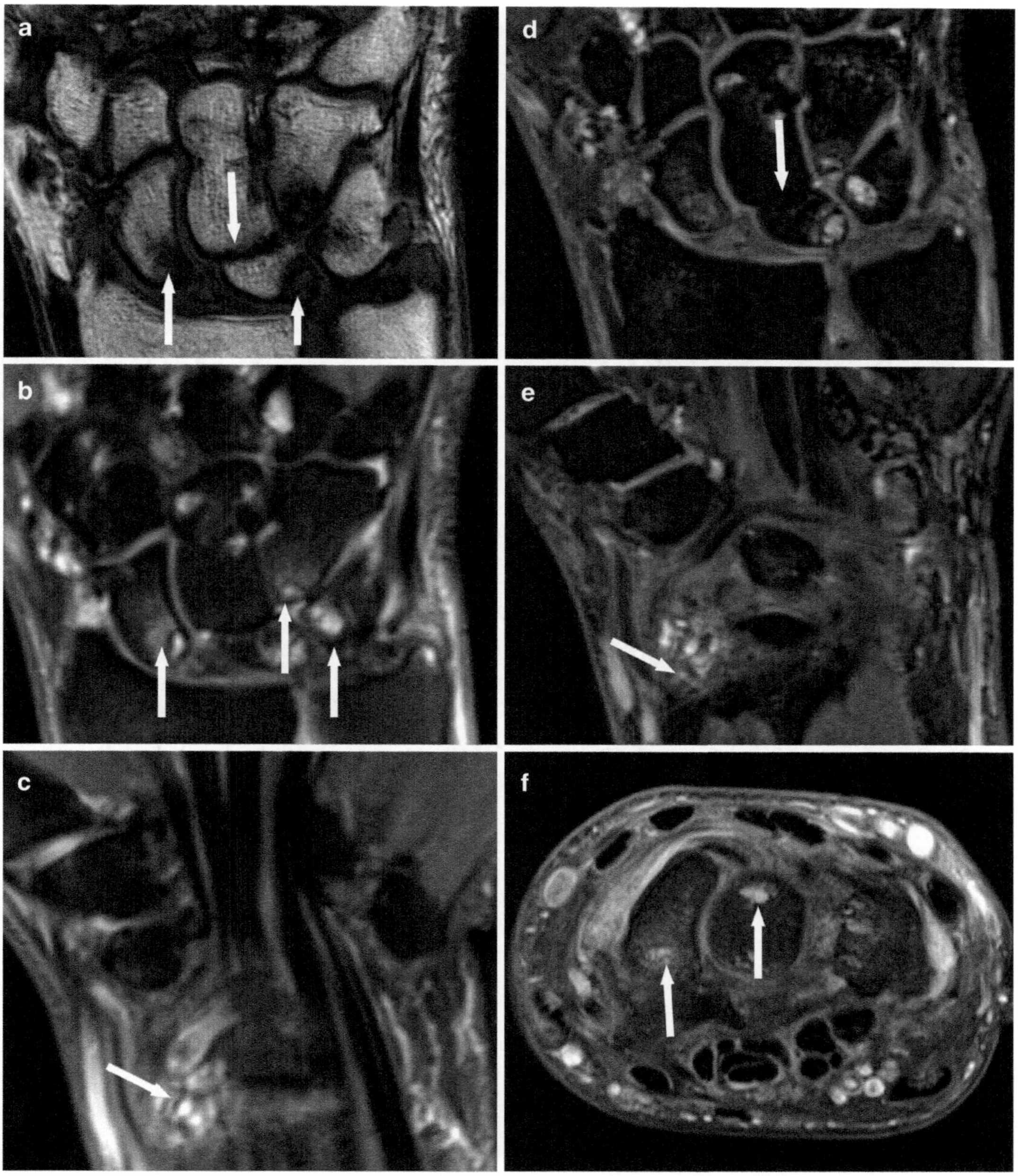

Fig. 21 Cor T1-WI (**a**), T2-WI FS (**b**, **c**) and 3D GRE (**d**, **e**); Ax T2-WI FS (**f**). Even STT and CL narrowing with sclerotic borders (**a**). Diffuse carpal subchondral cysts with BMO (**b**, **f**). Infiltration of the RSC and RLT ligament (**c**, **e**). Proximal migration of the C (**d**). SL widening and SLL destruction (**a**, **b**)

A complex regional pain syndrome (CRPS), previously called Reflex Sympathetic Dystrophy (RSD), may be a differential diagnosis as well. This acute and painful demineralisation (Fig. 32) may show on MRI (Fig. 33), BMO, IA fluid, oedema of the deeper soft tissues (muscles, connective tissues and periost), CE of a thickened skin, and peri-articular CE.

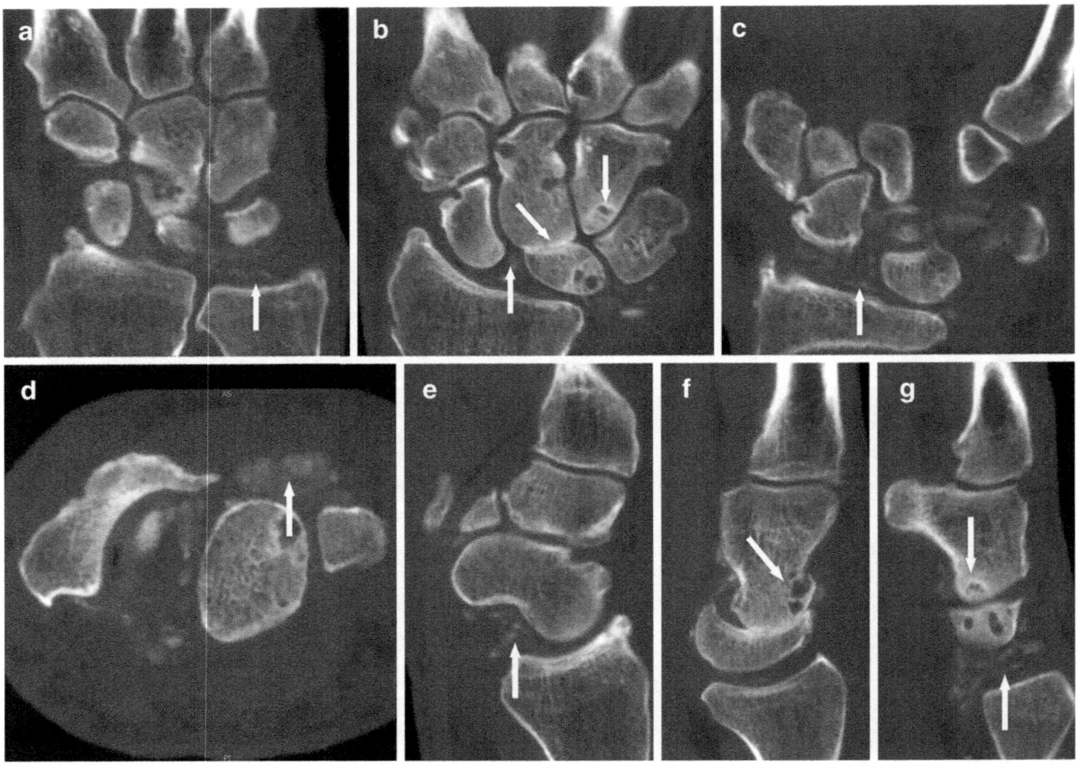

Fig. 22 Cor (**a**–**c**), Ax (**d**) and Sag (**e**–**g**) CT images. Diffuse calcification deposits: TFCC (**a**, **g**), SL pace (**b**, **c**), hyaline cartilage (**c**, **d**), RSC and RLT (**e**) with diffuse small cysts with sclerotic borders (**b**, **f**, **g**). Degenerative narrowed aspect of the STT and CL joint (**b**, **f**, **g**)

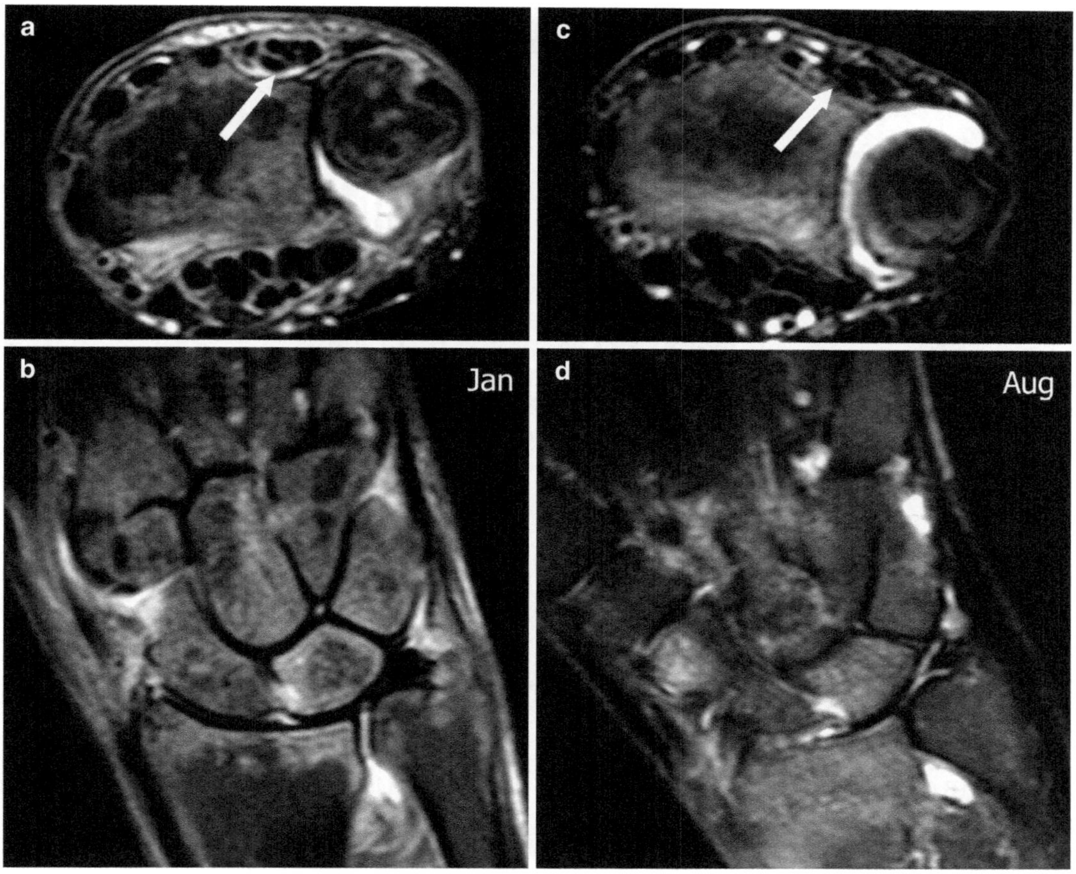

Fig. 23 Ax (**a**, **c**) and Cor (**b**, **d**) T2-WI FS. Tenosynovitis (**a**) and diffuse carpal BMO (**b**) regressing through therapy (**c**, **d**; **August**)

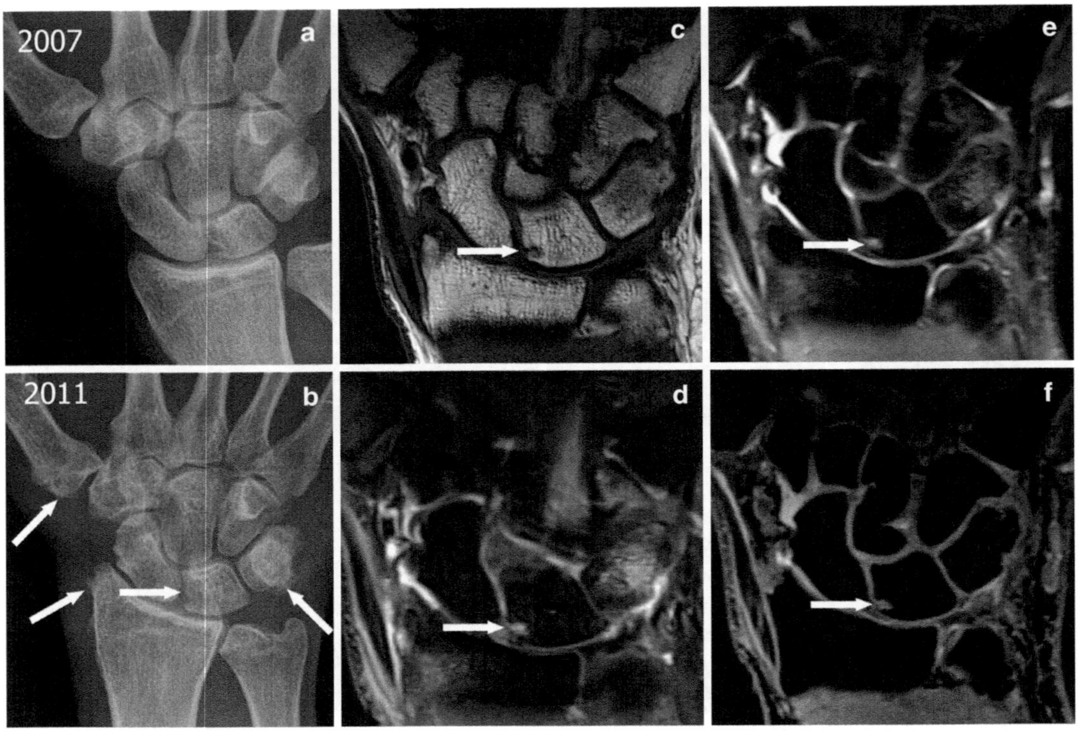

Fig. 24 Standard PA (**a**, **b**); Cor T1-WI (**c**) with FS CE (**d**), T2-WI FS (**e**) and 3D GRE (**f**). Occurence (**2007**; **a**, **c**, **e**) and development (**2011**; **b**, **d**, **f**) of lesions: small areas of osteoperiostitis develop (**a**, **b**). A small erosion of the L (**b–f**) becomes visible on standard views (**a**, **b**), while on the initial MRI it is already visible (**c**, **e**). The CE lesion is still active (**d**)

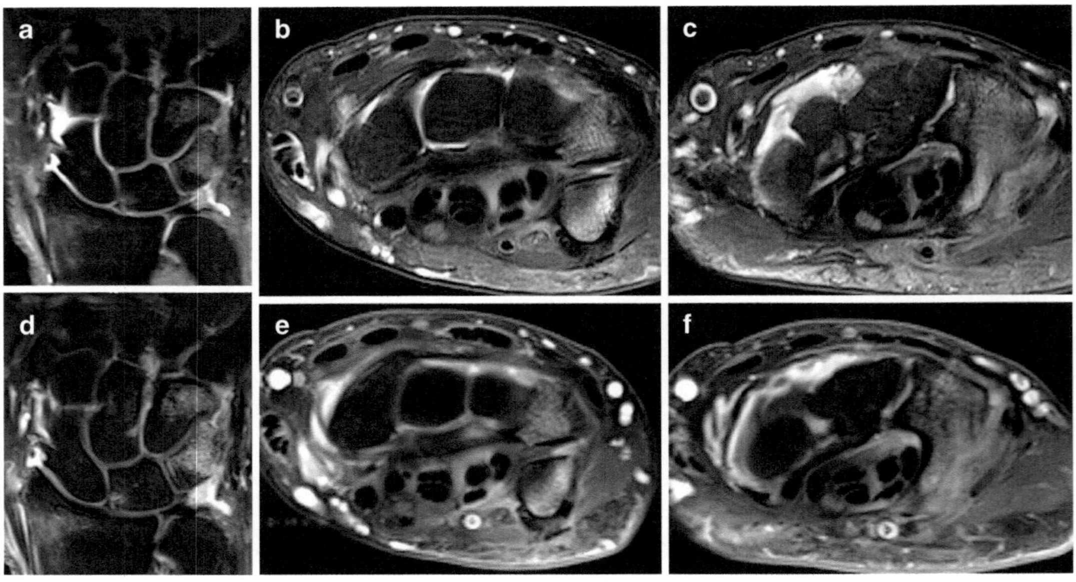

Fig. 25 Cor (**a**) and Ax (**b**, **c**) T2-WI; Cor (**d**) and Ax (**e**, **f**) T1-WI FS with CE. BMO of the H, Tri and P (**a–c**) with CE (**d–f**)

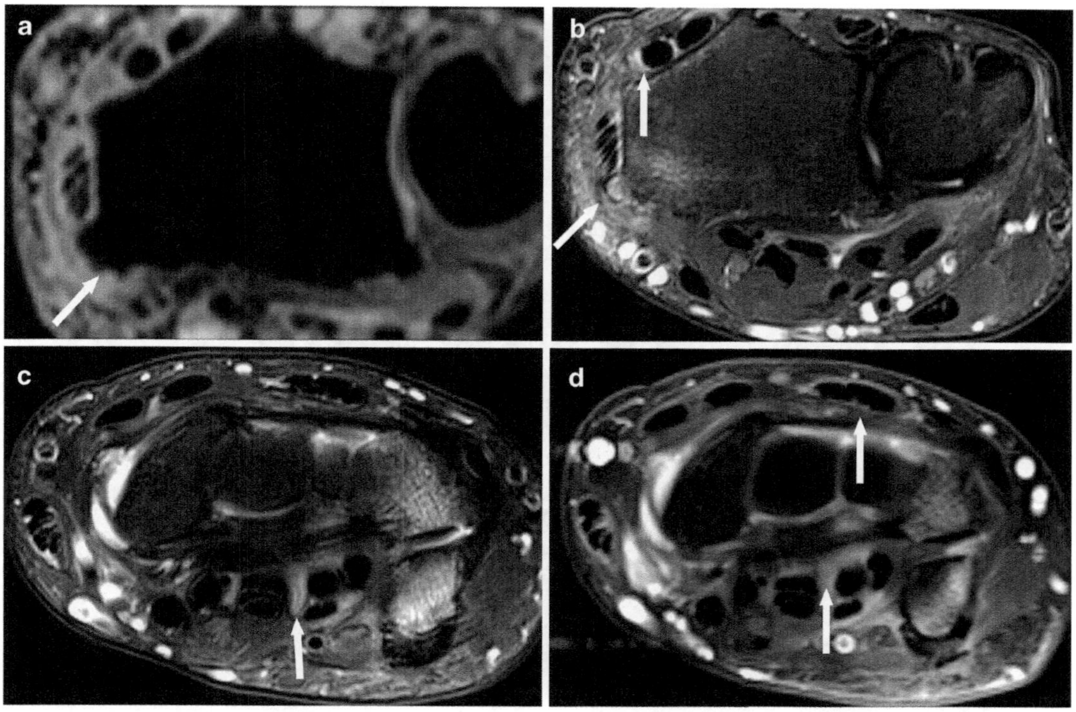

Fig. 26 Ax 3D GRE (**a**), T2-WI FS (**b**, **c**) and T1-WI FS with CE (**d**). Osteoperiostitis (**a**, **b**) and at tenosynovitis (**b**–**d**)

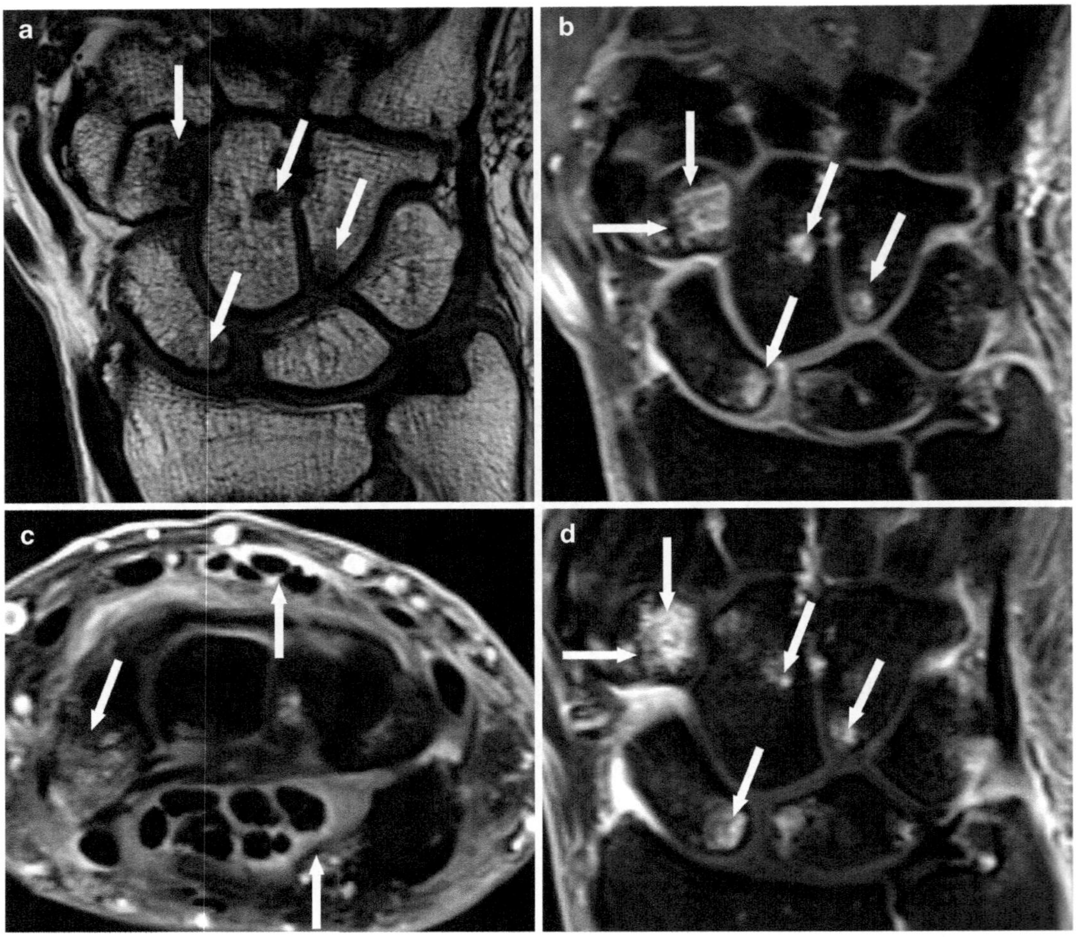

Fig. 27 Cor T1-WI (**a**); Cor (**b**) and Ax (**c**) T2-WI FS; Cor T1-WI FS with CE (**d**). Acute trauma in May with fracture of the tra and surrounding BMO (**a**, **b**). Discovery of several areas of BMO at the capitate, hamate and scaphoid (**a–c**) with CE (**d**) and tenosynovitis (IV, fcr and fd) (**c**); underlying inflammation suggested

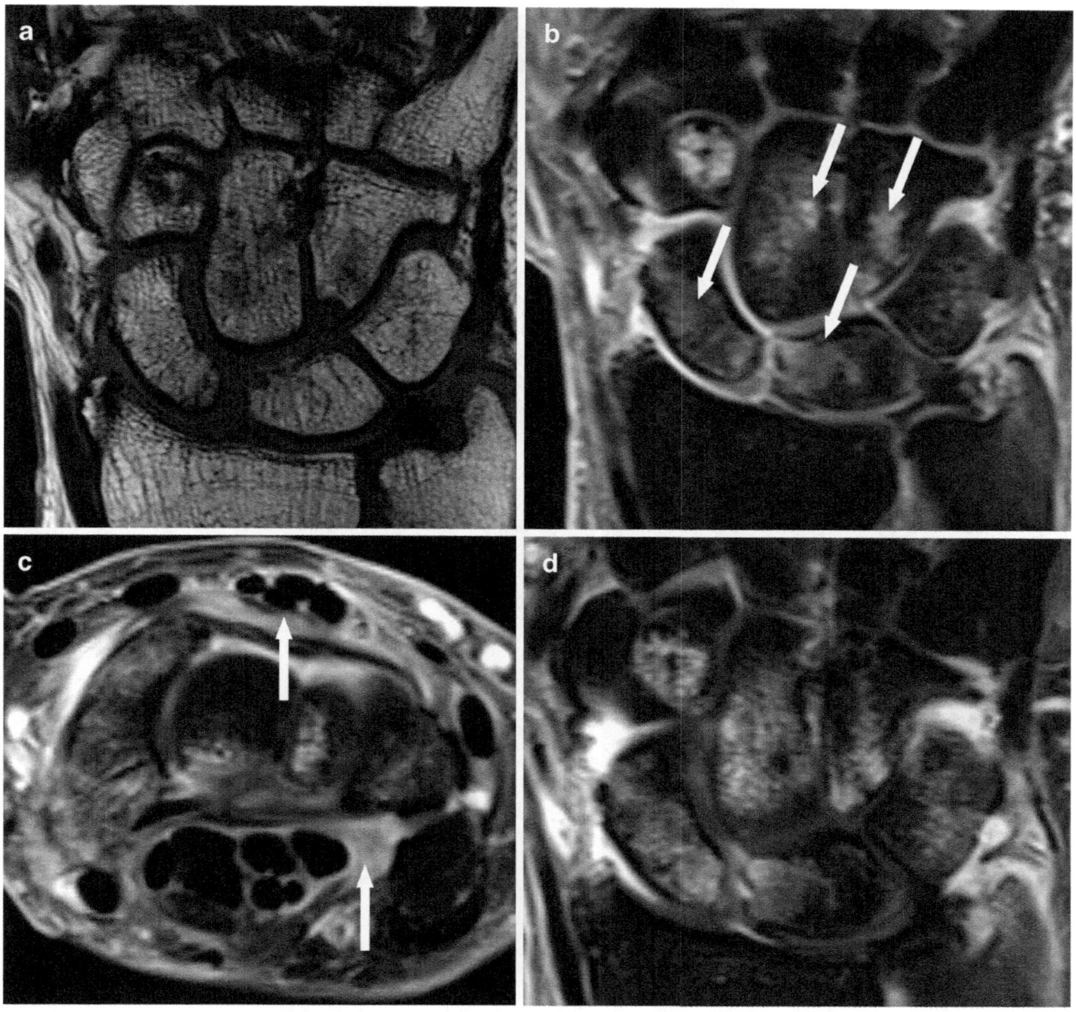

Fig. 28 Cor T1-WI (**a**); Cor (**b**) and Ax (**c**) T2-WI FS; Cor T1-WI FS with CE (**d**). Acute pain surges in September. Increased BMO (**a**, **b**), persisting tenosynovitis © and diffuse carpal CE (**d**) are visualised

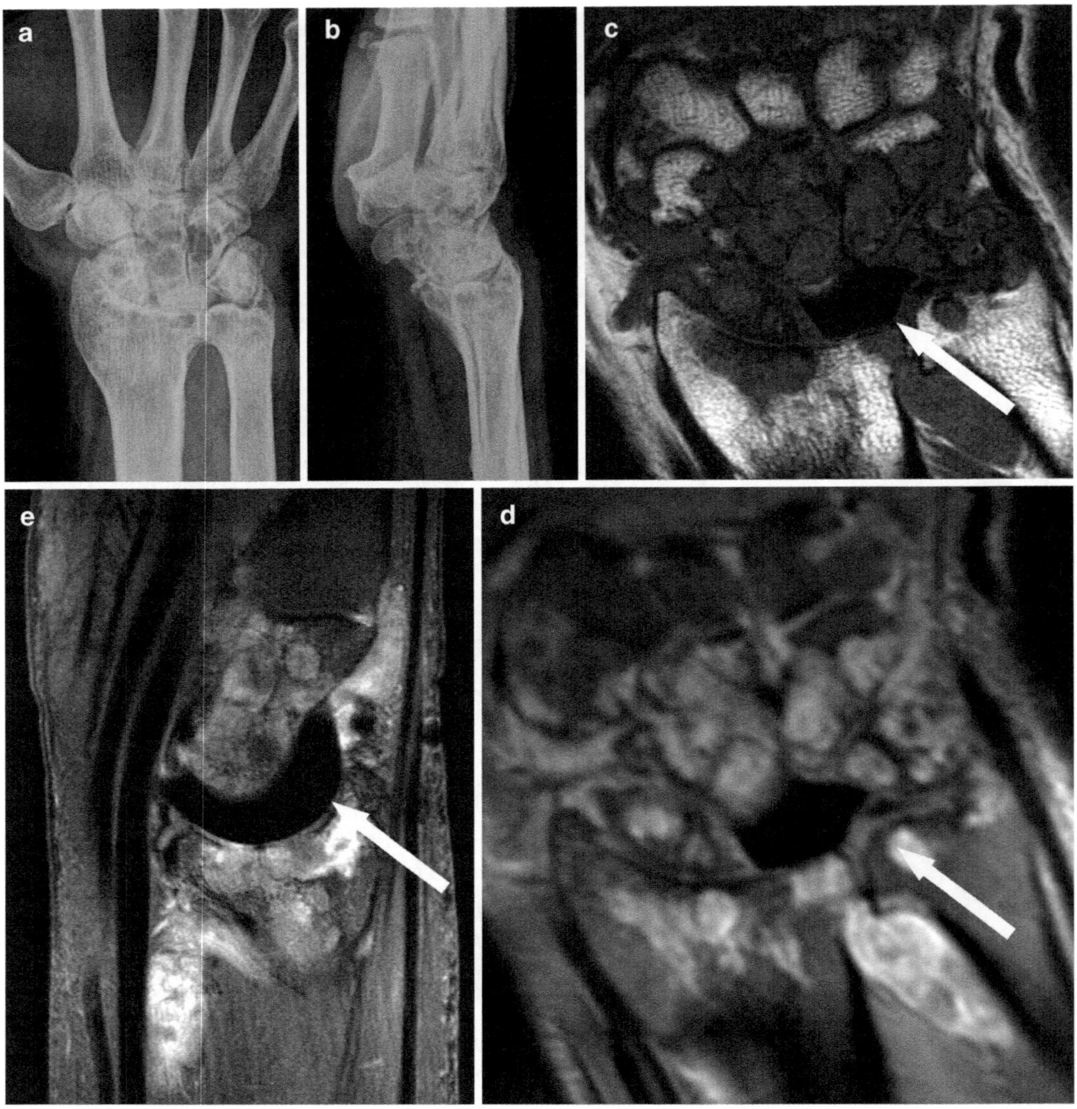

Fig. 29 Standard PA (**a**) and Lateral (**b**) views; Cor T1-WI (**c**) and T2-WI FS (**d**); Sag T1-WI FS with CE (**e**). A lunate silicone prosthesis surrounded by (peri)carpal BMO, CE synovial proliferation and erosions

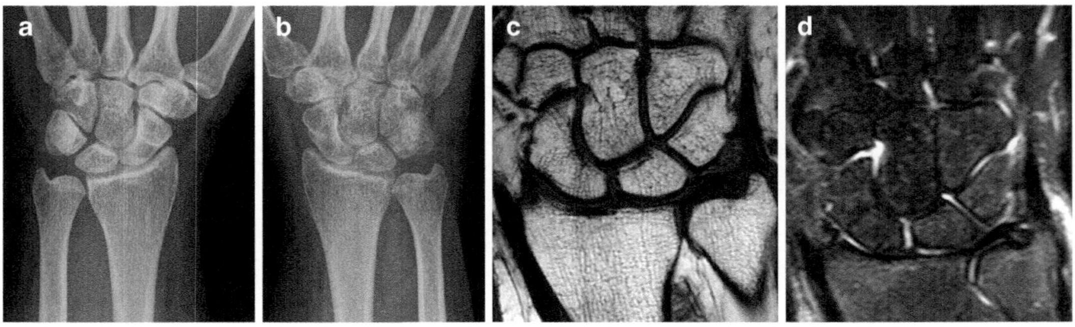

Fig. 30 Standard PA left (**a**) and right (**b**) views; Cor T1-WI (**c**) and T2-WI FS (**d**). Diffuse unilateral plain (peri)carpal demineralisation of the right wrist (**a**, **b**) without obvious BMO, erosive lesions nor synovial proliferation

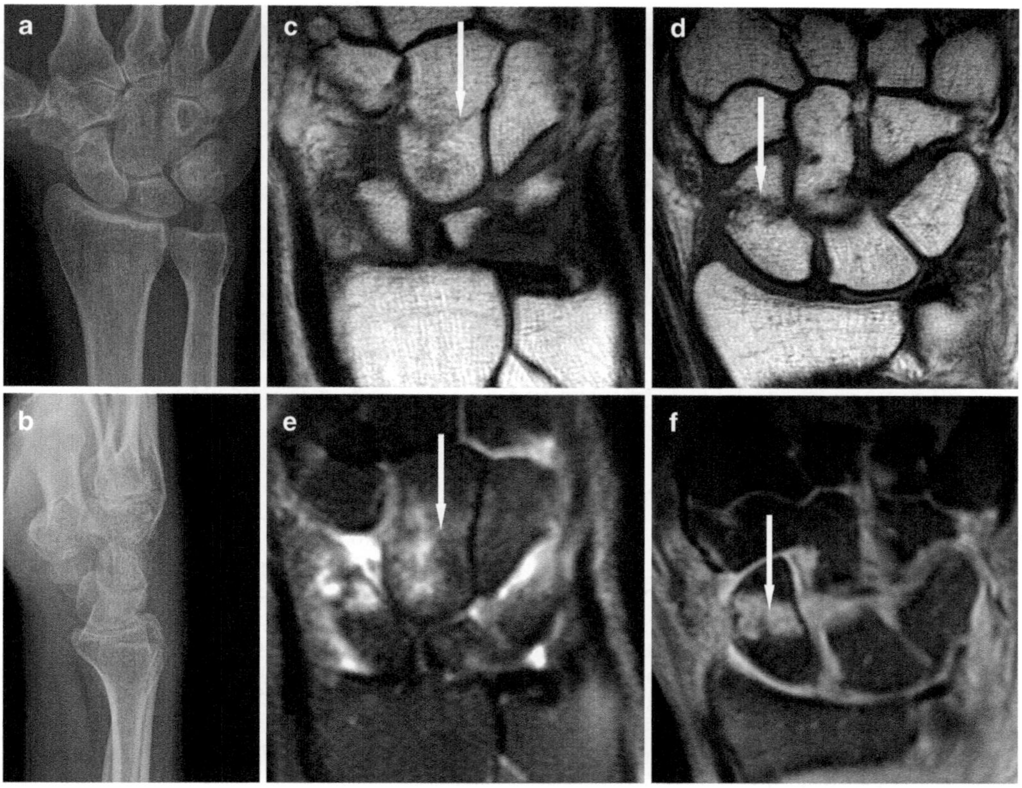

Fig. 31 Standard PA (**a**) and Lateral (**b**) views; Cor T1-WI (**c, d**) and T2-WI FS (**e, f**). Diffuse unilateral persisting pain and (peri)carpal demineralisation due to an accidentally discovered fracture of S and C

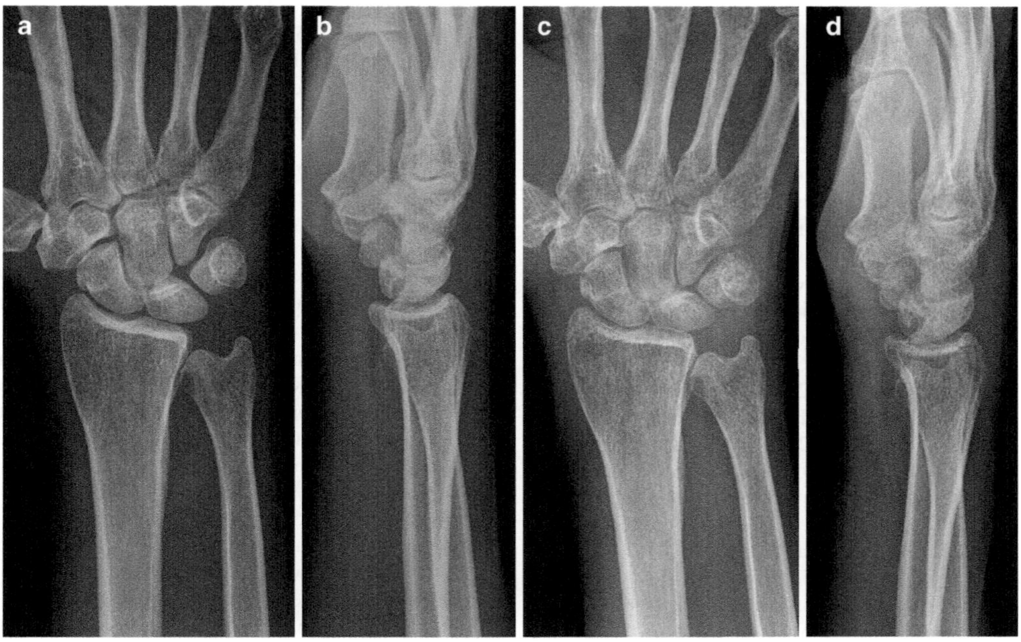

Fig. 32 Standard PA (**a**, **c**) and Lateral (**b**, **d**) views. Diffuse unilateral persisting pain and fast demineralisation (June–September)

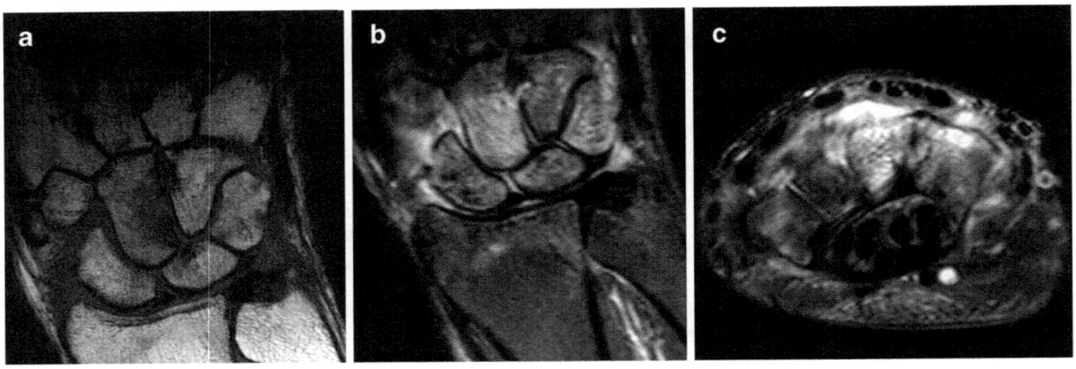

Fig. 33 Cor T1-WI (**a**); Cor (**b**) and Ax (**c**) T2-WI FS. Diffuse (peri) BMO, IA fluid and dorsal deep juxta-articular soft tissue oedema

References

Aizenberg E, Roex EAH, Nieuwenhuis WP, Mangnus L, van der Helm-van Mil AHM, Reijnierse M, Bloem JL, Lelieveldt BPF, Stoel BC (2018) Automatic quantification of bone marrow edema on MRI of the wrist in patients with early arthritis: a feasibility study. Magn Reson Med 79(2):1127–1134. https://doi.org/10.1002/mrm.26712. Epub 2017 May 7. Erratum in: Magn Reson Med. 2019 Jul;82(1):510. PMID: 28480581; PMCID: PMC5811824

Barbieri F, Parascandolo P, Vosilla L, Cesario L, Viano G, Cimmino MA (2013) Assessing MRI erosions in the rheumatoid wrist: a comparison between RAMRIS and a semiautomated segmentation software. Ann Rheum Dis 71(Suppl 3):709–709. https://doi.org/10.1136/annrheumdis-2012-eular.1253

Bennett RM, O'Connell DJ (1978) The arthritis of mixed connective tissue disease. Ann Rheum Dis 37(5):397–403. https://doi.org/10.1136/ard.37.5.397. PMID: 718271; PMCID: PMC1000265

Boeren AMP, Niemantsverdriet E, Verstappen M, Wouters F, Bloem JL, Reijnierse M, van der Helm-van Mil AHM (2023) Towards a simplified fluid-sensitive MRI protocol in small joints of the hand in early arthritis patients: reliability between modified Dixon and regular Gadolinium enhanced TSE fat saturated MRI-sequences. Skeletal Radiol 52(6):1193–1202. https://doi.org/10.1007/s00256-022-04238-8. Epub 2022 Nov 28. PMID: 36441238

Corzo P, Garcia-Duitama I, Agustí Claramunt A, Salman Monte TC, Monfort J (2020) Comparision of musculoskeletal involvement of wrist and hand by MRI in two systemic lupus erythematosous groups. Ann Rheum Dis 79(Suppl 1):664–665. https://doi.org/10.1136/annrheumdis-2020-eular.4825

Couzens G, Daunt N, Crawford R, Ross M (2014) Positive magnetic resonance imaging findings in the asymptomatic wrist. ANZ J Surg 84(7–8):528–532. https://doi.org/10.1111/ans.12552. Epub 2014 Feb 26. PMID: 24612468

Dakkak YJ, Matthijssen XME, van der Heijde D, Reijnierse M, van der Helm-van Mil AHM (2020) Reliability of magnetic resonance imaging (MRI) scoring of the metatarsophalangeal joints of the foot according to the rheumatoid arthritis MRI score. J Rheumatol 47(8):1165–1173. https://doi.org/10.3899/jrheum.190258. Epub 2019 Sep 15. PMID: 31523041; PMCID: PMC7115895

Ejbjerg B, McQueen F, Lassere M, Haavardsholm E, Conaghan P, O'Connor P, Bird P, Peterfy C, Edmonds J, Szkudlarek M, Genant H, Emery P, Østergaard M (2005) The EULAR-OMERACT rheumatoid arthritis MRI reference image atlas: the wrist joint. Ann Rheum Dis 64(Suppl 1):i23–i47. https://doi.org/10.1136/ard.2004.031823. PMID: 15647419; PMCID: PMC1766827

Eriksen EF, Ringe JD (2012) Bone marrow lesions: a universal bone response to injury? Rheumatol Int 32(3):575–584. https://doi.org/10.1007/s00296-011-2141-2. Epub 2011 Sep 8. PMID: 21901347

Eshed I, Feist E, Althoff CE, Hamm B, Konen E, Burmester GR, Backhaus M, Hermann KG (2009) Tenosynovitis of the flexor tendons of the hand detected by MRI: an early indicator of rheumatoid arthritis. Rheumatology (Oxford) 48(8):887–891. https://doi.org/10.1093/rheumatology/kep136. Epub 2009 May 27. PMID: 19474128

Fujimori M, Nakamura S, Hasegawa K, Ikeno K, Ichikawa S, Sutherland K, Kamishima T (2017) Cartilage quantification using contrast-enhanced MRI in the wrist of rheumatoid arthritis: cartilage loss is associated with bone marrow edema. Br J Radiol 90(1077):20170167. https://doi.org/10.1259/bjr.20170167. Epub 2017 Jul 14. PMID: 28707530; PMCID: PMC5858812

Gandjbakhch F, Conaghan PG, Ejbjerg B, Haavardsholm EA, Foltz V, Brown AK, Møller Døhn U, Lassere M, Freeston J, Bøyesen P, Bird P, Fautrel B, Hetland ML, Emery P, Bourgeois P, Hørslev-Petersen K, Kvien TK,

McQueen F, Ostergaard M (2011) Synovitis and osteitis are very frequent in rheumatoid arthritis clinical remission: results from an MRI study of 294 patients in clinical remission or low disease activity state. J Rheumatol 38(9):2039–2044. https://doi.org/10.3899/jrheum.110421. PMID: 21885514

Gornitzky AL, Carrigan RB (2016) The diagnostic utility of MRI in the painful wrist: when to reconsider advanced imaging in the pediatric patient. Pediatrics (Evanston) 137(Suppl 3):596–596A. https://doi.org/10.1542/peds.137.Supplement_3.596A

Hetland ML, Ejbjerg B, Hørslev-Petersen K, Jacobsen S, Vestergaard A, Jurik AG, Stengaard-Pedersen K, Junker P, Lottenburger T, Hansen I, Andersen LS, Tarp U, Skjødt H, Pedersen JK, Majgaard O, Svendsen AJ, Ellingsen T, Lindegaard H, Christensen AF, Vallø J, Torfing T, Narvestad E, Thomsen HS, Ostergaard M, CIMESTRA Study Group (2009) MRI bone oedema is the strongest predictor of subsequent radiographic progression in early rheumatoid arthritis. Results from a 2-year randomised controlled trial (CIMESTRA). Ann Rheum Dis 68(3):384–390. https://doi.org/10.1136/ard.2008.088245. Epub 2008 Apr 3. PMID: 18388160

Hsu CY, Lu HC, Shih TT (2004) Tuberculous infection of the wrist: MRI features. AJR Am J Roentgenol 183(3):623–628. https://doi.org/10.2214/ajr.183.3.1830623. PMID: 15333346

Jans L, Chen M (2021) Arthritis imaging. Arthritis Imaging Publishing, Ghent. https://www.arthritisimaging.com

Kamp SH, Christensen R, Bliddal H, Østergaard M, Bouert R, Boesen M (2013) Prediction of clinical response to biologics in rheumatoid arthritis by baseline magnetic resonance imaging (MRI) of the wrist: a cohort study associating MRI synovitis score with clinical outcome. Ann Rheum Dis 72(Suppl 3):A758–A759. https://doi.org/10.1136/annrheumdis-2013-eular.2247

Matthews GS, Kiani B, Wuertzer SD, Powell JA, Roller BL, Lenchik L, Torabi M (2019) MRI of the wrist: algorithmic approach for evaluating wrist pain. Radiographics 39(2):447–448. https://doi.org/10.1148/rg.2019180157. PMID: 30844354

McQueen FM, Doyle A, Reeves Q, Gao A, Tsai A, Gamble GD, Curteis B, Williams M, Dalbeth N (2014) Bone erosions in patients with chronic gouty arthropathy are associated with tophi but not bone oedema or synovitis: new insights from a 3 T MRI study. Rheumatology (Oxford) 53(1):95–103. https://doi.org/10.1093/rheumatology/ket329. Epub 2013 Sep 29. PMID: 24080252

Mysling P, Dam E, Zaim S, Genant HK, Fuerst T, Lillholm M (2013) An evaluation of a novel technique for fully automatic synovitis quantification from pre- and post-contrast wrist MRI. Ann Rheum Dis 71(Suppl 3):303–304. https://doi.org/10.1136/annrheumdis-2012-eular.2404

Nieuwenhuis WP, Krabben A, Stomp W, Huizinga TW, van der Heijde D, Bloem JL, van der Helm-van Mil AH, Reijnierse M (2015) Evaluation of magnetic resonance imaging-detected tenosynovitis in the hand and wrist in early arthritis. Arthritis Rheumatol 67(4):869–876. https://doi.org/10.1002/art.39000. PMID: 25510520

Nusman CM, Rosendahl K, Maas M (2016) MRI protocol for the assessment of juvenile idiopathic arthritis of the wrist: recommendations from the OMERACT MRI in JIA working group and health-e-child. J Rheumatol 43(6):1257–1258. https://doi.org/10.3899/jrheum.160094. PMID: 27252505

Nusman CM, van den Berg JM, Nassar-Sheikh Rashid A, Ntailiani K, Karantanas A, Kuijpers TW, Maas M, Schonenberg-Meinema D (2019) Consider the wrist: a retrospective study on pediatric connective tissue disease with MRI. Rheumatol Int 39(12):2095–2101. https://doi.org/10.1007/s00296-019-04353-1. Epub 2019 Jun 20. PMID: 31222439

Ording Muller LS, Boavida P, Avenarius D, Damasio B, Eldevik OP, Malattia C, Lambot-Juhan K, Tanturri L, Owens CM, Rosendahl K (2013) MRI of the wrist in juvenile idiopathic arthritis: erosions or normal variants? A prospective case-control study. Pediatr Radiol 43(7):785–795. https://doi.org/10.1007/s00247-012-2575-z. Epub 2013 Jan 3. PMID: 23283407

Palosaari K, Vuotila J, Takalo R, Jartti A, Niemelä RK, Karjalainen A, Haapea M, Soini I, Tervonen O, Hakala M (2006) Bone oedema predicts erosive progression on wrist MRI in early RA – a 2-yr observational MRI and NC scintigraphy study. Rheumatology (Oxford) 45(12):1542–1548. https://doi.org/10.1093/rheumatology/kel137. Epub 2006 May 2. PMID: 16670155

Rubin DA (2019) MRI and ultrasound of the hands and wrists in rheumatoid arthritis. I. Imaging findings. Skeletal Radiol 48(5):677–695. https://doi.org/10.1007/s00256-019-03179-z. Epub 2019 Feb 23. PMID: 30796506

Savnik A, Malmskov H, Thomsen HS, Graff LB, Nielsen H, Danneskiold-Samsøe B, Boesen J, Bliddal H (2002) MRI of the wrist and finger joints in inflammatory joint diseases at 1-year interval: MRI features to predict bone erosions. Eur Radiol 12(5):1203–1210. https://doi.org/10.1007/s003300101114. Epub 2001 Sep 25. PMID: 11976868

Shabshin N, Schweitzer ME (2009) Age dependent T2 changes of bone marrow in pediatric wrist MRI. Skeletal Radiol 38(12):1163–1168. https://doi.org/10.1007/s00256-009-0752-4. Epub 2009 Aug 7. PMID: 19662404

Tehranzadeh J, Ashikyan O, Anavim A, Shin J (2008) Detailed analysis of contrast-enhanced MRI of hands and wrists in patients with psoriatic arthritis. Skeletal Radiol 37(5):433–442. https://doi.org/10.1007/s00256-008-0451-6. Epub 2008 Feb 20. PMID: 18286282

Valeri G, Ferrara C, Ercolani P, De Nigris E, Giovagnoni A (2001) Tendon involvement in rheumatoid arthritis of the wrist: MRI findings. Skeletal Radiol 30(3):138–143. https://doi.org/10.1007/s002560100322. PMID: 11357451

Xiao F, Griffith JF, Ko JKL, Yue J, Leung JCS, Yeung DKW, Tam LS (2021) MRI wrist in early rheumatoid arthritis: reduction in inflammation assessed quantitatively during treatment period correlates best with clinical improvement. Skeletal Radiol 50(7):1337–1345. https://doi.org/10.1007/s00256-020-03669-5. Epub 2020 Nov 26. PMID: 33244616

Yang H, Rivoire J, Hoppe M, Srikhum W, Imboden J, Link TM, Li X (2015) Computer-aided and manual quantifications of MRI synovitis, bone marrow edema-like lesions, erosion and cartilage loss in rheumatoid arthritis of the wrist. Skeletal Radiol 44(4):539–547. https://doi.org/10.1007/s00256-014-2059-3. Epub 2014 Dec 10. PMID: 25488101

Yuen M, Friedman L, Orr W, Cockshott WP (1992) Proliferative periosteal processes of phalanges: a unitary hypothesis. Skeletal Radiol 21(5):301–303. https://doi.org/10.1007/BF00241768. PMID: 1502582

Carpal Tunnel Syndrome

Contents

1 General

The carpal tunnel is defined from the pisiform bone proximally (Fig. 1a) until the level of the hamulus of the hamate bone distally (Fig. 1b). Squeezing of the median nerve during this pathway may give rise to a carpal tunnel syndrome (Chammas 2014; Chammas et al. 2014; Falkiner and Myers 2002; Martinoli et al. 2000; Newington et al. 2015). The diameter of the median nerve will increase at the P level and the nerve will be flattened at the H level.

The axial standard view of the carpal tunnel (Fig. 2a) is not routinely realised due to the difficult positioning, but also does not give us a lot of information. US (Gitto and Draghi 2016; Lee et al. 2019) on the other hand may be used as a first approach (Fig. 2b–d).

M. Mespreuve, K. Waked, *MRI of the Wrist*, Medical Radiology,
https://doi.org/10.1007/978-3-031-63973-9_14

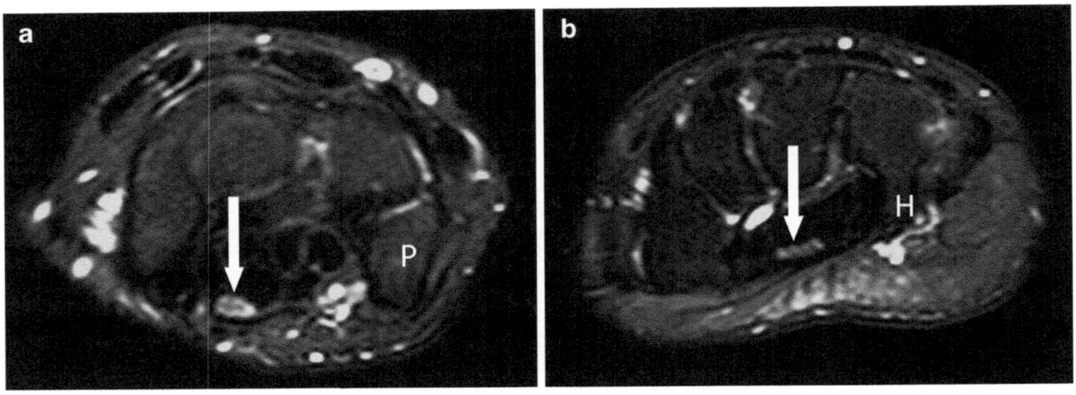

Fig. 1 Ax T2-WI FS (**a**, **b**). The median nerve with high signal at the entrance (**a**) and the exit of the carpal tunnel (**b**)

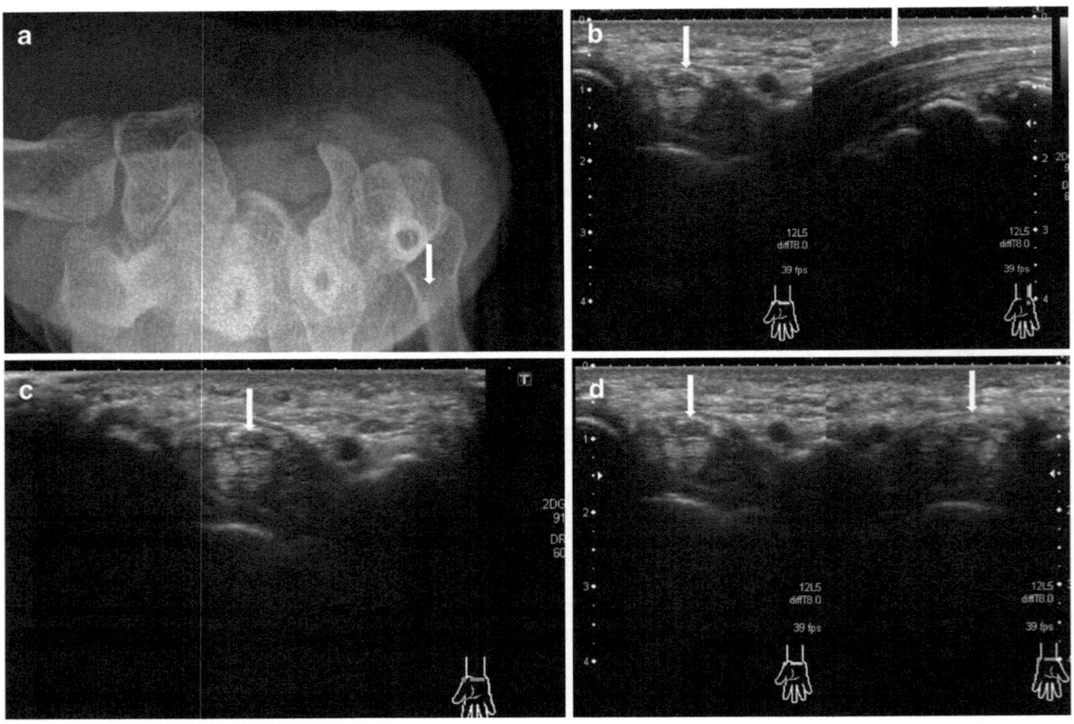

Fig. 2 Standard axial view (**a**); US of the CT in longitudinal and transverse direction (**b**–**d**)

2 MRI Findings

Additionally, on MRI, the signal intensity increases on T2-WI and fasciculation appears in case of progressive CTS (Figs. 1, 3, 4, 5, 6, 7, and 8). The median nerve is swollen at the level of the pisiform bone (Fig. 6a) and flattened at the level of the hamulus of the hamate bone (Figs. 3a, 4, and 6d). The flexor retinaculum forms a slight concave arch over the tunnel (Figs. 3a and 6). The signal intensity of the nerve has increased (3–8). The individual nerve bundles are also clearly visible (Figs. 3a, 4, and 6), even beyond the carpal tunnel (Fig. 3b). The width of the median nerve is compared distally to the reduced height (Fig. 4) and an index of more than 3 is considered abnormal (Lee et al. 2019; Park et al. 2020). Bowing of the fairly horizontal flexor retinaculum exceeding 3–4 mm is also considered abnormal (Fig. 4). The median nerve (Fig. 5 green arrow) is particularly compressed against the retinaculum by the flexor tendons in flexion (Phalen test) due to repositioning of the tendons (Fig. 5 red arrows) in the carpal tunnel. In a classical CTS, the nerve is involved with a high signal over the whole trajectory and beyond (Fig. 6). Moreover, the nerve is swollen proximally (Fig. 6a) and compressed distally (Fig. 6c).

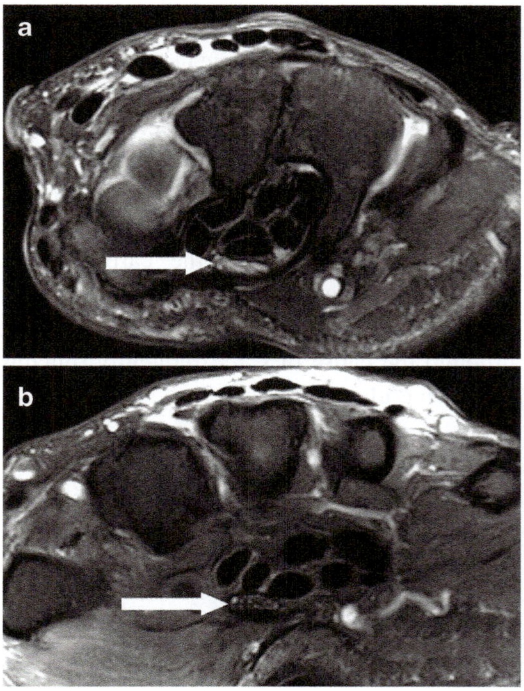

Fig. 3 Ax T2-WI FS (**a**, **b**). The median nerve is flattened at the level of the hamulus and the flexor retinaculum is arched (**a**). The signal intensity has increased (**a**, **b**). The individual nerve bundles are clearly visible (**a**) even beyond the carpal tunnel (**b**)

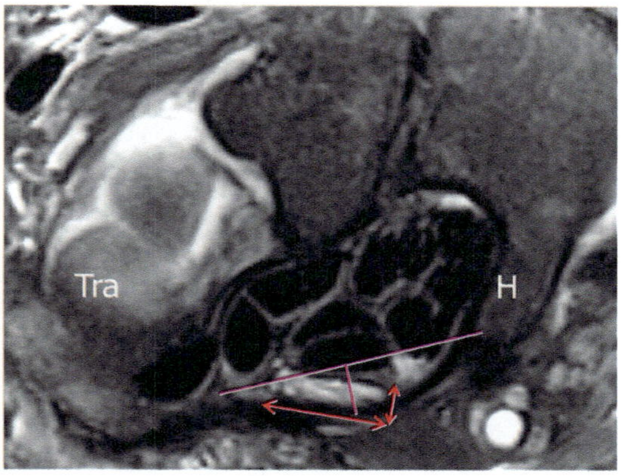

Fig. 4 Ax T2-WI FS. The median nerve is flattened at the level of the hamulus of the H with an index >3 (red arrows). The flexor retinaculum is arched more than 2.5–4 mm (pink lines)

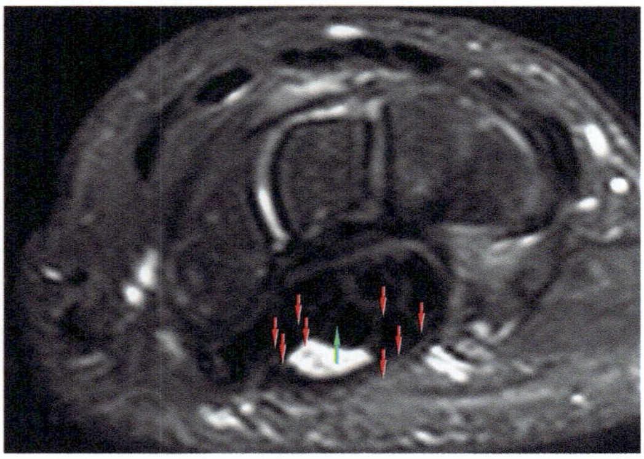

Fig. 5 Ax T2-WI FS. Compression of the median nerve (green arrow) between the flexor retinaculum and the flexor tendons (red arrows)

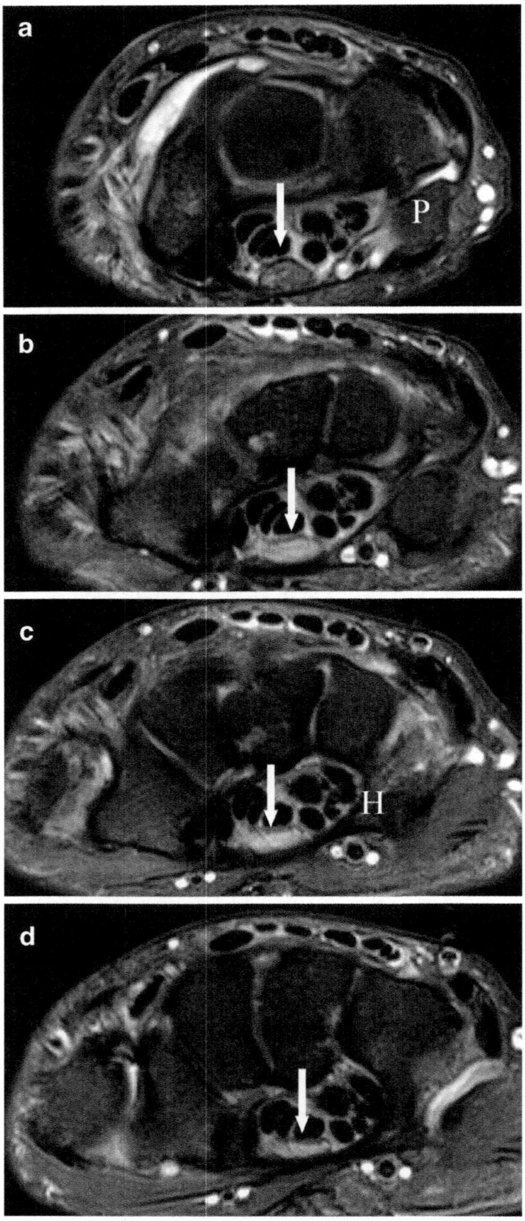

Fig. 6 Ax T2-WI FS. Diffuse higher signal and fasciculation (**a–d**) of the swollen nerve proximally (**a**) and flattened distally (**d**)

Variants of the median nerve are frequent and should be noticed to inform the surgeon in case of a planned intervention. The nerve splits early at the entrance of the carpal tunnel in about 3% in a vertical (Fig. 7) or horizontal way (Fig. 8). A more vertical orientation may be combined with a deeper trajectory (Fig. 9). Near the median nerve, an arterial anomaly with persisting a. mediana or an a. interossea may be found (Fig. 10), eventually combined with a deep vertical and a superficial horizontal component (Fig. 11). Splitting of the nerve distally in the carpal tunnel should be noticed as well (Fig. 12). Giant median nerves (without symptoms) in the wrist of craftsman are rare (Fig. 13). The need for a comparative MRI seems rather irrelevant (Fig. 14). Measurements of the nerve and the curved retinaculum can be done without MRI and comparison of the (moreover not always increased) signal can easier be done with the ulnar nerve on the same image and sequence (Fig. 8).

Eventual causal abnormal structures (Khaled and Drapé 2015; Kostakoğlu et al. 1997; Pirola et al. 2009; Schön et al. 1992; Sookur et al. 2008; Teh and Whiteley 2007; Zeiss and Guilliam-Haidet 1996) in the carpal tunnel should also be identified (such as enlarged lumbrical muscles or fibrosis of the tenosynovium), although the cause of CTS frequently remains unknown ("idiopathic").

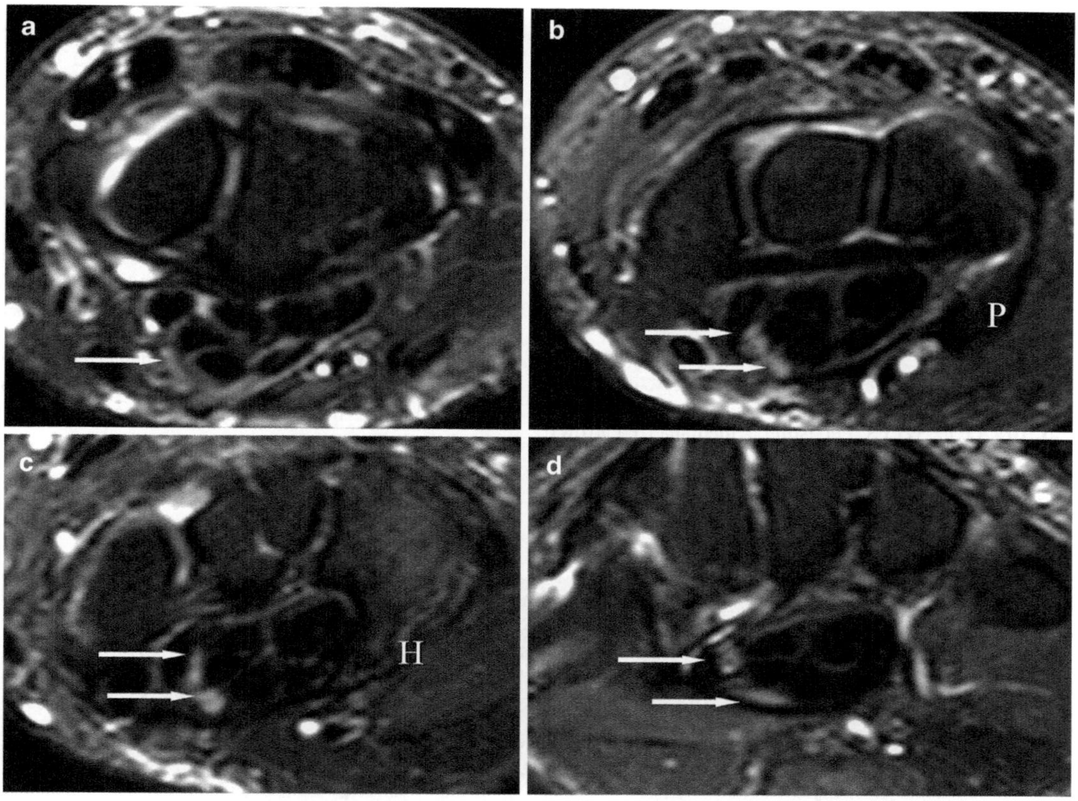

Fig. 7 Ax T2-WI FS (**a**–**d**). Early vertical splitting of the median nerve at the entrance of the carpal tunnel

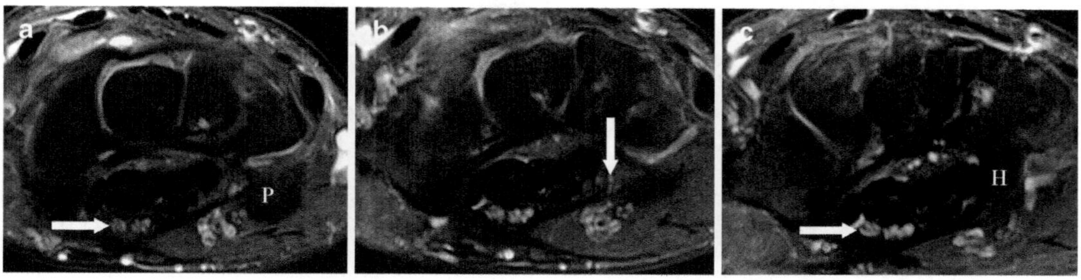

Fig. 8 Ax T2-WI FS. Early horizontal splitting of the median nerve (**a**–**c**) with a convex retinaculum and a higher signal compared to the ulnar nerve (**b**)

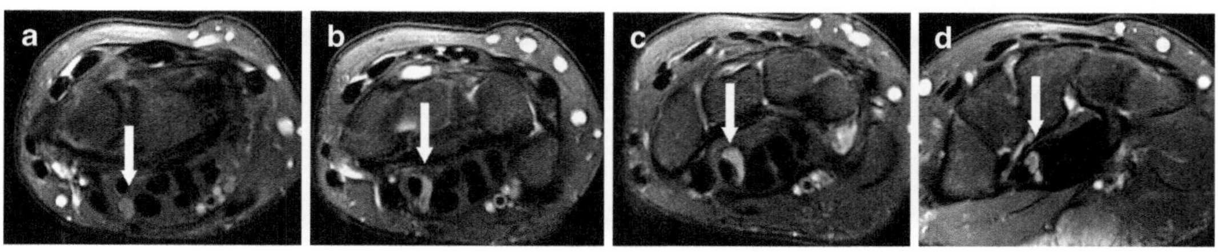

Fig. 9 Ax T2-WI FS (**a**–**d**). Vertical orientation with deep trajectory

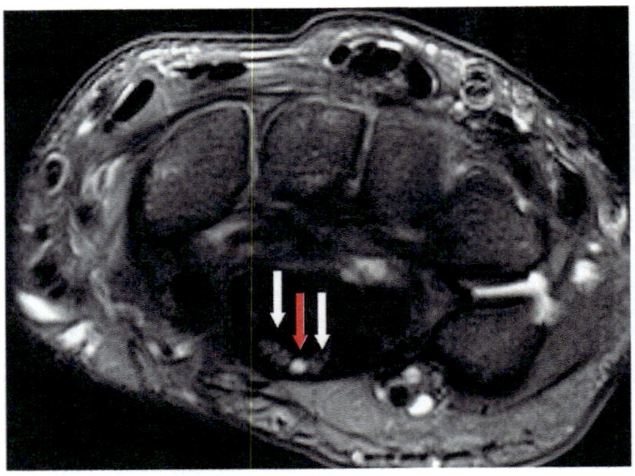

Fig. 10 Ax T2-WI FS. Persisting a. mediana (red arrow) between a split median nerve (white arrows)

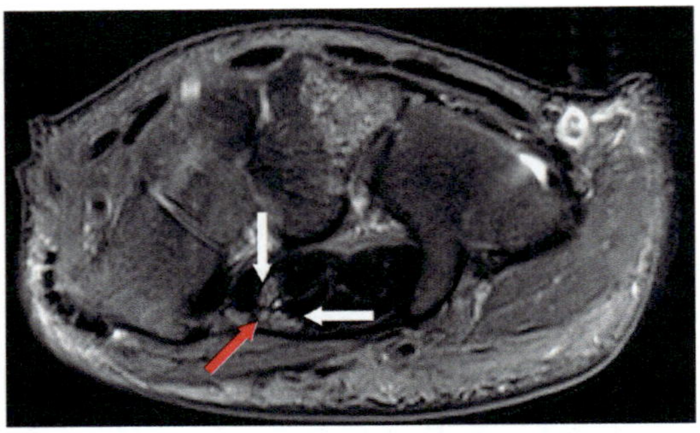

Fig. 11 Ax T2-WI FS. Persisting a. mediana (red arrow) between a split median nerve (white arrows) with a deep vertical and a superficial horizontal component

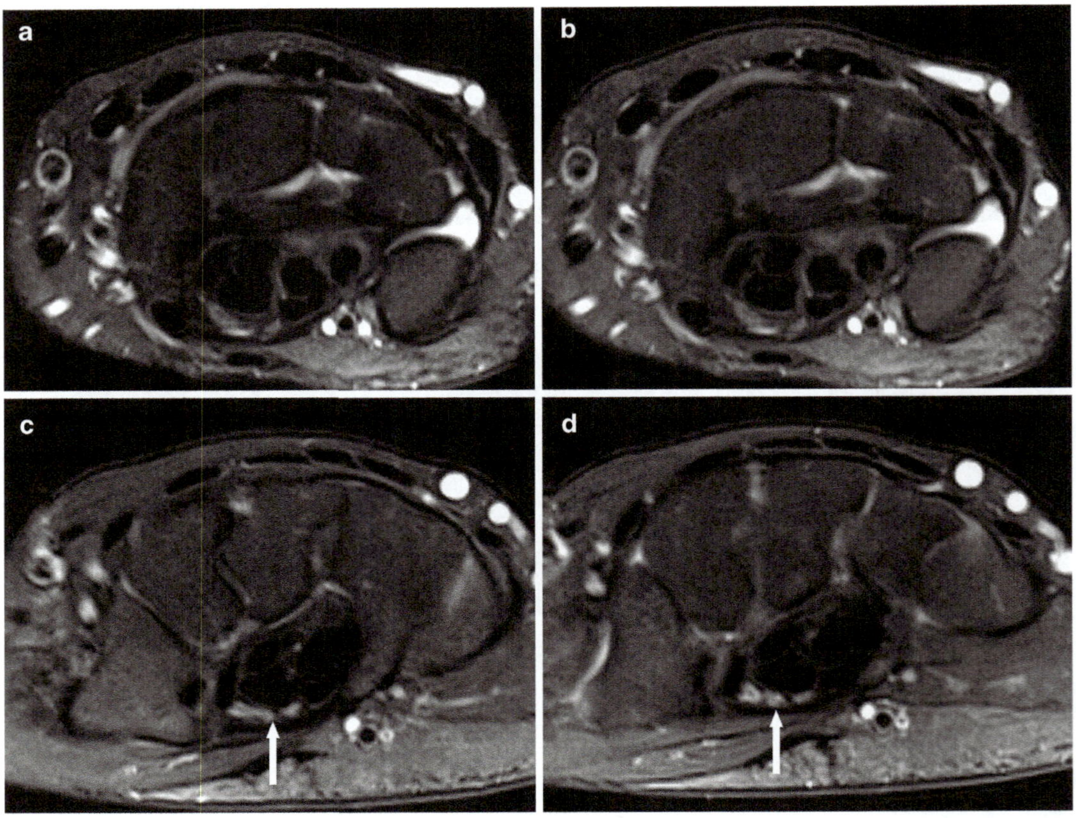

Fig. 12 Ax T2-WI FS (**a**–**d**).The median nerve splits distally in the carpal tunnel

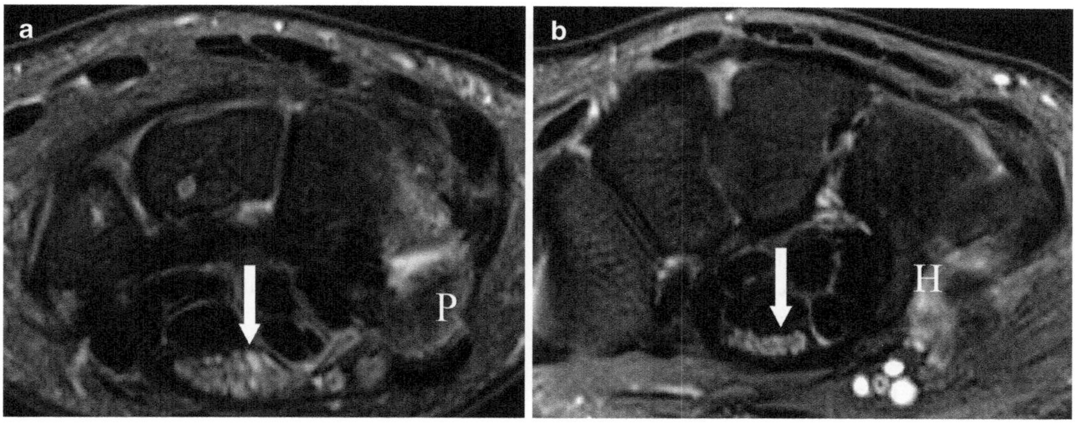

Fig. 13 Ax T2-WI FS (**a–b**). Giant median nerve with fasciculation

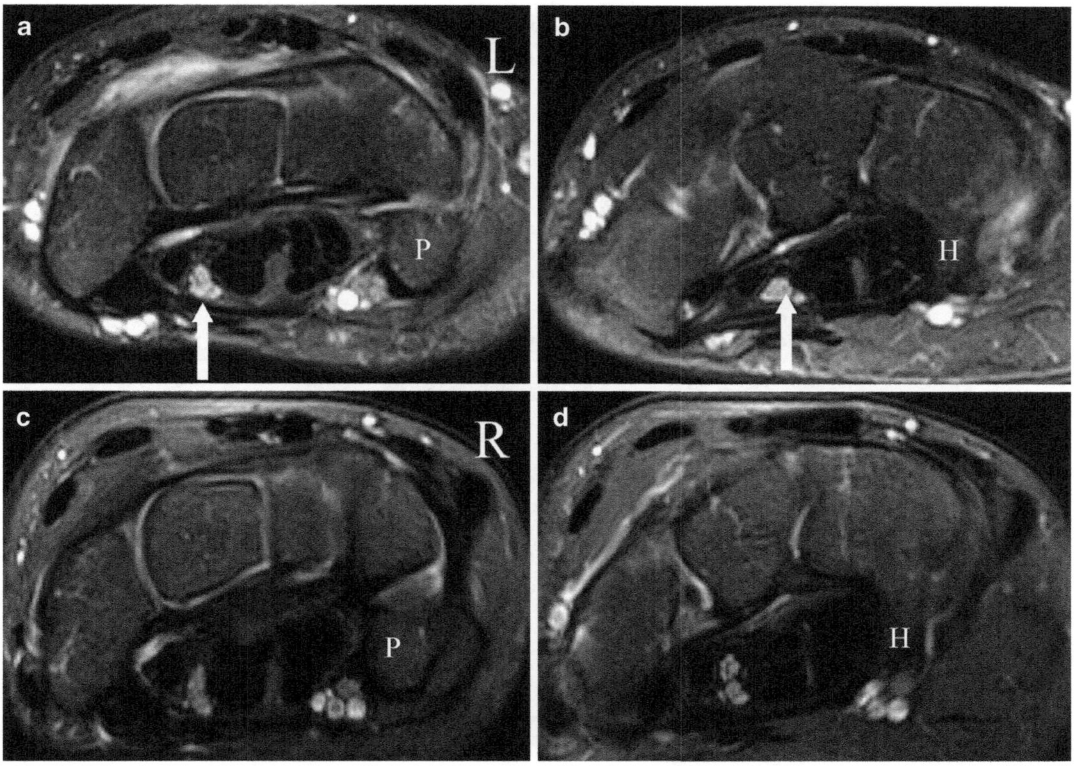

Fig. 14 Ax T2-WI FS. Bilateral MRI. The mirrored (pathological) left side (**a**, **b**) is compared with the (normal) right side (**c**, **d**)

3 Causal Abnormalities

Hypertrophic callus formation after carpal arthrodesis narrows the carpal tunnel with displacement of the content and substantial compression of the median nerve (Fig. 15). A displaced carpal prosthesis towards the carpal tunnel compresses the content and induces a CTS (Fig. 16), eventually in combination with flexor tenosynovitis. In RA (Eshed et al. 2009), extensive pannus and/or fibrosis formation narrows the carpal tunnel (Fig. 17). A lunate bone in a DISI configuration tilted into the carpal tunnel narrows the kinked channel (Fig. 18). The extreme tilt of the lunate in a SLAC wrist grade III with an elongated and thickened RLT ligament provokes a CTS (Fig. 19). Substantial musculotendinous variants (Schön et al. 1992; Sookur et al. 2008; Zeiss and Guilliam-Haidet 1996; Stein et al. 2011) or ruptures accompanied by a seroma and/or hematoma narrow the tunnel and may give also rise to a CTS (Fig. 20). An arthrosynovial cyst under tension extending in the carpal tunnel may squeeze (part(s) of) the median nerve (Fig. 21).

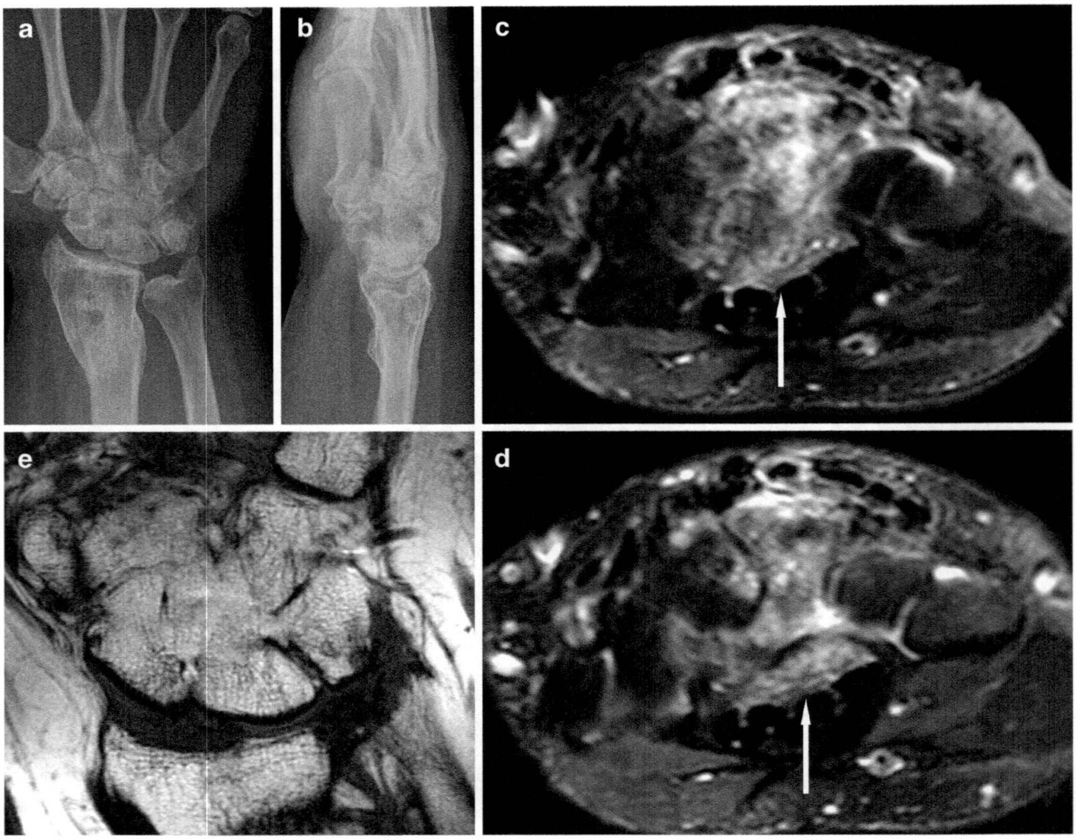

Fig. 15 Standard PA (**a**) and Lateral views (**b**); Ax T2-WI FS (**c**, **d**); Cor T1-WI (**e**). Hypertrophic callus after carpal arthrodesis with narrowing of the carpal tunnel

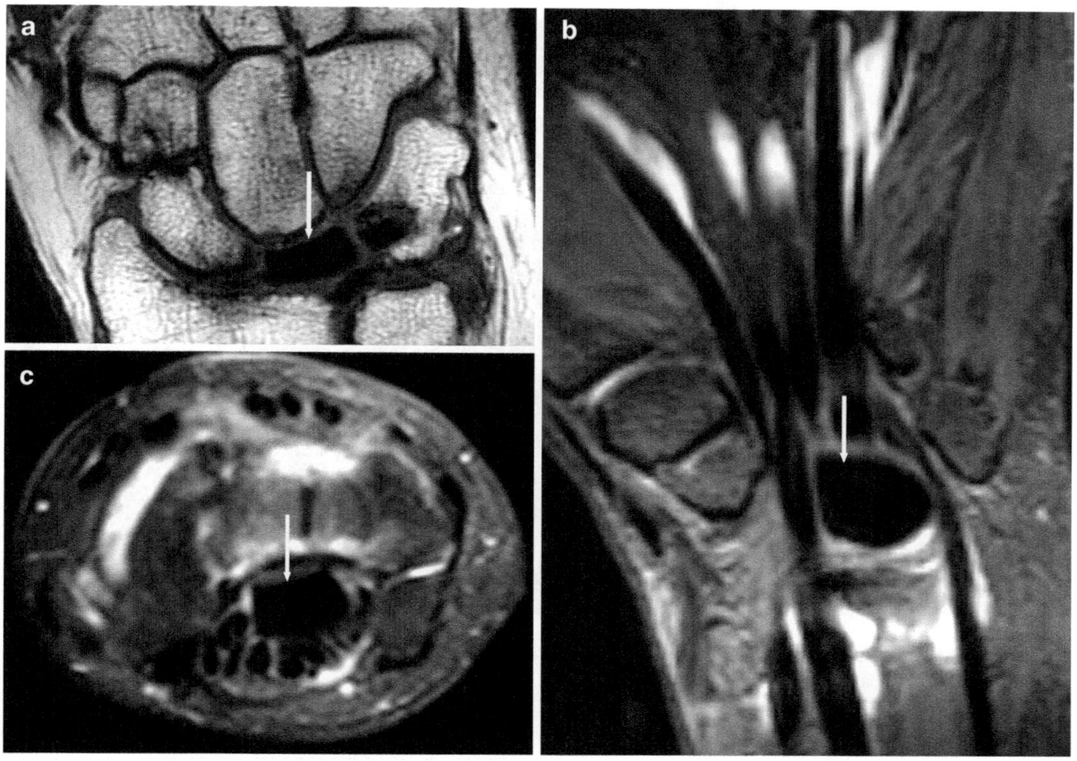

Fig. 16 Cor T1-WI (**a**) and T2-WI FS (**b**); Ax T2-WI FS (**c**). L prosthesis (**a–c**) tilted in the carpal tunnel (**b, c**) with compression on the content and additional tenosynovitis. High signal of the median nerve and bowed retinaculum (**c**)

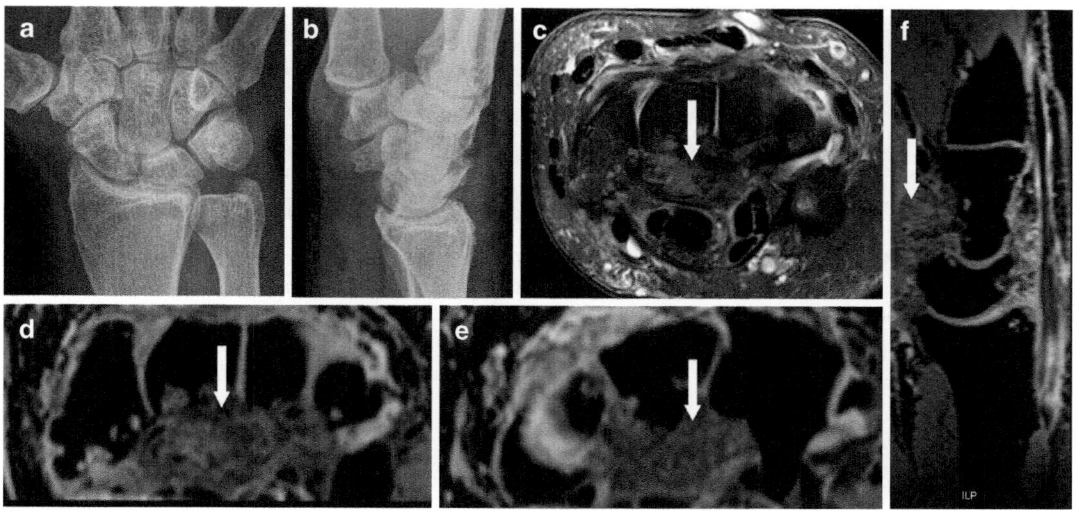

Fig. 17 Standard PA (**a**) and Lateral views (**b**); Ax T2-WI FS (**c**); Ax (**d, e**); and Sag (**f**) 3D GRE. RA with extensive pannus and fibrosis formation narrowing the carpal tunnel

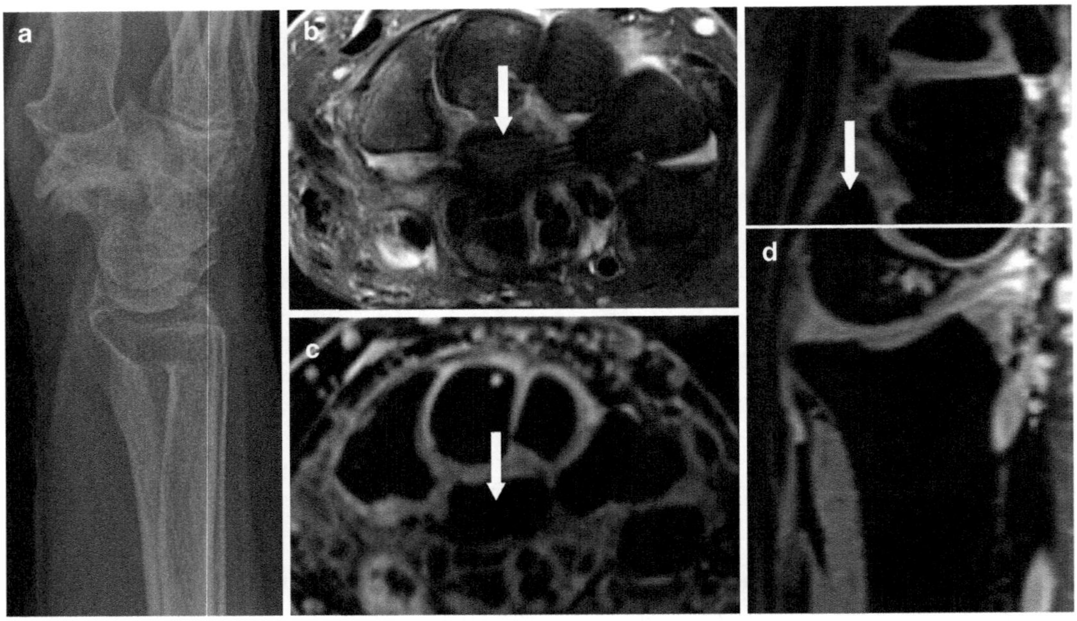

Fig. 18 Standard Lateral view (**a**); Ax T2-WI FS (**b**); Ax (**c**); and Sag (**d**) 3D GRE. DISI configuration (**a**) with tilting of the L (**b–d**) in the carpal tunnel

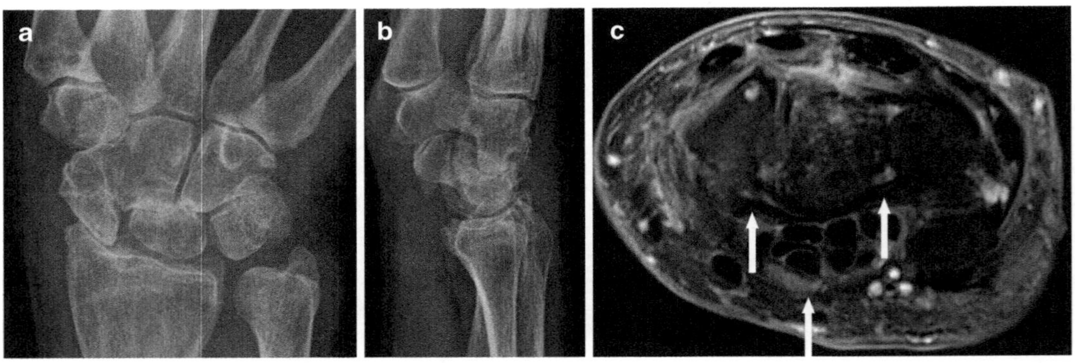

Fig. 19 Standard PA (**a**) and Lateral (**b**) views; Ax T2-WI FS (**c**). SLAC grade III with pronounced DISI configuration (**a**, **b**), elongation and thickening of the RLT ligament (**c**) and tilting of the L in the carpal tunnel resulting in a curved retinaculum and flattening of the median nerve (**c**)

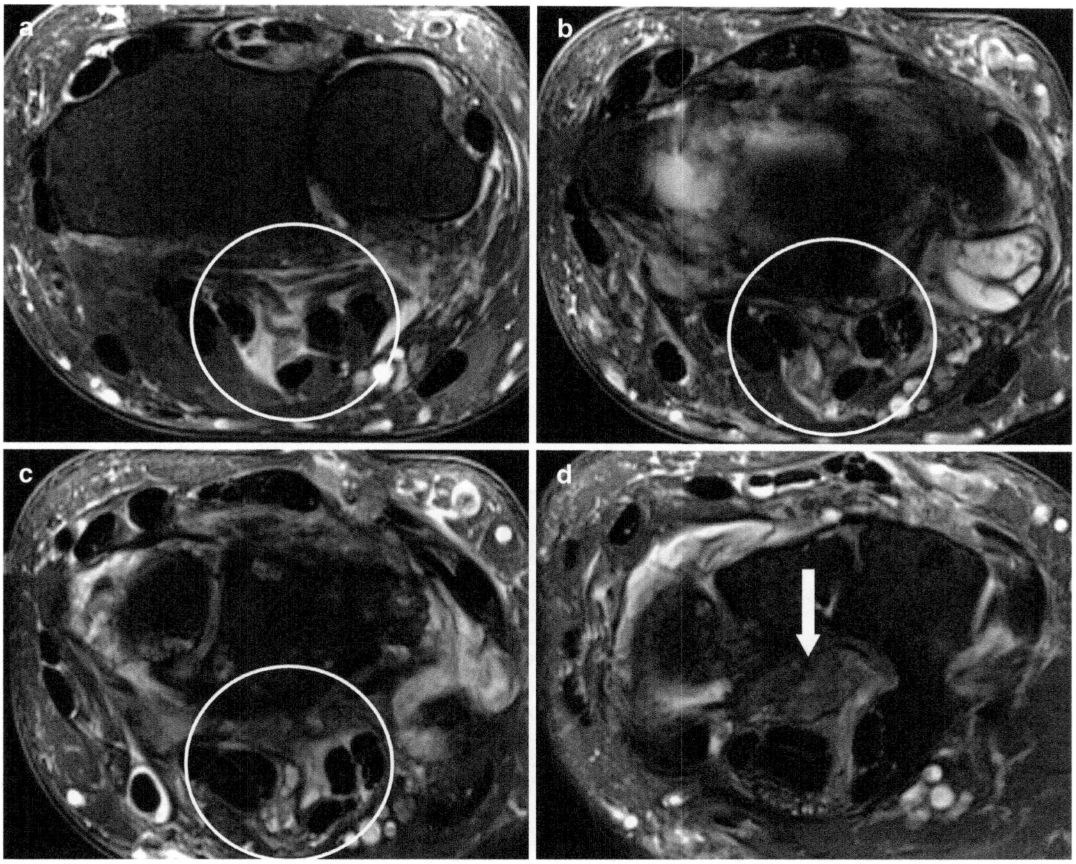

Fig. 20 Ax T2-WI FS. Musculotendinous rupture (**a–c**) with seroma/hematoma (**d**) narrowing the carpal tunnel

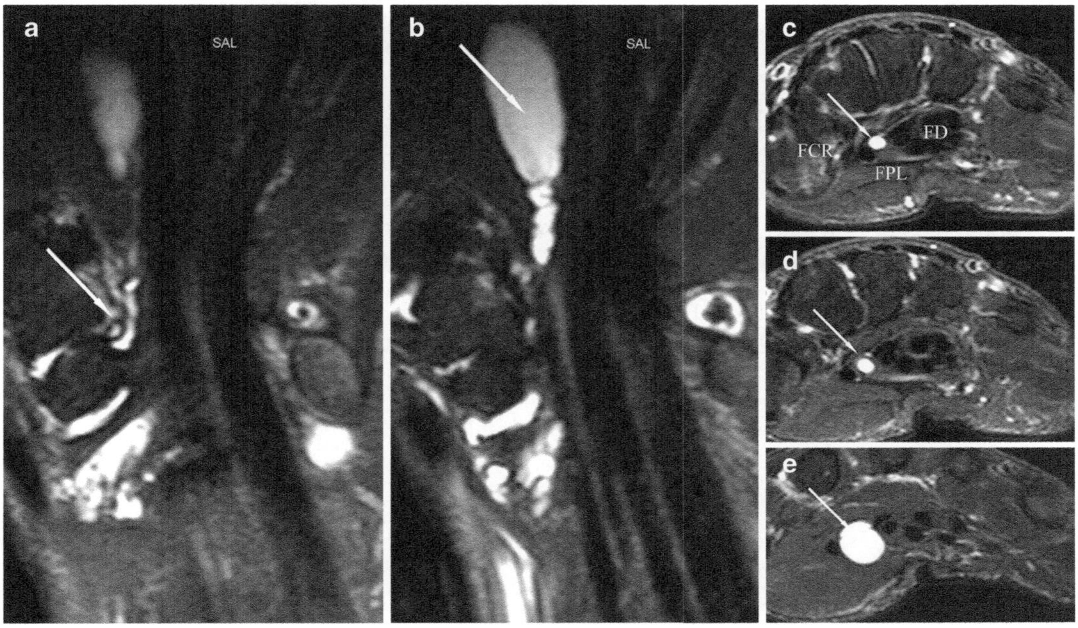

Fig. 21 Cor 3D GRE (**a**, **b**); Ax T2-WI FS (**c–e**). Arthrosynovial cyst extending in the carpal tunnel

4 Post-Operative Status

The post-operative status after CTS surgery shows a defect of the flexor retinaculum proximally (Fig. 22a, b) and (eventually) distally (Fig. 22c, d) depending on the type of surgery. Persisting symptoms after CTS surgery may be due to hematoma, seroma, insufficient resection of the flexor retinaculum (proximally and/or distally) or fibrous "repair" of the flexor retinaculum, which can all be demonstrated by MRI. Fibrous repair of the retinaculum varies: complete, only proximally (Fig. 23) or distally (Fig. 24). Recurrence of a mass (Khaled and Drapé 2015; Kostakoğlu et al. 1997; Pirola et al. 2009; Teh and Whiteley 2007; Girgis and Epstein 2000) (Fig. 24) or fibrosis around the median nerve may cause the symptoms. However, the MRI findings are not always in accordance with the symptoms. Despite a normal status after surgery (Fig. 25); symptoms persist, and the EMG is positive for CTS which may warrant the need for surgical re-exploration.

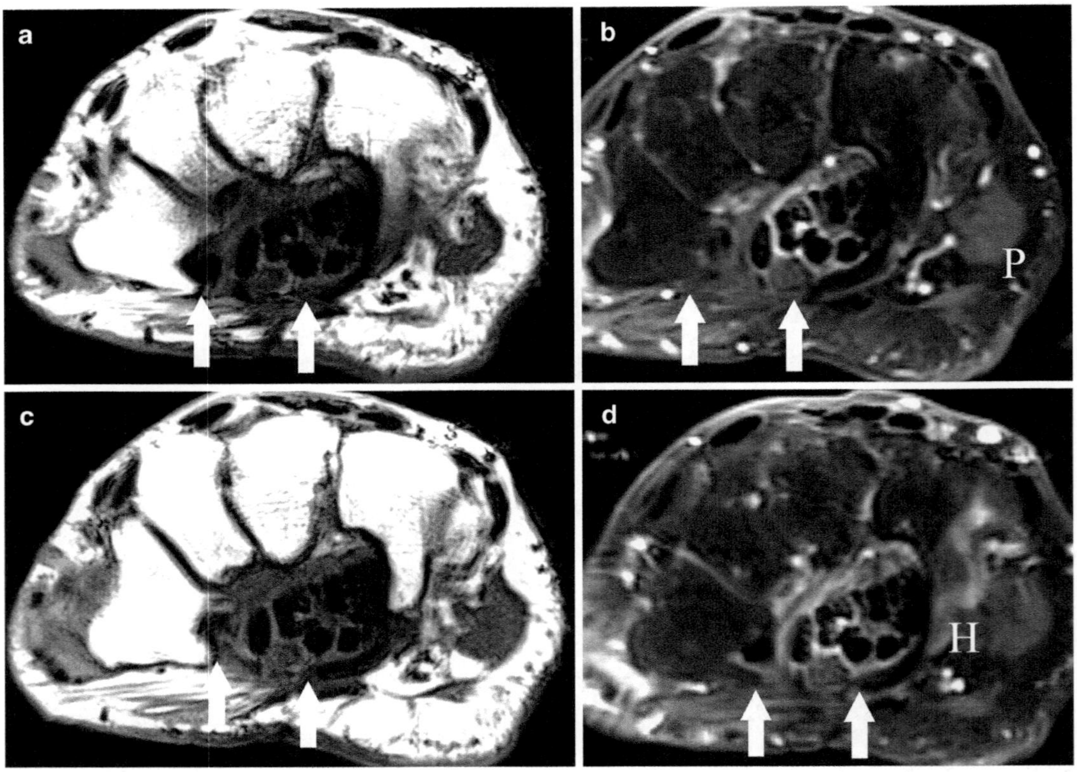

Fig. 22 Axial T1-WI (**a**, **c**) and T2-WI FS (**b**, **d**). Status after CTS surgery with clear defect proximally (**a**, **b**) and distally (**c**, **d**) of the flexor retinaculum

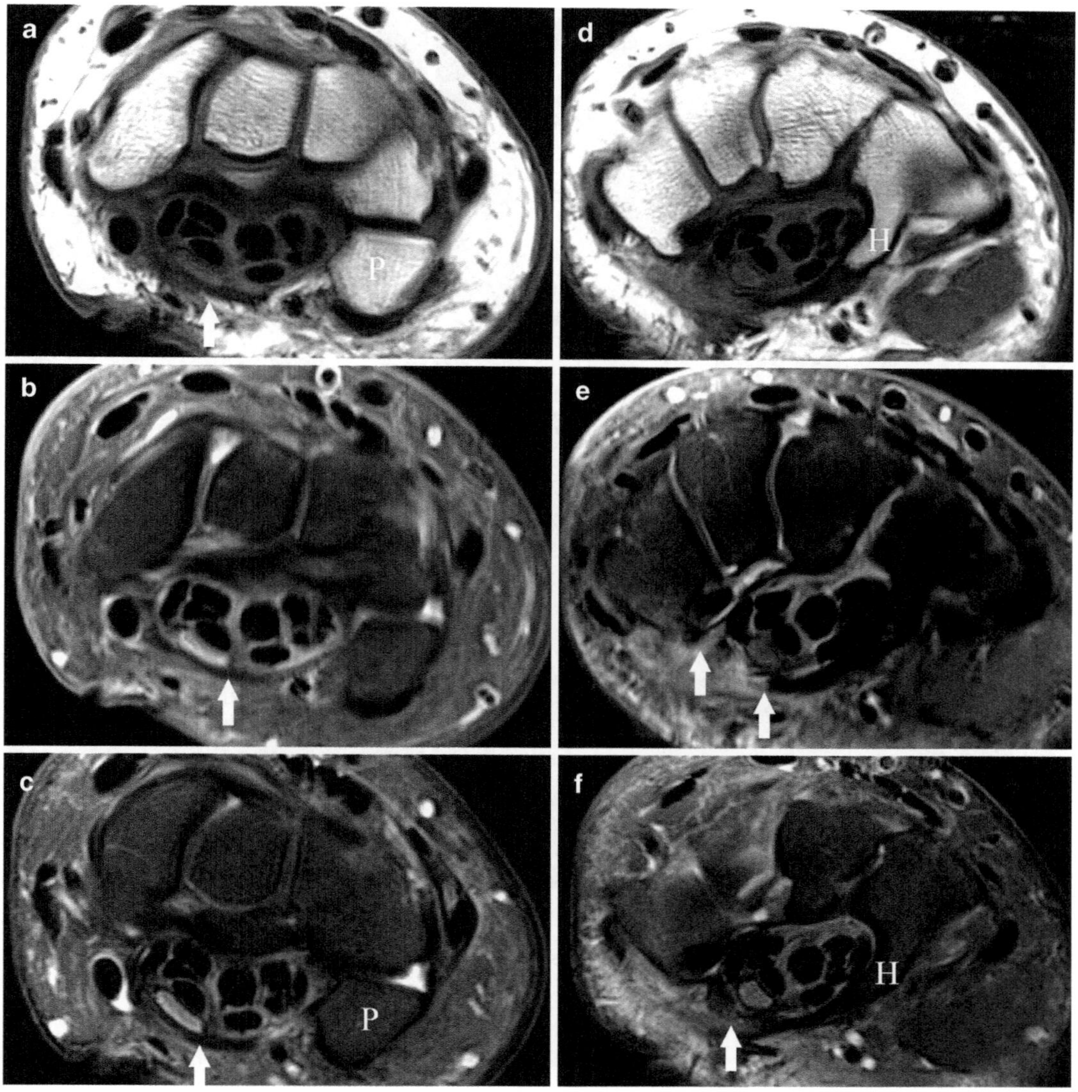

Fig. 23 Axial T1-WI (**a**, **d**); Axial T1-WI FS with CE (**b**, **e**); and T2-WI FS (**c**, **f**). Status after CTS surgery with fibrous repair proximally (**a**–**c**) and normal status distally (**d**–**f**) with a flexor retinaculum defect and slight migration of the tunnel content to palmar

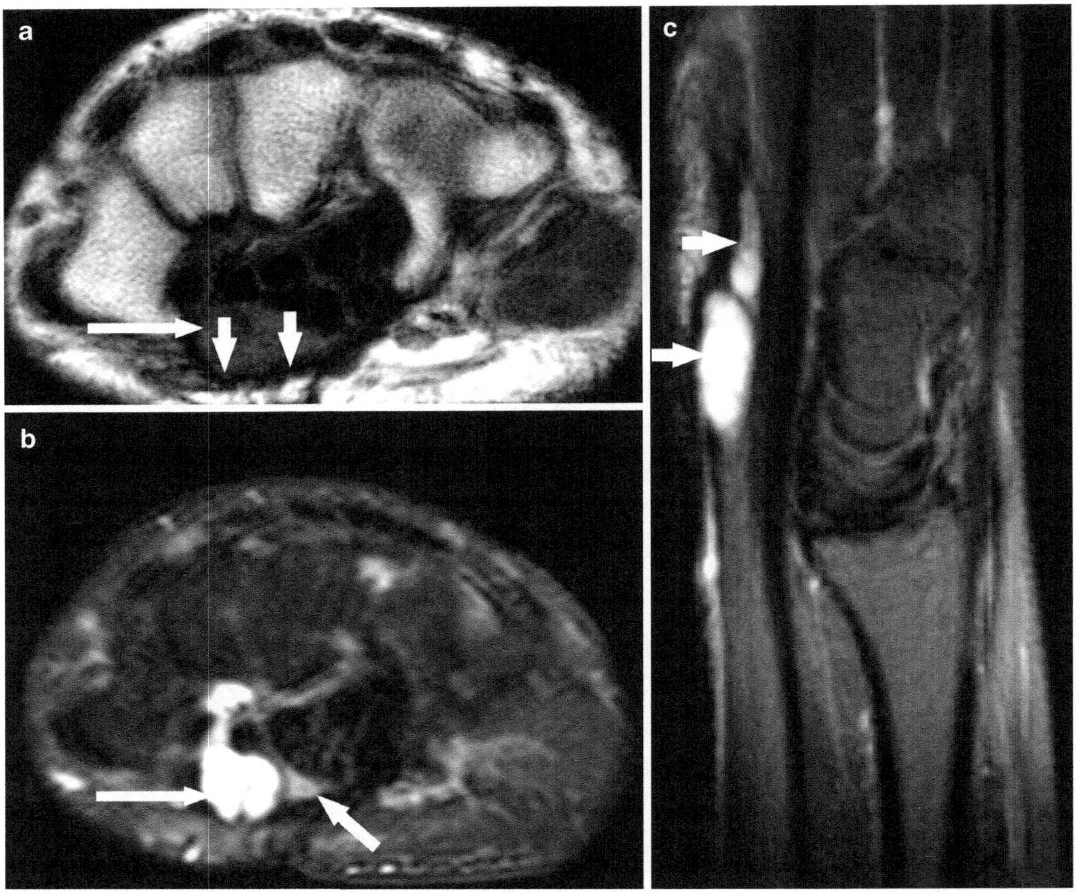

Fig. 24 Axial T1-WI (**a**); Ax (**b**) and Sag (**c**) T2-WI FS. Status after CTS surgery with fibrous repair distally (**a**) and recurrence of the arthrosynovial cyst (**a–c**) with compression on the median nerve (**b**)

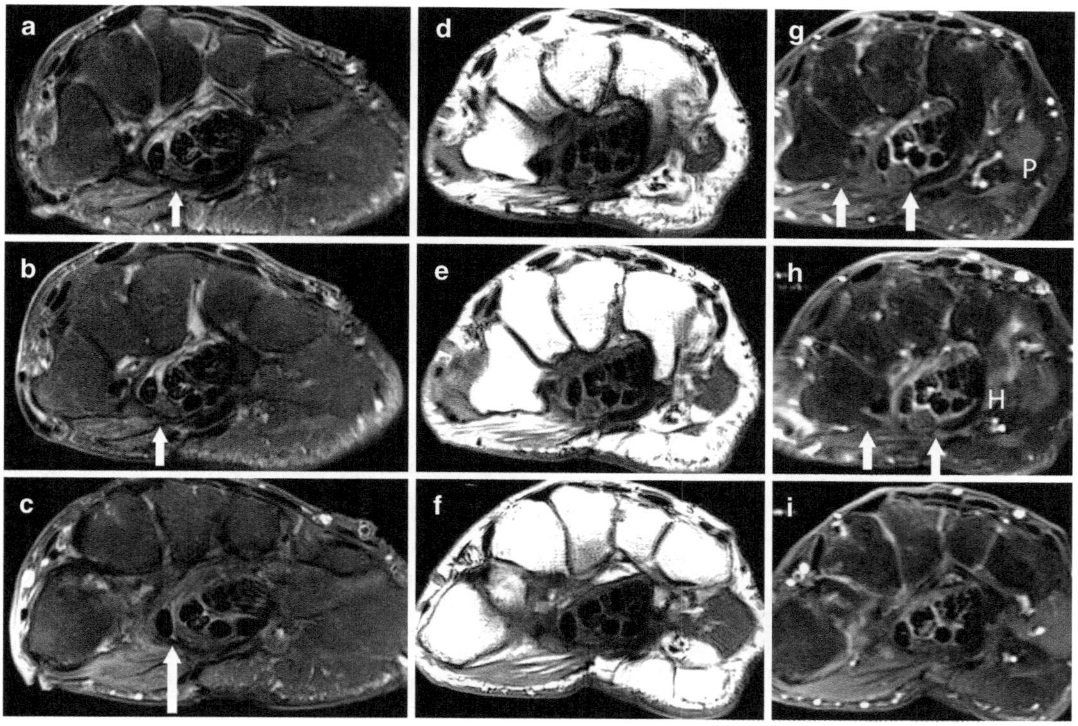

Fig. 25 Axial T2-WI FS (**a–c**); Ax T1-WI (**d–f**); and T2-WI FS (**g–i**) after surgery. Continuous aspect of the flexor retinaculum before surgery (**a–c**). Persistent symptoms and positive EMG despite a post-operative correct discontinuous flexor retinaculum (**d–i**)

5 Kiloh-Nevin Syndrome

The anterior interosseous branch (Gyftopoulos et al. 2010) splits of the median nerve in the forearm about 2–8 cm below the medial epicondyle. Isolated pathology involving this branch (neuritis, fracture, tumour, pronator teres tendinitis, bicipital bursitis, thrombus of ulnar collateral vessels) may result in a high signal on T2-WI of several muscles at the forearm (fdp, fpl) and at the wrist specifically of the m. pronator quadratus (Gyftopoulos et al. 2010) (Fig. 26).

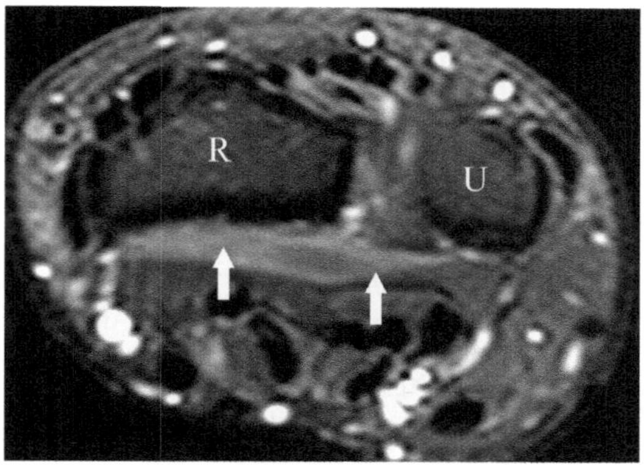

Fig. 26 Axial T2-WI FS. Isolated higher signal in the m. pronator quadratus

References

Chammas M (2014) Carpal tunnel syndrome. Chir Main 33(2):75–94. https://doi.org/10.1016/j.main.2013.11.010. Epub 2014 Feb 15. PMID: 24646612

Chammas M, Boretto J, Burmann LM, Ramos RM, Dos Santos Neto FC, Silva JB (2014) Carpal tunnel syndrome – part I (anatomy, physiology, etiology and diagnosis). Rev Bras Ortop 49(5):429–436. https://doi.org/10.1016/j.rboe.2014.08.001. PMID: 26229841; PMCID: PMC4487499

Eshed I, Feist E, Althoff CE, Hamm B, Konen E, Burmester GR, Backhaus M, Hermann KG (2009) Tenosynovitis of the flexor tendons of the hand detected by MRI: an early indicator of rheumatoid arthritis. Rheumatology (Oxford) 48(8):887–891. https://doi.org/10.1093/rheumatology/kep136. Epub 2009 May 27. PMID: 19474128

Falkiner S, Myers S (2002) When exactly can carpal tunnel syndrome be considered work-related? ANZ J Surg 72(3):204–209. https://doi.org/10.1046/j.1445--2197.2002.02347.x. PMID: 12071453

Girgis WS, Epstein RE (2000) Magnetic resonance imaging of the hand and wrist. Semin Roentgenol 35(3):286–296. https://doi.org/10.1053/sroe.2000.7339. PMID: 10939130

Gitto S, Draghi F (2016) Normal sonographic anatomy of the wrist with emphasis on assessment of tendons, nerves, and ligaments. J Ultrasound Med 35(5):1081–1094. https://doi.org/10.7863/ultra.15.06105. Epub 2016 Apr 1. PMID: 27036166

Gyftopoulos S, Rosenberg ZS, Petchprapa C (2010) Increased MR signal intensity in the pronator quadratus muscle: does it always indicate anterior interosseous neuropathy? AJR Am J Roentgenol 194(2):490–493. https://doi.org/10.2214/AJR.09.2361. PMID: 20093614

Khaled W, Drapé JL (2015) MRI of wrist and hand masses. Diagn Interv Imaging 96(12):1238–1246. https://doi.org/10.1016/j.diii.2015.10.005. Epub 2015 Nov 10. PMID: 26564613

Kostakoğlu N, Borman H, Keçik A (1997) Anomalous flexor digitorum superficialis muscle belly: an unusual case of mass in the palm. Br J Plast Surg 50(8):654–656. https://doi.org/10.1016/s0007-1226(97)90515-4. PMID: 9613412

Lee RKL, Griffith JF, Ng AWH, Tipoe GL, Chan AWH, Wong CWY, Tse WL, Ho PC (2019) Cross-sectional area of the median nerve at the wrist: comparison of sonographic, MRI, and cadaveric measurements. J Clin Ultrasound 47(3):122–127. https://doi.org/10.1002/jcu.22647. Epub 2018 Dec 29. PMID: 30597562

Martinoli C, Bianchi S, Gandolfo N, Valle M, Simonetti S, Derchi LE (2000) US of nerve entrapments in osteofibrous tunnels of the upper and lower limbs. Radiographics 20(Spec):S199–S213. https://doi.org/10.1148/radiographics.20.suppl_1.g00oc08s199; discussion S213–S217. Erratum in: Radiographics 2000;20(6):1818 PMID: 11046171

Newington L, Harris EC, Walker-Bone K (2015) Carpal tunnel syndrome and work. Best Pract Res Clin Rheumatol 29(3):440–453. https://doi.org/10.1016/j.berh.2015.04.026. Epub 2015 May 27. PMID: 26612240; PMCID: PMC4759938

Park JS, Won HC, Oh JY, Kim DH, Hwang SC, Yoo JI (2020) Value of cross-sectional area of median nerve by MRI in carpal tunnel syndrome. Asian J Surg 43(6):654–659. https://doi.org/10.1016/j.asjsur.2019.08.001. Epub 2019 Aug 28. PMID: 31473048

Pirola E, Hébert-Blouin MN, Amador N, Amrami KK, Spinner RJ (2009) Palmaris profundus: one name, several subtypes, and a shared potential for nerve compression. Clin Anat 22(6):643–648. https://doi.org/10.1002/ca.20848. PMID: 19644968

Schön R, Kraus E, Boller O, Kampe A (1992) Anomalous muscle belly of the flexor digitorum superficialis associated with carpal tunnel syndrome: case report. Neurosurgery 31(5):969–970. https://doi.org/10.1227/00006123-199211000-00026; discussion 970–971. PMID: 1436428

Sookur PA, Naraghi AM, Bleakney RR, Jalan R, Chan O, White LM (2008) Accessory muscles: anatomy, symptoms, and radiologic evaluation. Radiographics 28(2):481–499. https://doi.org/10.1148/rg.282075064. PMID: 18349452

Stein JM, Cook TS, Simonson S, Kim W (2011) Normal and variant anatomy of the wrist and hand on MR imaging. Magn Reson Imaging Clin N Am 19(3):595–608. https://doi.org/10.1016/j.mric.2011.05.007; ix. PMID: 21816333

Teh J, Whiteley G (2007) MRI of soft tissue masses of the hand and wrist. Br J Radiol 80(949):47–63. https://doi.org/10.1259/bjr/53596176. Epub 2006 May 10. PMID: 16687461

Zeiss J, Guilliam-Haidet L (1996) MR demonstration of anomalous muscles about the volar aspect of the wrist and forearm. Clin Imaging 20(3):219–221. https://doi.org/10.1016/0899-7071(95)00013-5. PMID: 8877177

Canal of Guyon

Contents

1 General

The canal of Guyon (or ulnar tunnel) is a small palmar tunnel at the ulnar side (Dimitriou and Natsis 2007; Martinoli et al. 2000), located in between the flexor retinaculum (deep) and the superficial palmar ligament (superficial). It starts at the pisiform bone (ulnar side) and reaches till the hamulus of the hamate bone (radial side). It only contains the ulnar nerve, artery, and veins. Local squeezing of the ulnar nerve during this pathway may give rise to a specific motor and/or sensory neuritis (Dimitriou and Natsis 2007; Gornitzky and Carrigan 2016). The diameter of the median nerve increases. US may be useful as a first medical imaging approach (Fig. 1).

M. Mespreuve, K. Waked, *MRI of the Wrist*, Medical Radiology,
https://doi.org/10.1007/978-3-031-63973-9_15

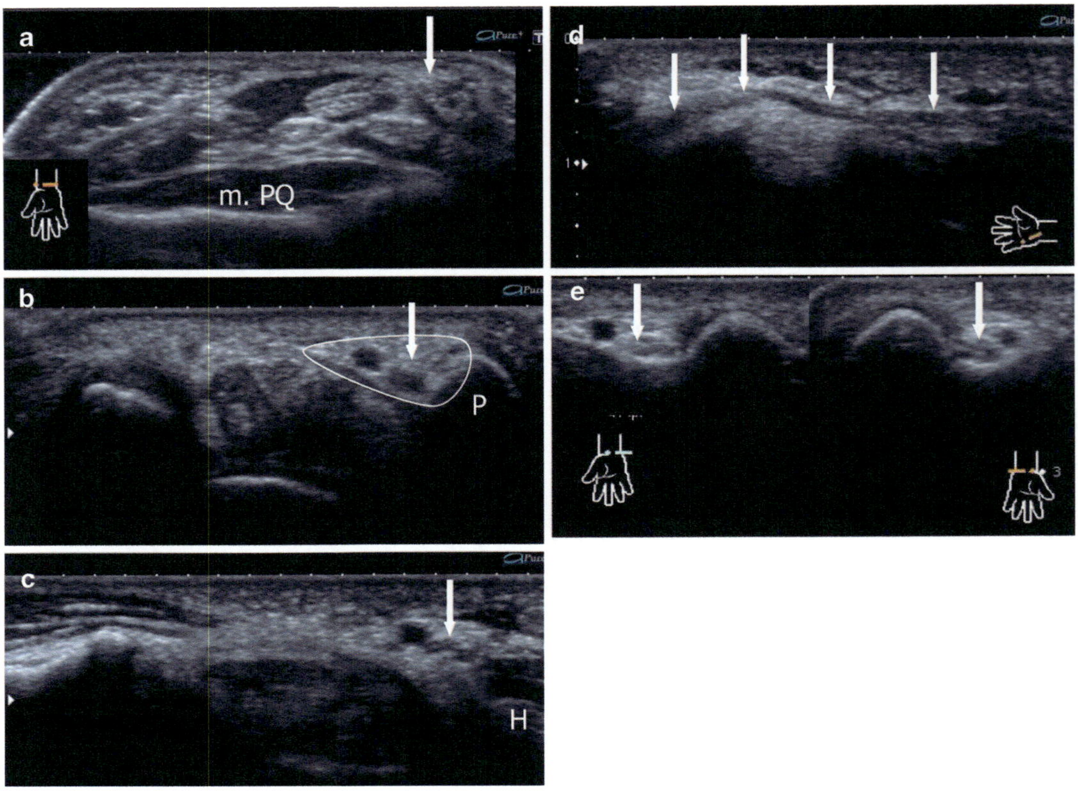

Fig. 1 Transverse (**a**–**c**); longitudinal (**d**); and comparative transverse (**e**) US. The ulnar nerve (**a**–**e**) in the Guyon canal (**b**)

2 MRI findings

Additionally, on MRI, the signal intensity increases on T2-WI (Fig. 2). The ulnar nerve is swollen (Fig. 3) and fasciculation appears (Fig. 4).

Eventual causal abnormal structures in the carpal tunnel should also be identified, although the cause of CTS frequently remains unknown ("idiopathic").

The three clinical types depend on the location of the squeezing of the nerve (Martinoli et al. 2000) (Fig. 5). Type 1 defined by motor and sensory deficiency is caused by a compression proximal of or near the pisiform bone (proximal to the splitting of the ulnar nerve in a superficial sensory and deep motor branch). A type 2 with only motor deficiency is the result of compression distal from the split of the deep motor branch, along the fibrous arch of the hypothenar muscles. In type 3 with only sensory deficiency, the cause is located distal from the split at the superficial branch, along the hypothenar fascia.

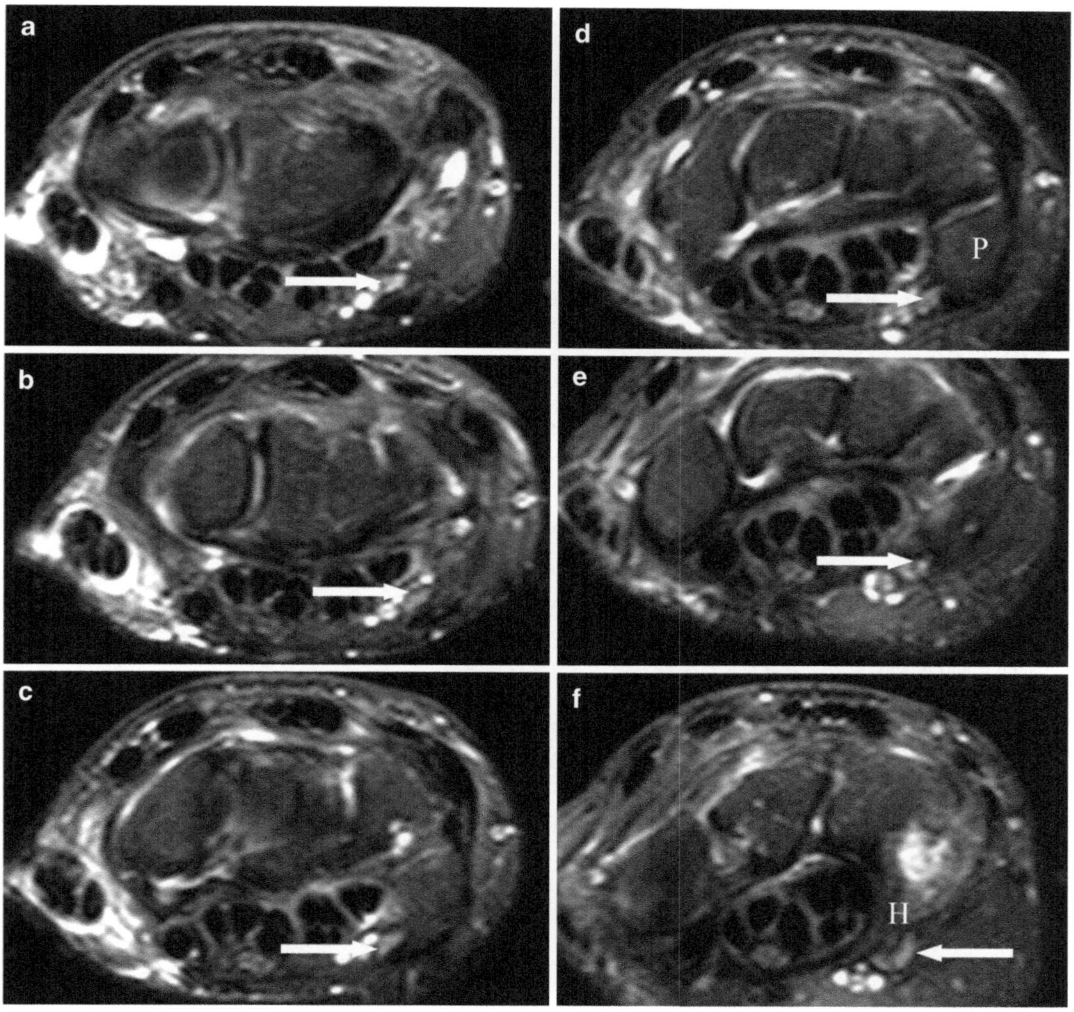

Fig. 2 Ax T2-WI FS. The ulnar nerve proximal from (**a**) and in the canal of Guyon (**b–d**), splits (**e–f**) and gives a superficial sensory and deep motor branch (H)

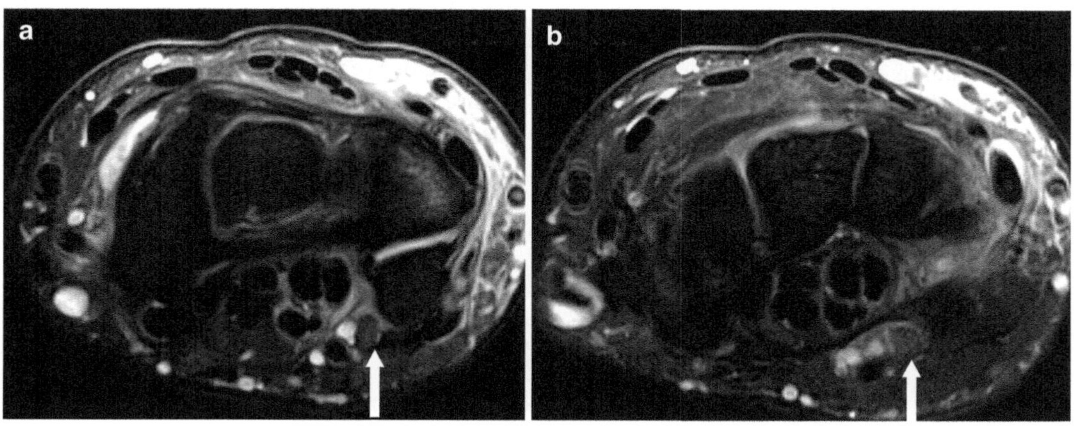

Fig. 3 Ax T2-WI FS (**a–b**). Swollen ulnar nerve

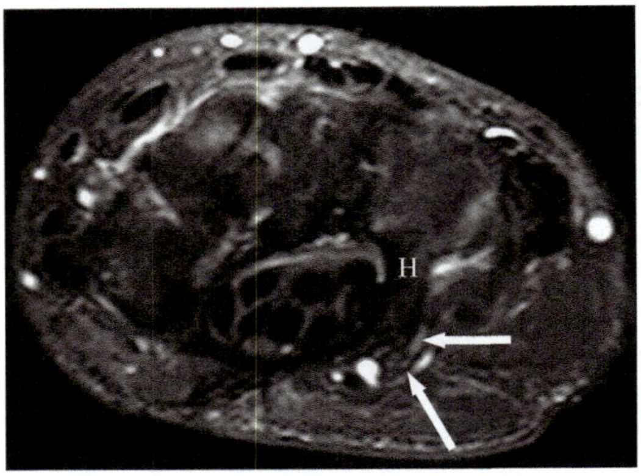

Fig. 4 Ax T2-WI FS. The branches of the ulnar nerve with high signal and fasciculation

Fig. 5 Standard PA with projected ulnar nerve trajectory. The ulnar nerve runs radially from the P, splits between P and h, and gives at the ulnar side of the h rise to a deep motor and a superficial sensory branch

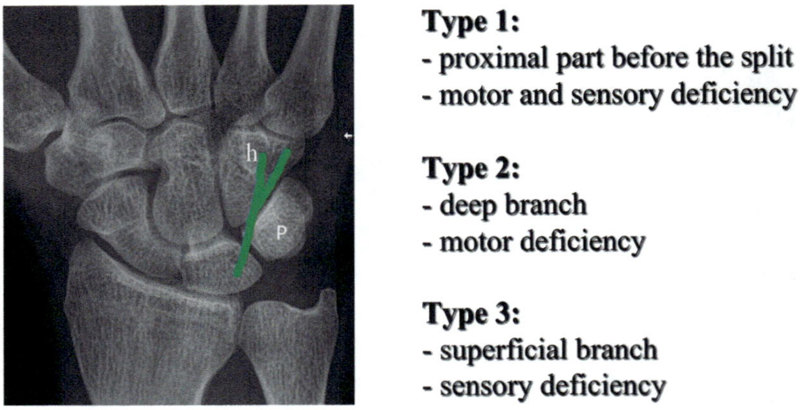

3 Causal abnormalities

Different pathologies may cause a local neuritis of the ulnar nerve. Cyst, trauma (Fig. 6), specific fracture of the hamulus (Fig. 7), repetitive microtrauma resulting in hypothenar hammer syndrome with ulnar artery dissection, stenosis, pseudo-aneurysm (Fig. 8) or thrombosis (Figs. 8 and 9), CTS (Fig. 10), (pseudo)tumour (Dimitriou and Natsis 2007; Harvie et al. 2003, 2004; Pirola et al. 2009; Spiess and Gursel 2006) (Fig. 11), ganglion cysts, or frequently "iatrogenic".

The Hypothenar Hammer Syndrome is a consequence of repeat blunt trauma of the ulnar palm, which may lead to direct nerve injury, fracture of the H or pseudo-aneurysm of the ulnar artery (Milling and Kinmonth 1977). In a patient with ulnar nerve neuritis and a history of Raynaud disease, thrombosis of the ulnar artery must be ruled out.

Surgical treatment by opening the canal of Guyon is often recommended in case of a type 1 or type 2 neuritis, in which the motor branch is involved.

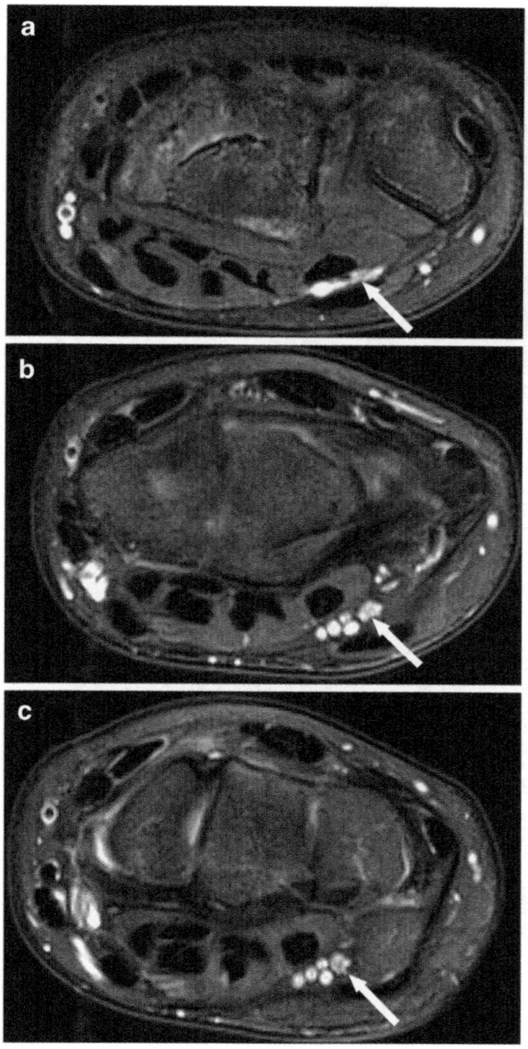

Fig. 6 Ax T2-WI FS. Fracture epiphysiolysis Salter-Harris type 2 and dorsal ulnar luxation (**a**) with neuritis of the ulnar nerve (**a–c**)

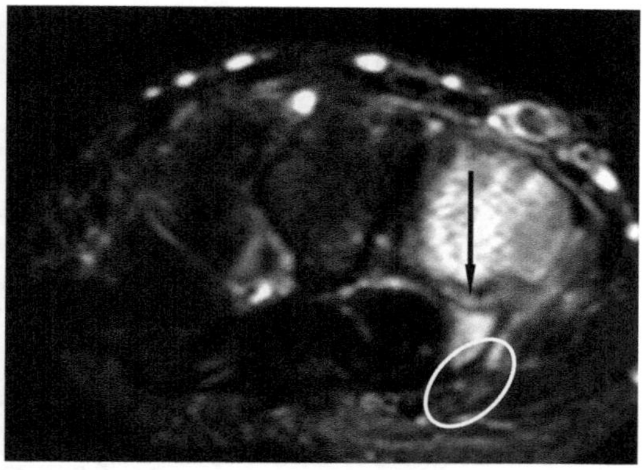

Fig. 7 Ax T2-WI FS. Fracture at the base of the hamulus with ulnar nerve neuritis

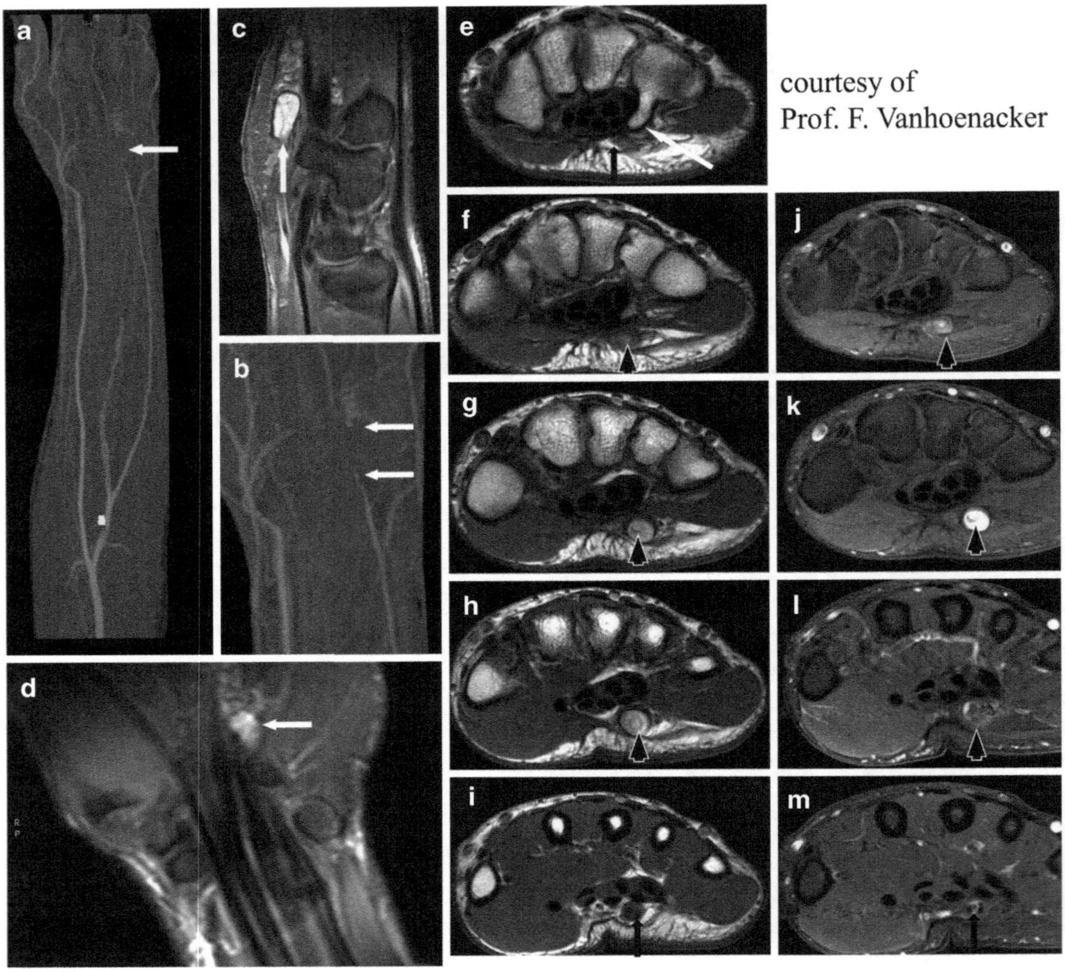

Fig. 8 MR angiography (**a**, **b**); Sag (**c**) and Cor (**d**) T2-WI FS; Ax T1-WI (**e**–**i**); and Ax T1-WI FS with CE (**j**–**m**). Pseudo-aneurysm of the ulnar artery close to the hamulus with further extending thrombus

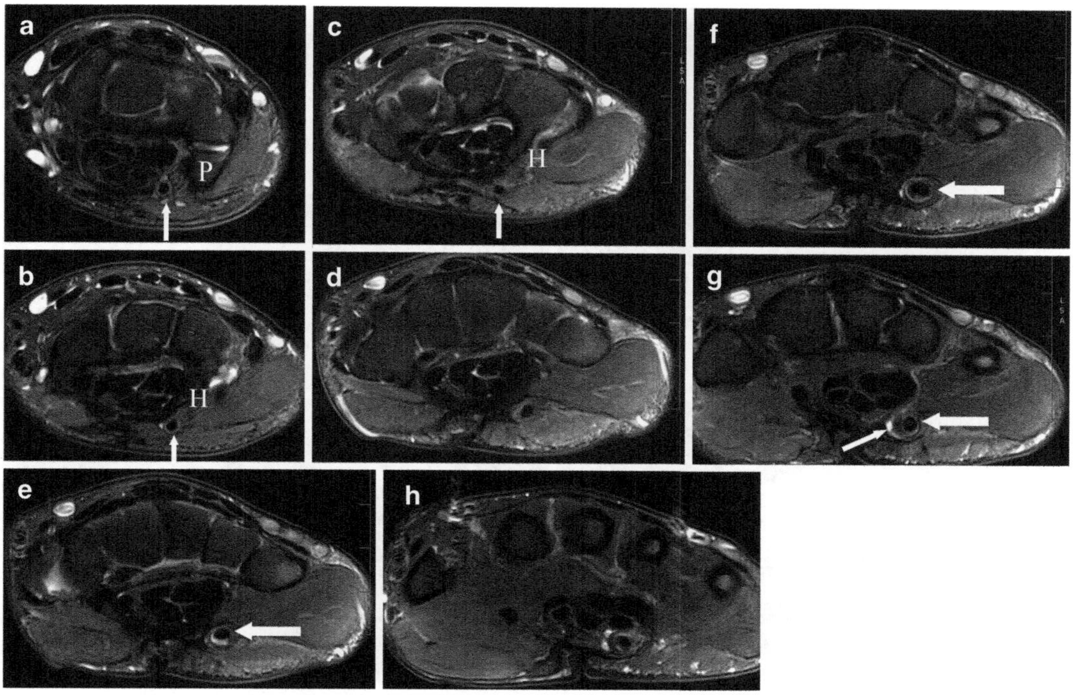

Fig. 9 Ax T2-WI FS. Old thrombus in the ulnar artery centred at the location of penetration of the palmar aponeurosis (**a**, **b**) and continuing in the superficial palmar arch (**c**–**h**)

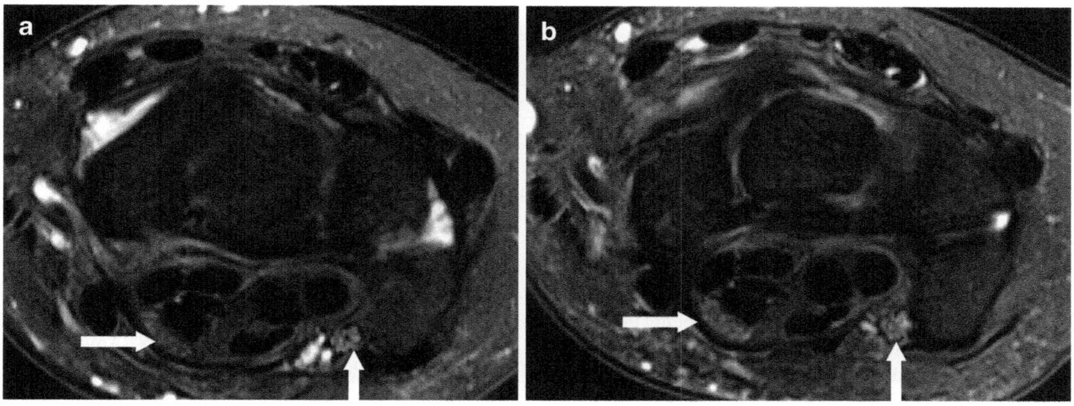

Fig. 10 Ax T2-WI FS (**a**–**b**). Fibrous repair of the flexor retinaculum with CTS and ulnar nerve neuritis

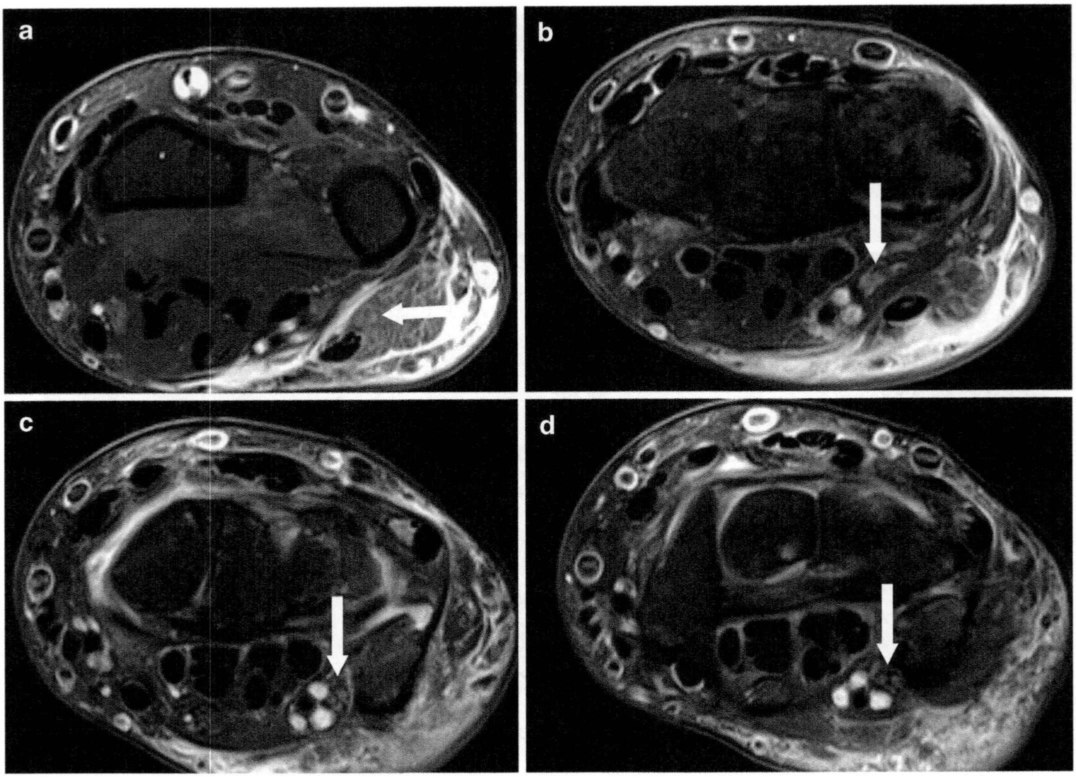

Fig. 11 Ax T2-WI FS. Crush trauma of the fcu (**a**) with hematoma and neuritis of the ulnar nerve (**b–d**)

References

Dimitriou C, Natsis K (2007) Accessory abductor digiti minimi muscle causing ulnar nerve entrapment at the Guyon's canal: a case report. Clin Anat 20(8):974–975. https://doi.org/10.1002/ca.20518. PMID: 17583589

Gornitzky AL, Carrigan RB (2016) The diagnostic utility of MRI in the painful wrist: when to reconsider advanced imaging in the pediatric patient. Pediatrics (Evanston) 137(Suppl 3):596–596A. https://doi.org/10.1542/peds.137.Supplement_3.596A

Harvie P, Patel N, Ostlere SJ (2003) Ulnar nerve compression at Guyon's canal by an anomalous abductor digiti minimi muscle: the role of ultrasound in clinical diagnosis. Hand Surg 8(2):271–275. https://doi.org/10.1142/s0218810403001819. PMID: 15002110

Harvie P, Patel N, Ostlere SJ (2004) Prevalence and epidemiological variation of anomalous muscles at Guyon's canal. J Hand Surg Br 29(1):26–29. https://doi.org/10.1016/j.jhsb.2003.08.004. PMID: 14734065

Martinoli C, Bianchi S, Gandolfo N, Valle M, Simonetti S, Derchi LE (2000) US of nerve entrapments in osteofibrous tunnels of the upper and lower limbs. Radiographics 20 Spec:S199–S213. https://doi.org/10.1148/radiographics.20.suppl_1.g00oc08s199; discussion S213–S217. Erratum in: Radiographics 2000 Nov-Dec;20(6):1818. PMID: 11046171

Milling MA, Kinmonth MH (1977) False aneurysm of the ulnar artery. Hand 9(1):57–59. https://doi.org/10.1016/s0072-968x(77)80033-8. PMID: 892625

Pirola E, Hébert-Blouin MN, Amador N, Amrami KK, Spinner RJ (2009) Palmaris profundus: one name, several subtypes, and a shared potential for nerve compression. Clin Anat 22(6):643–648. https://doi.org/10.1002/ca.20848. PMID: 19644968

Spiess AM, Gursel E (2006) Entrapment of the ulnar nerve at Guyon's canal by an accessory abductor digiti minimi muscle. Plast Reconstr Surg 117(3):1060–1061. https://doi.org/10.1097/01.prs.0000201226.25499.92. PMID: 16525331

Tumours and Tumour-Like Conditions

Contents

M. Mespreuve, K. Waked, *MRI of the Wrist*, Medical Radiology,
https://doi.org/10.1007/978-3-031-63973-9_16

1 General

Three groups are considered (Nguyen et al. 2004): bone, soft tissue (Yilmaz et al. 2022), and pseudotumours. Benign tumours of bone (Table 1) and soft tissue (Table 2) of various types are illustrated with a focus on specific details for the wrist. Malignant tumours of the wrist in general are extremely rare.

However, for more specialised information about this specific and complex topic in general, the reader should consult more dedicated publications (Nguyen et al. 2004; Yilmaz et al. 2022; Khaled and Drapé 2015).

Especially with tumours, always consider MRI combined with the standard views as a diagnostic unit.

Table 1 Summary of the most frequent bone tumours

Bone tumours	
Benign	
Fibrous cortical defect/non-ossifying fibroma	
Fibrous dysplasia	
Enostoma/sclerotic bone island	
Enchondroma	Most frequent
Solitary	
Multiple	Sometimes degeneration/ Ollier's disease/Maffucci's syndrome (+ soft tissue haemangiomata)
Bone haemangioma	
Bone cyst	
Intraosseous ganglion	
Osteochondroma	
Giant cell tumour	Locally aggressive
Malignant	
Very rare!	

Table 2 Summary of the most frequent soft tissue tumours

Soft tissue tumours	
Benign	
"Ganglioncyst"	MRI = /some are haemorrhagic
Synovial herniation: cyst	
Mucoid degeneration: ganglion	
Lipoma	
Neural fibrolipoma of median nerve	Hamartoma
Schwannoma/Neurinoma	
AVM/Haemangioma/ Aneurysm	
Synovial (osteo) chondromatosis	
Giant cell tumour:	
Local: nodular tenosynovitis	
Diffuse: extra-articular "PVNS"	50% relapse after surgery
Malignant	
Very rare!	

2 Bone: Benign Tumours

2.1 Fibrous Cortical Defect (FCD) and Non-ossifying Fibroma (NOF)

FCD are small lesions, primarily located in the cortex of the bone (Figs. 1 and 2). They are usually asymptomatic. NOF are larger, located eccentrically and protruding in the medullary cavity of the bone and often symptomatic (Fig. 3). They are both usually found in patients with an immature skeleton (Fig. 1), eccentrically located (in contrast with a central bone cyst), oriented according to the bone axis and do not contain internal calcifications (different from an enchondroma) (Figs. 1, 2, and 3). MRI shows a lesion with iso-signal intensity to muscle on T1-WI and high signal intensity on T2-WI. On both sequences, marginal sclerosis may result in a low signal intensity rim. MRI also shows eventual extension of the lesion in the soft tissues (Fig. 2c–e).

2.2 Fibrous Dysplasia (FD)

This benign developmental fibro-osseous process in the bone medulla (Fig. 4) is a lucent expansile mono- or polyostotic bone lesion affecting all ages. The borders are well-defined with a maintained external cortical contour, but endosteal scalloping and cortical thinning may be present. The lucent lesion has a typical ground glass appearance. The cystic lucent aspect may be mixed with

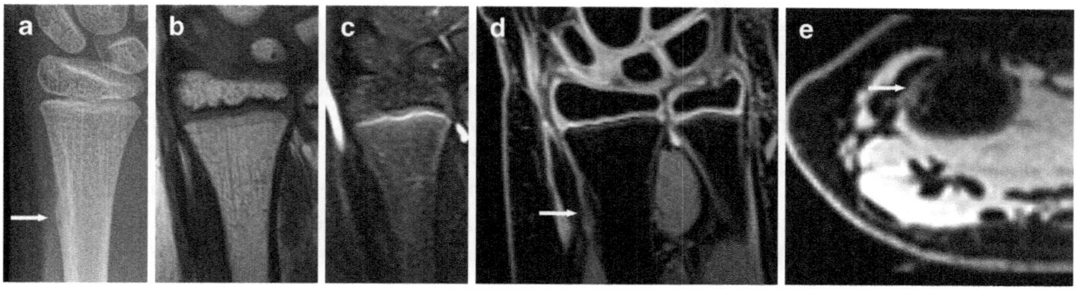

Fig. 1 Standard PA (**a**) view; Cor T1-WI (**b**), T2-WI FS (**c**); and 3D GRE (**d**); Ax 3D GRE (**e**). Immature skeleton with small FCD (**a**) hardly visible on fine MR images (**d, e**)

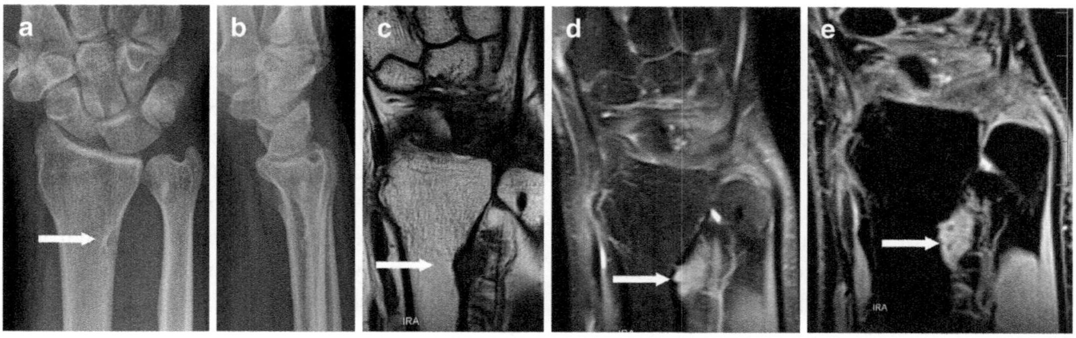

Fig. 2 Standard PA (**a**) and Lateral (**b**) views; Cor T1-WI (**c**), T2-WI FS (**d**); and 3D GRE (**e**). FCD in an adult centred on the cortex of the radius extending in the medullary cavity and the soft tissues

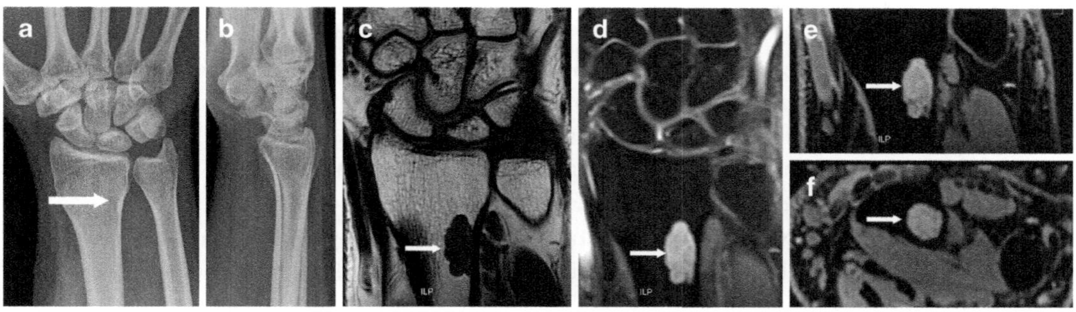

Fig. 3 Standard PA (**a**) and Lateral (**b**) views; Cor T1-WI (**c**), T2-WI FS (**d**); and 3D GRE (**e**); Ax 3D GRE (**f**). Larger NOF located eccentrically and protruding in the medullary cavity

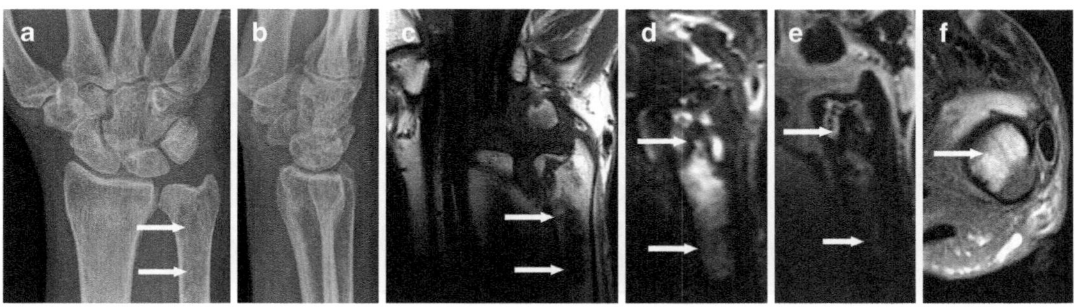

Fig. 4 Standard PA (**a**) and Lateral (**b**) views; Cor T1-WI (**c**), T2-WI FS (**d**); and 3D GRE (**e**); Ax T2-WI FS (**f**). Medullar heterogenous lucent fibrous dysplasia of the ulna with ground glass aspect (**a, b**) and variable signal intensity (**c–f**)

sclerotic zones of variable extent, resulting in an intermediate to low heterogenous signal on T1-WI and a variable signal on T2-WI. CE usually is moderate to intense. Thick reactive sclerotic bone surrounding the lesion (rind sign) may be present.

2.3 Bone Island (BI)/Enostosis

A bone island (Fig. 5) has a pathognomonic appearance in the bone medulla as a homogeneously dense, non-enhancing small and rounded lesion with low signal on all sequences.

2.4 Enchondroma

An enchondroma is the most frequent primary bone tumour of the hand. Fifty percent of all enchondromas are located in the hand and 90% of all hand tumours are diagnosed as enchondromas. This benign intramedullary tumour (Fig. 6) most often occurs in young patients within the proximity of the region of the (earlier) epiphysial plate. Although benign, evolution to a malignant chondroma is possible.

Radiologically, it is a lesion very similar to a low-grade chondrosarcoma. Fortunately, chondrosarcomata are extremely rare in the wrist. Arguments in favour of an enchondroma are an intact cortex, endosteal scalloping involving less than two-thirds of the cortex, absence of a soft tissue mass and a size of less than 5 cm. Pain may be due to a pathological fracture, which is often the first clinical sign and should warrant the clinician of a potential enchondroma. An enchondroma (Figs. 6 and 7) is a radiolucent, sharply defined (complex) lobulated (Fig. 6d, g) central medullary lesion with peripheral satellite foci (Fig. 6c). It shows an internal heterogeneous signal, intermediate to low on T1-WI (Figs. 6b and 7b) with internal foci of low signal (chondroid matrix) and is mainly hyperintense on T2-WI (Figs. 6c and 7c) without oedema of the bone marrow, nor of the surrounding soft tissues. CE is noted at the scalloped margins (Fig. 6e) and with intralesional curvilinear T1-hyperintensities (rings and arcs enhancement). Small lesions are difficult to differentiate, and the internal calcifications play a key role (Fig. 7a) in the diagnosis. The proximal phalanx of the fifth radius is most affected, followed by the MC joint and second phalanx.

Multiple enchondromas are found in Ollier's disease and in Maffucci's syndrome. Ollier's disease is characterised by multiple enchondromas within the body, often leading to skeletal deformities, limb discrepancy, and fractures. There is a 25% risk of malignant development. Maffucci's syndrome primarily affects the bones and skin and is characterised by multiple enchondromas, bone deformities, and soft tissue haemangiomas. The risk of malignant transformation to a chondrosarcoma is close to a 100%.

2.5 Haemangioma

This slow-growing asymptomatic vascular tumour located in the medullary cavity of the bone (Figs. 8, 9, and 10) may show the typical prominent trabeculation (Figs. 8a and 10c). Depending on their increasing lipid content, the signal on T1-WI is

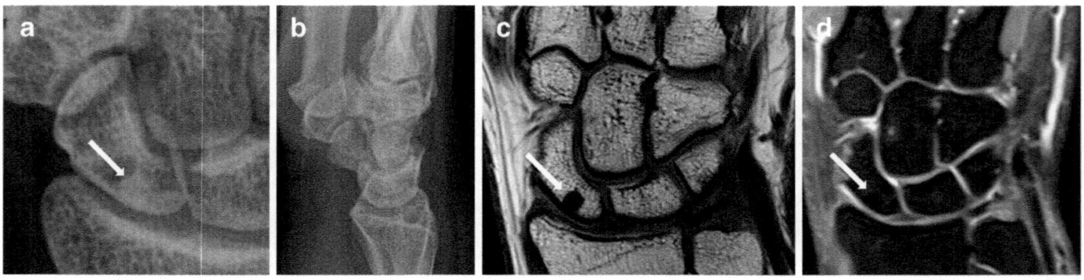

Fig. 5 Standard PA (**a**) and Lateral (**b**) views; Cor T1-WI (**c**) and T2-WI FS (**d**). Homogeneously dense, rounded BI (**a**, **b**) with low signal on all sequences (**c**, **d**)

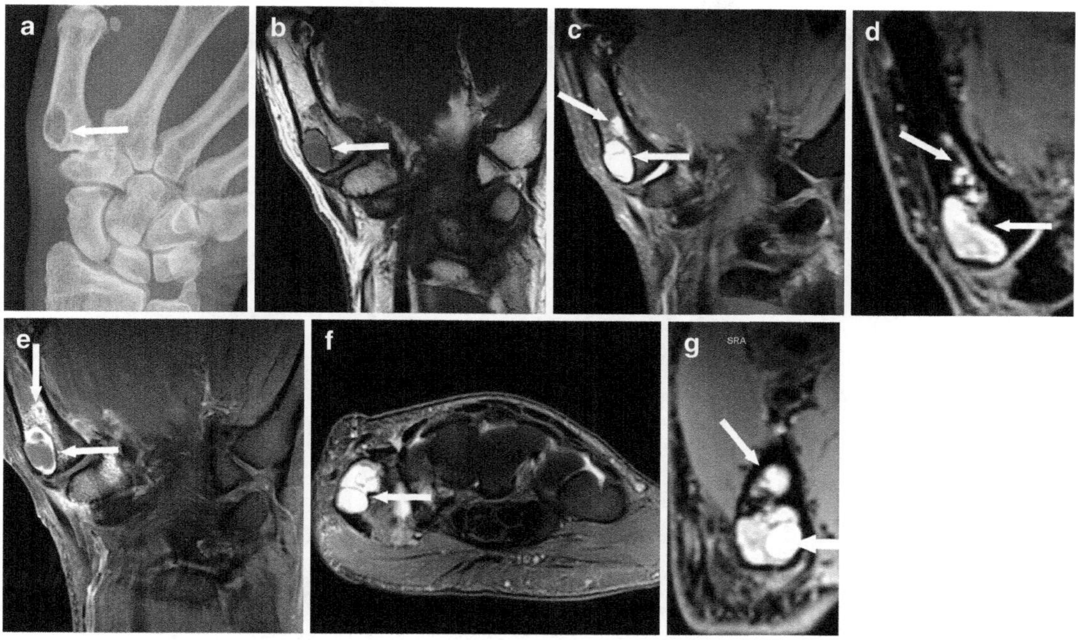

Fig. 6 Standard PA (**a**) view; Cor T1-WI (**b**); PD WI (**c**) and T2-WI FS (**d**); T1-WI FS with CE (**e**); Ax T2-WI FS (**f**); Sag 3D GRE (**g**). Radiolucency at the base of the thumb (**a**), sharply defined (complex) lobulated (**b–g**) with intermediate signal on T1-WI (**b**) and hyperintense on T2-WI (**c**). CE at the scalloped margins (**e**)

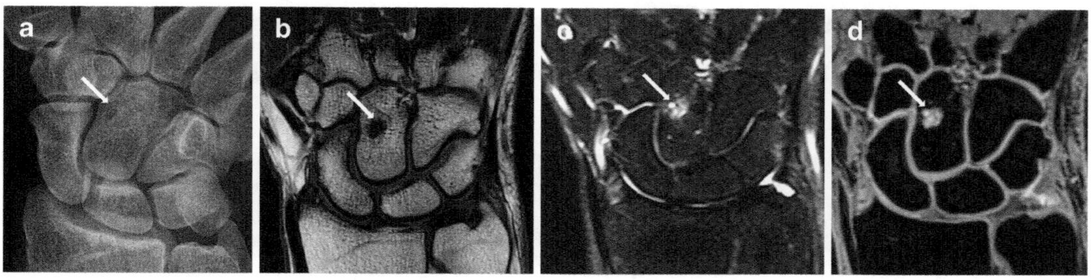

Fig. 7 Standard PA (**a**) view; Cor T1-WI (**b**); T2-WI FS (**c**); Cor 3D GRE (**d**). Small enchondroma of the C

from low (Figs. 8c and 10d) to intermediate (Fig. 9b) to high and on T2-WI the signal is high (Figs. 8d, 9c, and 10e). They are slightly irregularly delineated (Figs. 8e, f and 9d) (unlike a bone cyst), show no connection with the joint space(s) (Fig. 10f, g) (unlike an intraosseous ganglion), contain no calcifications (unlike an enchondroma) and scalloping is absent (unlike an enchondroma).

2.6 Bone Cyst (BC)

These relatively infrequent (Fig. 11) fluid-filled tumour develops in growing bones. They may disappear without leading to any symptoms. However, weakened bone due to a larger BC is more sensitive to a pathological fracture. This fracture may be indirectly noticed due to a so called “fallen bone fragment” or a “rising gas bubble”. A unicameral BC shows a sclerotic margin (Figs. 11 and 12a, b). The contour is sharply defined (Fig. 11c), the internal signal is determined by the fluid content: low on T1-WI (Figs. 12d and 13c, f), high on T2-WI (Figs. 12e and 13d, g) and GRE (Fig. 12f) and peripheral CE may be present (Fig. 13e, h). Rarely, they present as a multiloculated lesion (Fig. 14), but meticulous MRI analysis may reveal an even rare coincidence of two lesions. A BV

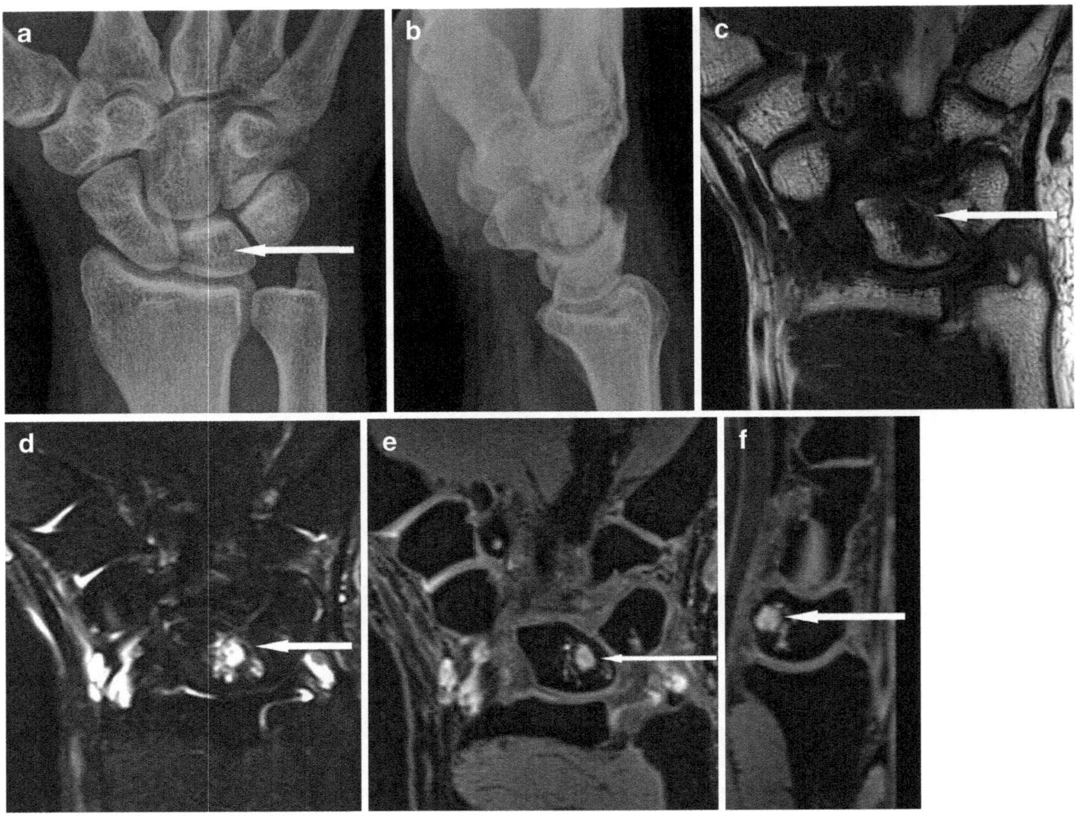

Fig. 8 Standard PA (**a**) and Lateral (**b**) view; Cor T1-WI (**c**); T2-WI FS (**d**); Cor (**e**) and Sag (**f**) 3D GRE. Hemangioma of the L

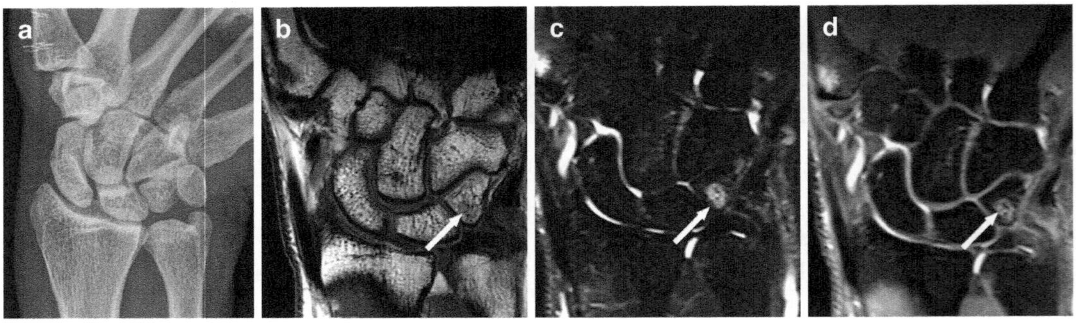

Fig. 9 Standard PA (**a**) view; Cor T1-WI (**b**); T2-WI FS (**c**); Cor (**d**) 3D GRE. Hemangioma of the Tri not visible on the standard view

does not give metastatic lesions but may be locally aggressive with extension into the surrounding soft tissue (visualised by perilesional oedema). Degenerative cysts have similar aspects, but the adjacent joint is obviously deformed by osteoarthrosis (Fig. 15).

2.7 Intraosseous Ganglion Cyst (IOG)

The small cystic uni- or multilocular IOG (Figs. 16 and 17) is situated adjacent to the joint, but without adjacent degenerative or inflammatory lesions. It

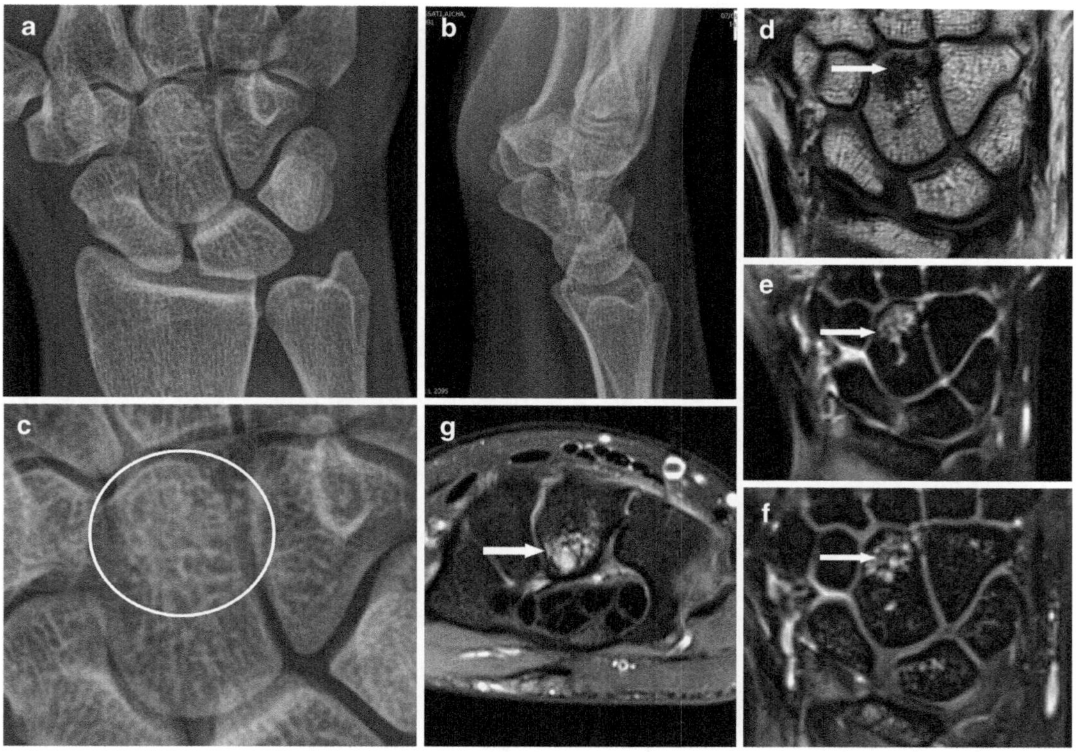

Fig. 10 Standard PA (**a**), lateral (**b**), and detail (**c**) views; Cor T1-WI (**d**), T2-WI (**e**), and 3D GRE (**f**). Ax T1-WI FS with CE (**g**). Coarse trabecular pattern (**c**). T1-WI low (**d**) and T2-WI high signal (**e**). Coarse trabeculation (**f**) and without connection with the adjacent joint spaces (**f**, **g**)

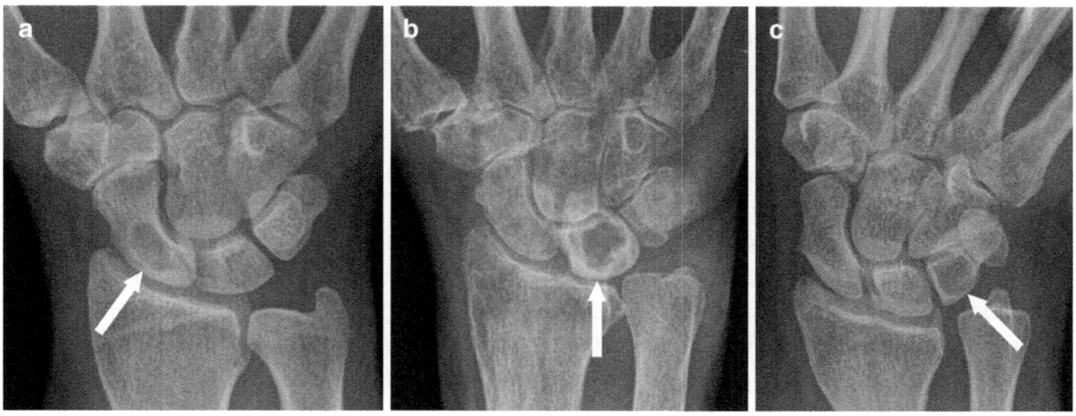

Fig. 11 Standard PA views. Bone cyst of the S (**a**), L (**b**), and Tri (**c**) with fine sclerotic margin (**a**, **c**). Denser and irregular aspect of the border of the BC due to a previous fracture (**b**)

is a well-defined cystic lesion with a blunt cortical defect and a sclerotic rim. Solitary or multiple lesions (Fig. 17) may appear as isointense on T1-WI and with high signal on T2-WI. The CE is rather heterogenous or as a peripheral rim. These "small" lesions may grow (Fig. 18) and become significantly larger (Fig. 18e, f) and eventually result in a pathologic fracture.

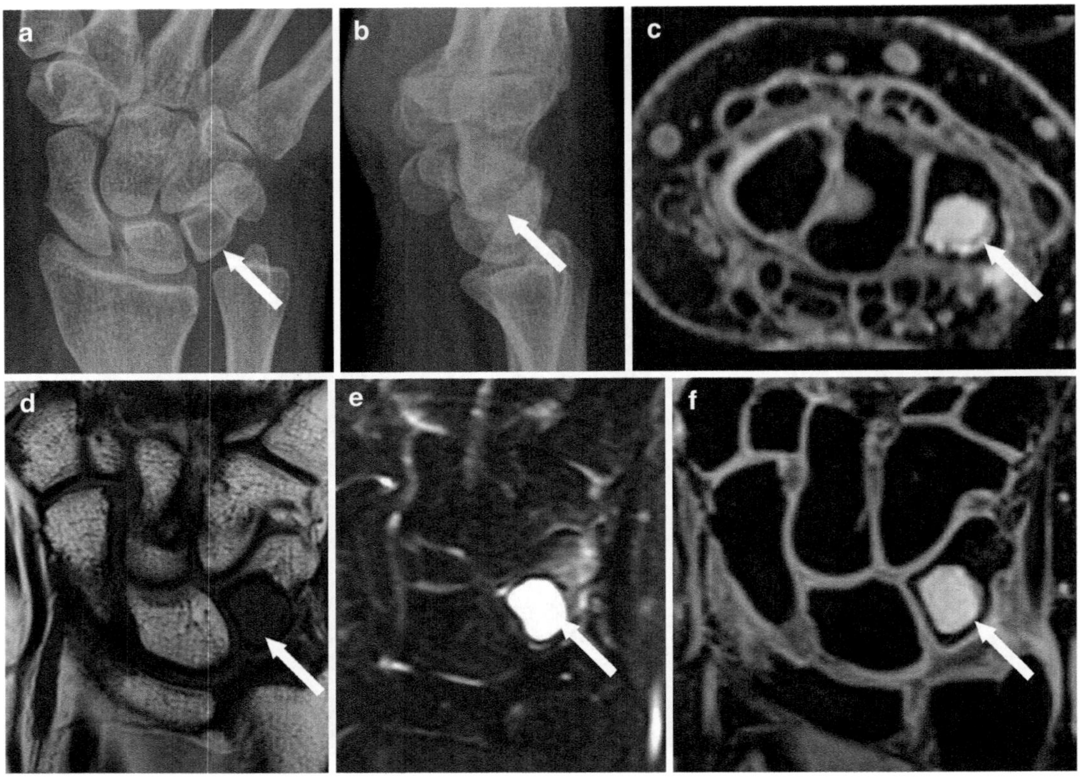

Fig. 12 Standard PA (**a**) and lateral (**b**) views; Ax 3D GRE (**c**); Cor T1-WI (**d**), T2-WI FS (**e**), and 3D GRE (**f**). Bone cyst of the Tri

2.8 Osteochondroma ("Osseocartilaginous Exostosis")

This benign, exophytic, osseous tumour (Chew and Weissleder 1991; Murphey et al. 2000) (Fig. 19) develops away from the bone during the skeletal growth period, mostly as a solitary lesion, unless in a multiple hereditary form (El-Sobky et al. 2018; Simmons et al. 1999; Vanhoenacker et al. 2001; Wuyts et al. 2002; Wuyts and Van Hul 2000). In adults they remain stable. On imaging, the cortex remains intact, with only a periosteal defect where the tumour develops. In the hand, the phalanx is mostly affected, where it is often associated with a tendon rupture, as it usually grows close to a tendon insertion. Paraosteal osteochondromatous proliferation is called Nora-lesion (Dhondt et al. 2006; Nora et al. 1983; Yuen et al. 1992). Malignant transformation of the covering cartilage cap into a chondrosarcoma is rare (Fei et al. 2018). Spontaneous resolution has been described (Claikens et al. 1998; Deprez et al. 2011).

2.9 Giant Cell Tumour (GCT)

GCT (Figs. 20 and 21) are "benign" bone tumours but with potentially an aggressive behaviour. They also have a high recurrence rate and exceptionally a capacity of metastasising (to the lungs). A CT is therefore mandatory in every case of GCT. The lytic lesion (Fig. 20a, b) is located around the earlier closed growth plate with trabecular and cortical destruction and breakthrough (Fig. 20c–e, f–h). It is located eccentrically and extends to the subchondral bone as a well-defined lesion but without surrounding sclerosis. Eventually, an aggressive periosteal reaction (Fig. 20h) and BMO (Fig. 20g, i) may develop. The tumour may

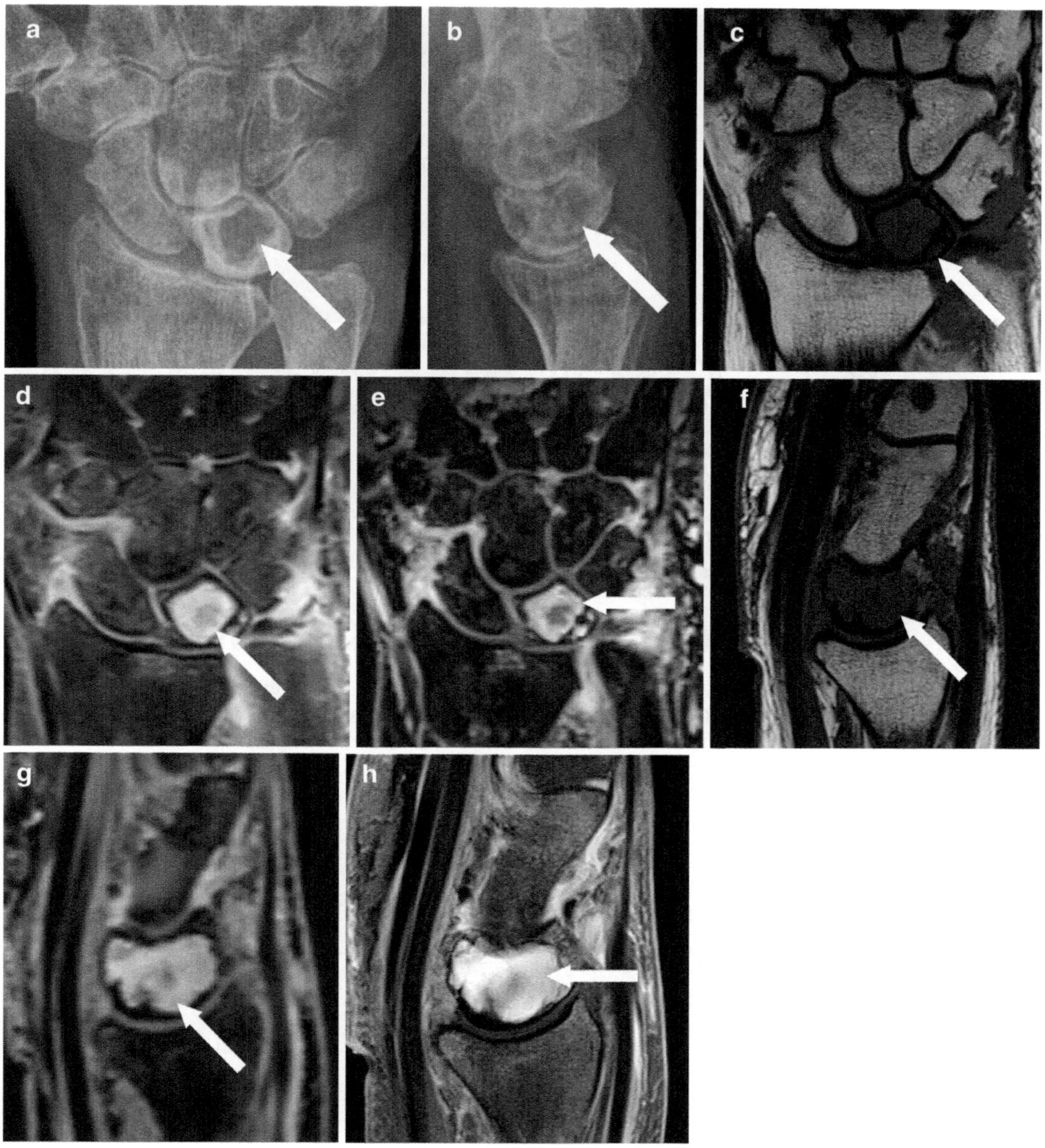

Fig. 13 Standard PA (**a**) and lateral (**b**) views; Cor T1-WI (**c**), T2-WI FS (**d**), and T1-WI FS wit CE (**e**); Sag T1-WI (**f**), T2-WI FS (**g**), and T1-WI FS wit CE (**h**). Bone cyst of the L with low signal on T1-WI (**c**, **f**), high on T2-WI (**d**, **g**), and peripheral CE (**e**, **h**)

extend in the soft tissues (Fig. 20f, j). Relapse (Fig. 21) is frequent (up to 50%), mainly determined by the original soft tissue extension (Fig. 20f, j). The Campanelli classification is based on the aspect of the lesion border and soft tissue expansion: type 1 involves a well-defined lesion with an intact, but thin cortex. Type 2 shows expansion of the thin cortex. Type 3 typically shows irregular borders and expansion into the soft tissues.

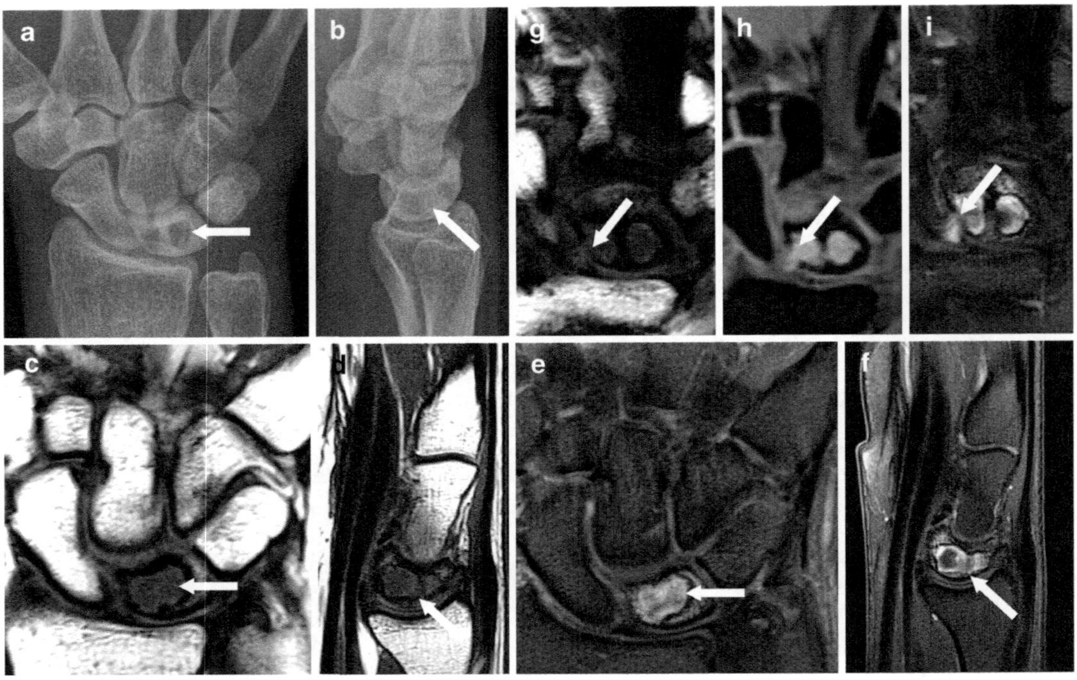

Fig. 14 Standard PA (**a**) and lateral (**b**) views; Cor (**c**) and Sag (**d**) T1-WI with CE (**e**, **f**); Cor T1-WI (**g**), 3D GRE (**h**), and T1-WI FS with CE (**i**). Bilocular "bone cyst" of the L (**a**, **b**) with low signal on T1-WI (**c**, **d**) and peripheral CE (**e**–**h**). However, broad cortical breach (**g**–**i**) with CE till in the SL ligament, which favours an intraosseous ganglion extending from a SLL lesion next to a BC

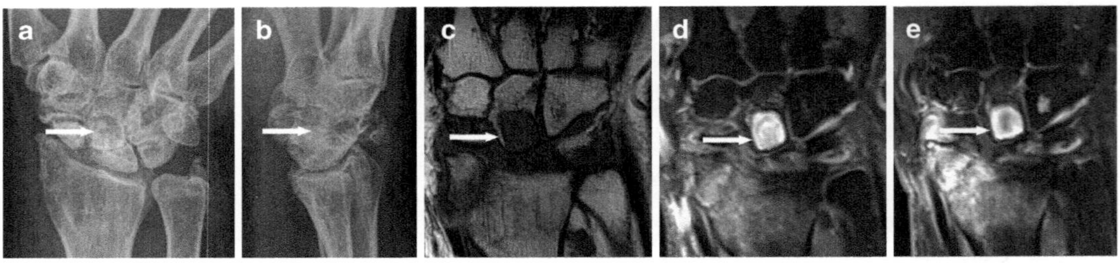

Fig. 15 Standard PA (**a**) and lateral (**b**) views; Cor T1-WI (**c**), T2-WI (**d**), and T1-WI FS with CE (**e**). Degenerative cyst in the C with extensive adjacent MC degeneration

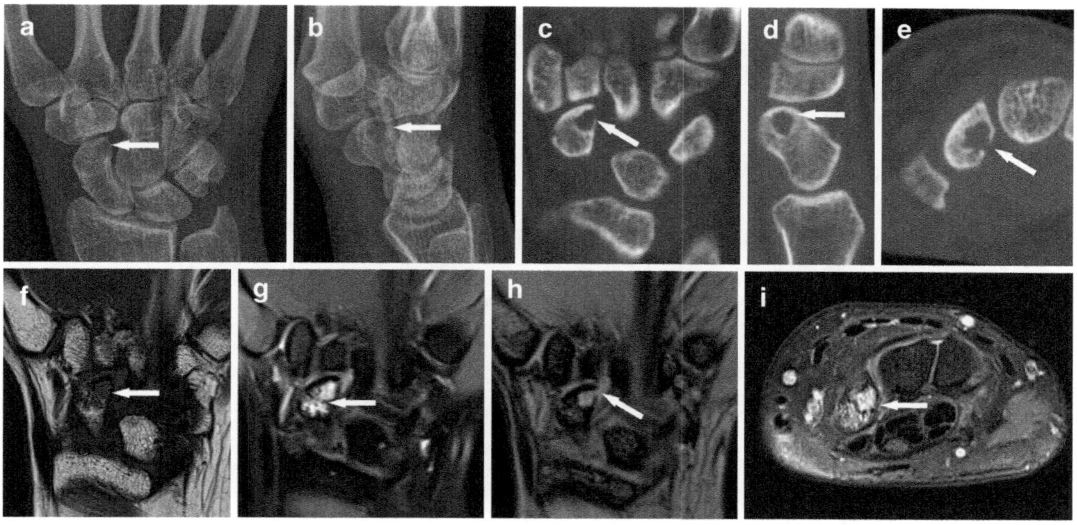

Fig. 16 Standard PA (**a**) and lateral (**b**) views; Cor (**c**), Sag (**d**), and Ax (**e**) CT images; Cor T1-WI FC), T2-WI (**g**), and 3D GRE (**h**); Ax T1-WI FS with CE. IOG of the S with a sclerotic margin (**a**, **b**). The typical cortical breach with blunt margins is best visualised by 3D-CT reconstructions (**c**–**e**). Low signal on T1-WI (**f**), high on T2-WI (**g**) with the small cortical breach on GRE (**h**). Heterogenous CE (**i**)

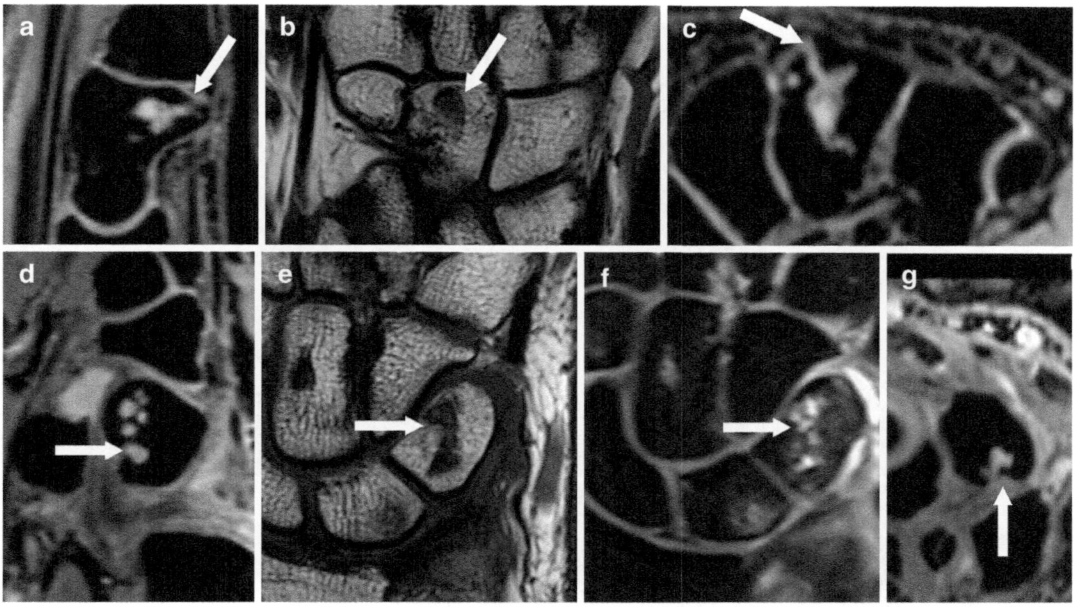

Fig. 17 Sag 3D GRE (**a**, **d**); Cor T1-WI (**b**, **e**); Cor T2-WI (**f**); Ax 3D GRE (**c**, **g**). Bifocal IOG o the C (**a**–**c**) and Tri (**d**–**g**) with a typical cortical breach to the adjacent joint

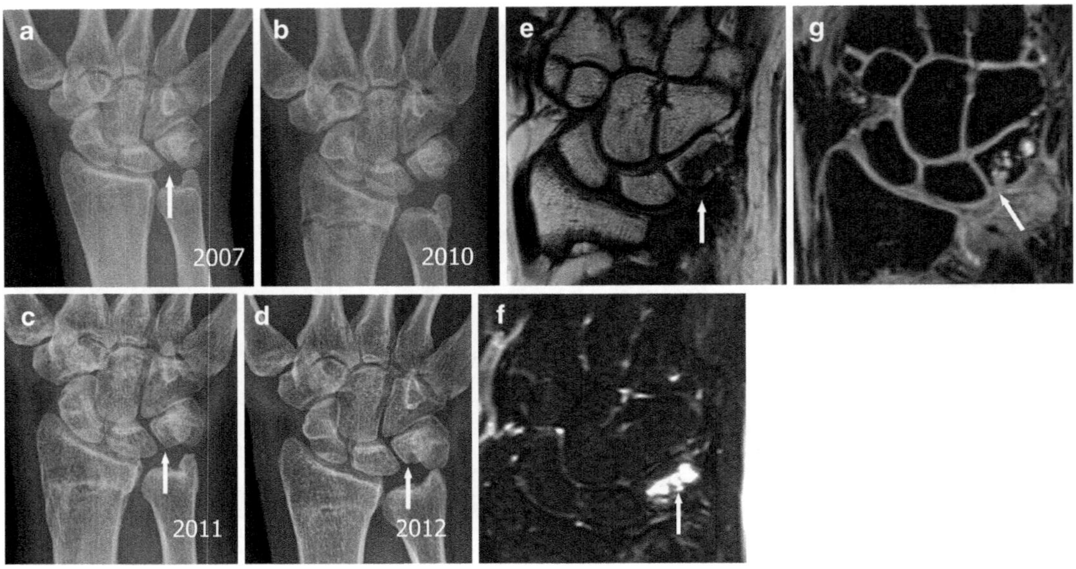

Fig. 18 Standard PA views (**a–d**); Cor T1-WI (**e**), T2-WI (**f**), and 3D GRE (**g**). No abnormality observed (**a**). Trauma (**b**) and follow-up (**c**, **d**) with appearance of a small lucent (**c**) growing (**d**) "small" lesion. Much larger lesion (IOG) shown at that moment by MRI (**e–g**)

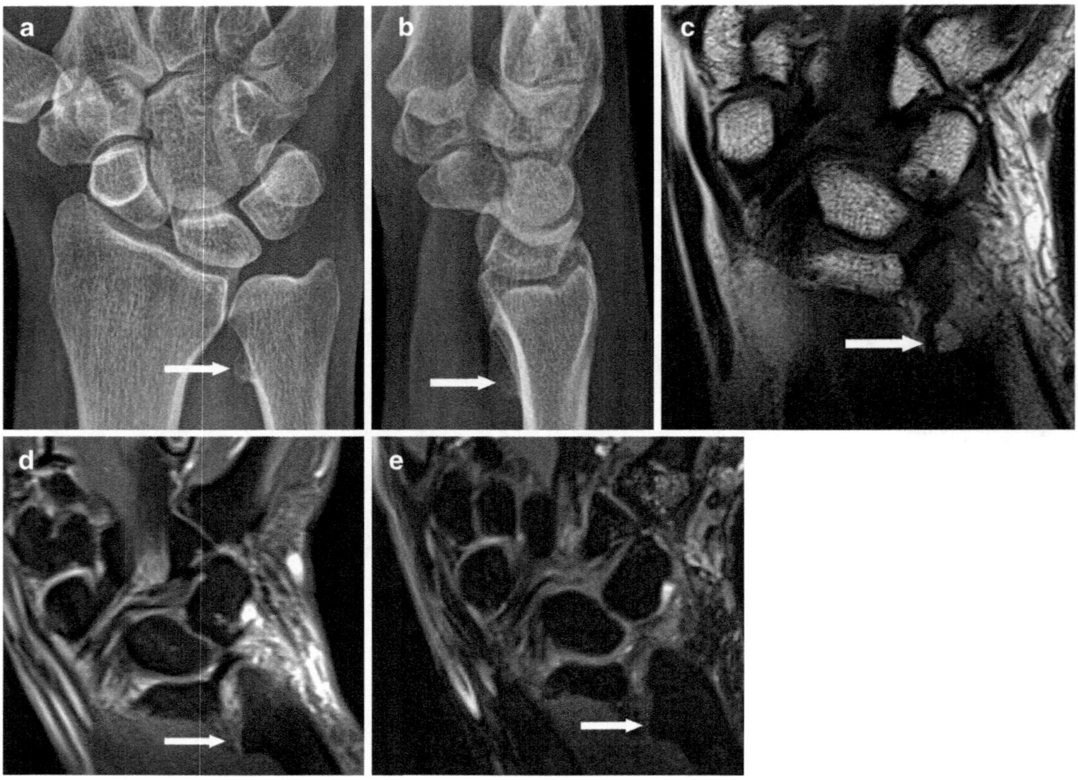

Fig. 19 Standard PA (**a**) and lateral (**b**) views; Cor T1-WI (**c**), T2-WI (**d**), and 3D GRE (**e**). A small sessile osteochondroma (adult form) in the metaphyseal region in continuity with the cortex and medulla of the U. The cartilage cap has disappeared

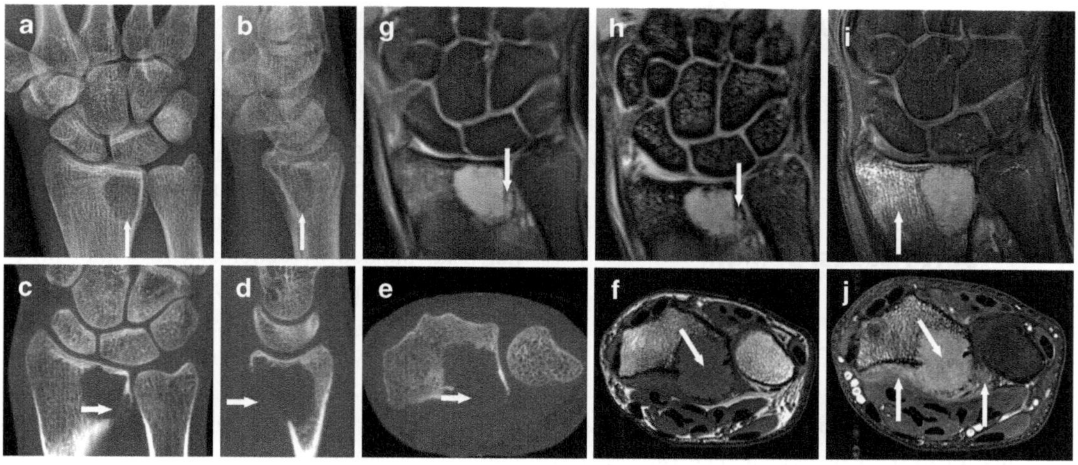

Fig. 20 Standard PA (**a**) and lateral (**b**) views; Cor (**c**), Sag (**d**), and Ax (**e**) CT images; Ax T1-WI (**f**) with FS and CE (**f**); Cor T2-WI (**g**), 3D GRE (**h**), and T1-WI FS with CE (**i**). Lytic GCT lesion around the earlier location of the growth plate of the R with trabecular and cortical destruction (**a**, **b**) and breakthrough (**c–e**). Intermediate signal on T1-WI (**f**) and high signal with zones of low signal (hemosiderin/fibrosis) and periosteal reaction (**g**, **h**). CE of the surrounding bone marrow (**j**), the lesion (**j**), and the extension to the soft tissues (**j**)

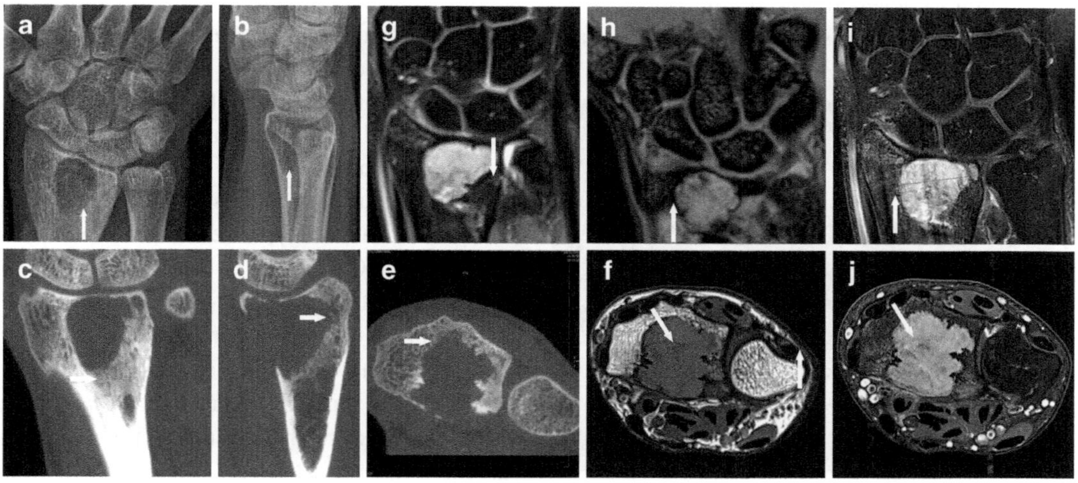

Fig. 21 Standard PA (**a**) and lateral (**b**) views; Cor (**c**), Sag (**d**), and Ax (**e**) CT images; Ax T1-WI (**f**) with FS and CE (**j**); Cor T2-WI (**g**), 3D GRE (**h**), and T1-WI FS with CE (**i**). GCT relapse 4 years after curettage. Larger and more radially located lytic and CE lesion with a residue of a bone graft (**g**)

3 Bone: Malignant Tumours

As they barely exist as an isolated lesion in the wrist, the reader should consult specific literature if ever needed.

4 Soft Tissues: Benign Tumours

4.1 (Ganglion) Cysts (GC)

The most frequent soft tissue tumours are grouped as "ganglion cysts" (Versteeg and Goyal 2019). A herniation of synovia is called a cyst and a mucoid degeneration a ganglion. The MRI image is identical. They are typical lesions of the wrist (Fig. 22) in connection with the joint capsule (Vo et al. 1995; Conway et al. 1985) or tendon sheath. In addition to degeneration, trauma and surgery are causal factors. US is the first method of imaging (Fig. 23). Most develop in the soft tissues, para- or sometimes intra-articular. The lesion can surface at a (long) distance from its origin (Fig. 24). The content of the regularly delineated cyst is low on T1-WI (increasing due to eventual high protein content or haemorrhage) and high on T2-WI. If ruptured, they are irregular and initially surrounded by oedema. CE of the rim or internal septa may occur. Typical locations may indicate the origin of the GC. SL lesions are associated with a typical dorsal (Fig. 22) and radiopalmar (Figs. 25 and 26) GC, extending from the SL through the space of Poirier. However, they may appear almost everywhere around the wrist (Fig. 27). Periosteal and intraosseous extension (Fig. 28) occurs. When present at the radial side, a pseudo-aneurysm of the radial artery is part of the differential diagnosis. When present on the ulnar side, compression of the ulnar nerve must be ruled out. An "occult cyst" is a millimetric cyst, difficult to visualise due to its small size, but clinically suspected in case of a painful dorsal lunate bone on palpation. If multiple GC are present, underlying inflammatory disease should be suspected and excluded or confirmed (Fig. 29). Atypical peri-ulnar locations of a GC may point to specific aetiology: meniscus homologue (Fig. 30), TFCC (Fig. 31) or ecu sheath (Figs. 32 and 33). Sometimes, an intra-osseous cyst can be located, often leading to chronic pain. A CT or scintigraphy may then be necessary for an accurate diagnosis. Surgical treatment may vary from needle aspiration with steroid injection to surgical excision. Unfortunately, recurrence is frequent and may be as high as 40% in case of a dorsal cyst.

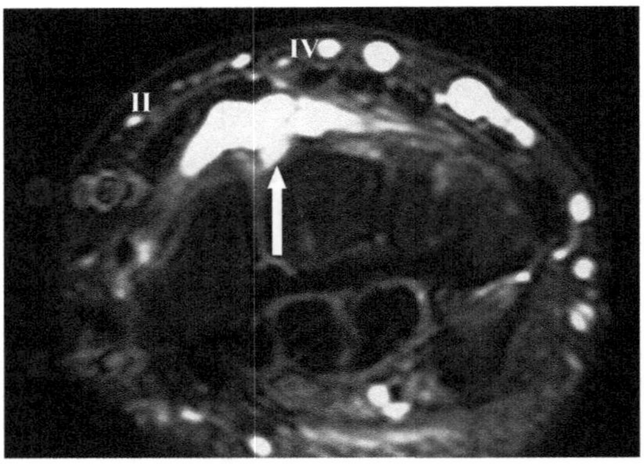

Fig. 22 Ax T2-WI FS. The classical high signal of a dorsal GC from the SL between the extensor tendons of compartment II and IV

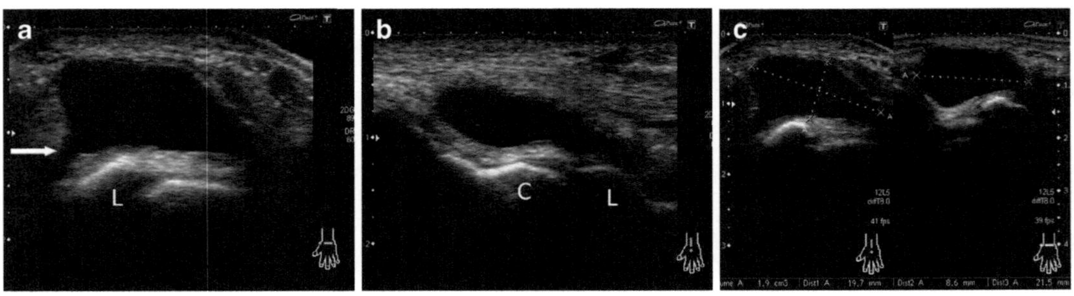

Fig. 23 Transverse and longitudinal US. The typical dorsal GC with the partial visualisation of the stalk

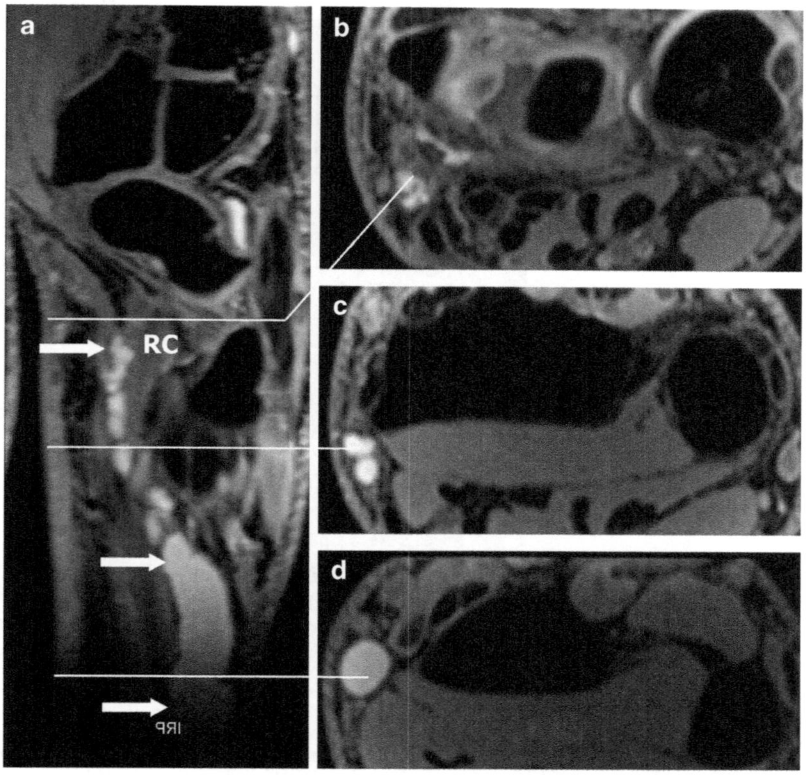

Fig. 24 Sag (**a**) and Ax (**b–d**) 3D GRE. GC surfacing at distance from the wrist with clear visualisation of the origin and the entire trajectory of the stalk

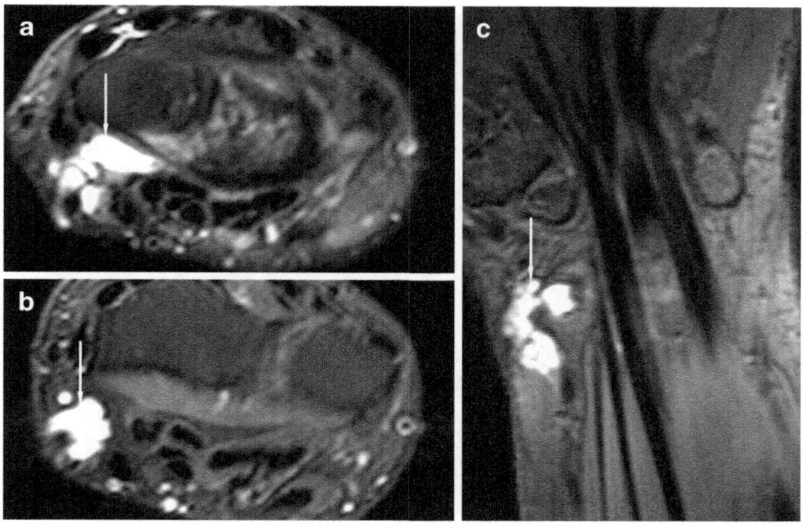

Fig. 25 Ax (**a**, **b**) and Cor (**c**) T2-WI FS. GC radiopalmar between the extensor compartment I and the flexor tendons

4.2 (Fibro)lipoma

The most common soft tissue tumour is composed of fat with or without other components influencing the high T2-WI signal (calcifications, fibrosis, necrosis, or inflammation) (Fig. 34). Symptoms may arise because of nerve compression. Macrodactyly is often present. At the location of the median nerve, the differential diagnosis with a fibro lipomatous hamartoma of the nerve is very important. The latter shows a typical fascicular pattern due to spreading of the nervous fibres. Malignant

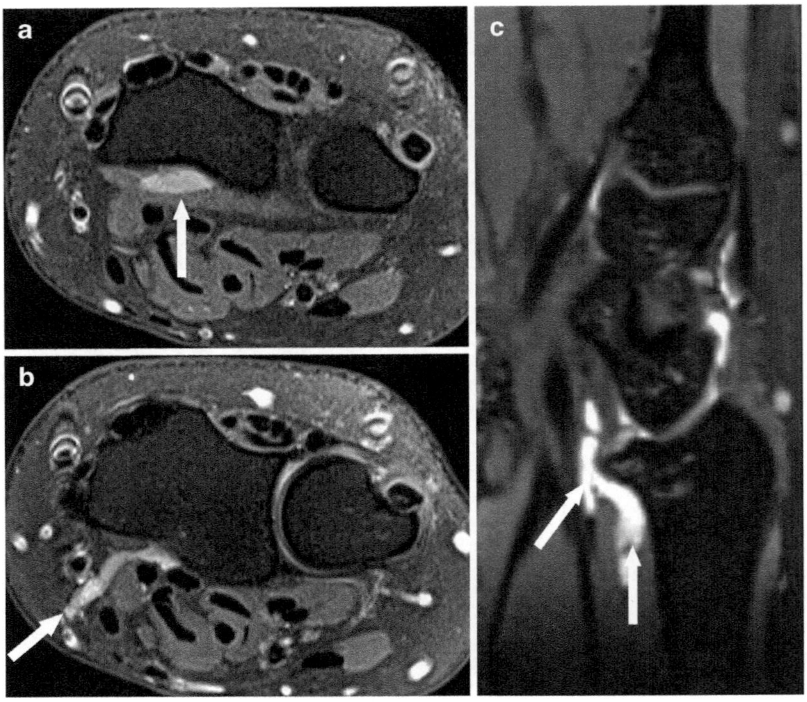

Fig. 26 Ax T2-WI FS. Radiopalmar GC between the fpl and fcr just distal from the PQ with a deep (**a**, **c**) and superficial (**b**, **c**) component

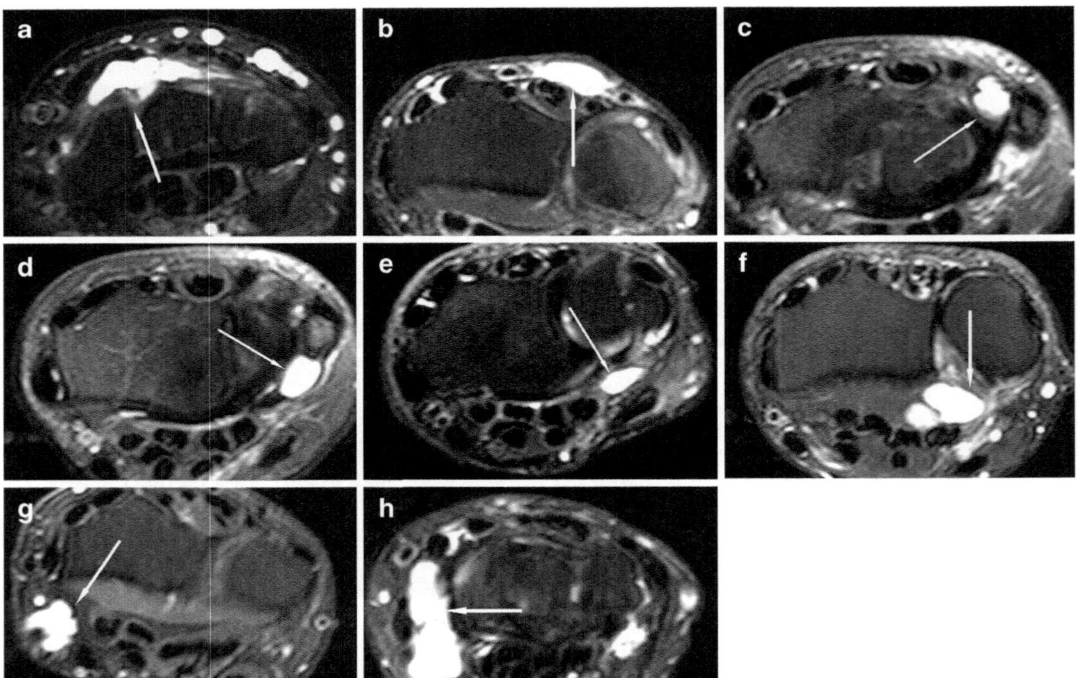

Fig. 27 Ax T2-WI FS. GC appear everywhere around the wrist: dorsal (**a**, **b**), periulnar dorsal (**c**) and ventral (**d**); ulnopalmar (**e**, **f**); radiopalmar (**g**); radial (**h**)

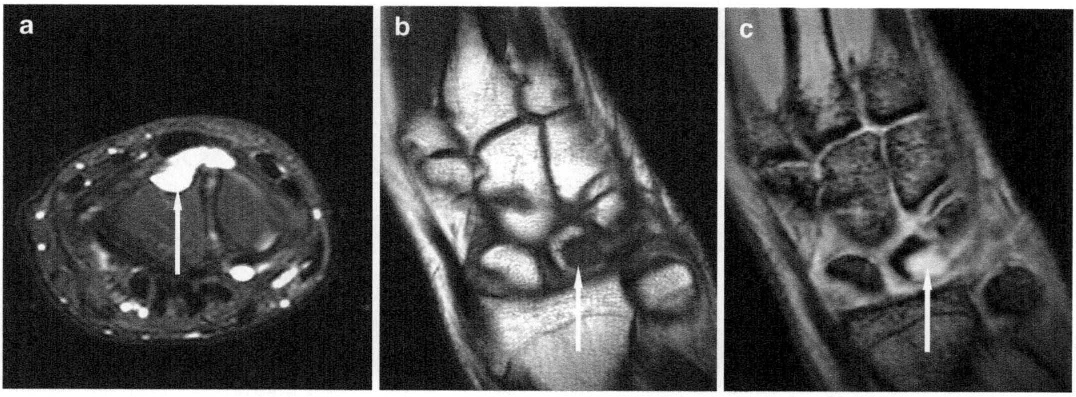

Fig. 28 Ax T2-WI FS (**a**); Cor T1-WI (**b**); Cor 2D GRE (**c**). GC with extension in the L

Fig. 29 Ax T2-WI FS (**a**–**c**); Standard PA view (**d**). Multiple GC (**a**–**c**) and RA erosions at the distal U and R

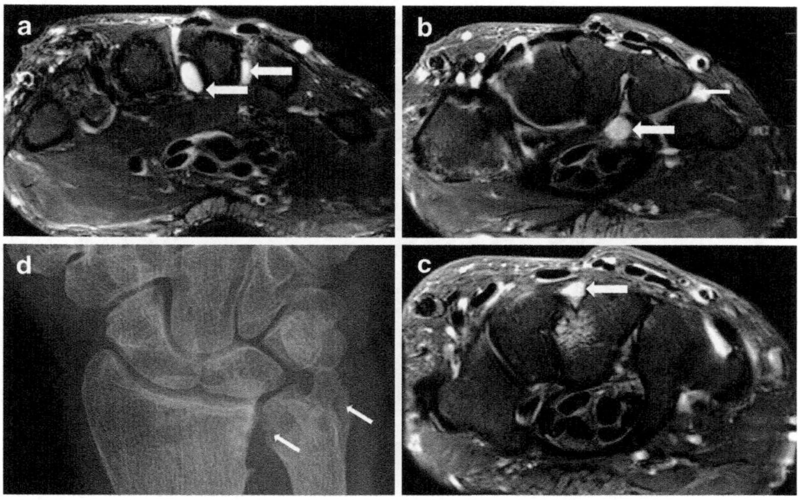

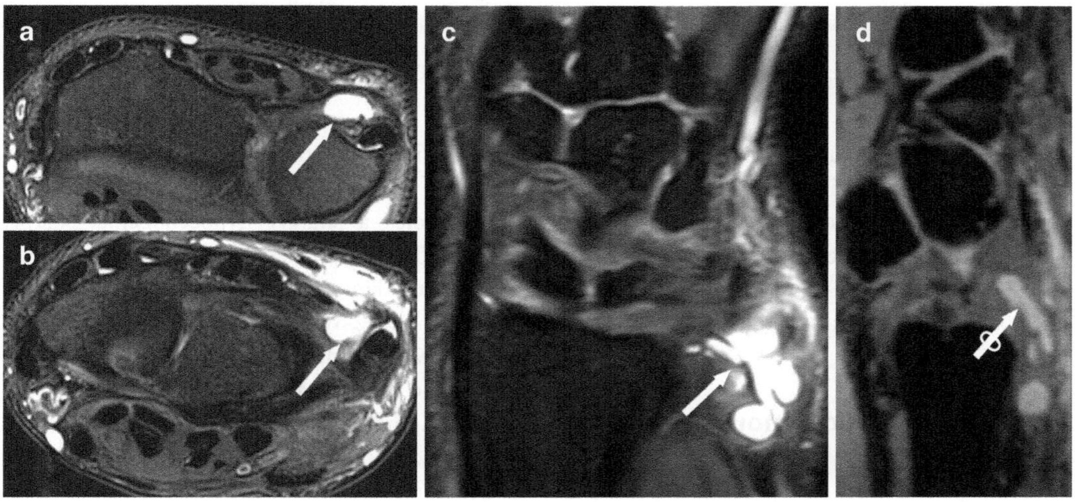

Fig. 30 Ax T2-WI FS (**a**, **b**); Cor (**c**) and Sag (**d**) 3D GRE. Dorso-ulnar GC of meniscus homologue

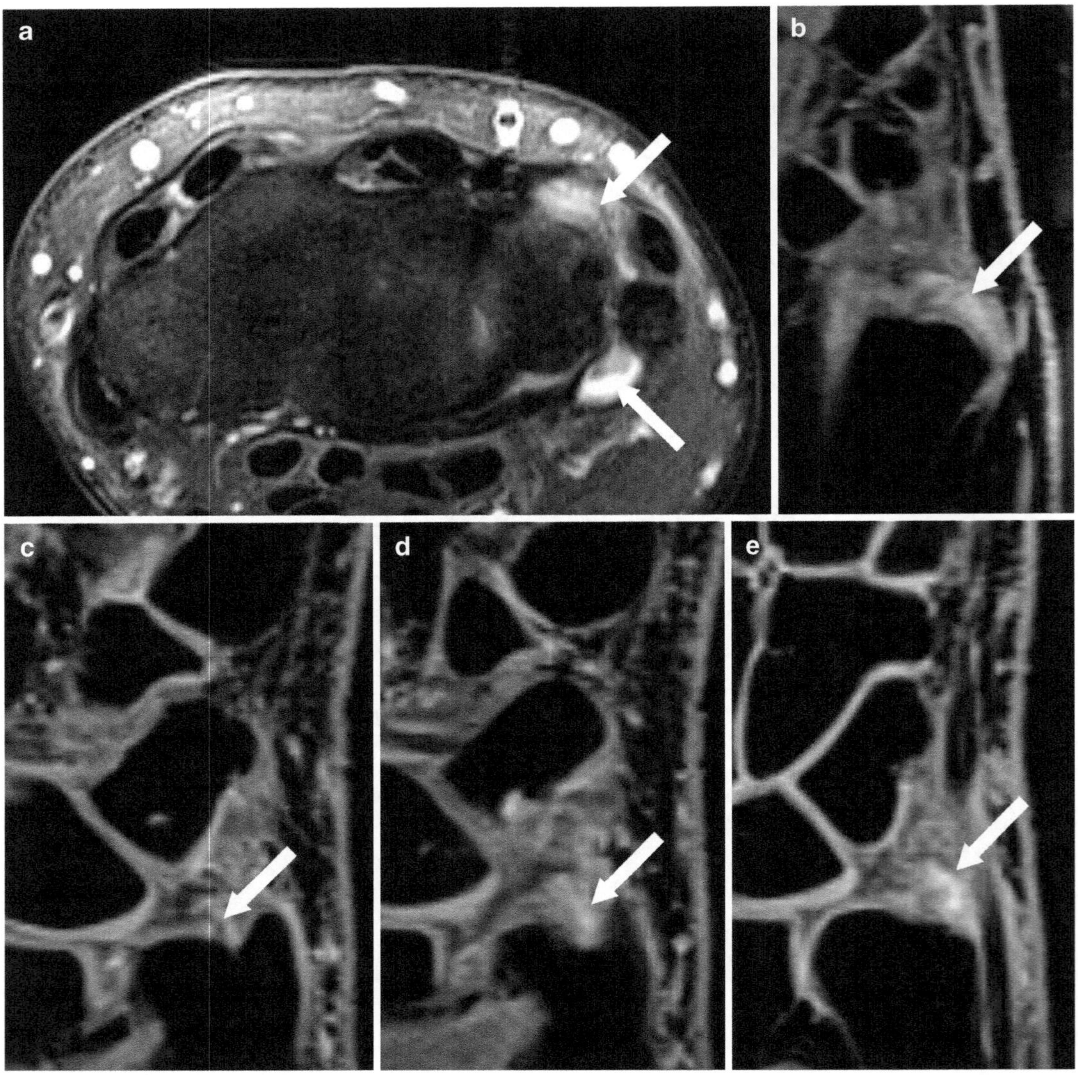

Fig. 31 Ax T2-WI FS (**a**); Sag (**b**) and Cor (**c–e**) 3D GRE. GC of TFCC

degeneration is rare (painful, rapid growth, invasion of surrounding tissue, size over 10 cm). When present in children, lipofibromatosis must be ruled out. This infiltrating, often congenital, lipoma does not have a clear capsule on imaging and is often growing around a nerve or vascular pedicle.

4.3 Neurogenic Tumour

Tumours arising from the peripheral nerves are rare. They are mostly benign and compress and/or invade the nerve and/or the surrounding soft tissues. Malignant tumours of the nerve sheaths however may cause destruction around the lesion. US demonstrates a slightly hypoechogenic, sharply delineated oval mass centred on the nerve (Fig. 35). MRI clearly demonstrates the low signal on T1-WI and high on T2-WI along the nerve trajectory. It also allows to evaluate the number of lesions, the extent, and the involvement of surrounding soft tissues (Fig. 36). Suspicious parts of tumour necrosis and adjacent soft tissue invasion are highlighted. A target sign (Fig. 37a, b) is in favour of a neurofibroma but does not exclude a schwannoma. CE is intense and rather heterogeneous (Fig. 37c, d).

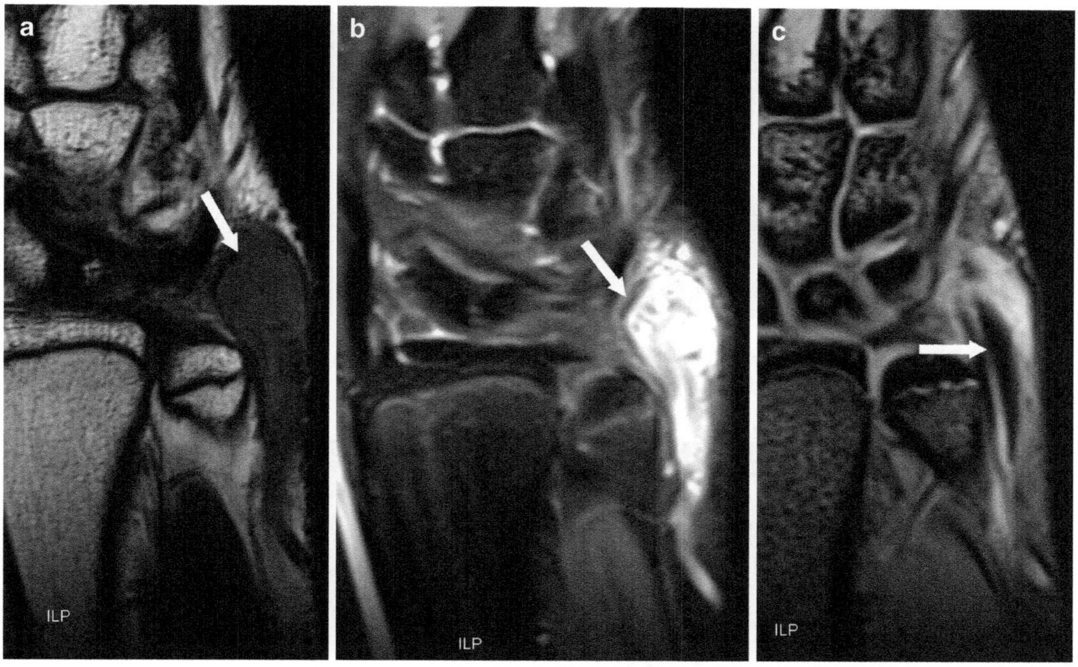

Fig. 32 Cor T1-WI (**a**); T2-WI FS (**b**); and 3D GRE (**c**). GC of ecu (compartment VI)

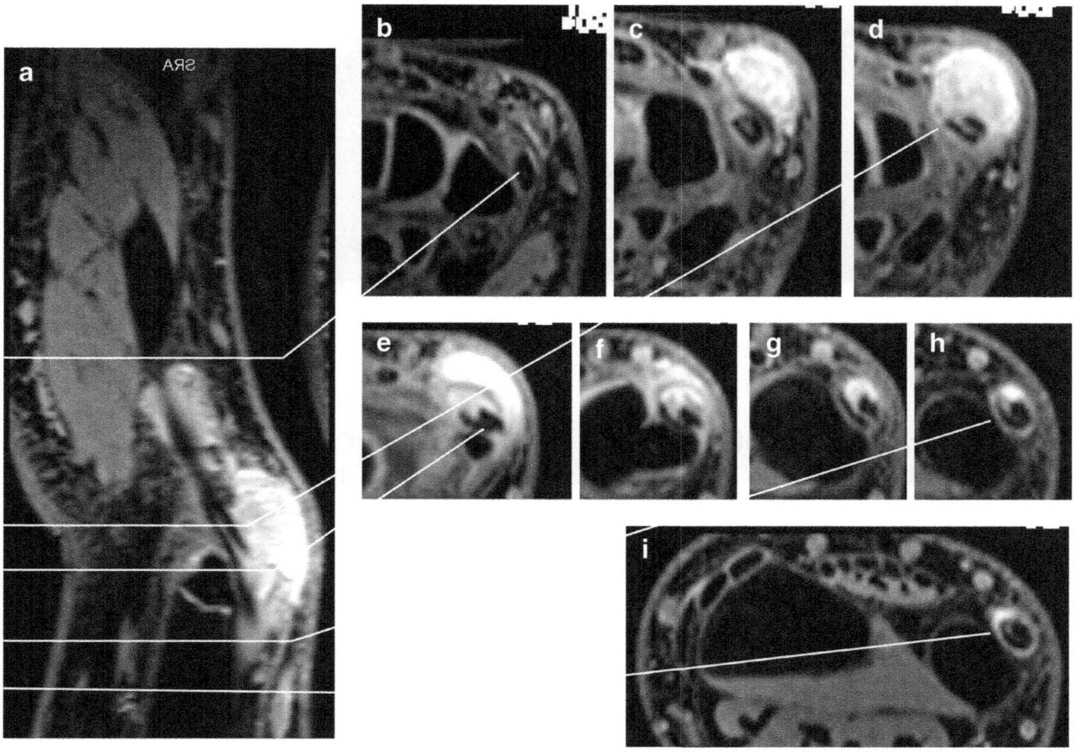

Fig. 33 Sag (**a**) and Cor (**b–i**) 3D GRE. GC of ecu (compartment VI) with extension, 3D location, and extent of the tendon fissuration

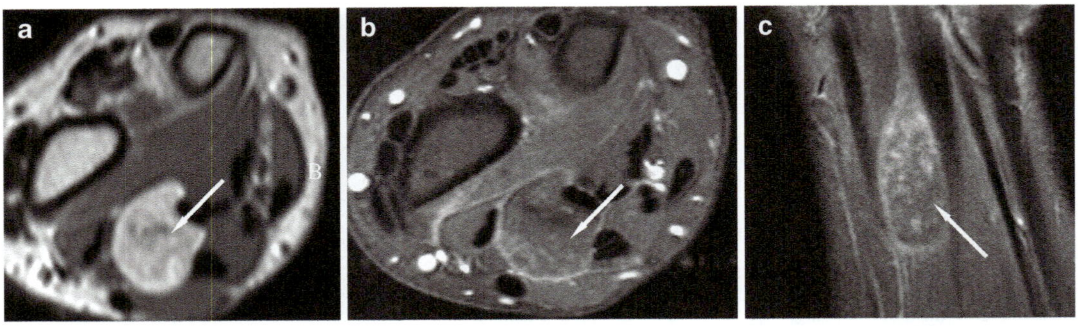

Fig. 34 T2-WI (**a**); Ax (**b**) and Cor (**c**) T1-WI with FS. Fibrolipoma at the median nerve region with slight heterogeneity of the high T2-WI signal (**a**) and fat suppression (**b**, **c**)

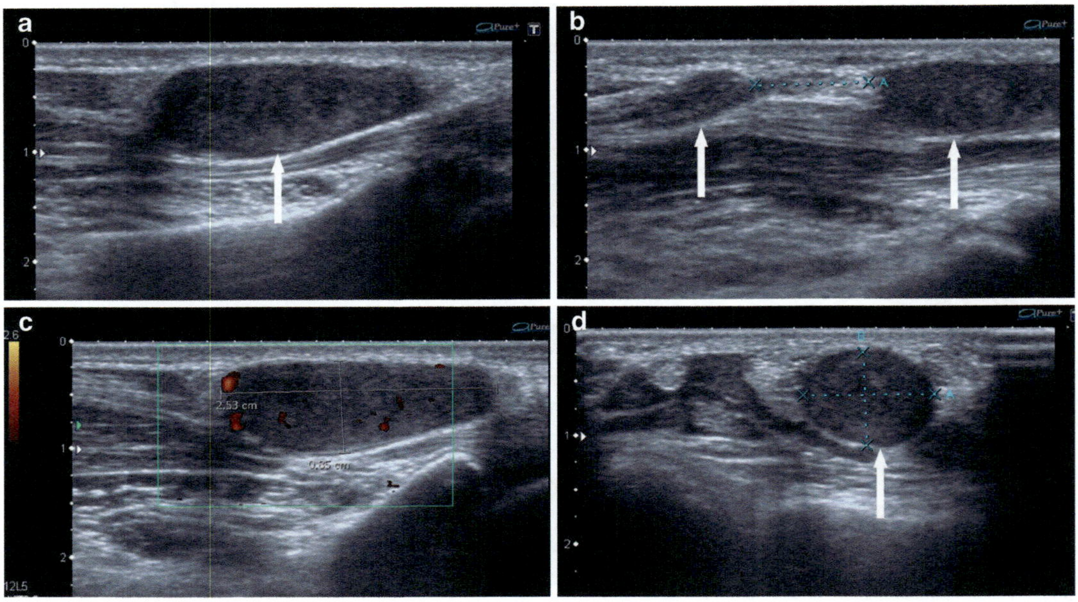

Fig. 35 US longitudinal (**a**, **b**) with colour Doppler (**c**) and transverse (**d**). Neurogenic tumour with bifocal involvement

4.4 Arteriovenous Malformation (AVM)

These congenital malformations are very uncommon. Often, they are an accidental finding (Fig. 38). They grow with age mostly in the soft tissues, seldomly in the joint or the bone. A post traumatic AVM may also arise. They are classified according to the affected part(s) (arteries, capillaries, veins, and/or lymphatics) and the vascular flow (low or high speed). They present as a well-defined lobulated mass with variable signal depending on the flow, with a signal often similar to muscle on T1-WI and high on T2-WI. The signal may be altered due to calcifications, thrombi, and high flow. CE depends on the type and the blood flow. MRI/MRA may be helpful to diagnose an AVM, determine the size and type, and in a follow-up setting.

4.5 (Primary) Synovial Osteochondromatosis

Due to a synovial metaplasia, rarely appearing in the wrist, multiple "bone" fragments (Fig. 39a) are deposited in a joint as loose cartilaginous bodies (Fig. 39). These may atrophy or enlarge depending on the synovial nourishment. They

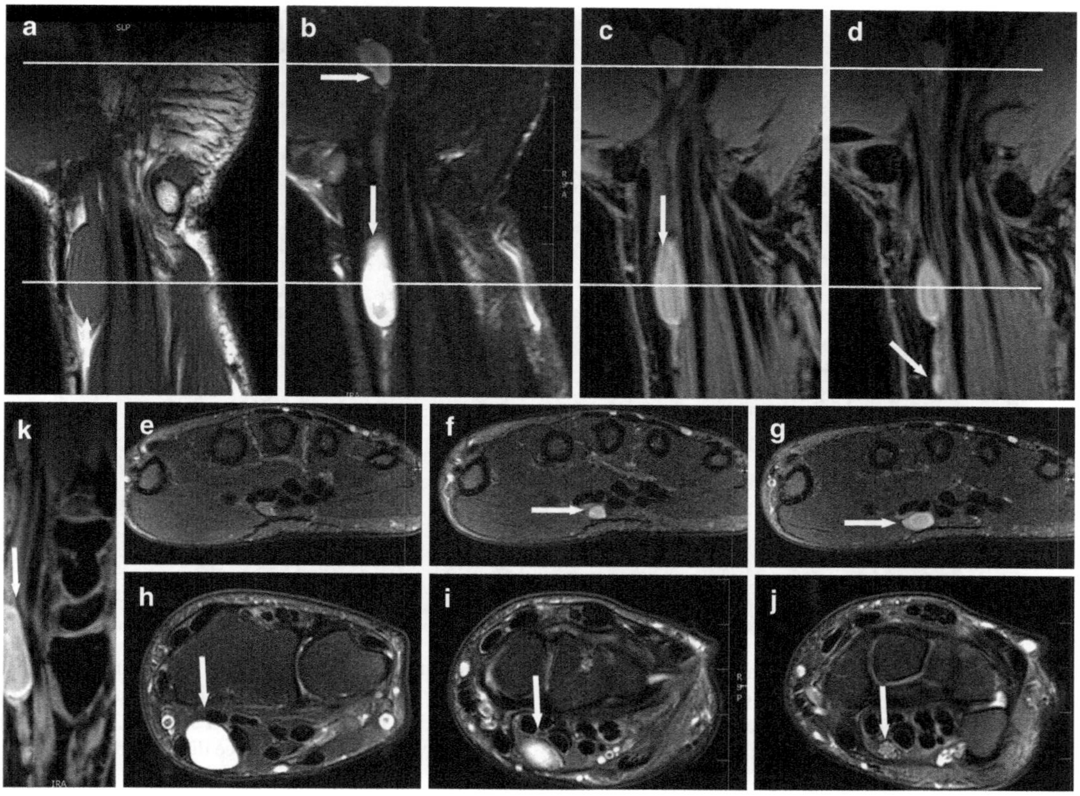

Fig. 36 Cor T1-WI (**a**), T2-WI FS (**b**), and 3D GRE (**c**, **d**); Ax T2-WI FS at the distal (**e–g**) and proximal (**h–j**) white line; and Sag 3D GRE (**k**). Neurogenic tumour with trifocal involvement (**a–k**): fasciculation of the median nerve between (**e**, **j**) the two lesions (**b**) of Fig. 35 and an additional small proximal lesion (**d**)

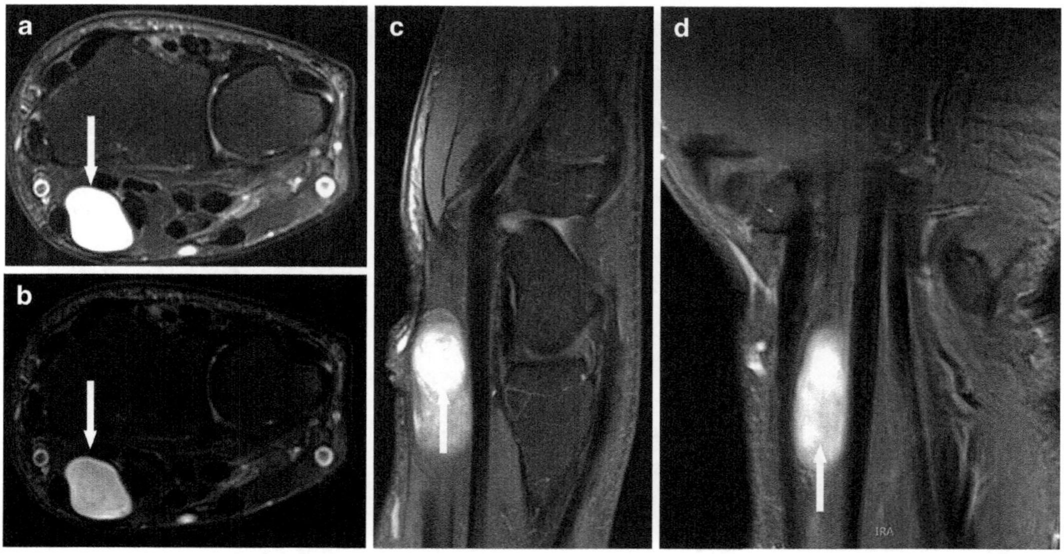

Fig. 37 Ax T2-WI FS (**a**, **b**); Sag (**c**) and Cor (**d**) T1-WI FS with CE. At first sight homogenous CE (**a**) may show a target sign at narrow windowing (**b**). Intensively heterogeneously enhancing neurogenic tumour (**c**, **d**) with sharp delineation in all directions

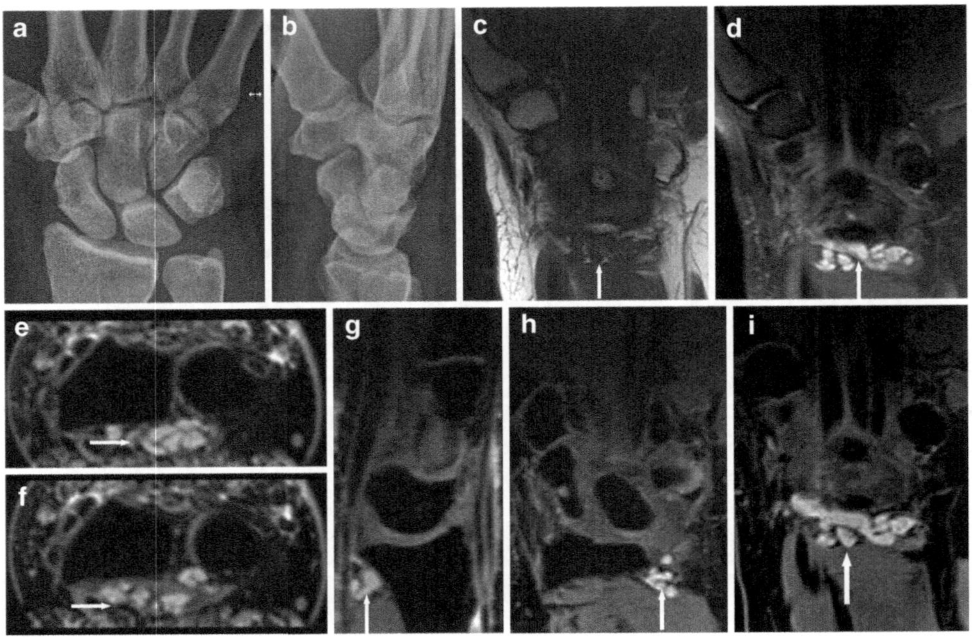

Fig. 38 Standard PA (**a**) and Lateral (**b**) views; Cor T1-WI (**c**) and T2-WI FS (**d**); Ax (**e**, **f**), Sag (**g**), and Cor (H-I) 3D GRE. No calcifications are observed on standard views (**a**, **b**). A well-defined lobulated mass infiltrating in the pronator quadratus muscle with variable signal depending on the flow, mainly with a signal similar to muscle on T1-WI (**c**) and high on T2-WI (**d**). The location and size are evaluated in the three dimensions (**e**–**i**)

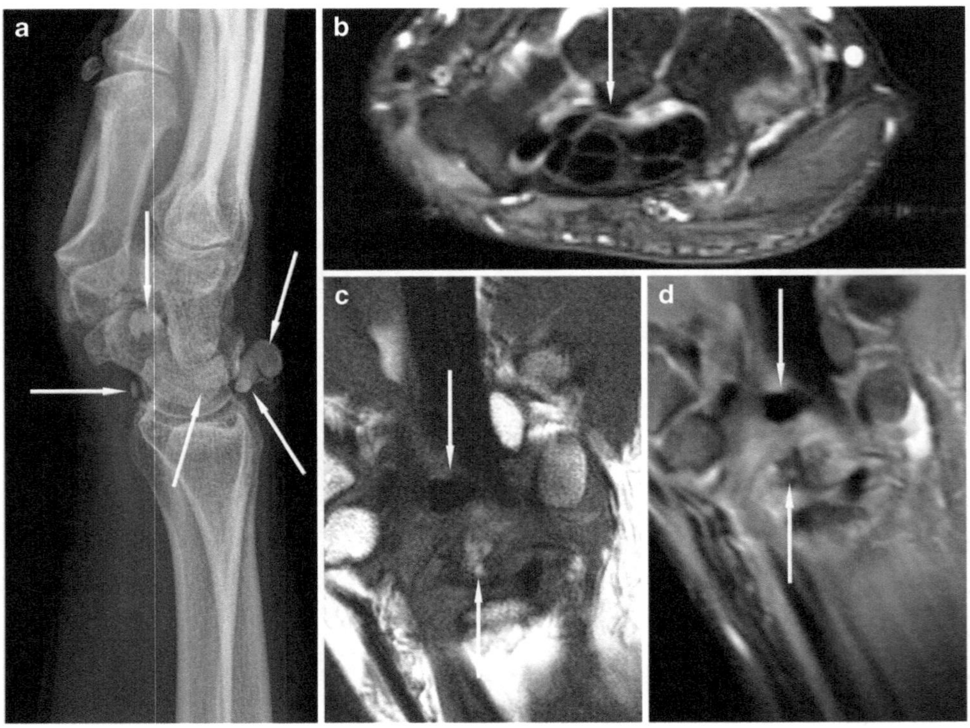

Fig. 39 Standard lateral view (**a**); Ax T2-WI FS (**b**); Cor T1-WI (**c**); Cor 2D GRE (**d**). Multiple, small osseous fragments of different size around a normal joint (**a**). Multiple homogeneously low (ossified) (**b**–**d**) and heterogenous (calcified) signal fragments (**c**, **d**)

also may calcify and/or ossify, resulting in a corresponding signal. Usually, they are small, numerous and more or less of the same size in a not degenerative altered joint of a young patient. The synovia shows CE irregularities. On the contrary, secondary synovial osteochondromatosis manifests as loose broken (larger) bone fragments in a clearly degenerative joint (Fig. 40).

4.6 Tenosynovial Giant Cell Tumour (tsGCT) ((Extraarticular) "pigmented villonodular synovitis"/PVNS)

These localised (soft tissue mass) or diffuse (with joint effusion and bone erosion) tumours arise from the synovium of the joints, bursae, and tendons (Okudaira et al. 2007). They are extra- (Fig. 41) or intra-articular (Fig. 42). The local form is the most frequent in the hand. Malignant forms are extremely rare.

An irregular nodular thickening of the synovia is combined with a joint effusion. Due to hemosiderin deposits, the (nodular thickened) synovia shows a low signal on T2-WI, especially on GRE (Figs. 41c and 42b) and adjacent bone erosion may be present (Fig. 42a, c).

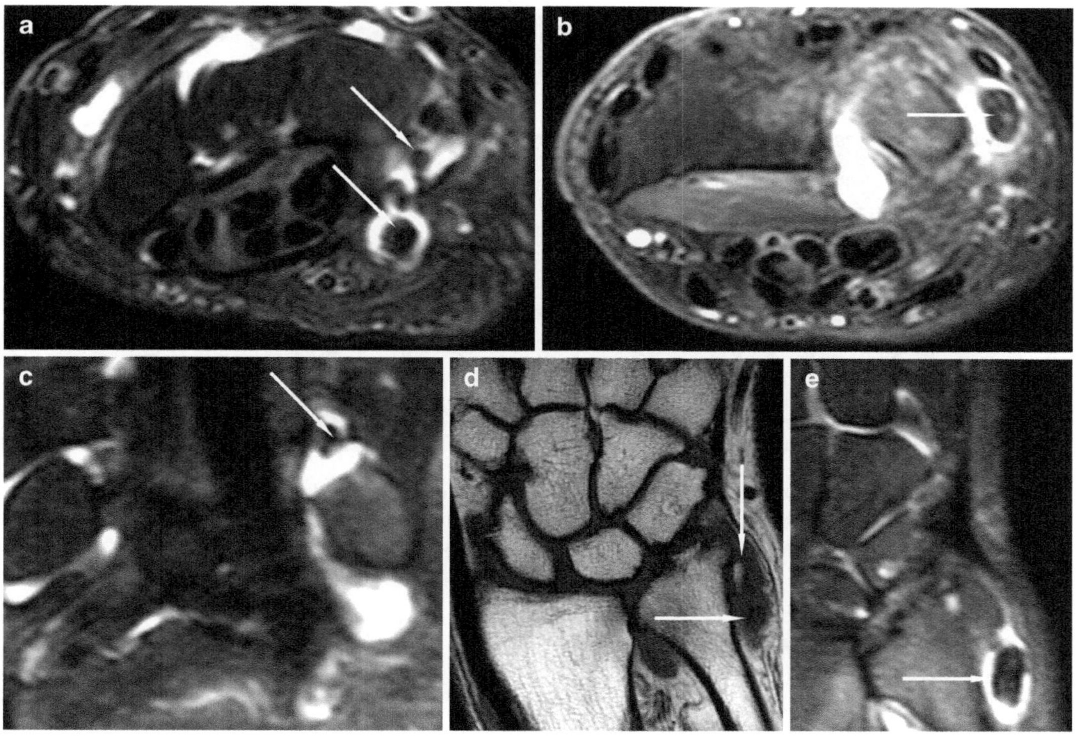

Fig. 40 Ax T2-WI FS (**a**, **b**); Cor T2-WI FS (**c**), T1-WI (**d**), and 2D GRE (**e**). Some fragments of different size in the largely distended TP- and DRU- (degenerative) joint capsule with a homogeneously low (ossified) signal

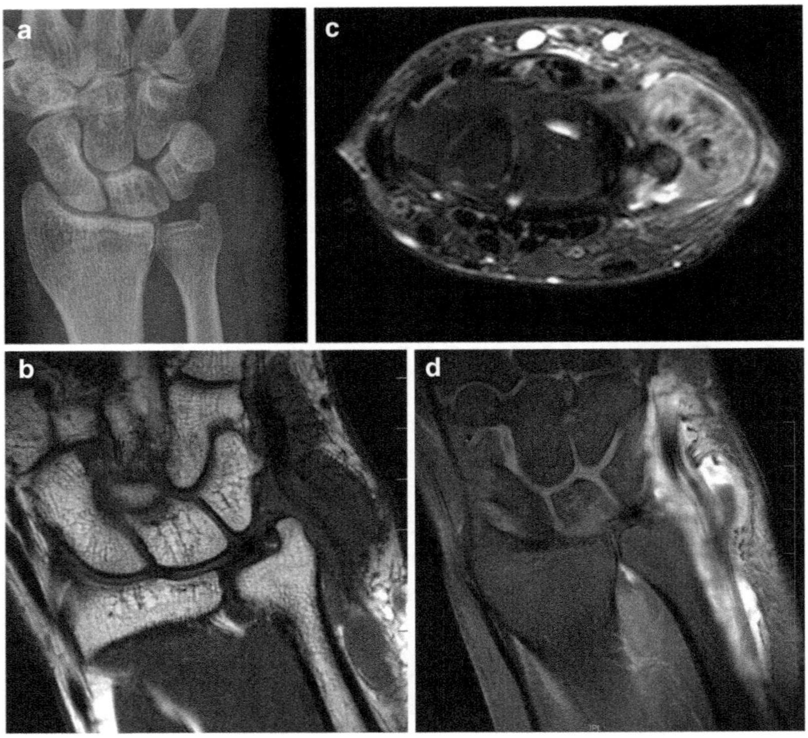

Fig. 41 Standard PA view (**a**); Cor T1-WI (**b**); Ax T2-WI FS (**c**); and Cor T1-WI FS with CE (**d**). Soft tissue swelling around the ulnar styloid (**a**). Heterogeneously low on T1-WI (**b**) and high on T2-WI (**c**) with CE (**d**)

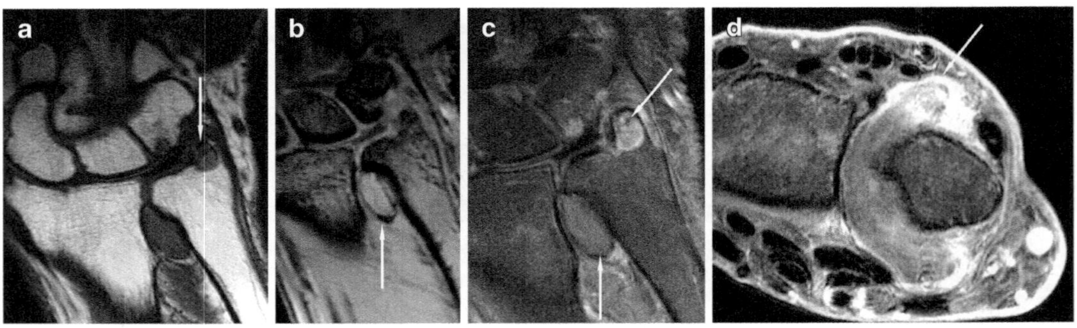

Fig. 42 Cor T1-WI (**a**) and 2D GRE (**b**); Cor (**c**) and Ax (**d**) T1-WI FS with CE. Erosion at the ulnar styloid (**a, c**) and erosive lesion of the distal radial cortex (**a, c**) due to a tsGCT (**c, d**). Hemosiderin deposit at the thickened synovial lining (**b**). CE of the erosion of the styloid (**c**) and the DRUJ synovial proliferation (**d**)

5 Soft Tissues: Malignant Tumours

As they barely exist in the wrist (Chung et al. 2016; Teh and Whiteley 2007), the reader should consult specific literature if ever needed.

6 Pseudotumours

6.1 Muscles

Overdeveloped muscles may simulate a "tumour" on US/MRI (Fig. 43) as does a solitary hypertrophic variant (Fig. 44).

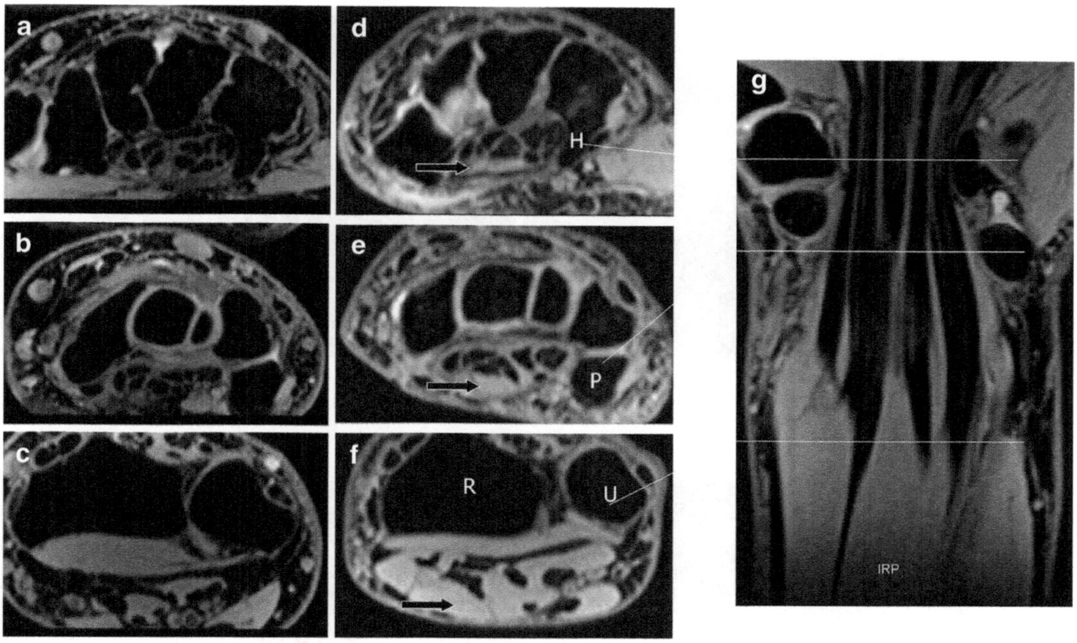

Fig. 43 Ax 3D GRE (**a**–**f**); Cor 3D GRE (**g**). Normal appearance (**a**, **c**). Athlete with "tumour" in the carpal tunnel due to hypertrophic forearm and lumbrical muscles (**d**–**g**)

Fig. 44 Ax T2-WI FS. A solitary pronounced flexor carpi ulnaris muscle (**a**) compared to a normal appearance (**b**)

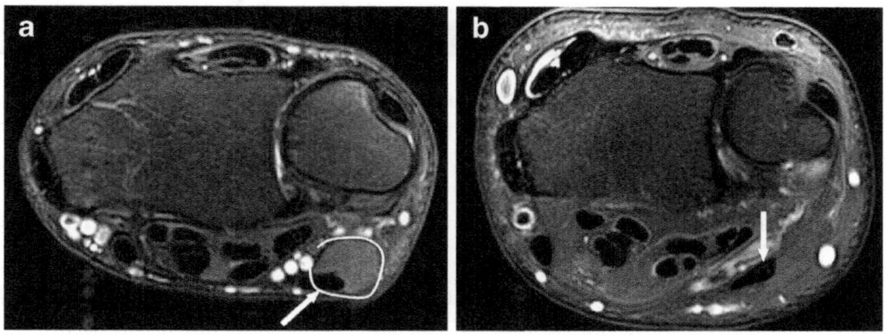

6.2 Traumatic Lesions

A "palpable tumour" due to a solitary soft tissue ossification is clearly diagnosed on standard views (Fig. 45). MRI (Fig. 46) may determine the exact spatial location, the cartilage component (potential growth), and the displacement and eventual compression of the soft tissue (tendons, vessels).

After a recent trauma, a painful "recent tumour-like swelling" (Fig. 47) is noted. MRI shows a loose bone fragment neo-articulating with the dorsally deformed triquetral bone, already secondary degenerative subcortical cysts, and BMO, indicating (also) previous traumatic sequelae.

Elective muscle contusion (Fig. 48), defined as a tumour on US, is due to a later (hetero)anamnestically confirmed crush trauma.

6.3 Infectious Lesions

The local swelling of an insidious infection is attributed to a Brodie abscess (Fig. 49). MRI illustrates the full extent of the pathology (Fig. 50).

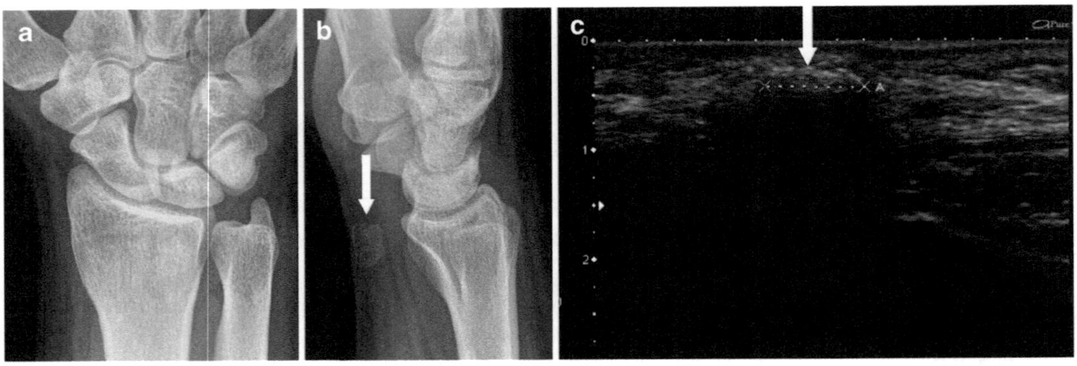

Fig. 45 Standard PA (**a**) and Lateral (**b**) views; US longitudinal (**c**). A "palpable tumour" due to a solitary soft tissue ossification (**b**, **c**)

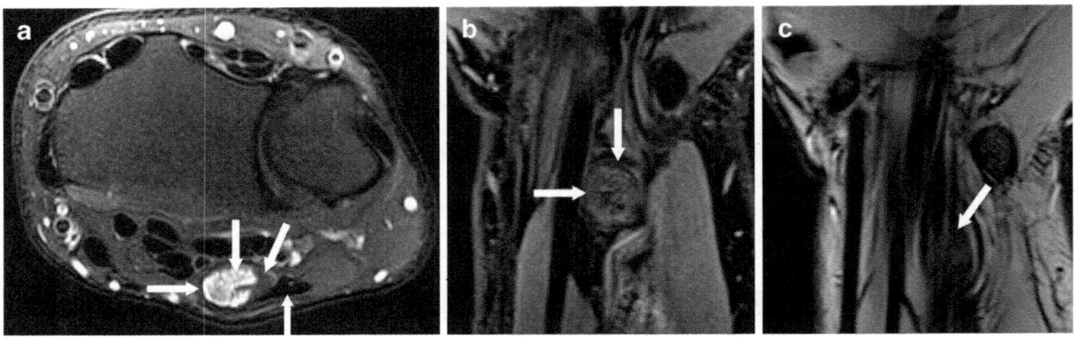

Fig. 46 Ax T2-WI FS (**a**); Cor 3D GRE (**b**, **c**). The exact location (**a**) and the cartilage component (**a**, **b**) are illustrated as is the effect of the interference with the flexor tendons (**b**, **c**)

6.4 Inflammatory Lesions

Silicone prosthesis may frequently cause extensive reactive synovitis on the long term (Fig. 51), sometimes presenting as a space occupying lesion.

Even extensive RA presents occasionally as a "silent local soft tissue lesion" (Figs. 52 and 53), epiphenomenon of extensive infiltration of intrinsic and extrinsic ligaments, small but diffuse and active CE erosions and synovial soft tissue swelling(s).

6.5 Degenerative Lesion

The dorsal tilting of the lunate bone in a DISI configuration results in a prominent aspect of the volar part in the carpal tunnel (Fig. 54) and may be confusing on US of the carpal tunnel in CTS if the radiologist is unaware of the degenerative status.

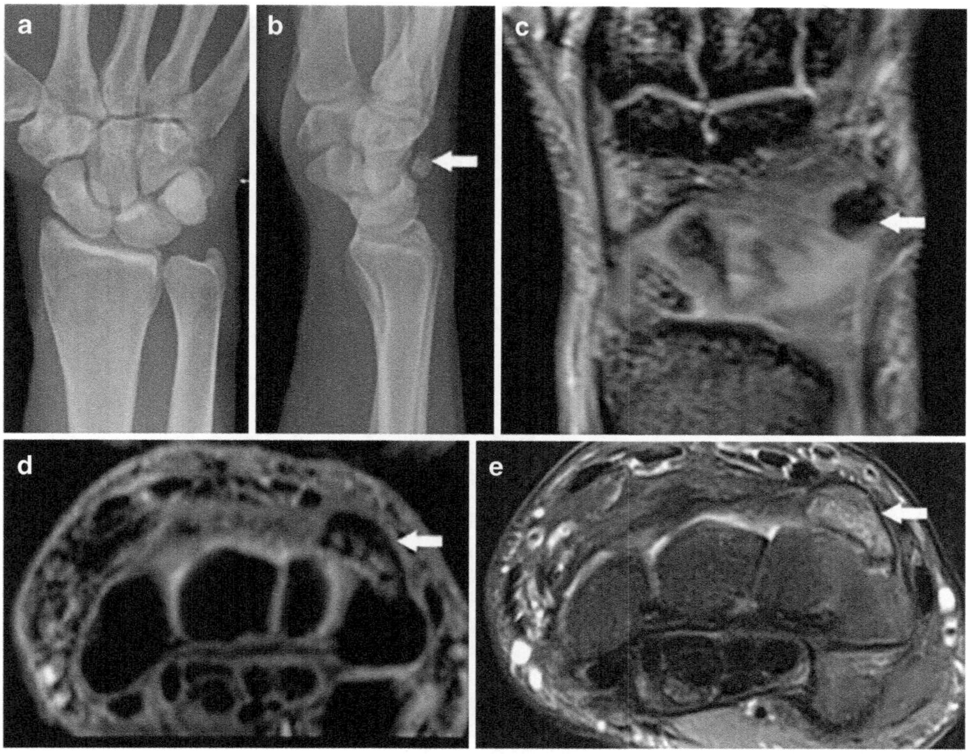

Fig. 47 Standard PA (**a**) and Lateral (**b**) views; Cor 2D GRE (**c**); Ax 3D GRE (**d**), and T2-WI FS (**e**). Ossification dorsal of carpus (**b**). The dorso-ulnar bone fragment (**c**) neo articulates with the dorsally deformed Tri with already adjacent degenerative changes (**d**) and BMO (**e**)

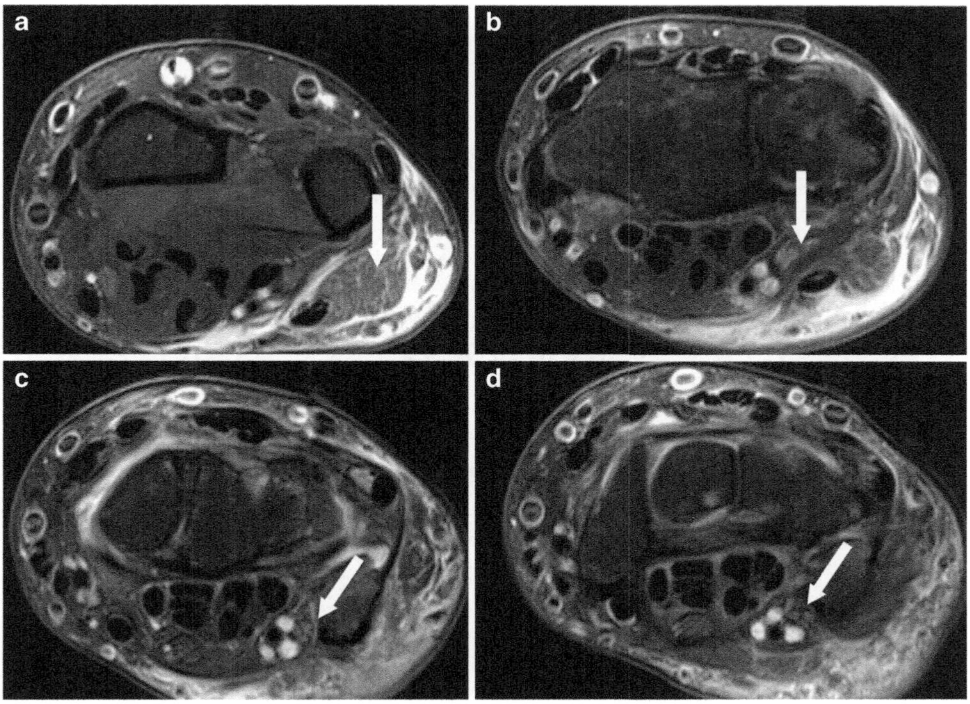

Fig. 48 Ax T2-WI FS (**a–d**). Crush trauma of the fcu with internal and surrounding oedema (**a**, **b**). Accompanying neuritis of the ulnar nerve (**c**, **d**)

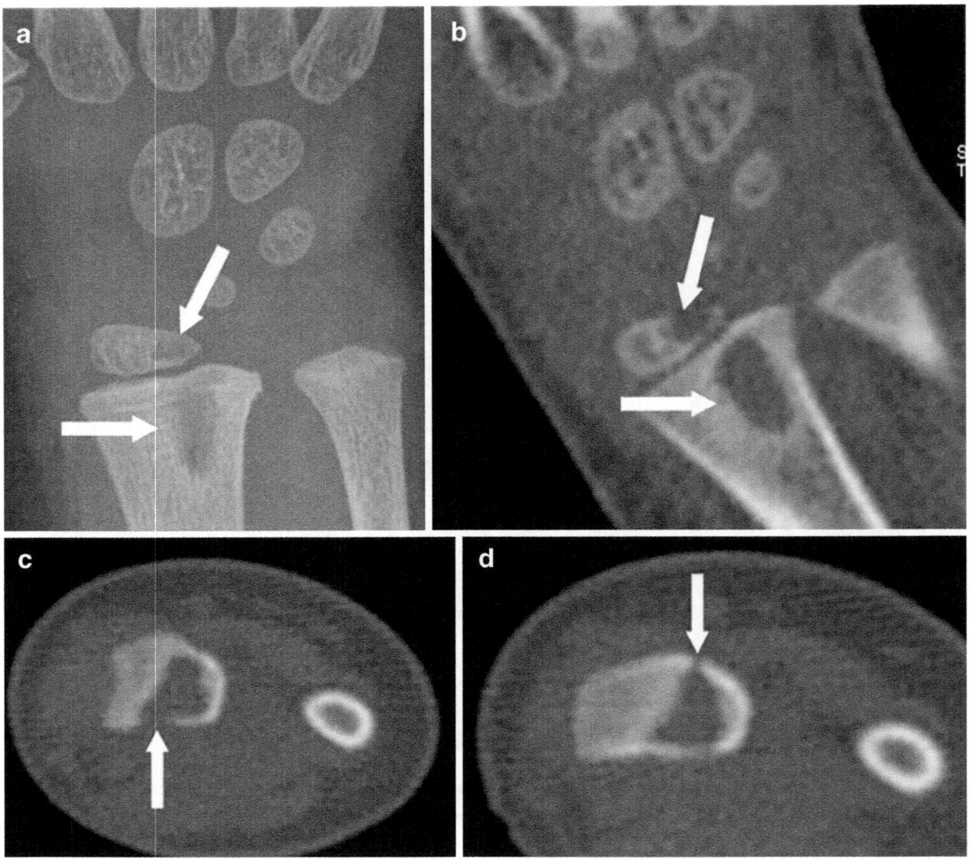

Fig. 49 Standard PA (**a**) view; Cor (**b**) and Ax (**c**, **d**) CT image. Swelling of the wrist: Brodie abscess of the radius

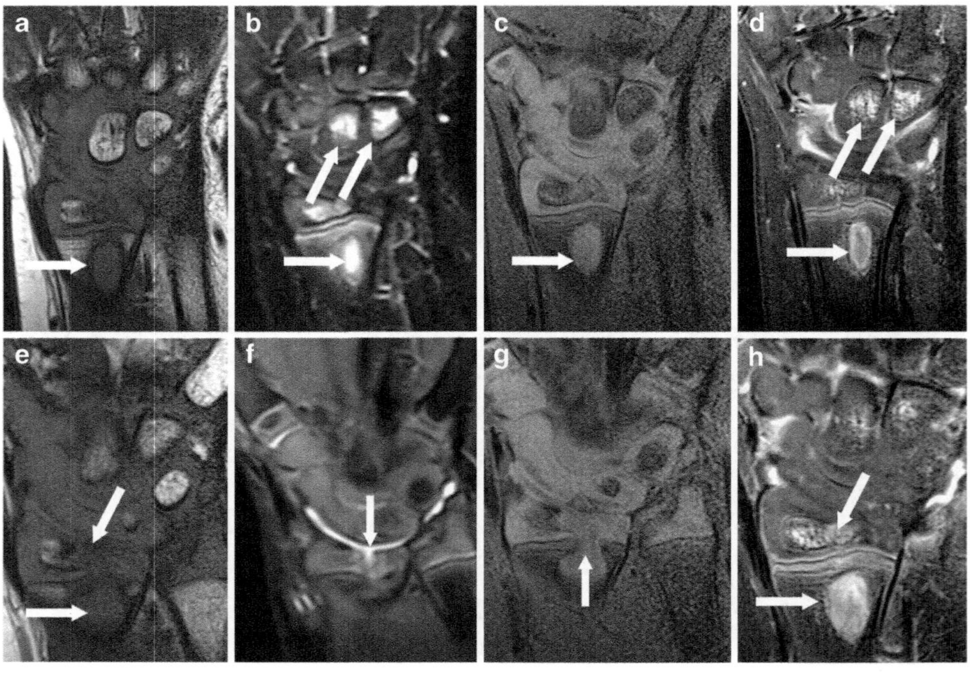

Fig. 50 Cor T1-WI (**a**, **e**), T2-WI FS (**b**), T1-WI-FS (**c**, **g**), T1-WI FS with CE (**d**, **h**), and PD-WI (**f**). Brodie abscess of radius (Fig. 47) with additional carpal lesions (**c** and **h**)

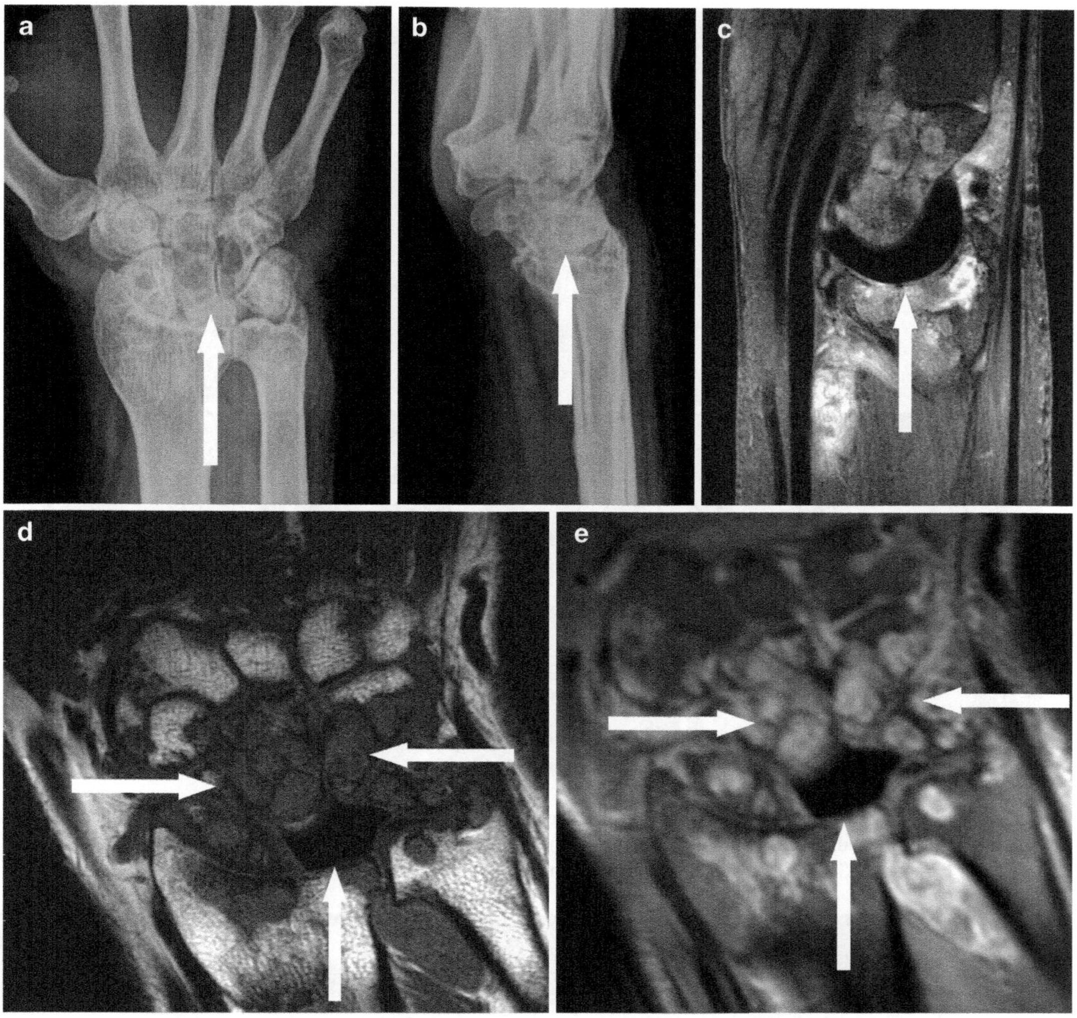

Fig. 51 Standard PA (**a**) and Lateral (**b**) views; T1-WI FS with CE (**c**, **e**); Cor T1-WI (**d**). Silicone prosthesis of the L (**a**–**e**) with extensive reactive synovitis (**d**, **e**)

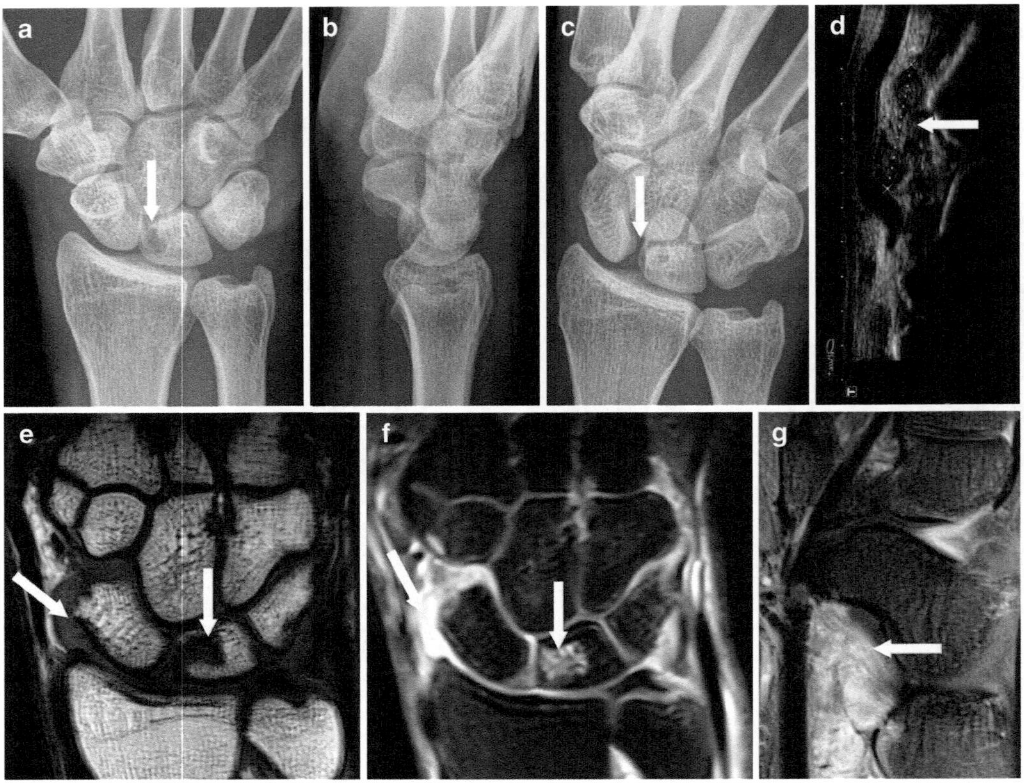

Fig. 52 Standard PA (**a**), Lateral (**b**), and PA with ulnar deviation (**c**); US longitudinal (**d**): Cor T1-WI (**e**); Cor (**f**) and Sag (**g**) T1-WI with FS and CE. Lytic lesion of S (**a**) with soft tissue swelling of the wrist region (**b**) and SL (dynamic) diastasis (**c**). Soft tissue lesion with vessel displacement (**d**). CE soft tissue proliferation and S bone erosion (**e–g**)

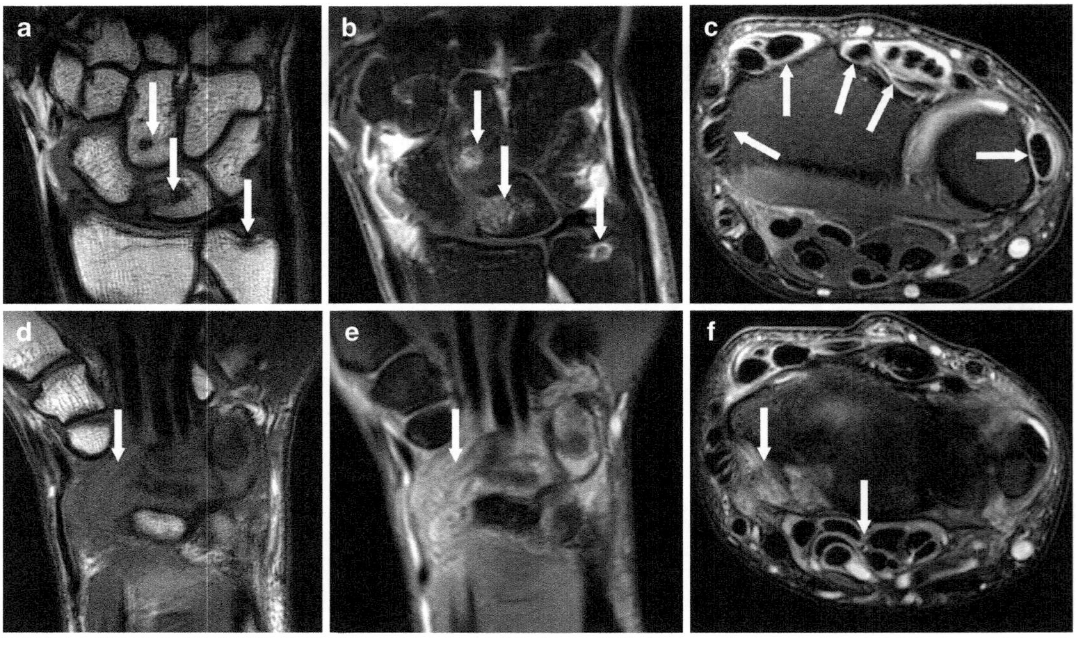

Fig. 53 Cor T1-WI (**a**, **d**), T1-WI with FS and CE (**b**, **e**); Ax T2-WI FS (**c**, **f**). CE erosion of C, S, and U (**a**, **b**). Tenosynovitis of extensor compartments (**c**) and flexors (**f**). Infiltration of extrinsic ligaments/carpal V with soft tissue proliferation and R bone erosion (**d–f**)

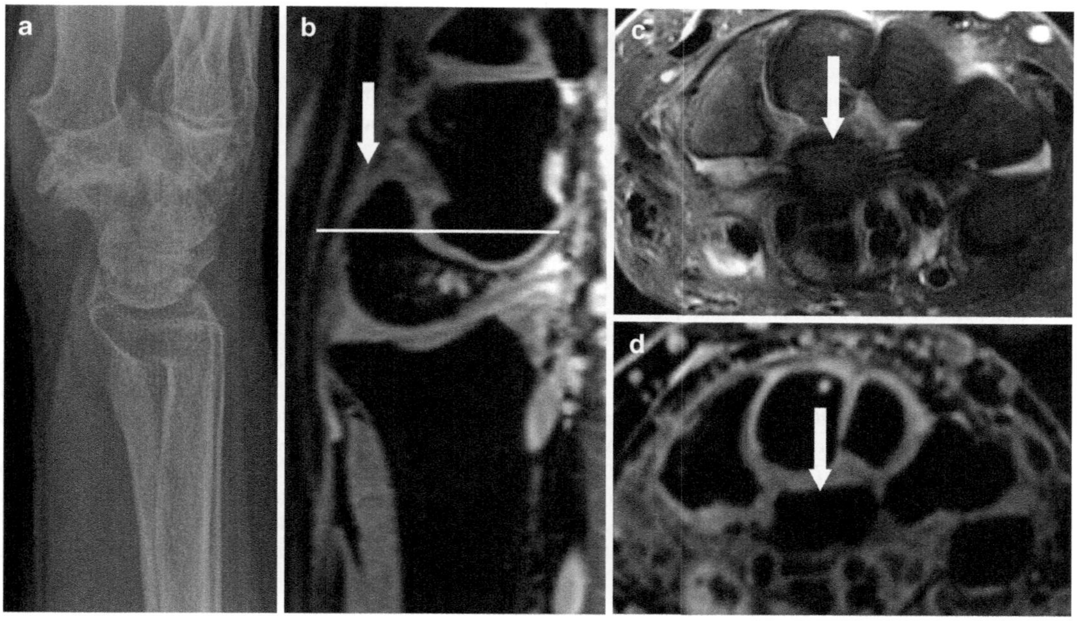

Fig. 54 Standard Later view (**a**); Sag 3D GRE (**b**); Ax T2-WI FS (**c**); and 3D GRE (**d**). DISI configuration (**a**) with tilting of volar part of the L in the carpal tunnel (**b–d**)

References

Chew FS, Weissleder R (1991) Radiation-induced osteochondroma. AJR Am J Roentgenol 157(4):792. https://doi.org/10.2214/ajr.157.4.1892038. PMID: 1892038

Chung BY, Lee SA, Choi J-A, Shim J-W (2016) Clear cell sarcoma of the wrist: MRI findings with diffusion-weighted image and histopathologic correlation. Investig Magn Reson Imaging 20(2):136–139

Claikens B, Brys P, Samson I, Baert AL (1998) Spontaneous resolution of a solitary osteochondroma. Skeletal Radiol 27(1):53–55. https://doi.org/10.1007/s002560050338. PMID: 9507614

Conway WF, Destouet JM, Gilula LA, Bellinghausen HW, Weeks PM (1985) The carpal boss: an overview of radiographic evaluation. Radiology 156(1):29–31. https://doi.org/10.1148/radiology.156.1.3923555. PMID: 3923555

Deprez FC, Beltrán-Marín M, Malghem J, Menten R, Clapuyt R (2011) Solitary osteochondroma: spontaneous regression. JBR-BTR 94(4):217. https://doi.org/10.5334/jbr-btr.635. PMID: 21980744

Dhondt E, Oudenhoven L, Khan S, Kroon HM, Hogendoorn PC, Nieborg A, Bloem JL, De Schepper A (2006) Nora's lesion, a distinct radiological entity? Skeletal Radiol 35(7):497–502. https://doi.org/10.1007/s00256-005-0041-9. Epub 2006 Apr 7. PMID: 16602017

El-Sobky TA, Samir S, Atiyya AN, Mahmoud S, Aly AS, Soliman R (2018) Current paediatric orthopaedic practice in hereditary multiple osteochondromas of the forearm: a systematic review. SICOT J 4:10. https://doi.org/10.1051/sicotj/2018002. Epub 2018 Mar 21. PMID: 29565244; PMCID: PMC5863686

Fei L, Ngoh C, Porter DE (2018) Chondrosarcoma transformation in hereditary multiple exostoses: a systematic review and clinical and cost-effectiveness of a proposed screening model. J Bone Oncol 13:114–122. https://doi.org/10.1016/j.jbo.2018.09.011. PMID: 30591865; PMCID: PMC6303411

Khaled W, Drapé JL (2015) MRI of wrist and hand masses. Diagn Interv Imaging 96(12):1238–1246. https://doi.org/10.1016/j.diii.2015.10.005. Epub 2015 Nov 10. PMID: 26564613

Murphey MD, Choi JJ, Kransdorf MJ, Flemming DJ, Gannon FH (2000) Imaging of osteochondroma: variants and complications with radiologic-pathologic correlation. Radiographics 20(5):1407–1434. https://doi.org/10.1148/radiographics.20.5.g00se171407. PMID: 10992031

Nguyen V, Choi J, Davis KW (2004) Imaging of wrist masses. Curr Probl Diagn Radiol 33(4):147–160. https://doi.org/10.1016/j.cpradiol.2004.01.002. PMID: 15306759

Nora FE, Dahlin DC, Beabout JW (1983) Bizarre parosteal osteochondromatous proliferations of the hands and feet. Am J Surg Pathol 7(3):245–250. https://doi.org/10.1097/00000478-198304000-00003. PMID: 6837834

Okudaira S, Takahashi S, Tsuda Y, Suzuki K, Kotoura Y (2007) Giant cell tumor of tendon sheath in the wrist: MRI, Thallium-201 and Gallium-67 scintigraphic findings. Jpn J Rheum Joint Surg 25(4):497–502. https://doi.org/10.11551/jsjd1982.25.497

Simmons AD, Musy MM, Lopes CS, Hwang LY, Yang YP, Lovett M (1999) A direct interaction between EXT proteins and glycosyltransferases is defective in hereditary multiple exostoses. Hum Mol Genet 8(12):2155–2164. https://doi.org/10.1093/hmg/8.12.2155. PMID: 10545594

Teh J, Whiteley G (2007) MRI of soft tissue masses of the hand and wrist. Br J Radiol 80(949):47–63. https://doi.org/10.1259/bjr/53596176. Epub 2006 May 10. PMID: 16687461

Vanhoenacker FM, Van Hul W, Wuyts W, Willems PJ, De Schepper AM (2001) Hereditary multiple exostoses: from genetics to clinical syndrome and complications. Eur J Radiol 40(3):208–217. https://doi.org/10.1016/s0720-048x(01)00401-6. PMID: 11731209

Versteeg G, Goyal K (2019) Radiologist identification of occult dorsal wrist ganglion cysts on MRI. J Wrist Surg 8(4):276–279. https://doi.org/10.1055/s--0039-1683847. Epub 2019 Mar 25. PMID: 31404246; PMCID: PMC6685734

Vo P, Wright T, Hayden F, Dell P, Chidgey L (1995) Evaluating dorsal wrist pain: MRI diagnosis of occult dorsal wrist ganglion. J Hand Surg Am 20(4):667–670. https://doi.org/10.1016/S0363-5023(05)80288-6. PMID: 7594299

Wuyts W, Van Hul W (2000) Molecular basis of multiple exostoses: mutations in the EXT1 and EXT2 genes. Hum Mutat 15(3):220–227. https://doi.org/10.1002/(SICI)1098-1004(200003)15:3<220::AID-HUMU2>3.0.CO;2-K. PMID: 10679937

Wuyts W, Bovée JV, Hogendoorn PC (2002) Van gen naar ziekte; hereditaire multipele exostosen [From gene to disease; hereditary multiple exostoses]. Ned Tijdschr Geneeskd 146(4):162–164. Dutch. PMID: 11845565

Yilmaz TF, Toprak H, Atasoy B, Sönmez FC, Aralasmak A, Gürkan V (2022) Radiological appearences of benign soft-tissue tumors of the hand and wrist with special emphasis on MRI. Bezmialem Sci 10(2):247–260. https://doi.org/10.14235/bas.galenos.2021.6398

Yuen M, Friedman L, Orr W, Cockshott WP (1992) Proliferative periosteal processes of phalanges: a unitary hypothesis. Skeletal Radiol 21(5):301–303. https://doi.org/10.1007/BF00241768. PMID: 1502582

Part IV

Section on Combined Pathology

Complex Cases

Contents

1 General

The isolated illustration of pathology types is rarely a reflection of reality. Two or more pathologies may often be discovered on the MRI images, which make the interpretation often difficult, but also challenging. An accurate analysis of all the elements is mandatory, before evaluating into which pathology or pathologies they fit. In doing so, a critical view on the accompanying clinical information is necessary to avoid bias. On the other hand, not all MRI abnormalities are (at the moment of the examination) clinically relevant. Therefore, discussing the MRI findings with the clinician is an integral part of the analysis of any MRI examination.

2 MRI Findings

The **"a"- images** (Figs. 1a, 2a, 3a, 4a, 5a, 6a, 7a, 8a, 9a, 10a, 11a, 12a, 13a, 14a, 15a, 16a, 17a, 18a, 19a, 20a, 21a, 22a, 23a, 24a, 25a, 26a, 27a, 28a, 29a, 30a, 31a, 32a, 33a, 34a, 35a, 36a, 37a, 38a, 39a, 40a, 41a, 42a, 43a, 44a, 45a, 46a, 47a, 48a, 49a, and 50a). In without arrow indications. A specific pathological finding at a location in the wrist is associated with a specific arrow, indicating direction in the different **"b"- images/sequences** (Figs. 1b, 2b, 3b, 4b, 5b, 6b, 7b, 8b, 9b, 10b, 11b, 12b, 13b, 14b, 15b, 16b, 17b, 18b, 19b, 20b, 21b, 22b, 23b, 24b, 25b, 26b, 27b, 28b, 29b, 30b, 31b, 32b, 33b, 34b, 35b, 36b, 37b, 38b, 39b, 40b, 41b, 42b, 43b, 44b, 45b, 46b, 47b, 48b, 49b, and 50b). In order to avoid "information overload", the specific pathology is only pointed out on the most important images. More details on the mentioned pathology can be reviewed in the previous chapters.

M. Mespreuve, K. Waked, *MRI of the Wrist*, Medical Radiology,
https://doi.org/10.1007/978-3-031-63973-9_17

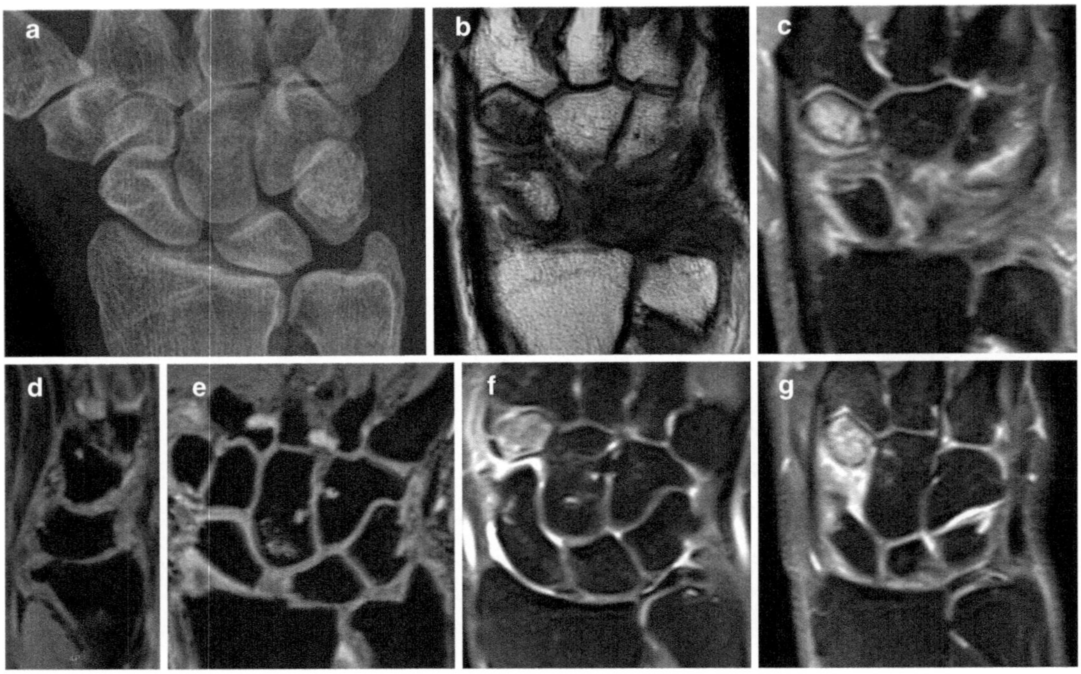

Fig. 1a Standard PA view (**a**); Cor T1-WI (**b**) and T2-WI FS (**c**); Sag (**d**) and Cor (**e**) 3D GRE; Cor T2-WI FS (**f**, **g**)

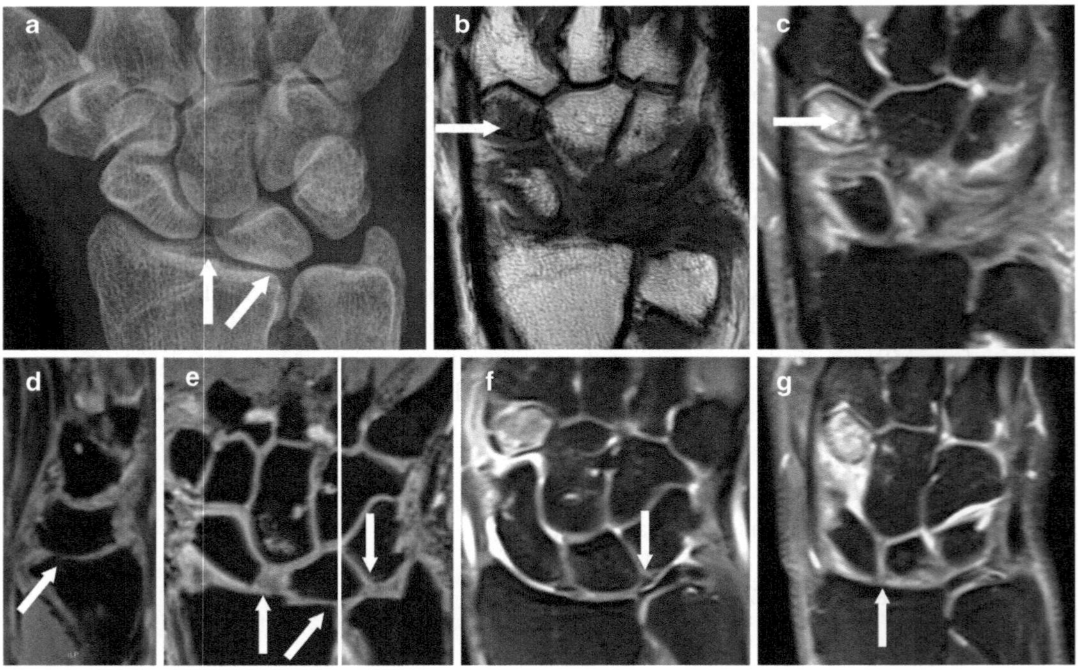

Fig. 1b Widening of the SL joint and narrowing of the R-L joint space (**a**); oedema of the tra with low signal fracture line (**b**, **c**); OA R-L (**a**, **d**, **e**); SLL tear (**a**, **e**, **g**); impaction of the R at the ulnar side of the RCJ (**e**); LTL tear (**e**, **f**)

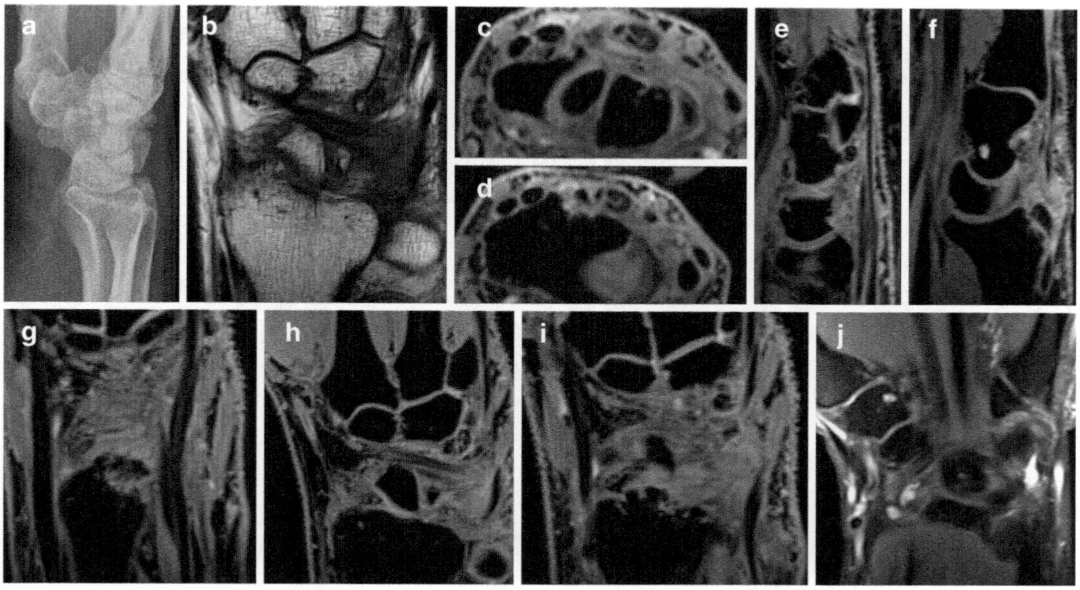

Fig. 2a Standard Lateral view (**a**); Cor T1-WI (**b**); Ax (**c**, **d**), Sag (**e**, **f**), and Cor (**g**–**i**) 3D GRE; Cor T2-WI FS (**j**)

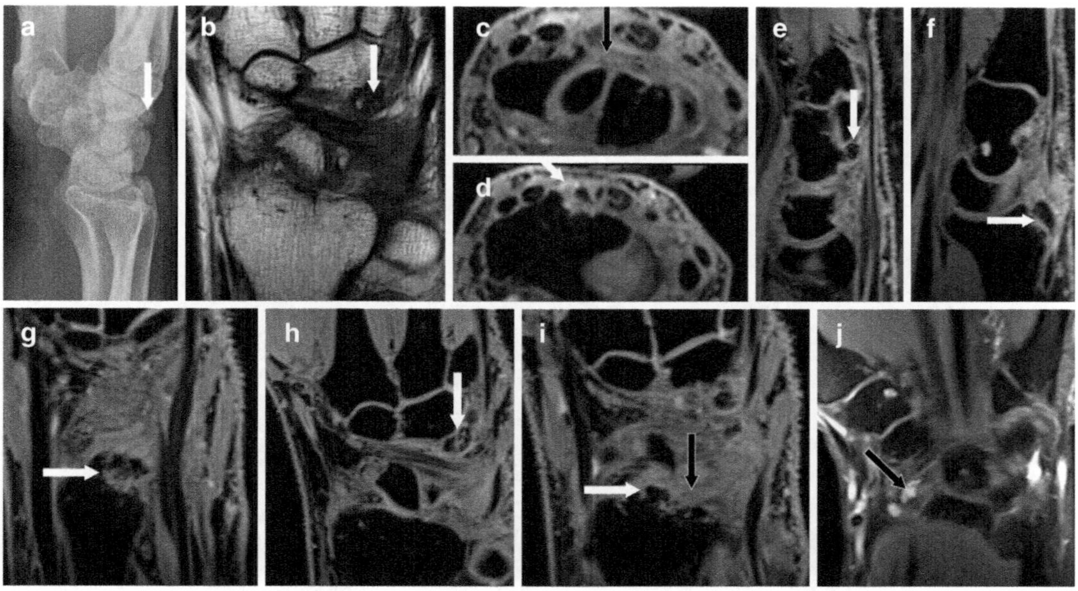

Fig. 2b Loose bone fragment dorsal of the second carpal row (**a**) from a dorsal H fracture (**b**, **e**, **h**); rupture of the extrinsic R-Tri ligament (**c**, **i**); rupture of the EPL (**d**); Fracture of the dorsal border of the R (**f**, **g**, **j**); radiopalmar ASC (**j**)

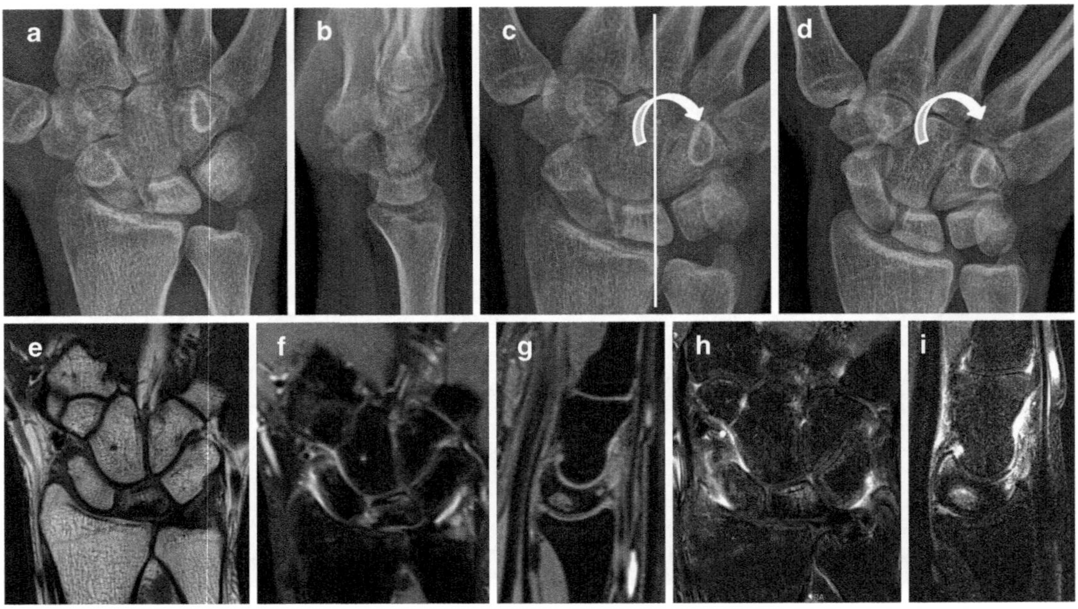

Fig. 3a Standard PA (**a**) and lateral (**b**) views; comparative PA view in ulnar deviation (**c**, **d**); Cor T1-WI (**e**), and T2-WI FS (**f**); Sag 3D GRE (**g**); Cor (**h**), and Sag (**i**) T1-WI FS with CE

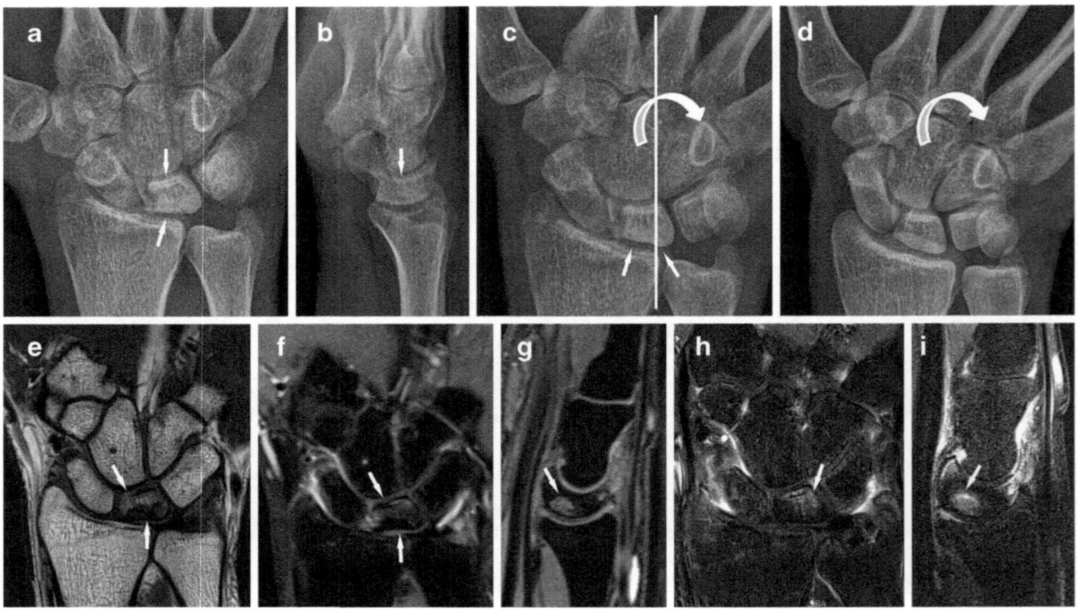

Fig. 3b Dense L (**a**, **b**) with flattened radial-proximal part (**a–c**); limited ulnar deviation (**c**, **d**); proximal necrotic part (**e**, **f**, **h**), and distal oedematous part (**e–h**) of the L; CE viable bone marrow (**h**, **i**)

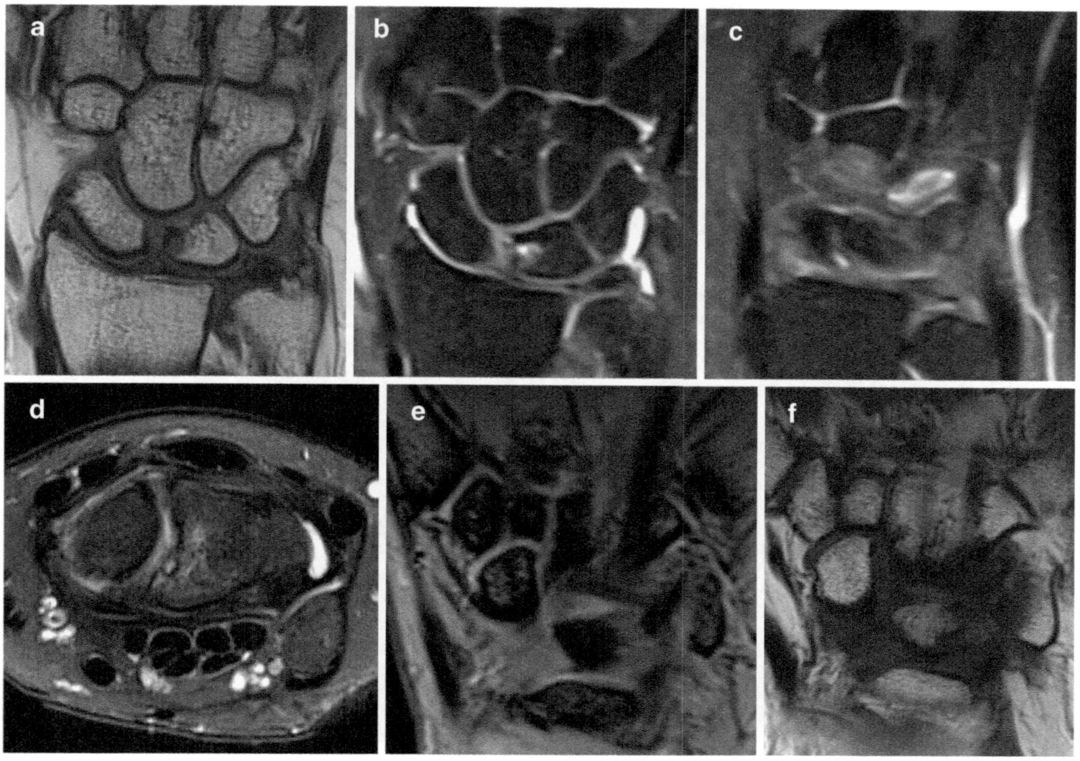

Fig. 4a Cor T1-WI (**a**), T2-WI FS (**b**), and PG-WI (**c**); Ax T2-WI FS (**d**); Cor 2D GRE (**e**), and T1-WI (**f**)

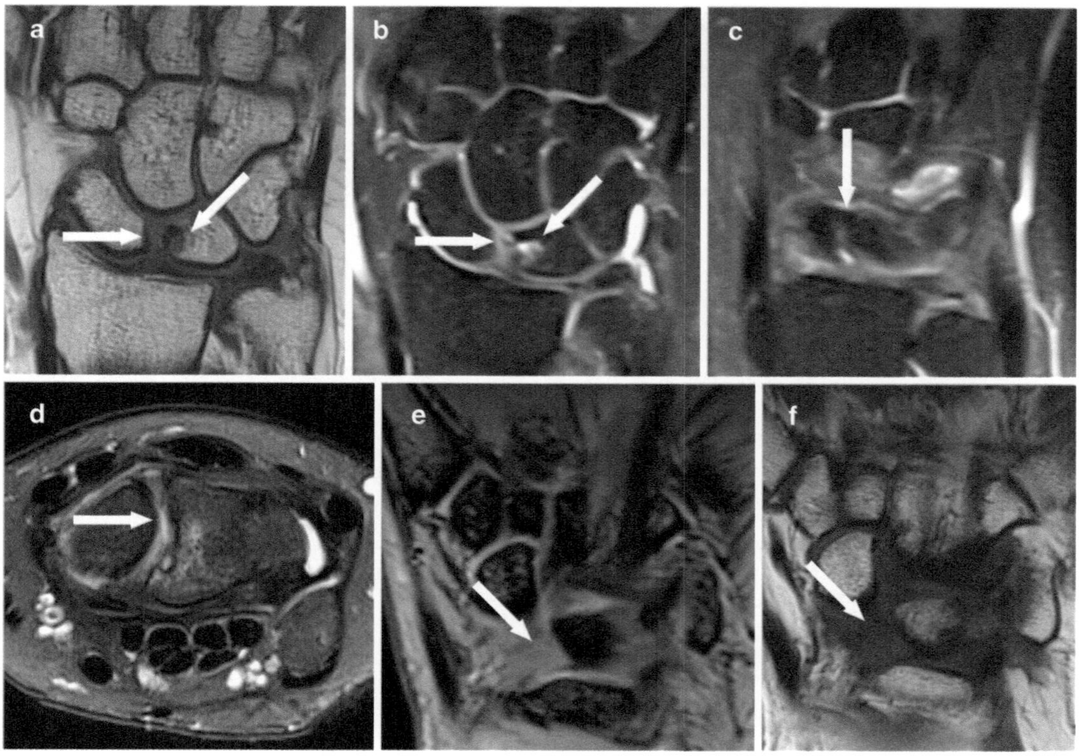

Fig. 4b Recent SL tear (**a**–**c**) with widening of the SL joint (**b**), fluid in the SL joint (**d**), and BMO of the L (**a**, **b**); intact dorsal part of SL (**c**); extrinsic RLT laceration (**e**, **f**)

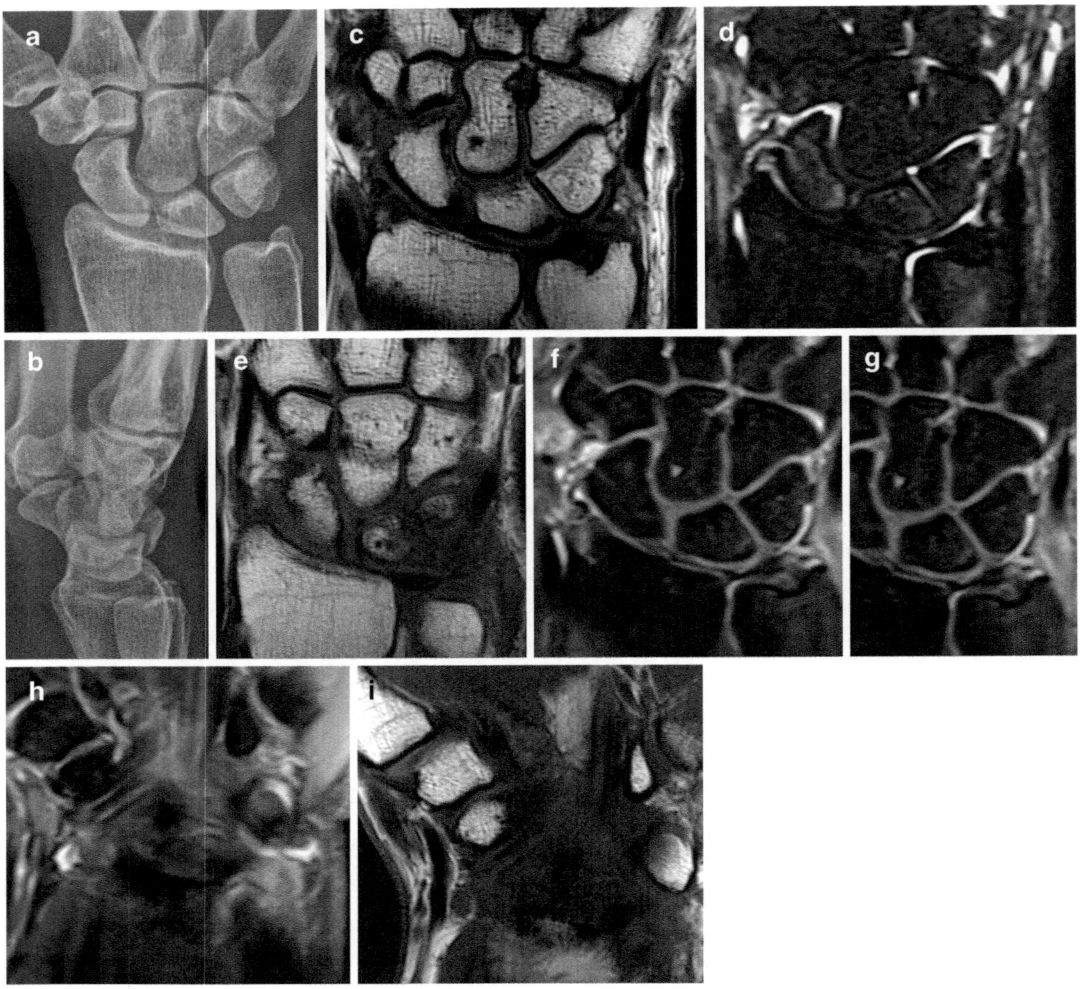

Fig. 5a Standard PA (**a**) and lateral (**b**) views; Cor T1-WI (**c**, **e**, **i**) and T2-WI FS (**d**, **f**–**h**)

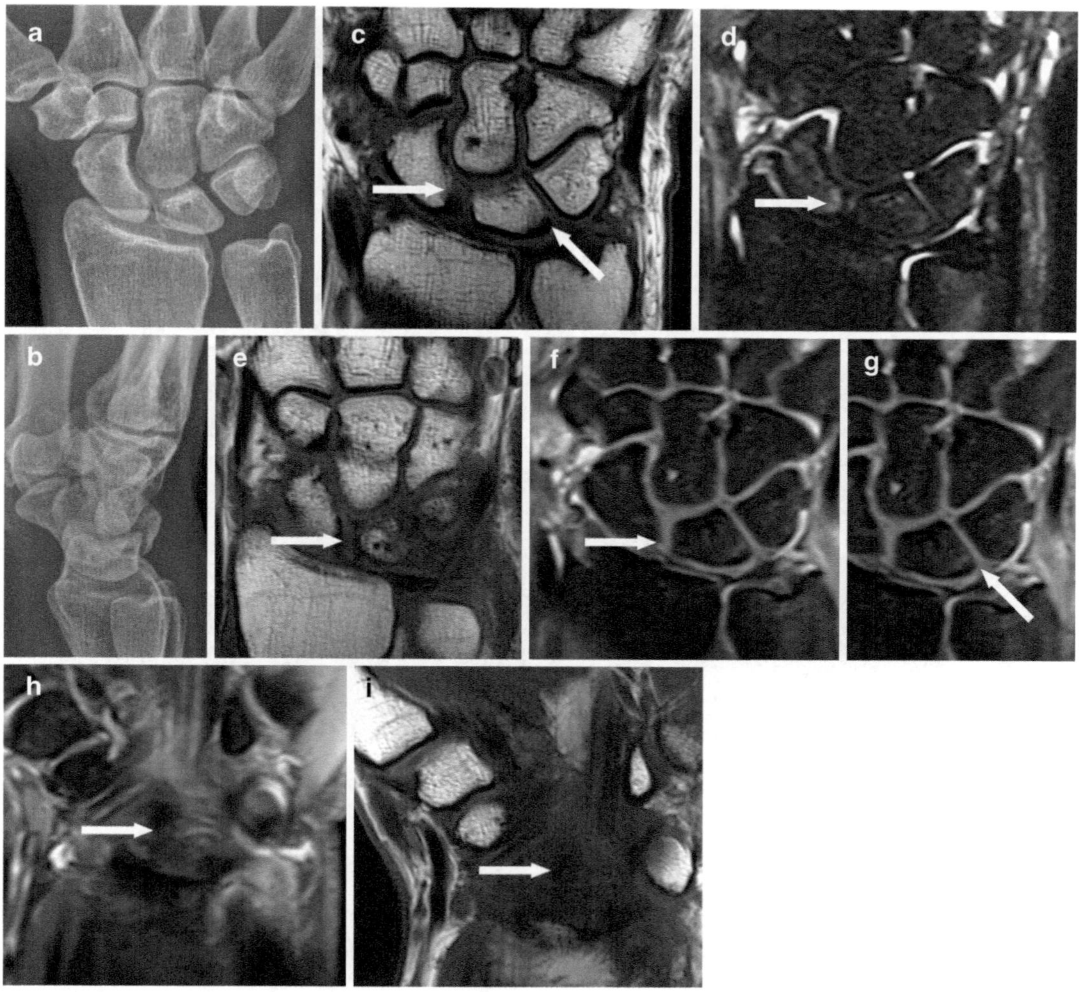

Fig. 5b Normal standard views (**a**, **b**), SLL tear with oedema at the adjacent S side (**c**–**f**); LTL tear (**c**, **g**); laceration of the radial component of the palmar V (RSC/RLT) (**h**, **i**)

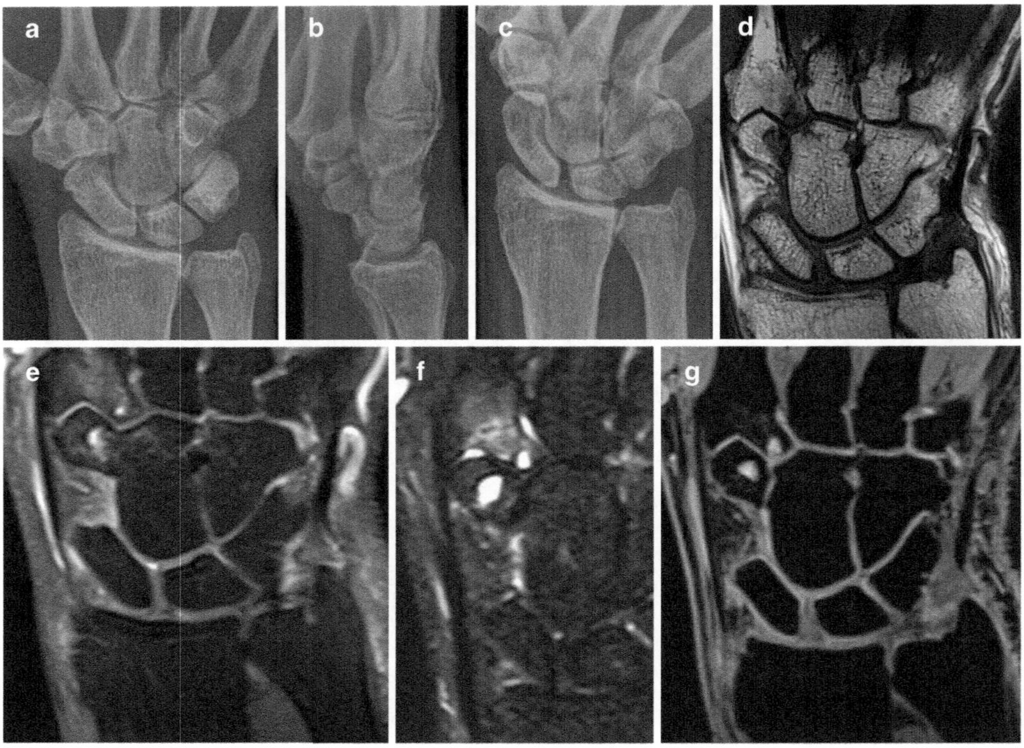

Fig. 6a Standard PA (**a**) and lateral (**b**) views; Standard PA view with clenched fist (**c**); Cor T1-WI (**d**), T2-WI FS (**e**, **f**), and 3D GRE (**g**)

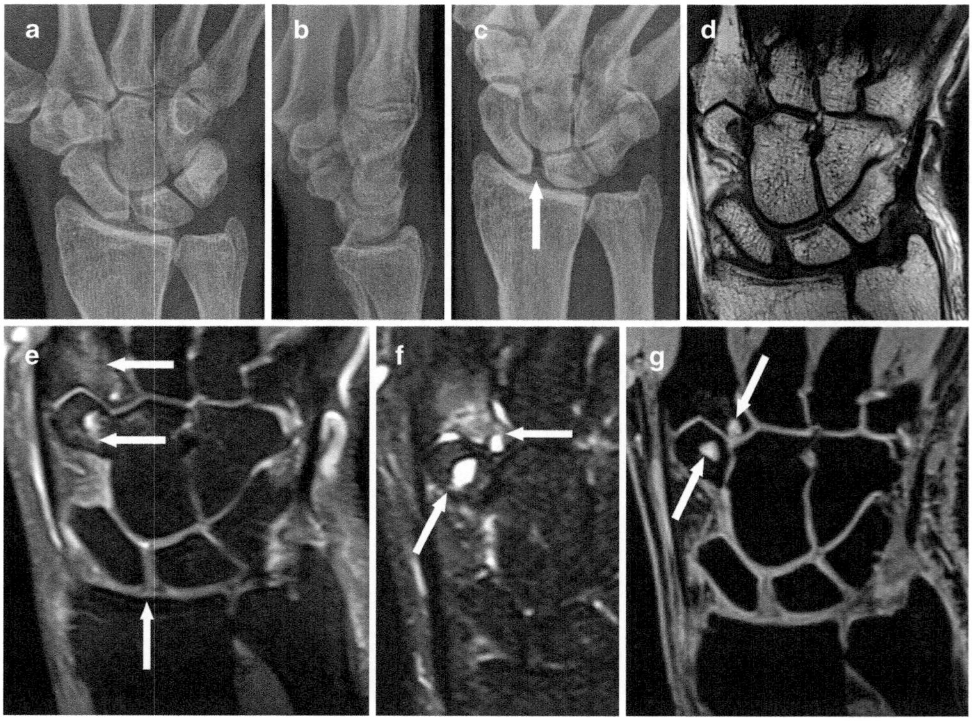

Fig. 6b Normal standard views (**a**, **b**); SL joint widening (**c**); SL tear (**d**, **e**); carpal boss CMC II with narrowing of the ulnar side of the joint space, subchondral cyst, and kissing BMO (**e–g**)

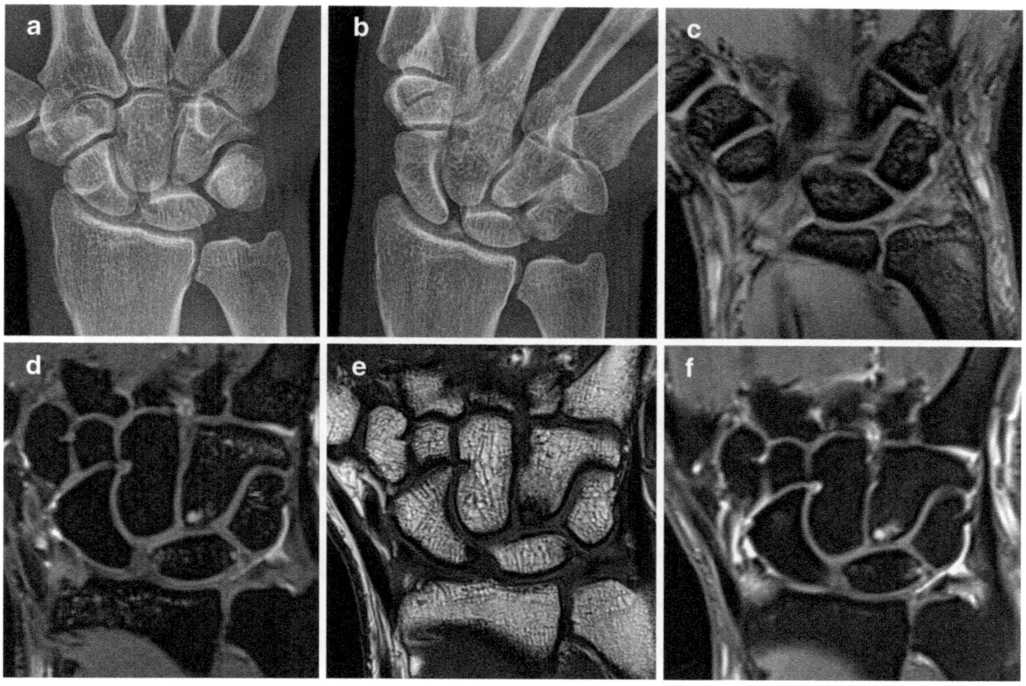

Fig. 7a Standard PA view (**a**), and PA view with clenched fist (**b**); Cor 2D GRE (**c**), 3D GRE (**d**), T1-WI (**e**), and T2-WI FS (**f**)

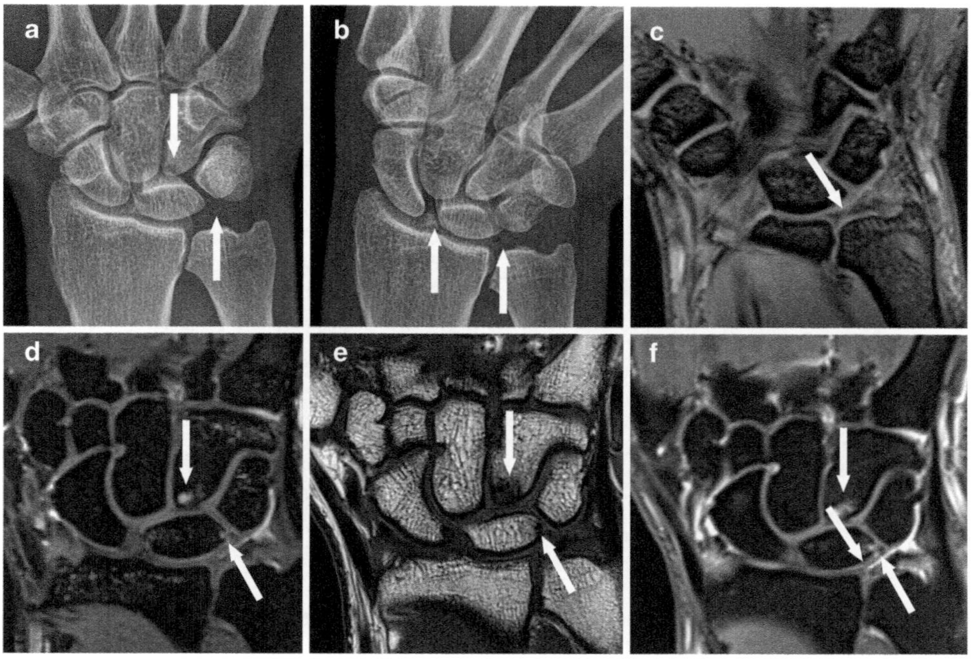

Fig. 7b Translucent proximal tip of the H (**a**); calcium deposits on the TFC and the hyaline cartilage of the SL- and LT joint (**a, b**) suggestive of crystal arthropathy, type CPPD; oblique fine central tear of the TFCC (**c**) with small step off at the surface (**f**), Palmer lesion I A; subchondral cyst (**d**) with surrounding BMO at the proximal tip of the H (**d–f**) with a L type 2 (**b**), compatible with HLA; small subchondral cyst starting chondromalacia at the proximal-ulnar corner of the L (**d–f**) pointing at initiating UA

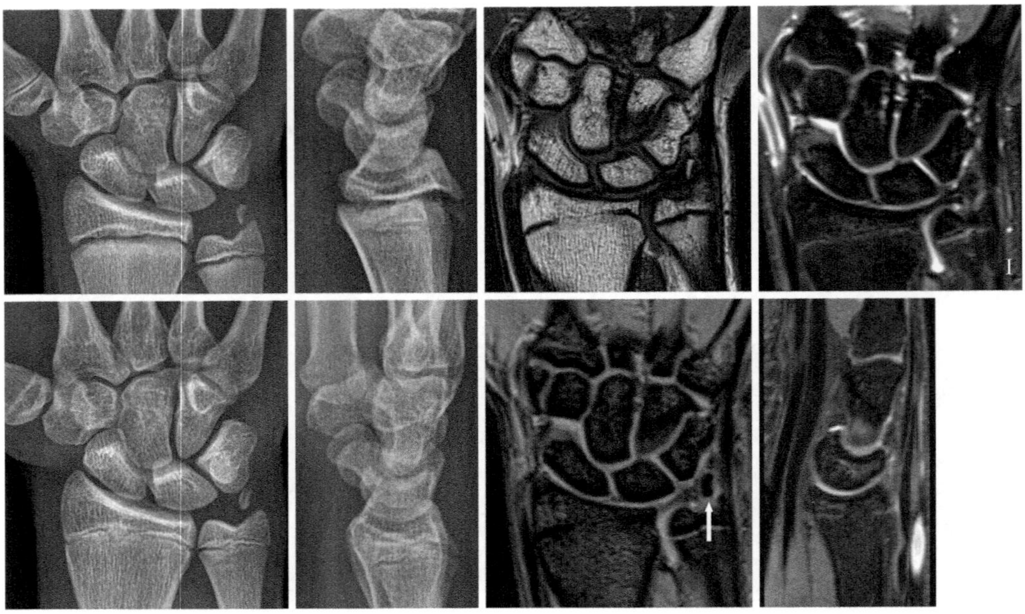

Fig. 8a Standard PA (**a**, **c**), and Lateral (**b**, **d**) views; Cor T1-WI (**e**), and T2-WI FS (**f**); Cor (**g**), and Sag (**h**) 3D GRE

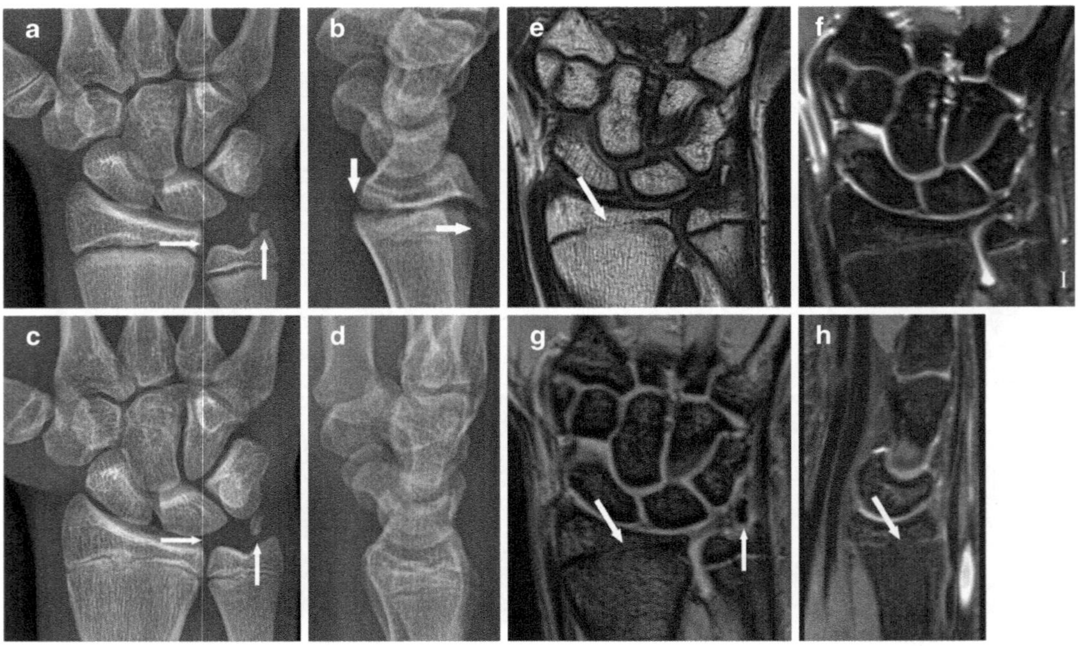

Fig. 8b Displaced fracture of the styloid process Gaulke type IIb and negative ulnar variance (**a**); Salter-Harris type II fracture—epiphysiolysis of the R (**b**); positive ulnar variance (**c**–**d**) after premature closure of the radial growth plate (**e**–**h**); non-union of the styloid fragment (**c**) with unstable TFFC (**g**)

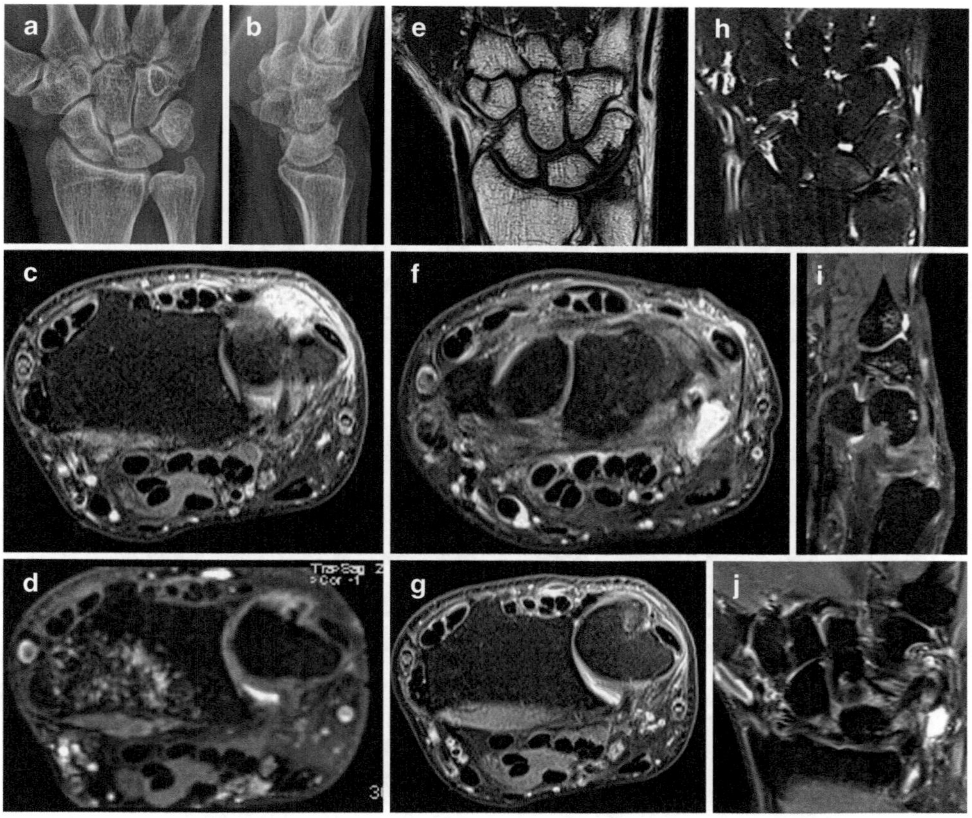

Fig. 9a Standard PA (**a**), and lateral (**b**) views; Ax T2-WI FS (**c**), and 3D GRE (**d**); Cor T1-WI (**e**), and T2-WI FS (**h**); Ax T2-WI FS (**f–g**); Sag (**i**), and Cor (**j**) 3D GRE

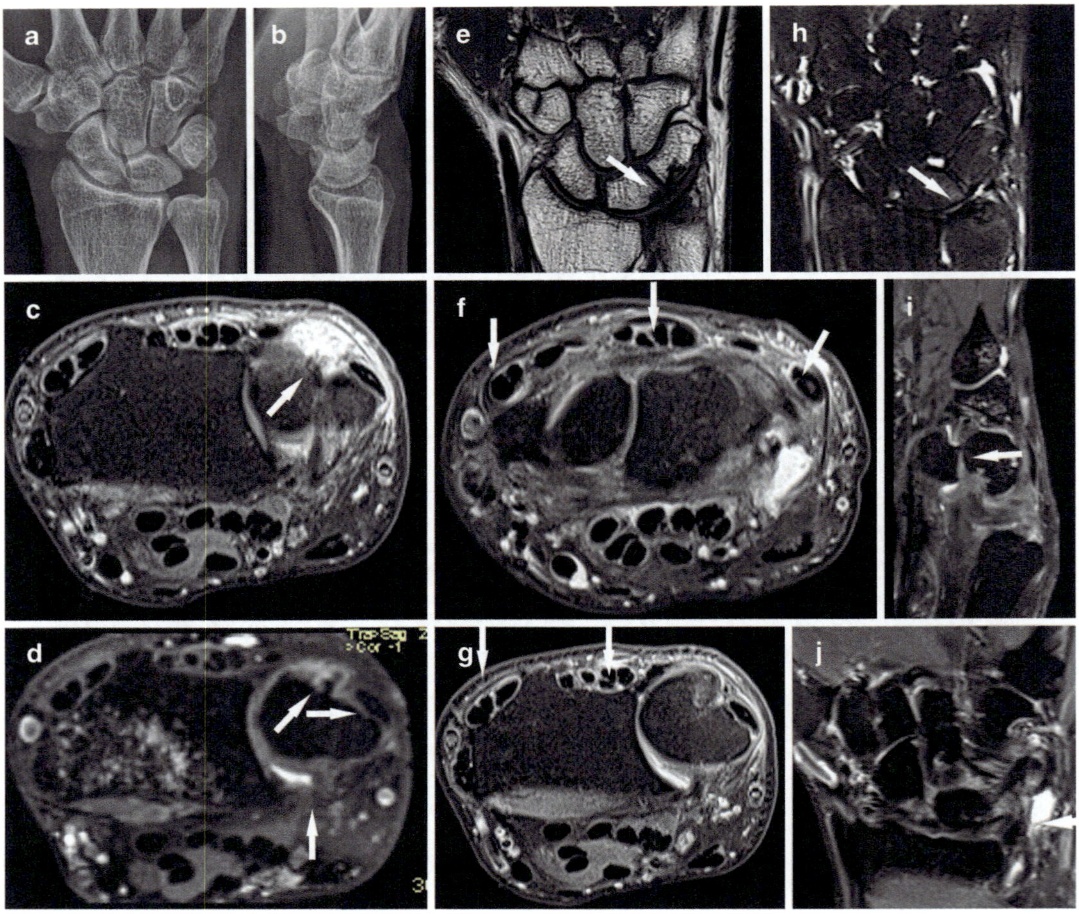

Fig. 9b Normal standard views (**a**, **b**). Second ulnar groove sign (**c**) witnessing a previous anterior ulnar luxation (**c**, **d**); laceration of the ventral distal RU ligament (**d**); subluxation of the ECU (**d**); oedema at the proximal-ulnar corner of the L and the adjacent Tri: starting UA? (**e**, **h**); mild tenosynovitis of extensor compartment II, IV and VI (**f**, **g**); OA of the TriP joint with osteophytes, hydrops in the proximal recess and distal narrowing of the joint (**i**, **j**)

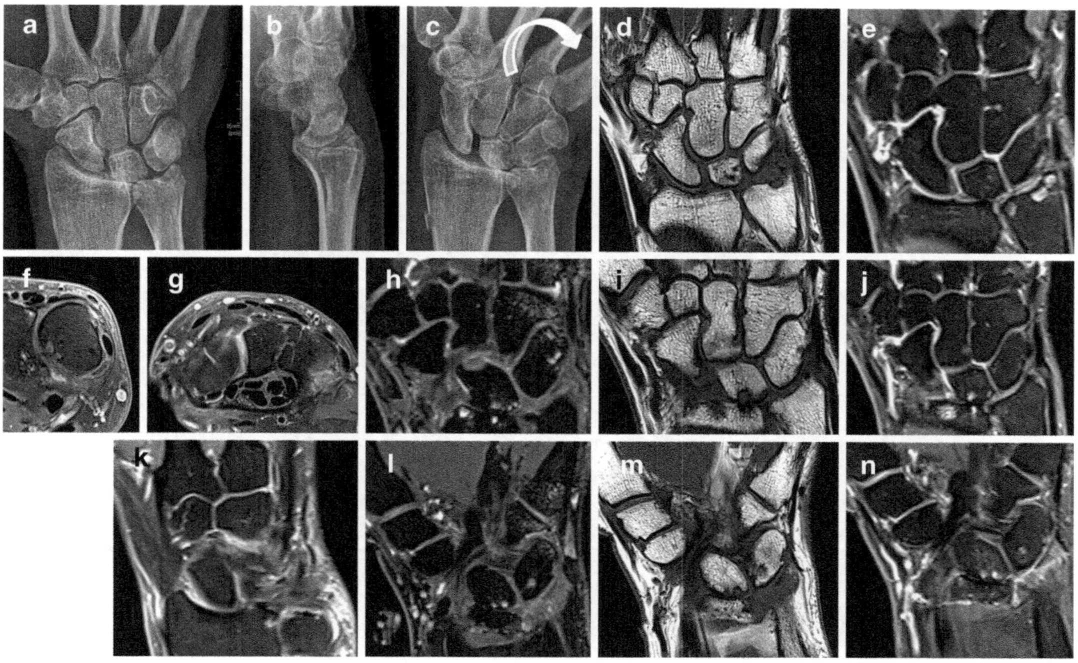

Fig. 10a Standard PA (**a**) and lateral (**b**) views, and PA view in ulnar deviation (**c**); Cor T1-WI (**d**, **i**, **m**), and T2-WI FS (**e**, **j**, **k**, **n**); Ax T2-WI FS (**f**, **g**); Cor 3D GRE (**h**, **l**)

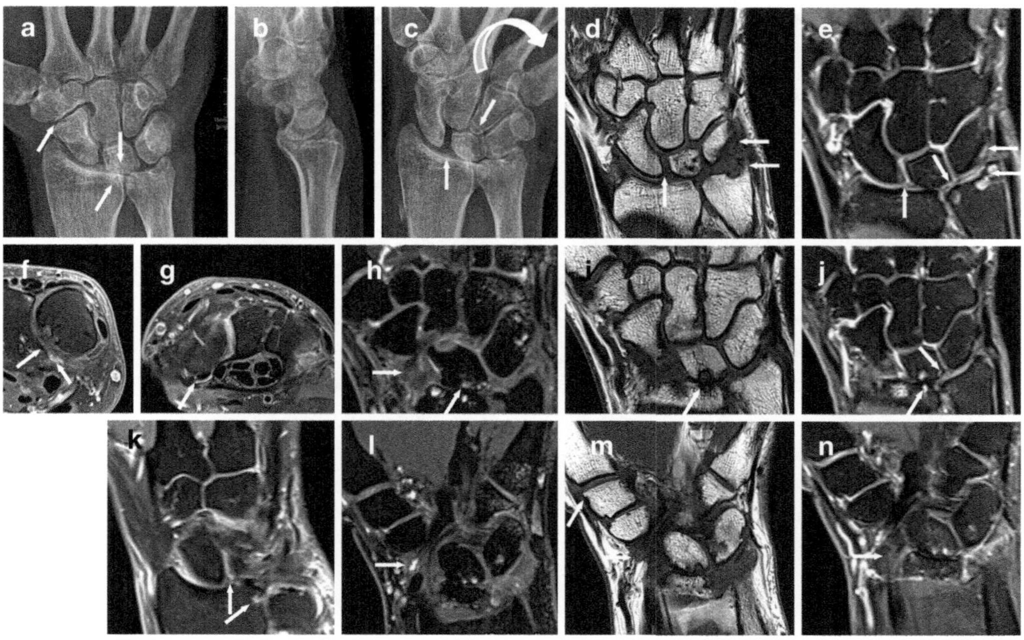

Fig. 10b OA STT (**a–b**, **m**) and RC joint (**a**, **i**, **j**); widening of the SL joint (**c**); narrowing of the HL joint and L Viegas type 2 (**c**). SL tear **d–e**, **k**); stylotriquetral abutment (**d**, **e**); UA (**e**, **j**); OA DRUJ (**f**, **k**); laceration of the anterior distal RU ligament (**f**); tenosynovitis of the FCR (**g**); partial laceration of the RSC (**h**, **l**, **n**)

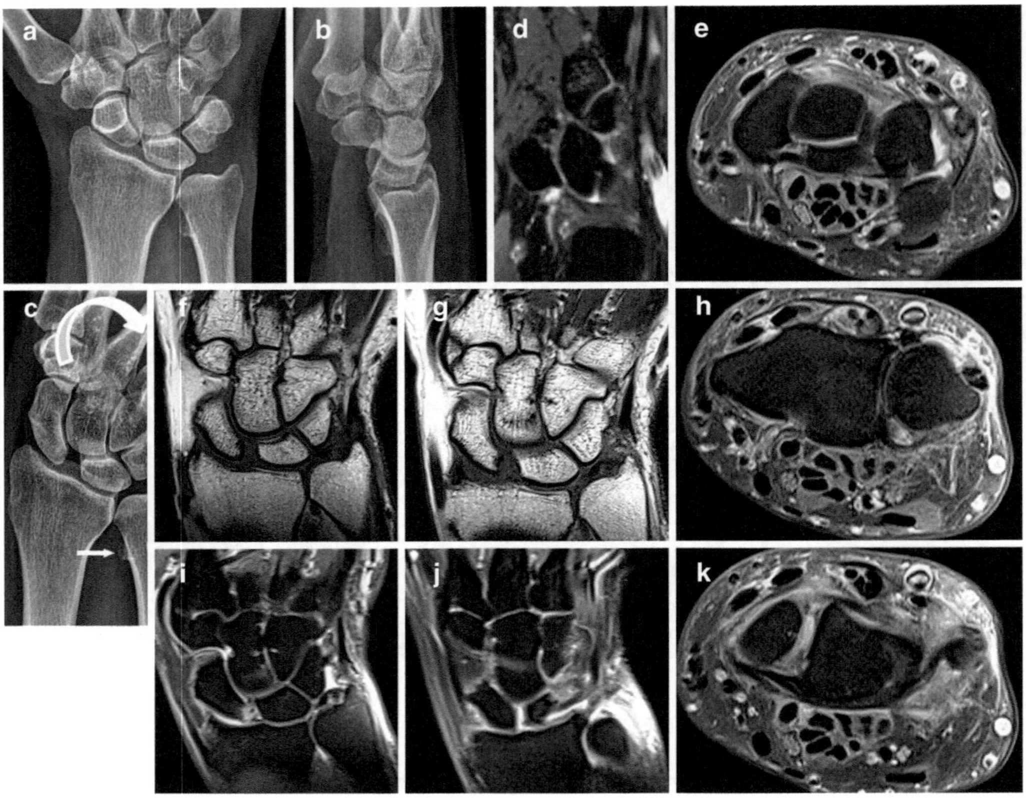

Fig. 11a Standard PA (**a**), and lateral (**b**) views, and AP view in ulnar deviation (**c**); Sag 3D GRE (**d**); Ax T2-WI FS (**e**, **h**, **k**); Cor T1-WI (**f**, **g**), and T2-WI FS (**i**, **j**)

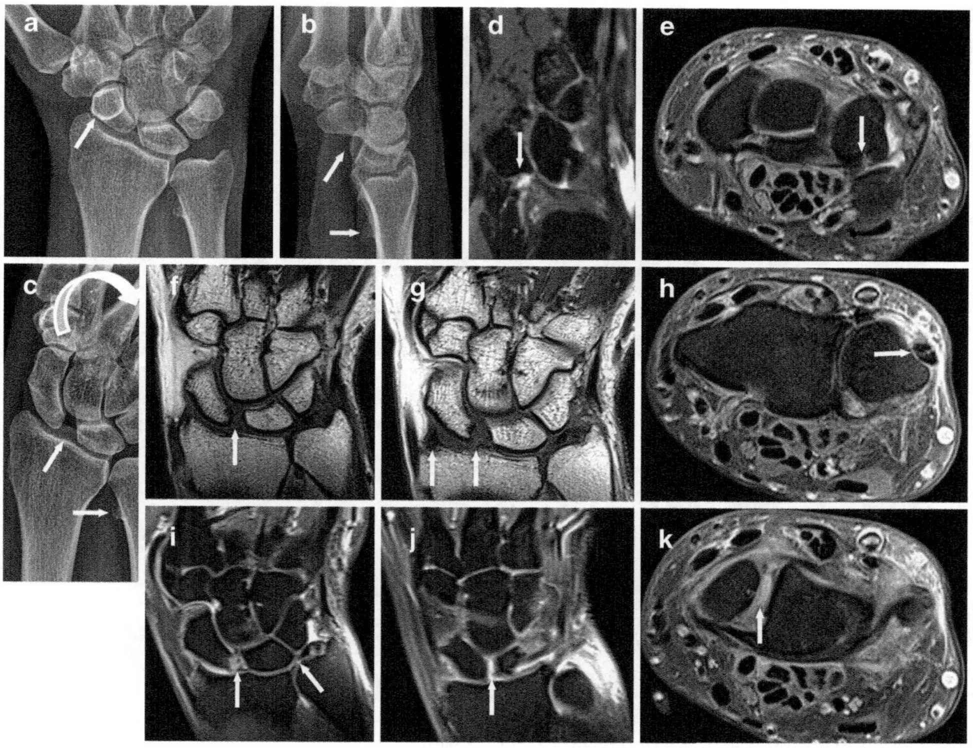

Fig. 11b Signet ring sign (**a**) and SL angle of >70° (**b**); small sessile osteochondroma (adult form) (**b**); OA TP joint (**d**, **e**); SL joint widening (**c**) and SL ligament tear (**f**, **g**, **i**–**k**); fissuration of the ECU tendon (**h**)

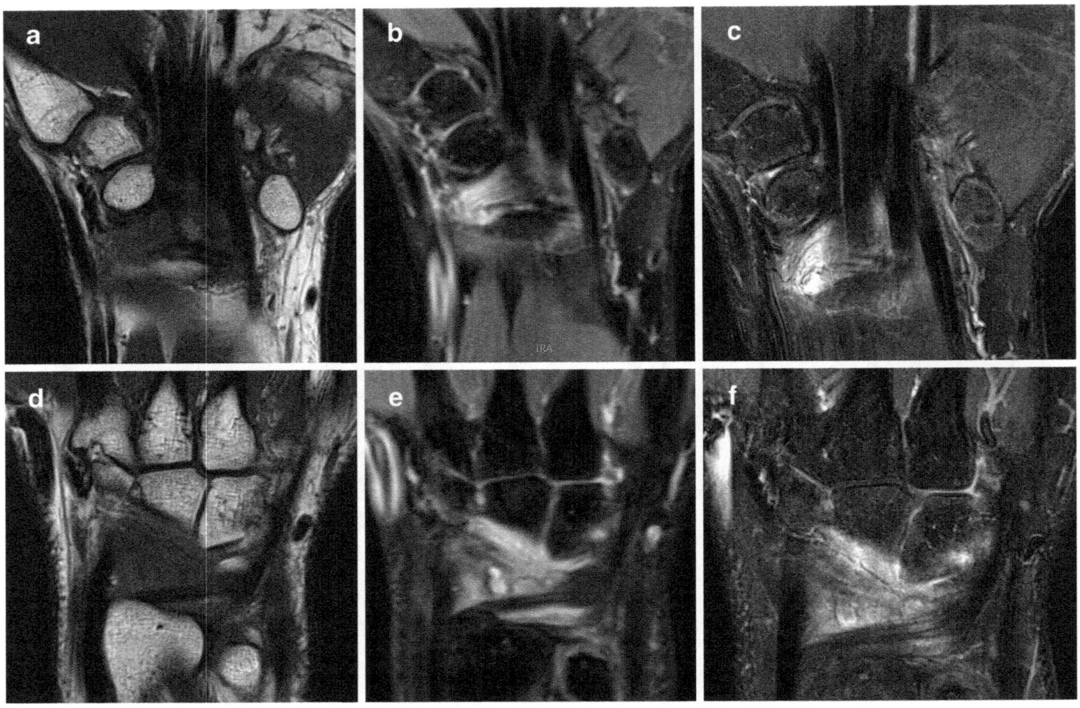

Fig. 12a Cor T1-WI (**a**, **d**), T2-WI FS (**b**, **e**), and T1-WI FS with CE (**c**, **f**)

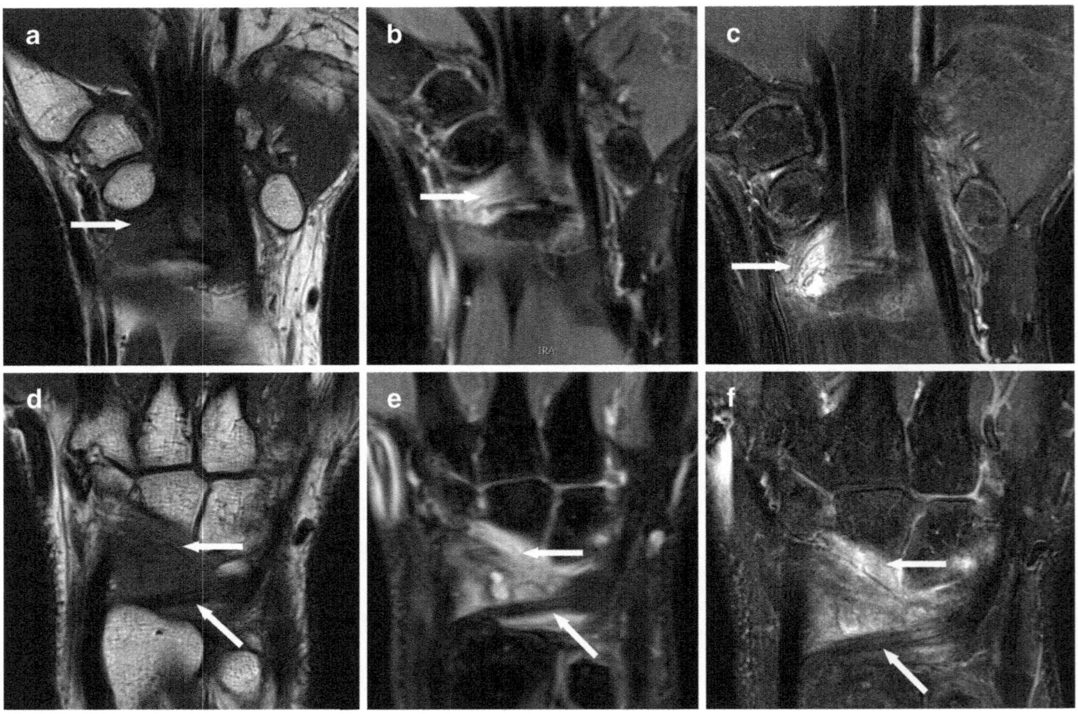

Fig. 12b Oedema/infiltration of the palmar RSC/RLT (**a**–**c**), and dorsal R-Tri (**d**–**f**) ligament. Intact dorsal R-Tri ligament (**d**–**f**)

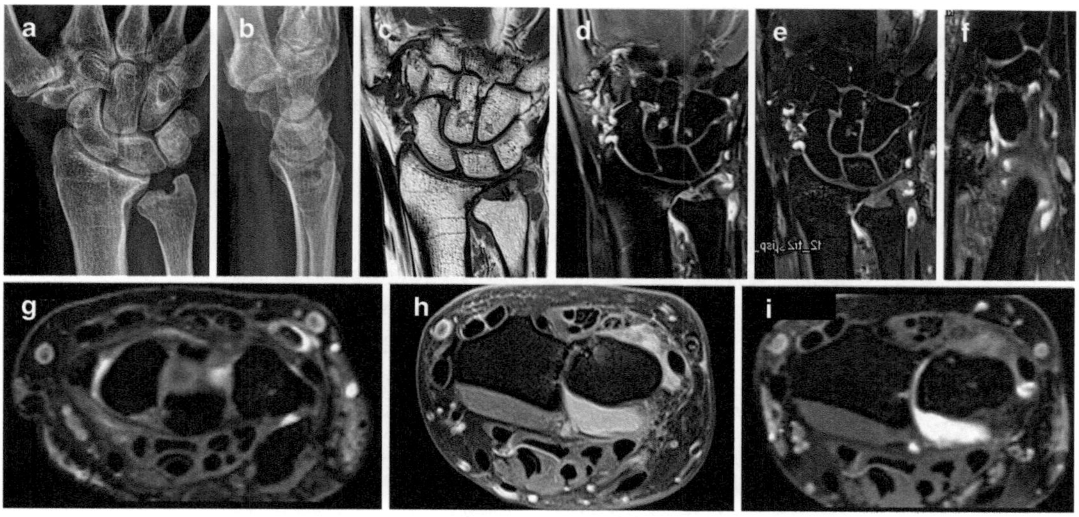

Fig. 13a Standard PA (**a**), and Lateral (**b**) views; Cor T1-WI (**c**), T2-WI FS (**d**); Cor (**e**), Sag (**f**), and Ax (**g**) 3D GRE; Ax T1-WI FS (**h**), and T2-WI FS (**i**)

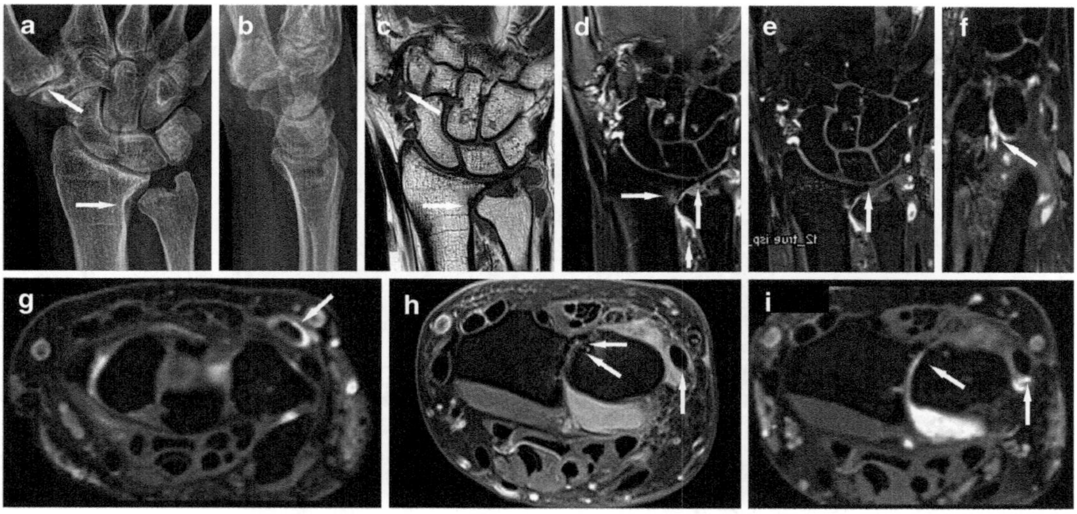

Fig. 13b OA of the STT joint (**a**–**c**); ulnar impingement (**c**, **d**, **h**, **i**); central TFCC tear type IC (**d**, **e**); OA of the TP joint (**f**); tenosynovitis of the EDM (**g**); deformed dorsal distal RU ligament (**h**); luxation of the ECU (**h**, **i**)

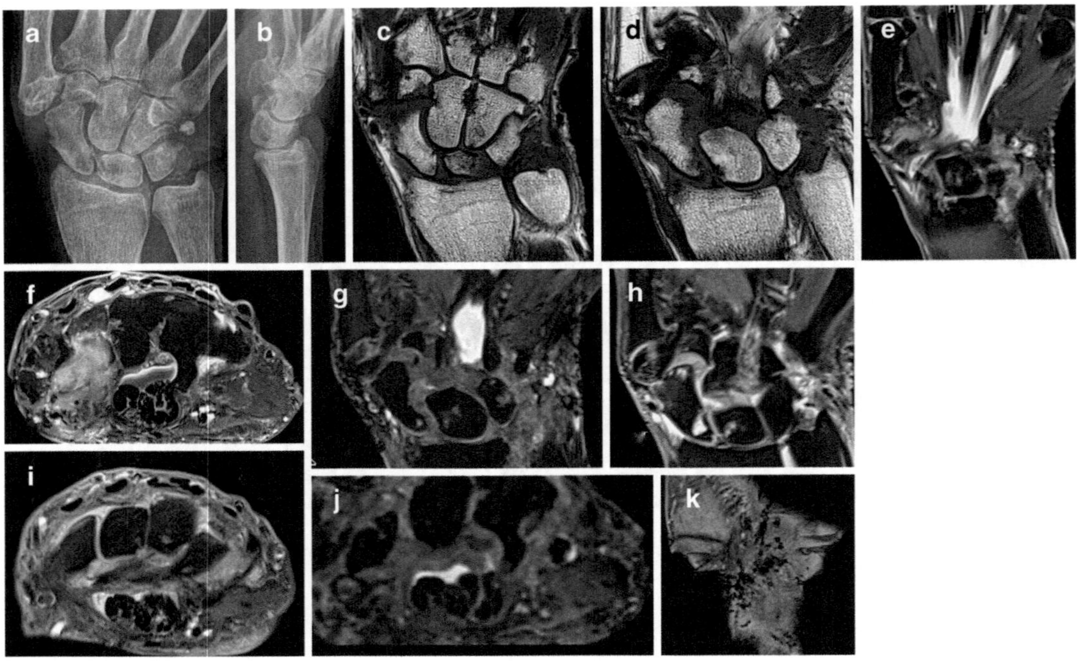

Fig. 14a Standard PA (**a**), and Lateral view (**b**); Cor T1-WI (**c–d**), and T2-WI FS (**e**); Ax T1-WI FS with CE (**f**); Cor 3D GRE (**g**), and T2-WI FS (**h**); Ax T2-WI FS (**i**), and 3D GRE (**j**); Cor 2D GRE (**k**)

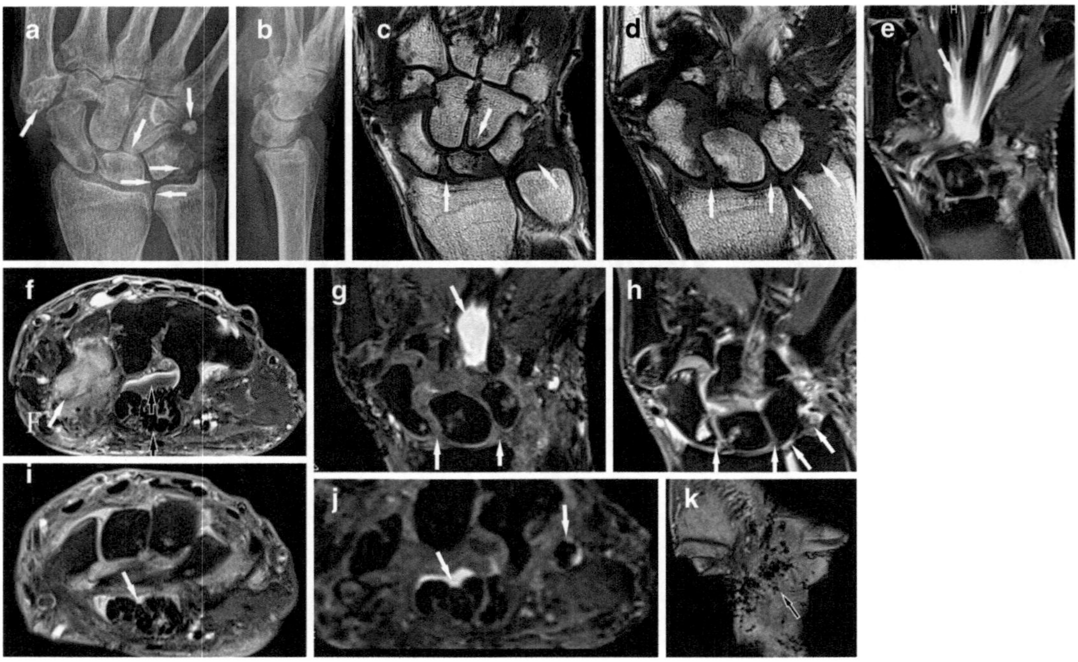

Fig. 14b Calcium deposits on the TFC and the hyaline cartilage of the DRU joint (**a–b**) suggestive of crystal arthropathy, type CPPD; positive ulnar variance (**a**); soft tissue calcification (**a**, **j**). HLA (**a**, **c**); resection of Tra with proximal migration of MC-I (**a**, **c**, **d**, **f**); signal alterations SL, LT and TFCC (**c**, **d**, **g**, **h**): CPPD and/or degenerative and/or laceration; susceptibility artefacts (**k**); status after surgery for CTS (**f**); tenosynovitis (**e**, **g**, **i–j**)

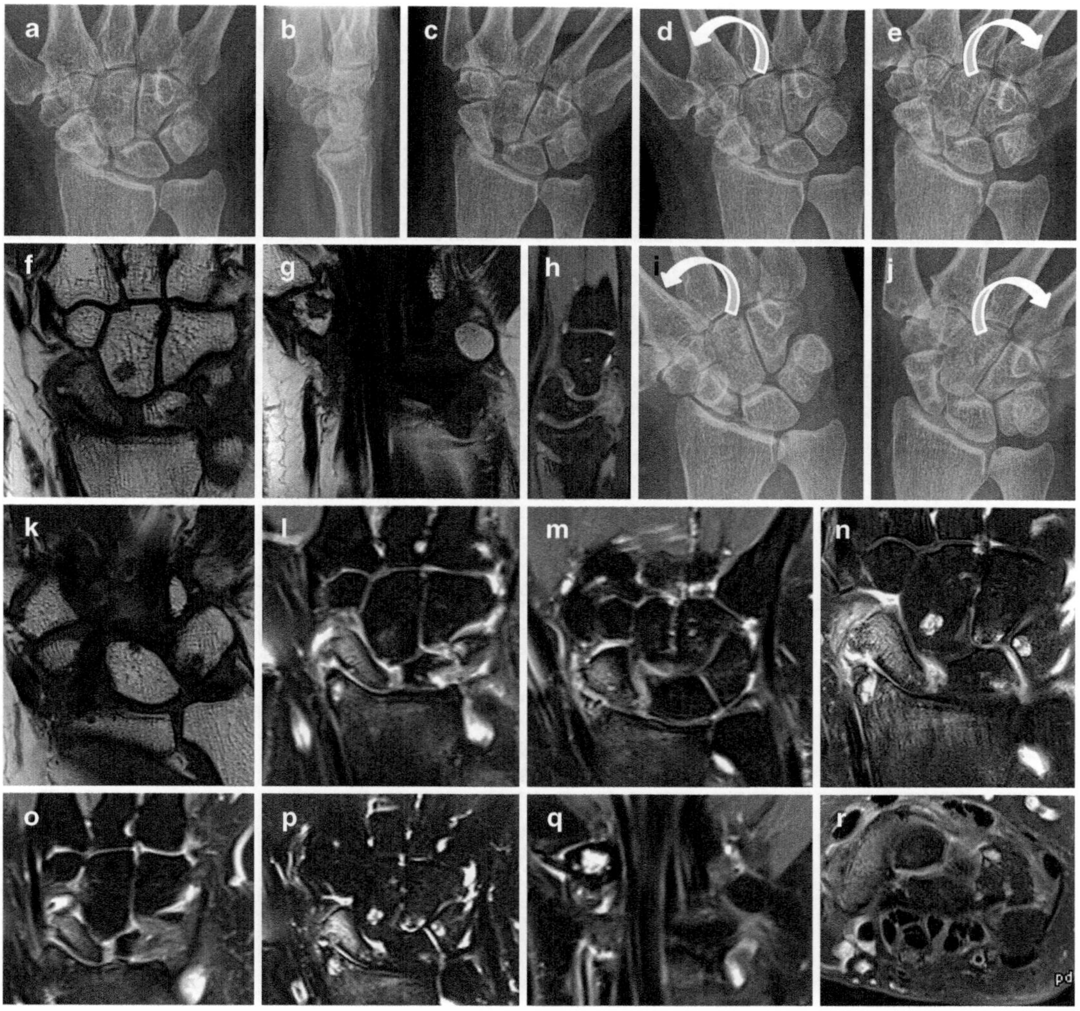

Fig. 15a Standard PA (**a**) and lateral (**b**) views; PA view with clenched fist (**c**), PA view—compared to the other side—in radial (**d**, **i**) and ulnar (**e**, **j**) deviation; Cor T1-WI (**f**, **g**, **k**); Sag 3D GRE (**h**); Cor T2-WI FS (**l**, **m**, **o**–**q**); Cor T1-WI FS with CE (**n**); Ax T2-WI FS (**r**)

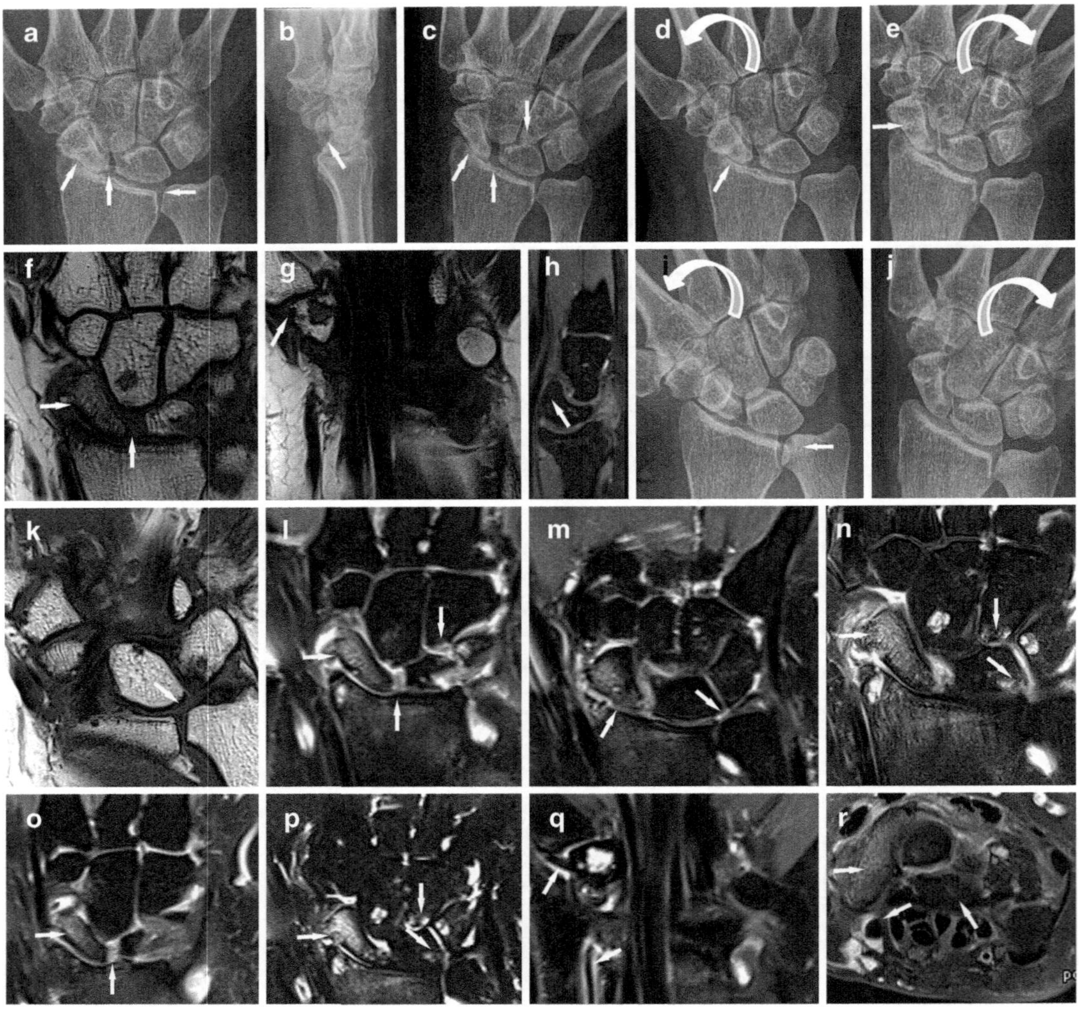

Fig. 15b Positive ulnar variance (**a**); rotatory subluxation of the S, and OA of the RCJ and MCJ (SLAC grade 3) (**a**, **c**, **d**, **h**, **m**); SL diastasis (**a**) increasing in UD (**c**) with SL lesion (**f**, **l**, **o**); static DISI with SL angle >70° (**b**, **h**); HLA (**c**, **l**); limited mobility in RD (**d**) and UD (**e**, **j**); OA of the CMC-1 joint (**g**) and at the other side DRUJ (**i**); TFCC lesion type II E (**k**, **m**, **n**); UA (**k**, **m**, **n**); tenosynovitis FCR (**q**, **r**); AVN of the S (**f**, **l**, **n**, **o**, **p**)

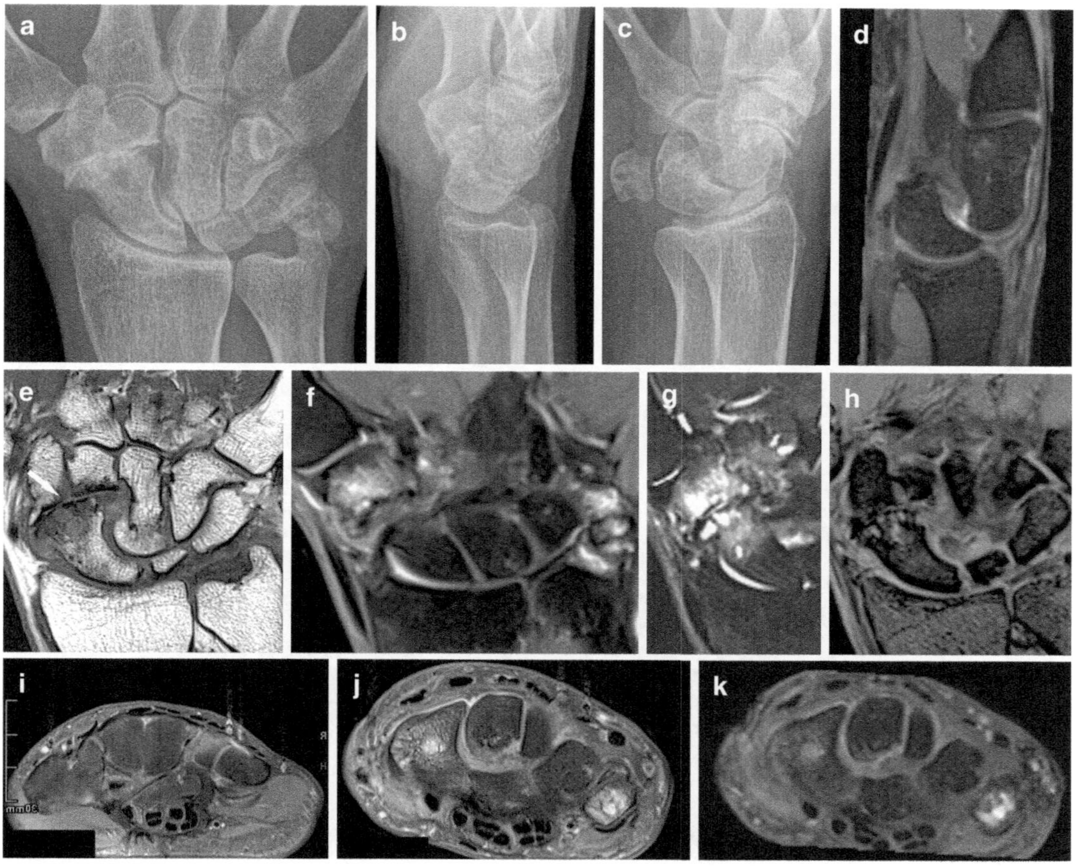

Fig. 16a Standard PA (**a**), and Lateral (**b**) views with 30° pronation (**c**); Sag 3D GRE (**d**); Cor T1-WI (**e**), T2-WI FS (**f**, **g**), 2D GRE (**h**); Ax T2-WI FS (**i**, **k**), and T1-WI FS with CE (**j**)

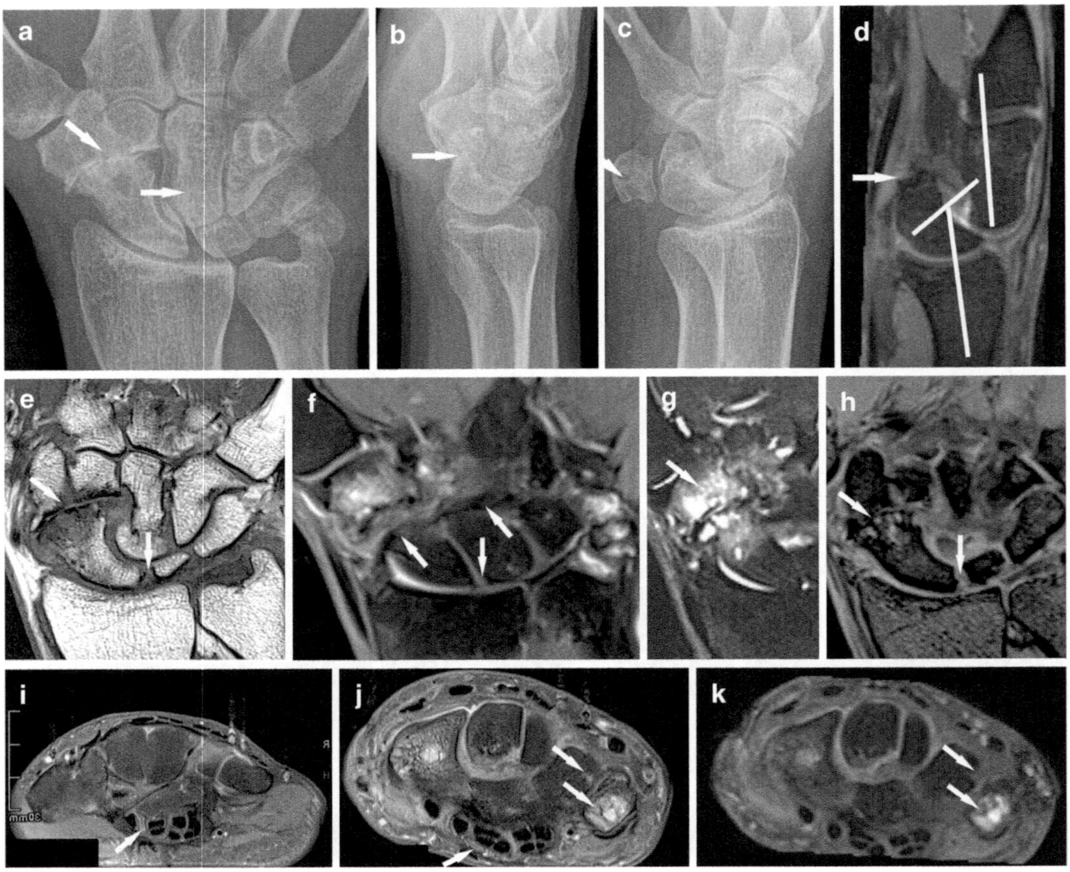

Fig. 16b CPPD typical at the STT joint (**a**, **e**, **g**, **h**) and TP (**c**, **j**, **k**); DISI with Z-configuration of the R-L-C axis (**b**, **d**); SL tear (**e**, **f**, **h**); midcarpal instability with proximal migration of the C (**a**, **d**) and prominent L tilted in the carpal tunnel (**b**, **d**) compressing the flexor tendons and the median nerve (**i**, **j**); deformed extrinsic palmar RSC ligament (**f**)

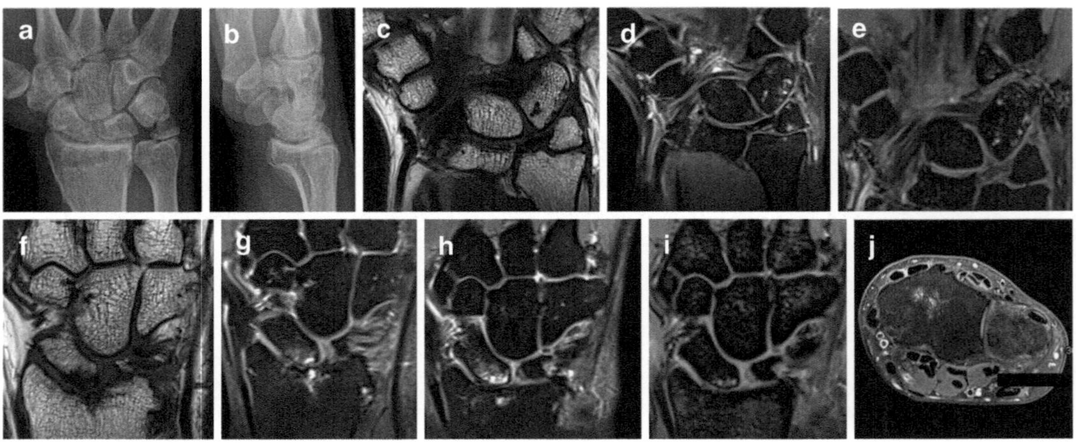

Fig. 17a Standard PA (**a**) and lateral (**b**) views; Cor T1-WI (**c**, **f**), 3D GRE (**d**, **e**, **i**), T2-WI FS (**g**, **h**); and Ax T2-WI FS (**j**)

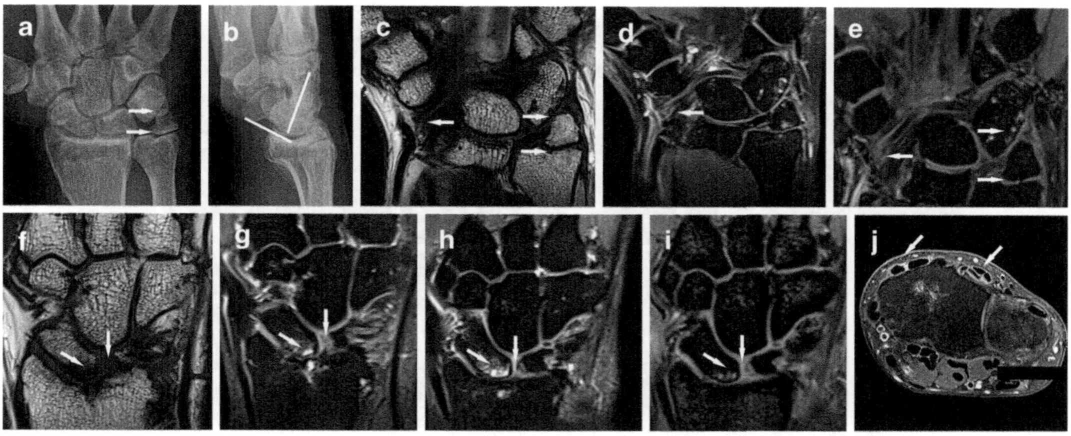

Fig. 17b Neo-articulation at the base of the ulnar styloid process (**a**, **c**, **e**); stylotriquetral abutment (**a**, **c**, **e**); DISI configuration (**b**);oedematous infiltration of the RSC ligament (**c**–**e**); SL tear (**f**–**i**); R-S abutment (**f**–**i**); tenosynovitis extensor compartment 2 and 4 (**j**)

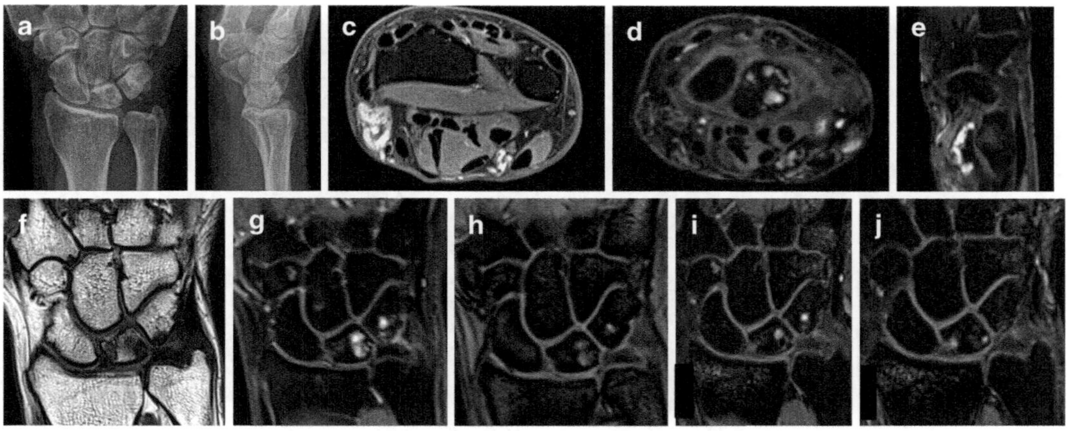

Fig. 18a Standard PA (**a**) and lateral (**b**) views; Ax T2-WI FS (**c**); AX (**d**) and Sag (**e**) 3D GRE; Cor T1-WI (**f**), T2-WI FS (**g**), and 3D GRE (**h**–**j**)

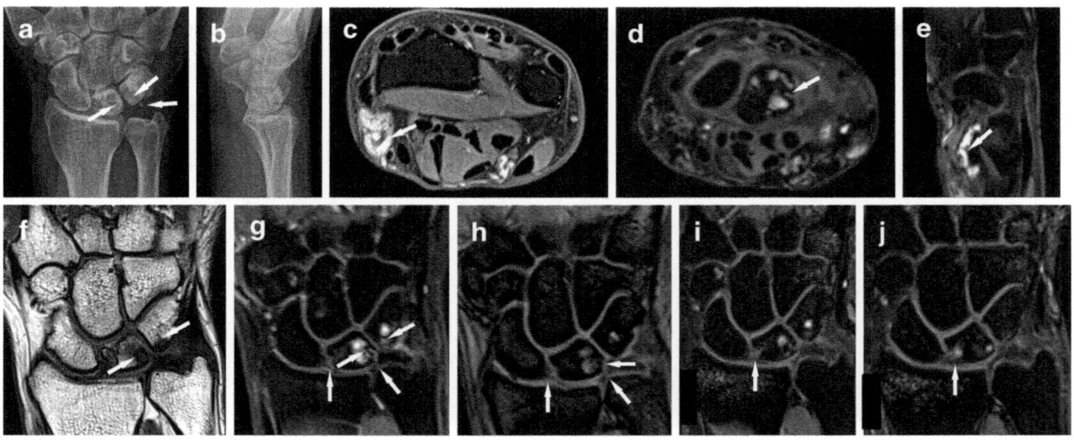

Fig. 18b LT tear with subchondral cysts (**a**–**b**, **d**, **f**, **g**), and loose and displaced fragment at the insertion (**a**, **h**); palmar ASC (**c**, **e**), SL tear with scar tissue (**g**–**j**); central degenerative TFCC lesion II C (**h**)

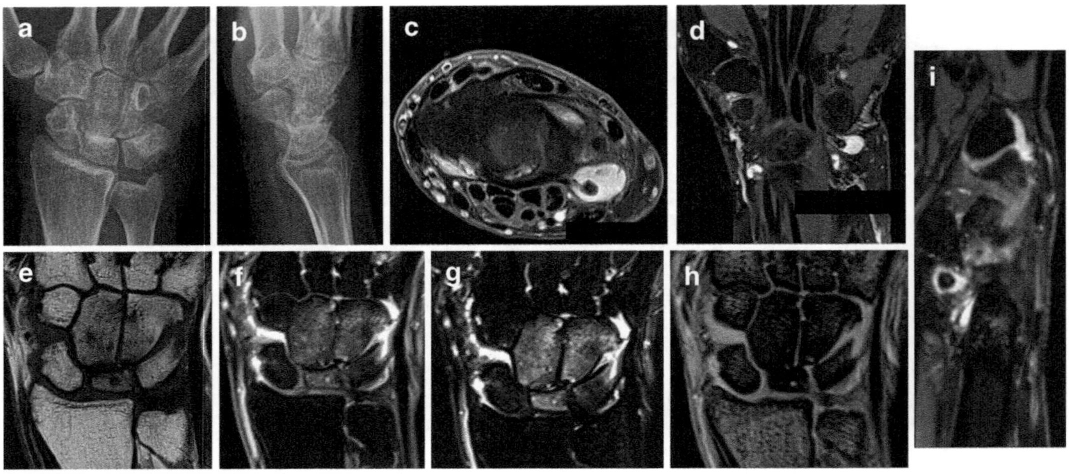

Fig. 19a Standard PA (**a**) and lateral (**b**) views; Ax T2-WI FS (**c**); Cor 3D GRE (**d**), T1-WI (**e**), T2-WI FS (**f**, **g**), and 2D GRE (**h**); Sag 3D GRE (**i**)

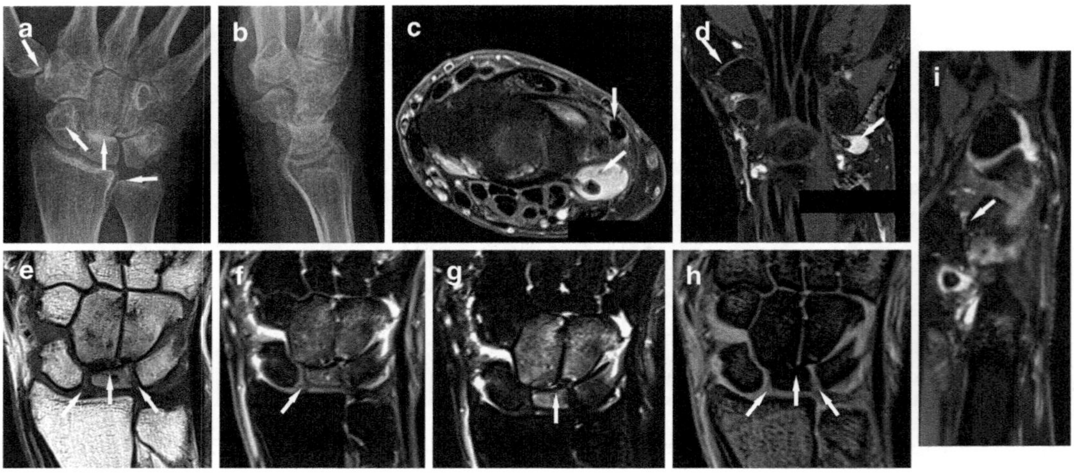

Fig. 19b negative ulnar variance (**a**); rotatory subluxation of the S (**a**–**b**); OA of the MedC-J (**a**, **e**, **g**, **h**) and CMC-I (**a**, **d**); tenosynovitis ECU (**c**); hydrops, subluxation and tilting of the P, and OCM at the Tri-P joint (**c**, **d**, **i**); SL (**e**, **f**) and LT (**e**, **h**) tear; step off at the 1st and 2nd line of Gilula (**a**, **h**)

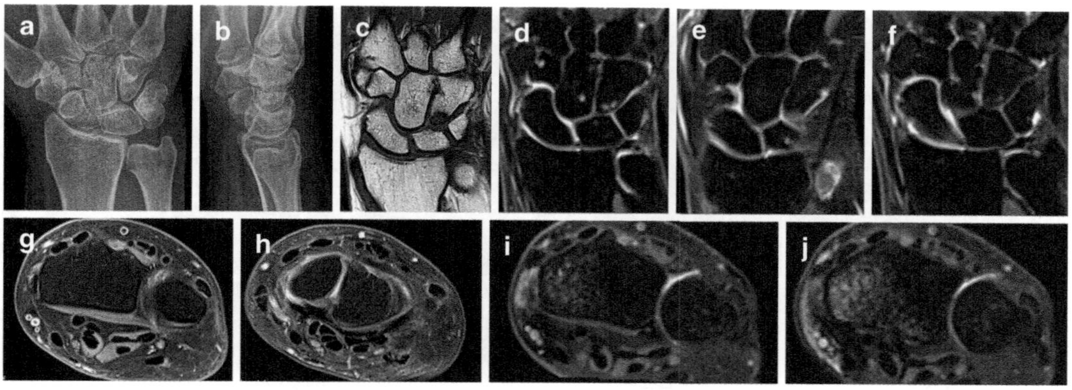

Fig. 20a Standard PA (**a**) and lateral (**b**) views; Cor T1-WI (**c**), T2-WI FS (**d–f**); Ax T2-WI FS (**g**, **h**), and 3D GRE (**i**, **j**)

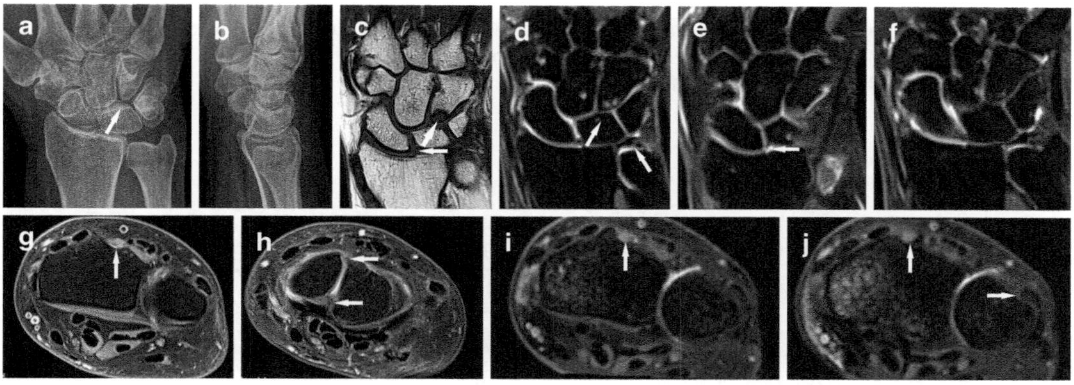

Fig. 20b Viegas type 2 L with HLA (**a**, **c**, **d**); SL tear with DISI (**b**, **e–f**, **h**); TFCC tear type Ib proximal insertion (**d**); rupture EPL (**g**, **i**, **j**); subluxation ECU (**j**); mild tenosynovitis extensor compartment 1–2, and 4–6 (**g**, **h**)

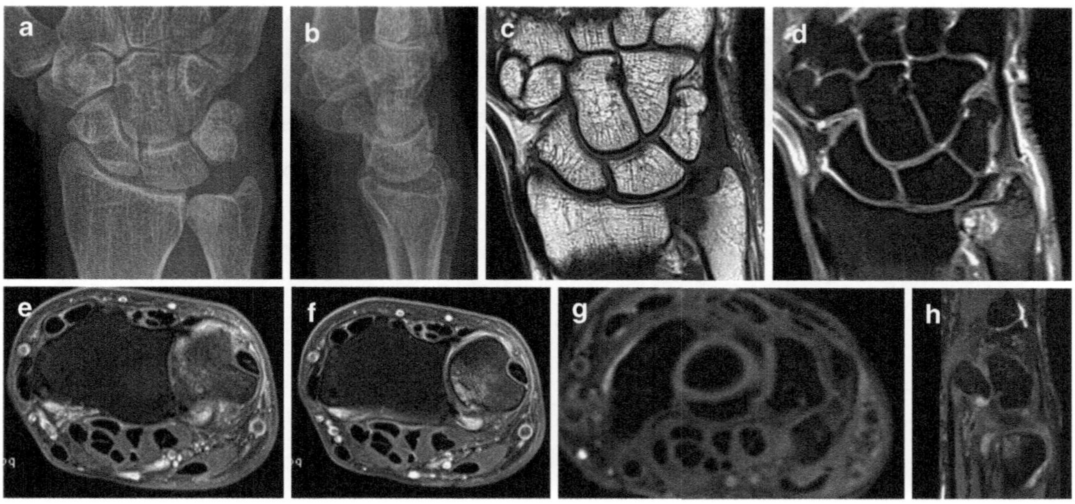

Fig. 21a Standard PA (**a**), and Lateral (**b**) views; Cor T1-WI (**c**), T2-WI FS (**d**); Ax T2-WI FS (**e**, **f**); Ax (**g**), and Sag (**h**) 3D GRE

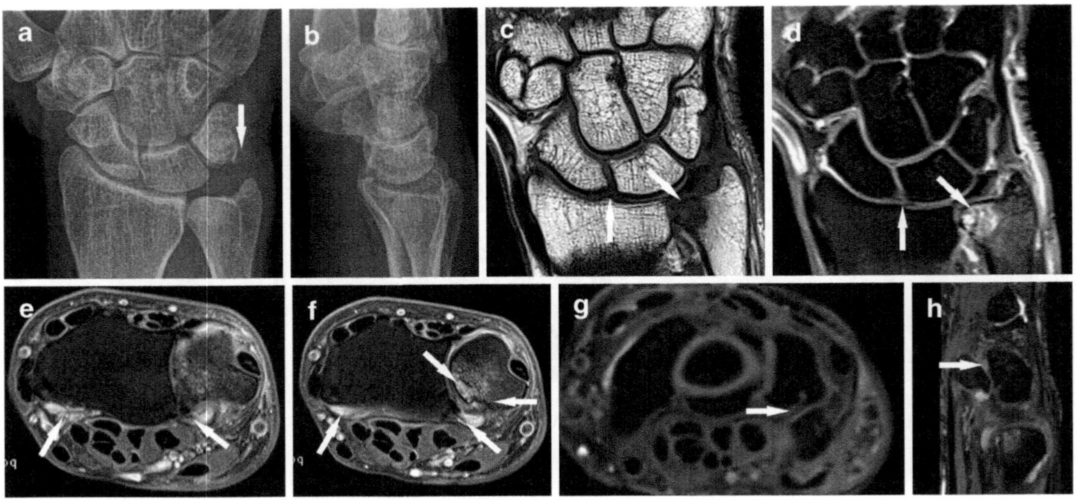

Fig. 21b Calcification at the ECU insertion (**a**–**b**); SL tear (**c**, **d**); small radiopalmar ASC (**e**, **f**); sequel dorsal U luxation with palmar RU ligament lesion (**e**, **f**) and oedema (**c**, **f**) and cortical impression at the U head (**f**); OA Tri-P joint (**g**, **h**)

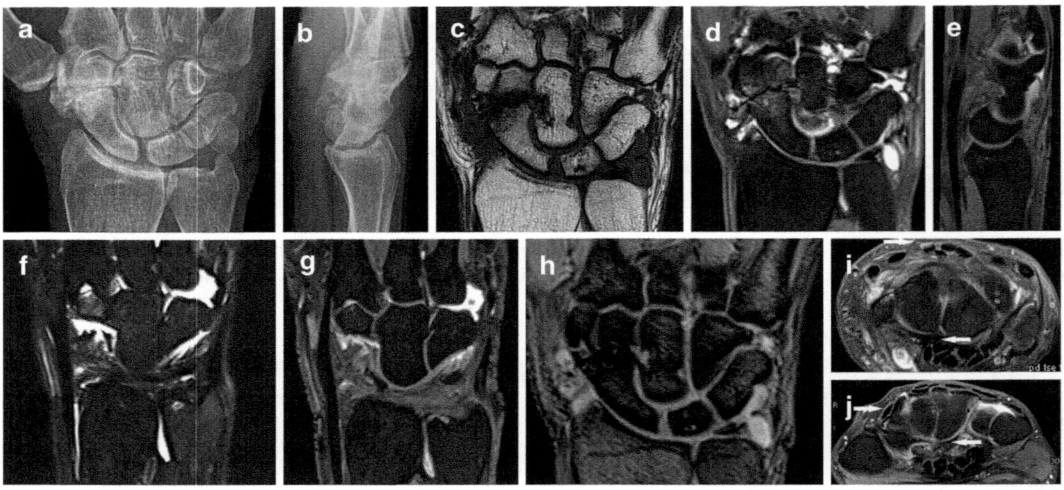

Fig. 22a Standard PA (**a**) and lateral (**b**) views; Cor T1-WI (**c**), T2-WI FS (**d**); Sag 3D GRE (**e**); Cor T2-WI FS (**f**, **g**); Ax t2-WI FS (**i**, **j**)

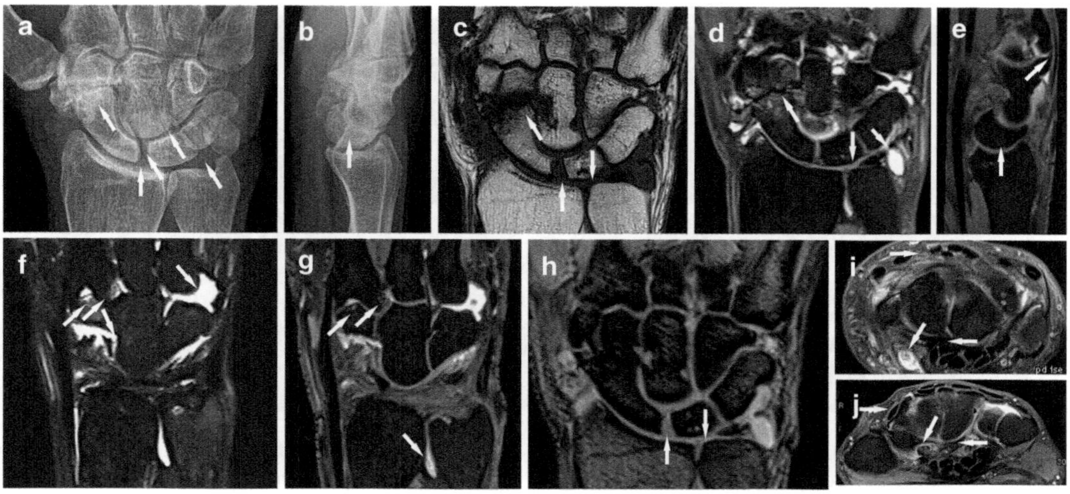

Fig. 22b Vacuum phenomenon at the SL joint (**a**); CPPD at the STT joint (**a**, **c**, **d**) with calcium deposits MCJ and at SL and TFCC (**a**); hydrops prestyloid recess RCJ (**d**), MCJ and CMC joint (**f**, **g**), and DRUJ (**g**); SL tear (**a**, **c**, **h**); DISI (**b**, **e**); CB CMC 2–3 (**e–g**); tenosynovitis FCR (**i**, **j**); debris space of Parona after CTS release (**i**, **j**); mild tenosynovitis extensor compartment 2 and 4 (**i**, **j**)

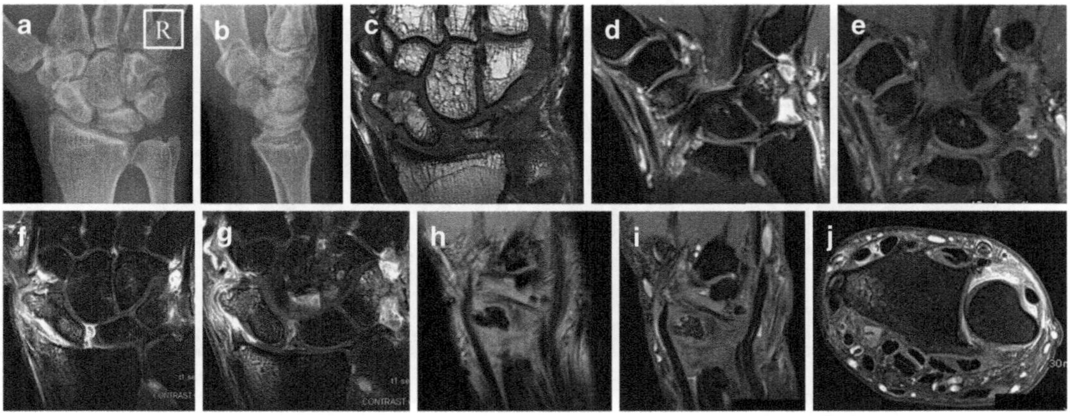

Fig. 23a Standard PA (**a**), and Lateral (**b**) views; Cor T1-WI (**c**), T2-WI FS (**d**), 3D GRE (**e**, **h**, **i**); Cor T1-WI FS with CE (**f**, **g**); Ax T2-WI FS (**j**). (Note: same patient as Fig. 23/right side)

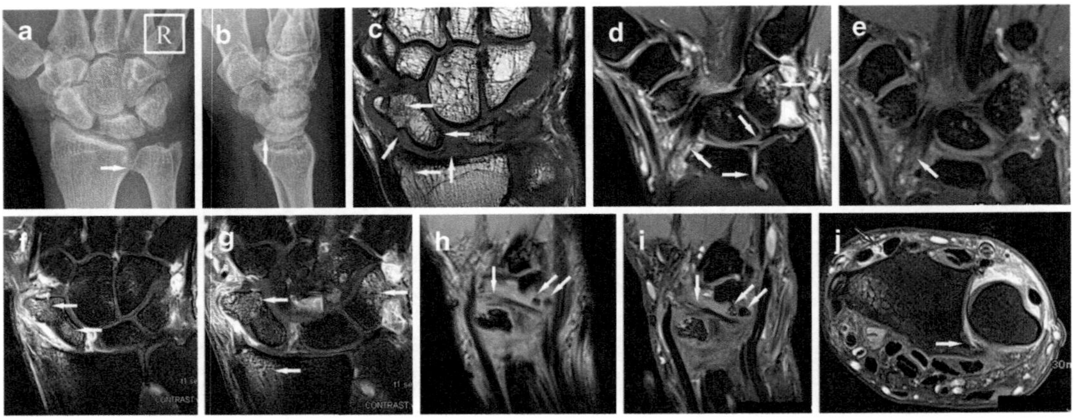

Fig. 23b OA DRUJ (**a**); DISI (**b**); old S waist # with cortical step off and more recent # of the tuberculum (**c**, **f**, **g**); SL tear (**c**); TFCC tear type I A (**d**); hydrops DRUJ (**d**); tear extrinsic RSC/RLT (**d**, **e**); dorsal fragments after recent Tri fracture (**d**, **g**, **h**, **i**); CE synovial proliferation around the S (**f**, **g**); rupture of the extrinsic dorsal S-Tri ligament (**h**, **i**); tenosynovitis extensor compartment 2 (**j**)

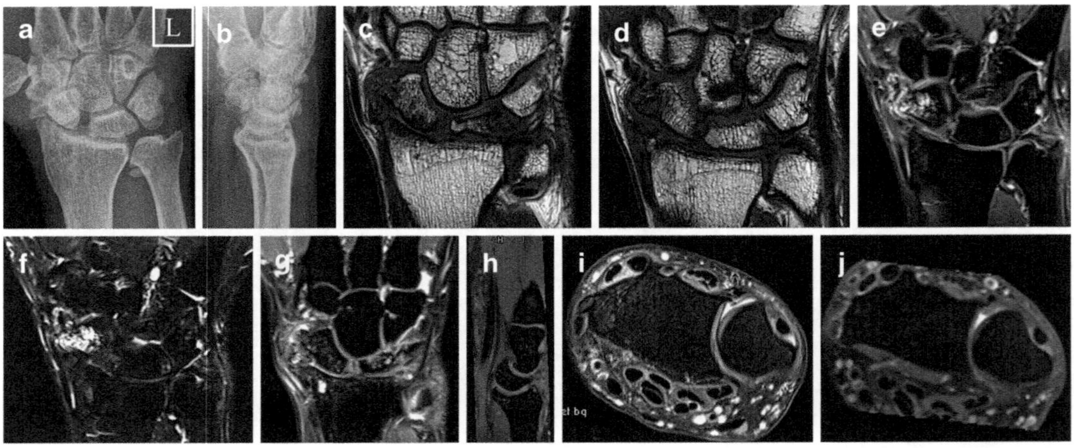

Fig. 24a Standard PA (**a**) and lateral (**b**) views; Cor T1-WI (**c**, **d**), T2-WI FS (**e**, **f**), 3D GRE (**g**); Sag 3D GRE (**h**); Ax T2-WI FS (**i**), and 3D GRE (**j**) (Note: same patient as Fig. 22/left side)

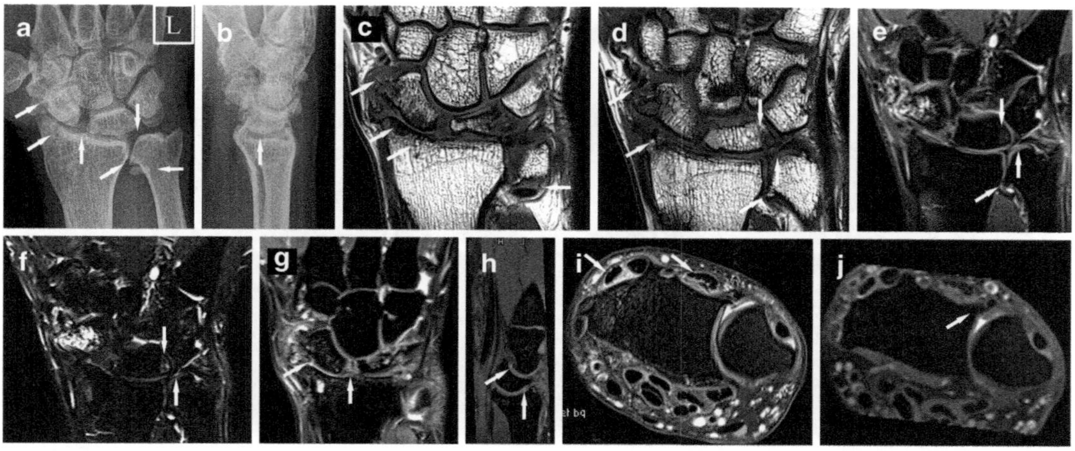

Fig. 24b SL diastasis (**a**) with DISI (**b**, **h**), and SL tear (**g**); OA at the R-S (**a**, **c**, **d**), STT (**a**, **c**, **d**), DRU (**a**, **e**), and MC (**h**) joint; positive ulnar variance (**a**) with starting UA (**a**, **d**, **e**), and TFCC lesion type II E (**e**, **f**); loose bony fragment anterior of the U (**a**, **c**); tenosynovitis especially extensor compartment 2 and 4 (**i**); loose fragment at the dorsal rim of the DRUJ (**j**)

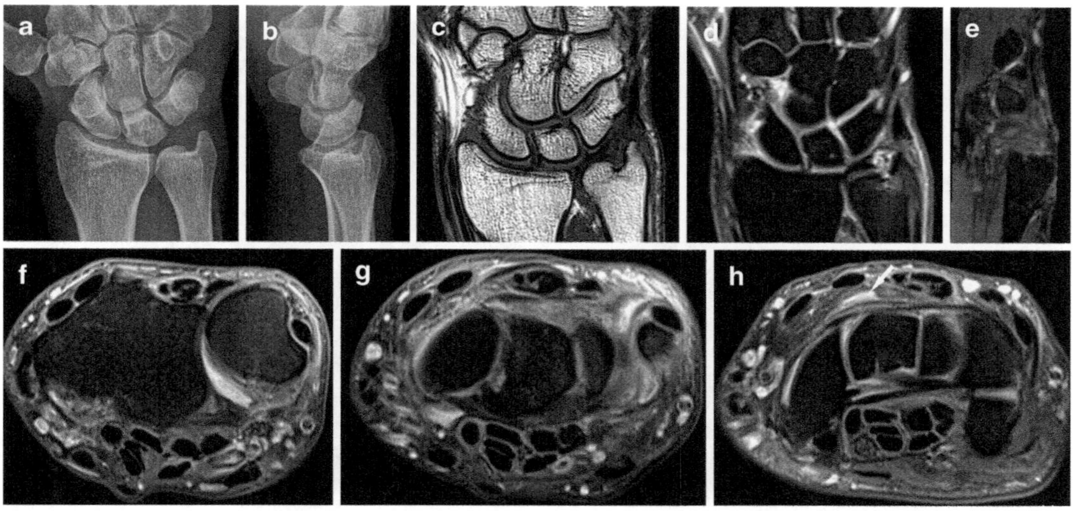

Fig. 25a Standard PA (**a**), and Lateral (**b**) views; Cor T1-WI (**c**), and T2-WI FS (**d**); Sag 3D GRE (**e**); Ax T2-WI FS (**f**–**h**)

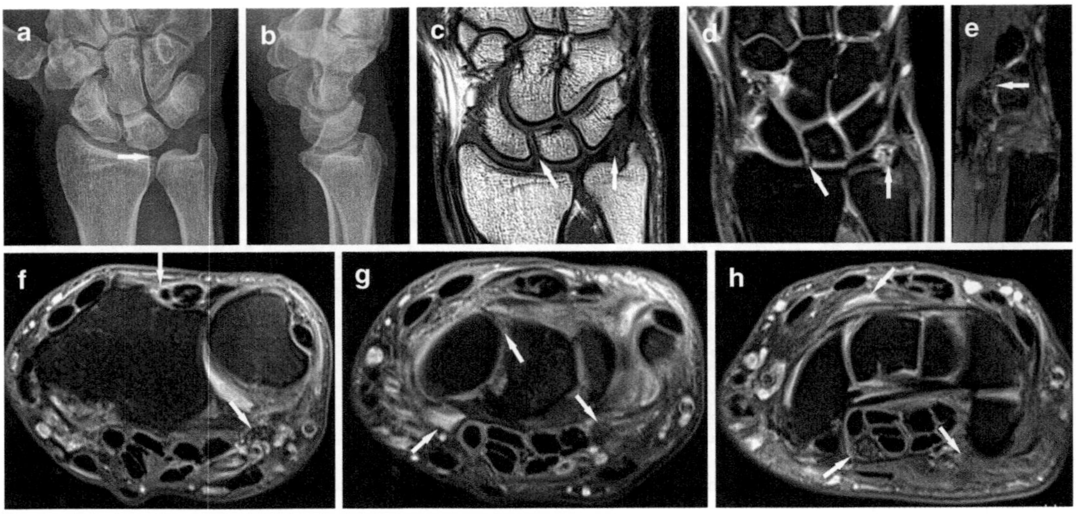

Fig. 25b Positive ulnar variance (**a**); TFCC tear type I B (**c**, **d**); SL tear (**c**, **d**, **g**) with palmar (**g**) and dorsal (**h**) ASC; distal # of the P (**e**); tenosynovitis ED compartment 4 (**f**); ulnar (**f–h**), and median (**h**) nerve neuritis

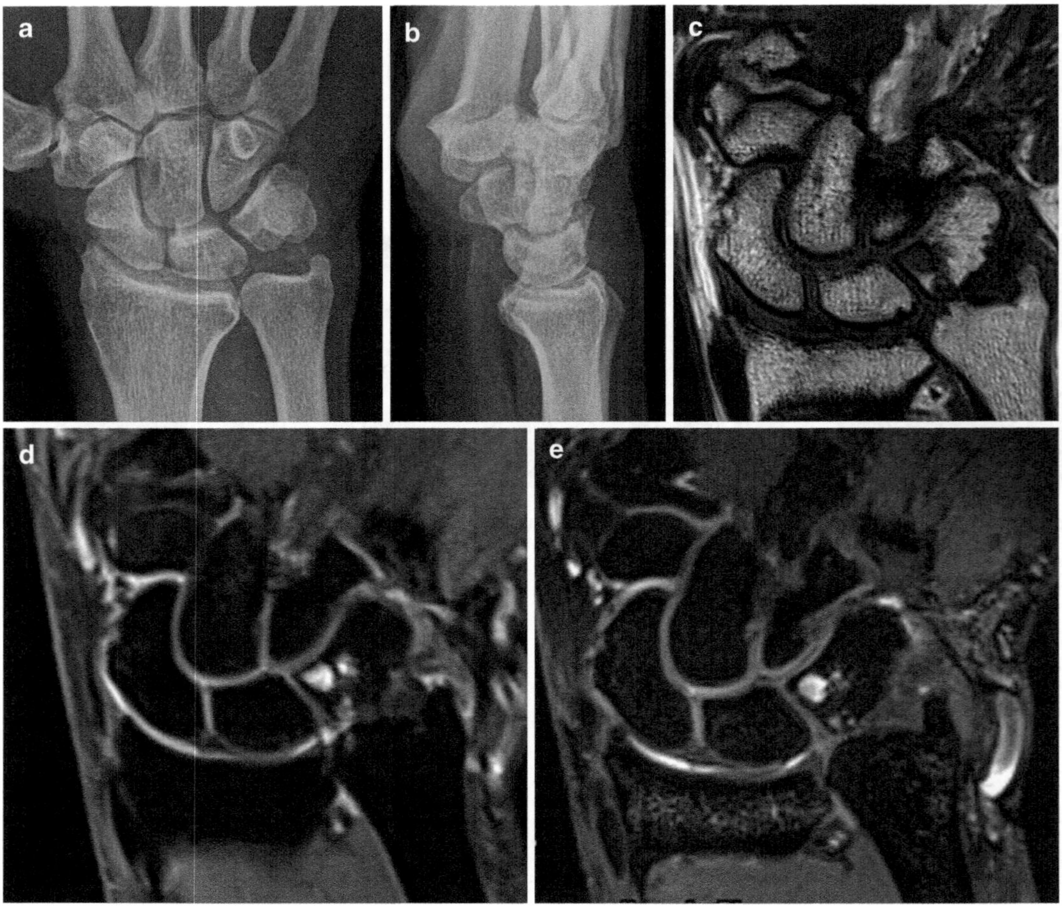

Fig. 26a Standard PA (**a**) and lateral (**b**) views; Cor T1-WI (**c**), T2-WI FS (**d**), and 3D GRE (**e**)

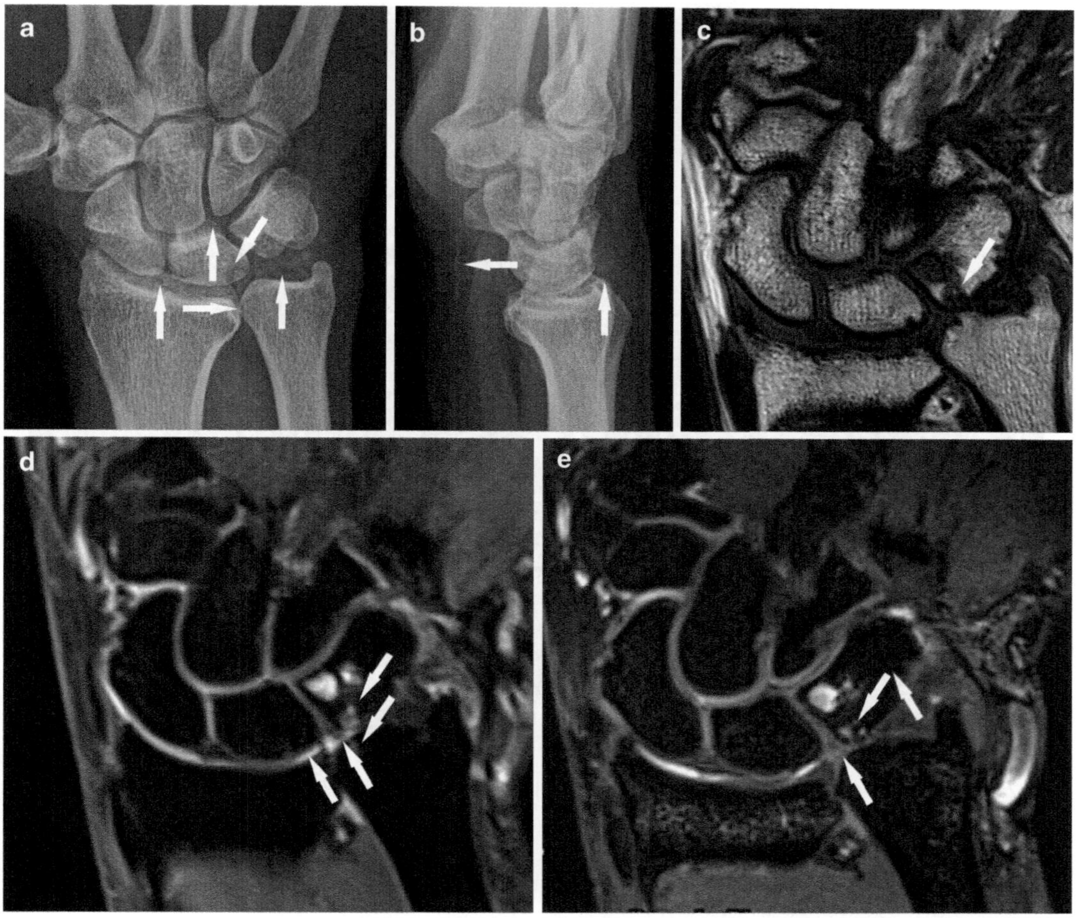

Fig. 26b Positive ulnar variance (**a**); CPPD with calcium deposits at the MC-, RC-, and DRUJ, SL, and TFCC (**a**); UA (**a**, **c**–**e**); atheromatous radial artery (**b**); degenerative TFCC type 2E (**d**, **e**)

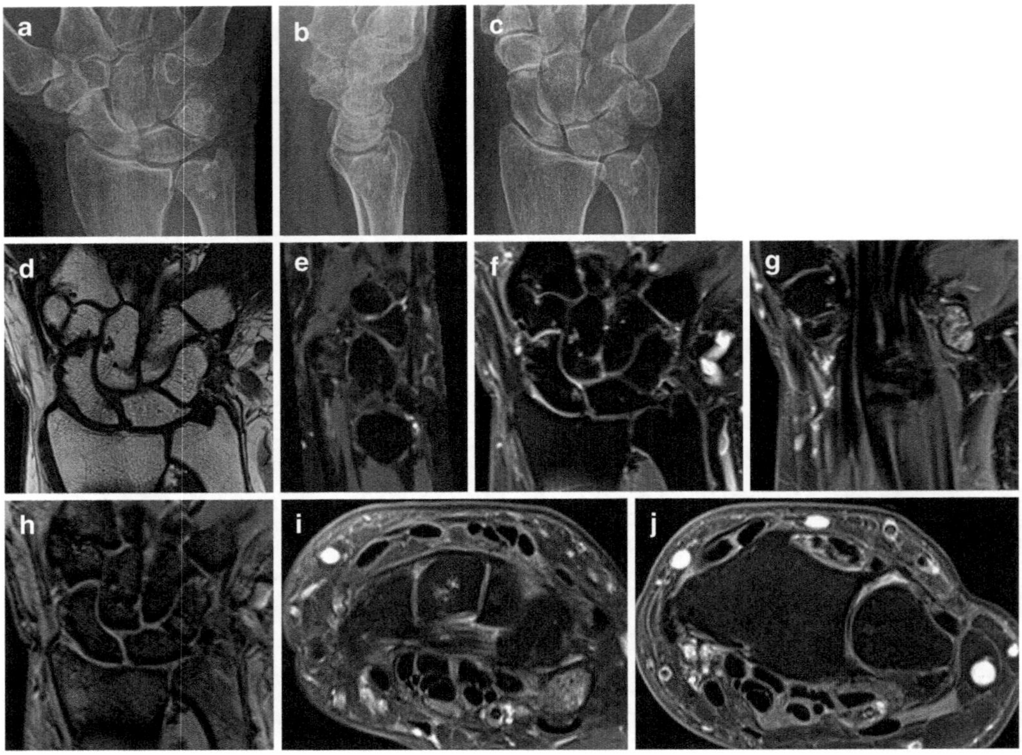

Fig. 27a Standard PA (**a**) and Lateral (**b**) views with clenched fist (**c**); Cor T1-WI (**d**); Sag 3D GRE (**e**); Cor T2-WI FS (**f–g**), and 2D GRE (**h**); Ax T2-WI FS (**i–j**)

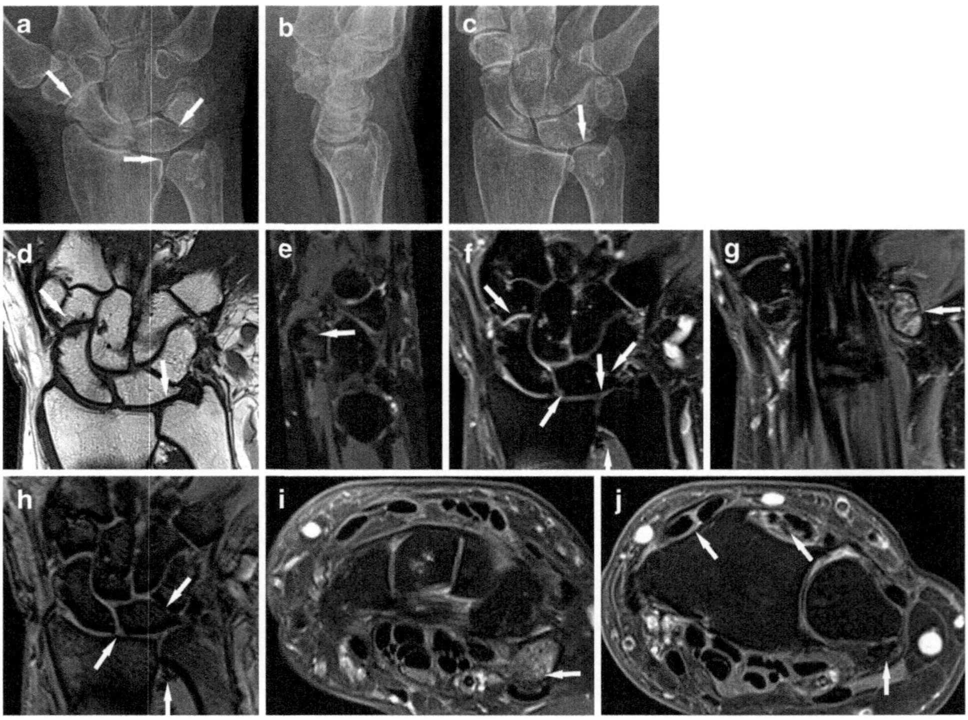

Fig. 27b Positive ulnar variance (**a**); OA STT (**a**, **d**); chondromalacia LT (**a**, **f**, **h**); UA (**c**, **d**, **f**); degenerative TFCC type 2E (**d**, **f**); # P (**e**, **g**, **i**): SL tear (**f**, **h**); OCM DRUJ (**h**, **j**); tenosynovitis extensor compartment 2 and 4 (**j**)

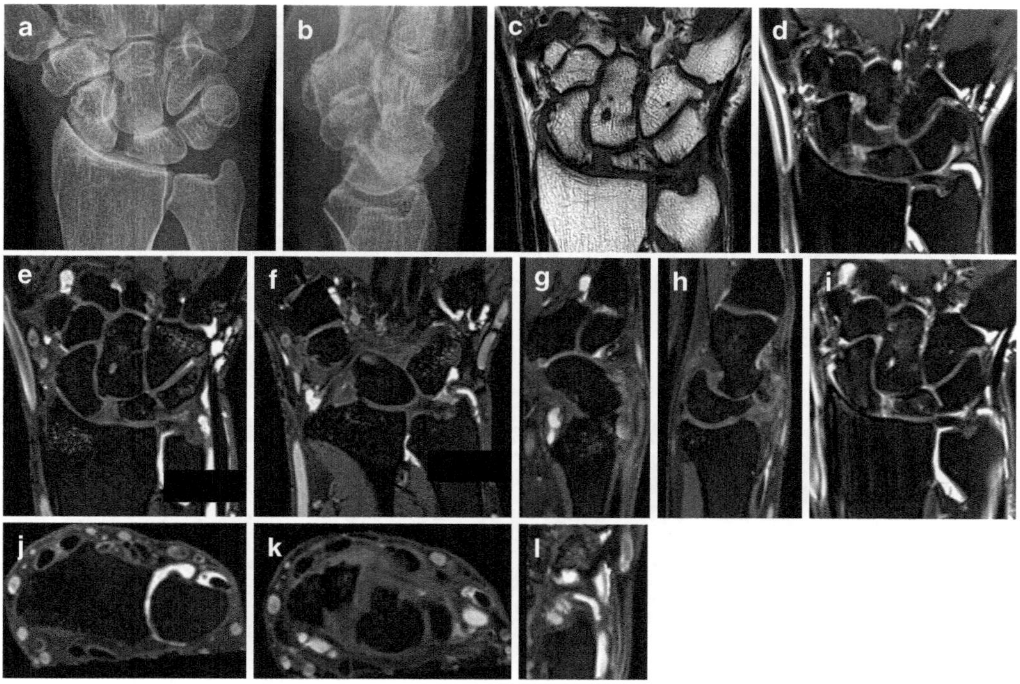

Fig. 28a Standard PA (**a**) and lateral (**b**) views; Cor T1-WI (**c**), T2-WI FS (**d**, **i**), and 3D GRE (**e**, **f**); Sag (**g**, **h**, **l**), and Ax 3D GRE (**j**, **k**)

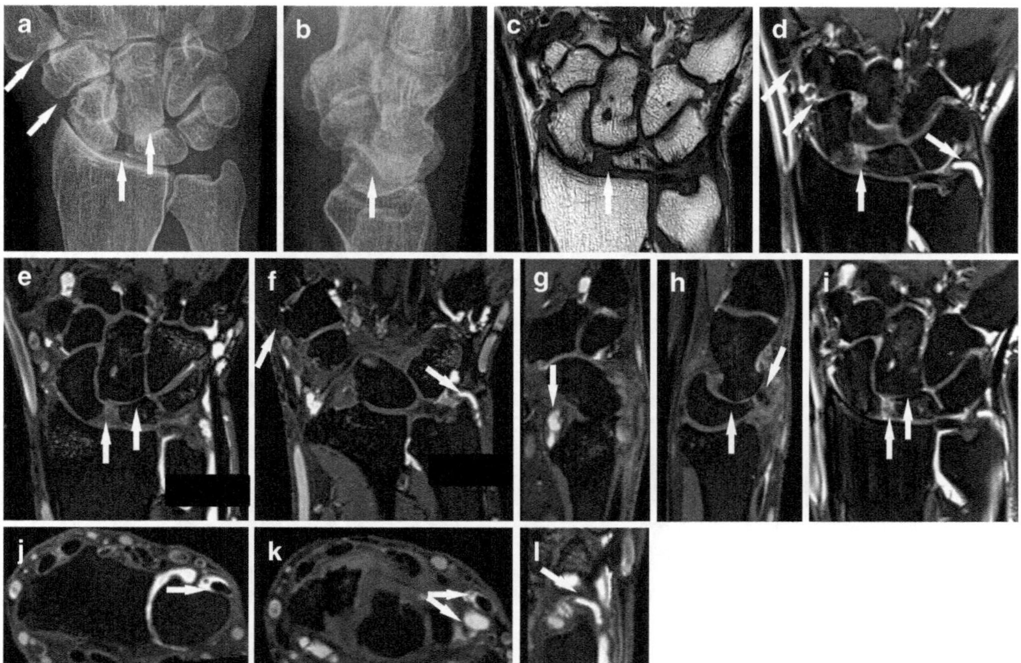

Fig. 28b OA CMC-I and STT Eaton-Littler grade 4 (**a**, **d**); SL (**a**, **c**–**e**, **i**); static CID (**a**), and DISI (**b**); SLAC grade III with OA RC-, and MCJ (**a**, **e**, **h**, **i**); peristyloidal neo bursa (**d**, **f**, **k**, **l**); radiopalmar ASC (**g**); midcarpal OCM (**h**); tenosynovitis ECU (**j**, **k**)

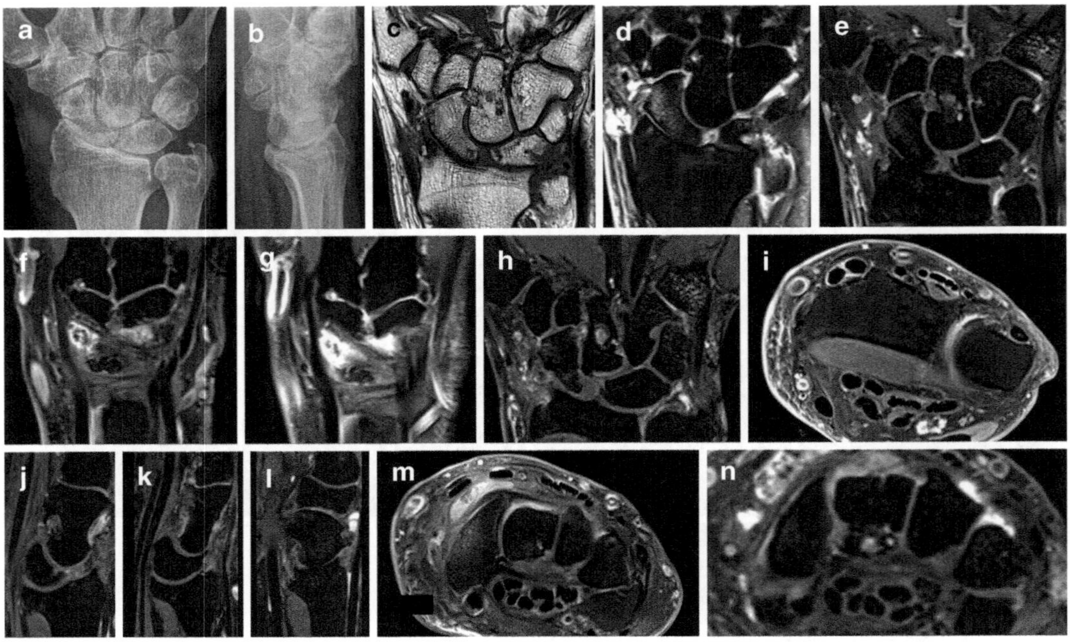

Fig. 29a Standard PA (**a**), and Lateral (**b**) views; Cor T1-WI (**c**), T2-WI FS (**d**, **g**), and 3D GRE (**e**, **f**, **h**); Ax T2-WI FS (**i**, **m**); Sag (**j–l**), and Ax (**n**) 3D GRE

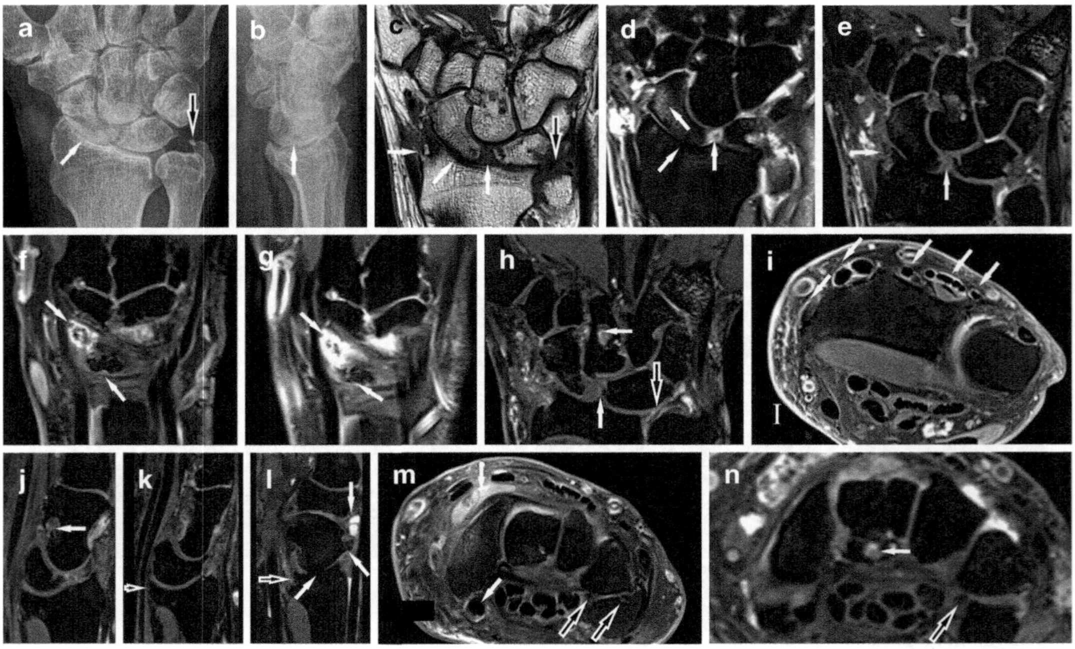

Fig. 29b OA R-S (**a**, **c**, **d**, **l**); small bone fragment (**a**) with TFCC I B (**c**), and II C (**h**); SL (**c–e**, **h**) with DISI (**b**); old # with loose fragment R styloid (**c**, **e**, **k**), P (**m**, **n**), and dorsal S (**d**, **f**, **l**); extrinsic S-Tri ligament tear (**f**, **g**); intraosseous ganglion C (**h**, **j**, **n**); tenosynovitis extensor compartment 2–5 (**i**), and FCR (**m**); small ASC (**l**, **m**)

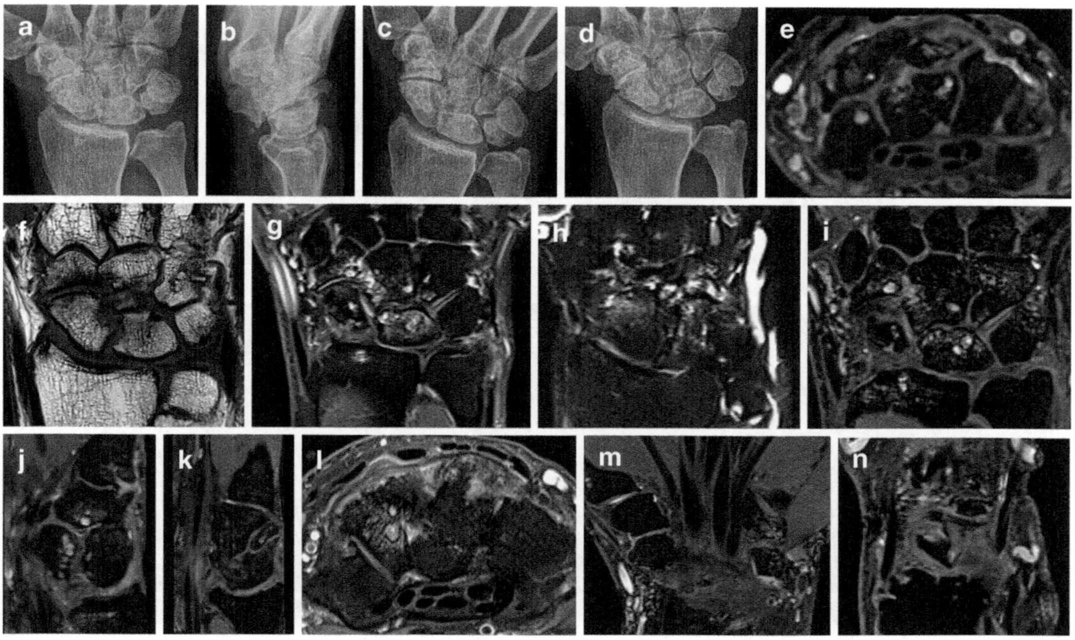

Fig. 30a Standard PA (**a**) and lateral (**b**) views; Standard PA in ulnar (**c**), and radial (**d**) deviation; Ax 3D GRE (**e**); Cor T1-WI (**f**), T2-WI FS (**g**, **h**), and 3D GRE (**i**, **m**, **n**); Sag 3D GRE (**j**, **k**); Ax T2-WI FS (**l**)

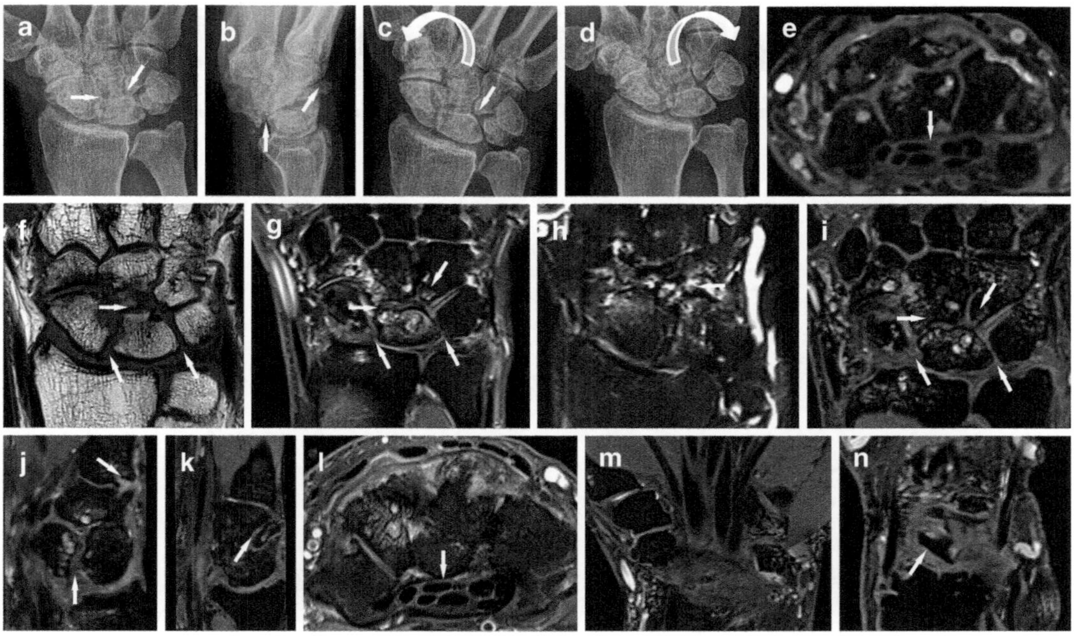

Fig. 30b HLA (**a**, **c–d**, **g**, **i**); mid carpal OA (**a**, **f**, **g**, **i**) with diffuse BMO (**h**); #S with pseudarthrosis (**b**, **j**); loose bone fragment dorsal of the C (**b**, **k**, **n**); narrow CT (**e**, **l–m**); SL, and LT tear with step off LT (**f**, **g**, **i**); degenerative CB CMC-II (**j**)

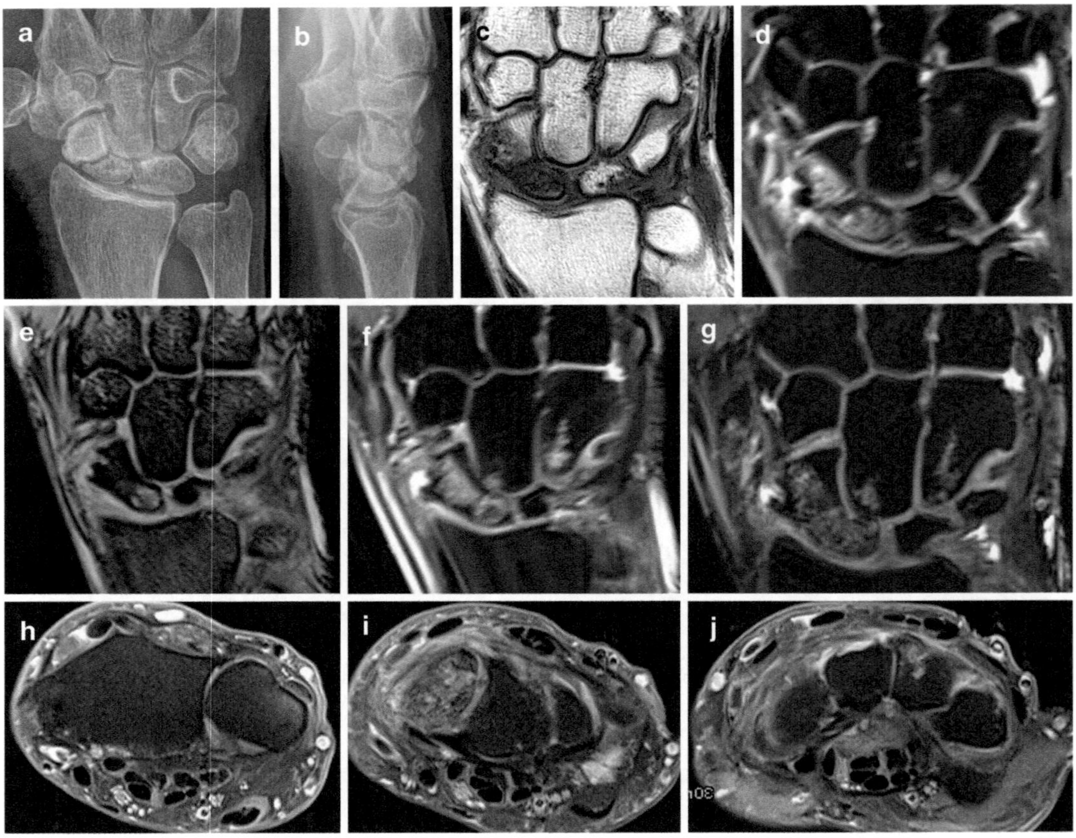

Fig. 31a Standard PA (**a**), and Lateral (**b**) views; Cor T1-WI (**c**), T2-WI FS (**d**, **f**, **g**), and 3D GRE (**e**); Ax T2-WI FS (**h**–**j**)

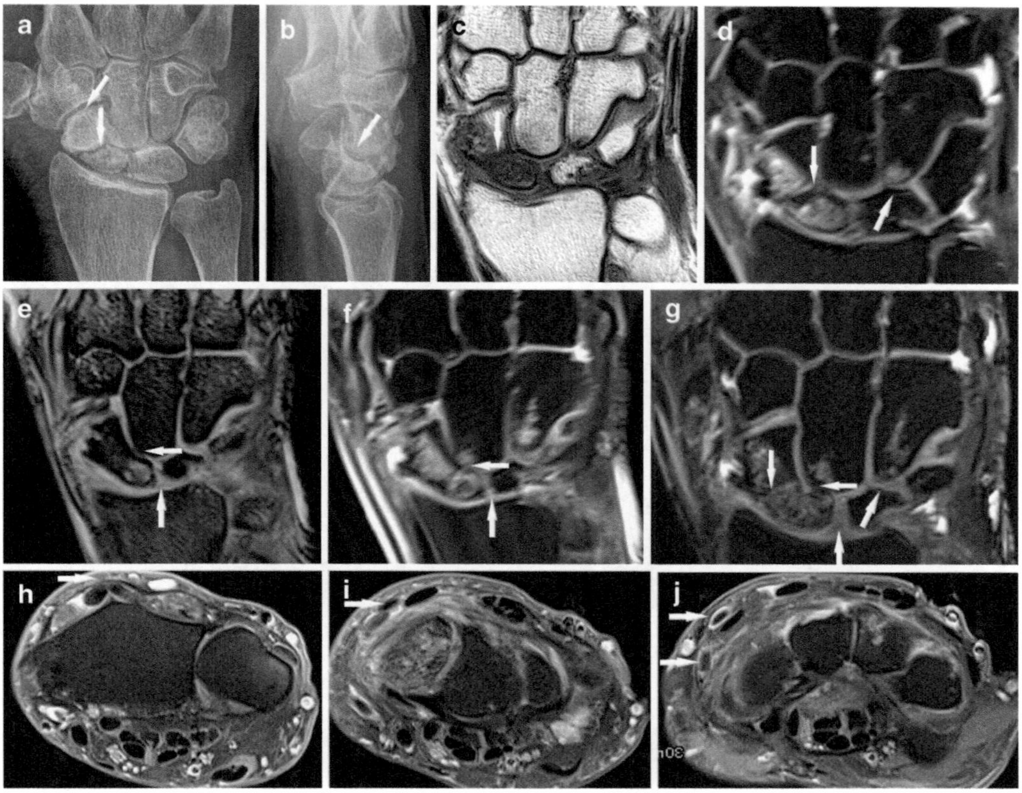

Fig. 31b S# with surrounding BMO (**a**, **c**, **d**, **g**); signet ring sign (**a**), and DISI (**b**); HLA (**d**, **g**); SL tear (**e–g**); OA MCJ (**e–g**); tenosynovitis due to distal cross over (epl over ecl, and ecb) (**h–j**)

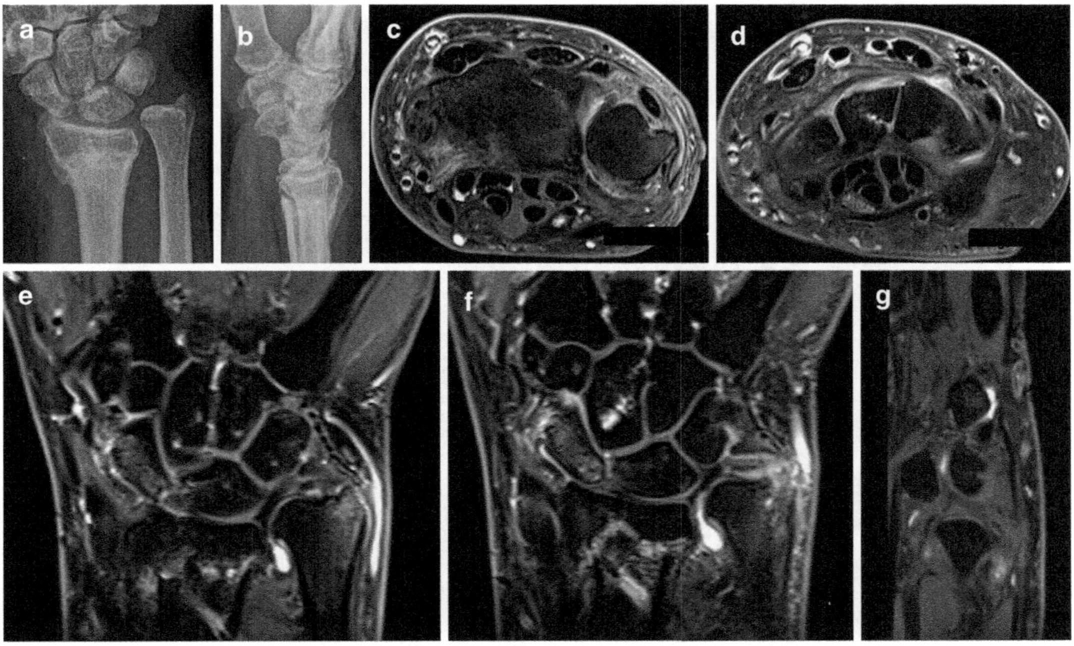

Fig. 32a Standard PA (**a**), and Lateral (**b**) views; Ax T2-WI FS (**c**, **d**); Cor T2-WI FS (**e**, **f**); Sag 3D GRE (**g**)

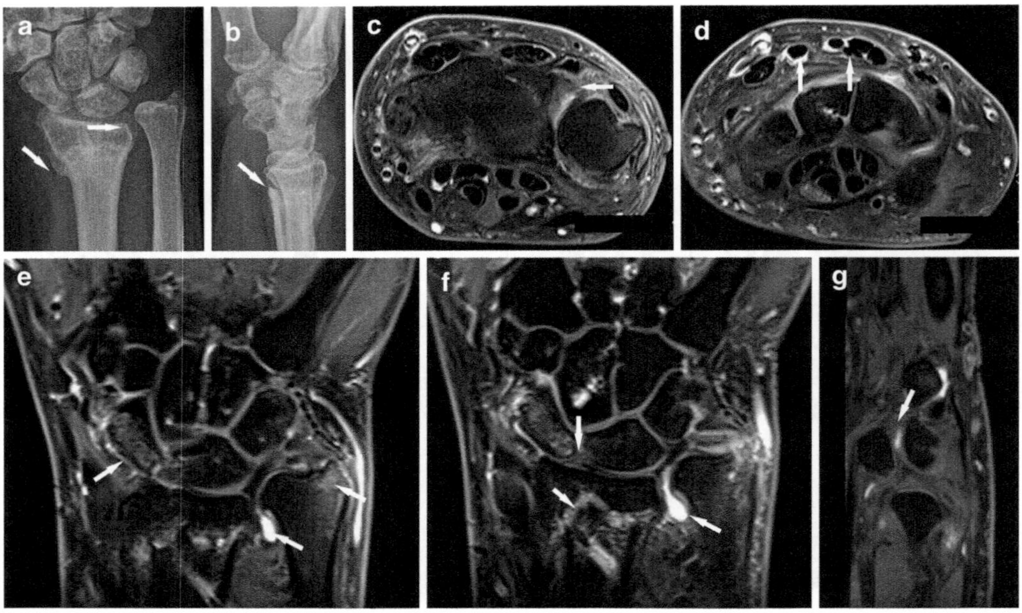

Fig. 32b Post-traumatic positive ulnar variance (**a**, **b**, **f**); tear dorsal RU ligament (**c**); tenosynovitis erb, and ed (**d**); BMO S, and styloid process U (**e**); hydrops DRUJ (**e**, **f**); SL tear (**f**); Tri-P subluxation (**g**)

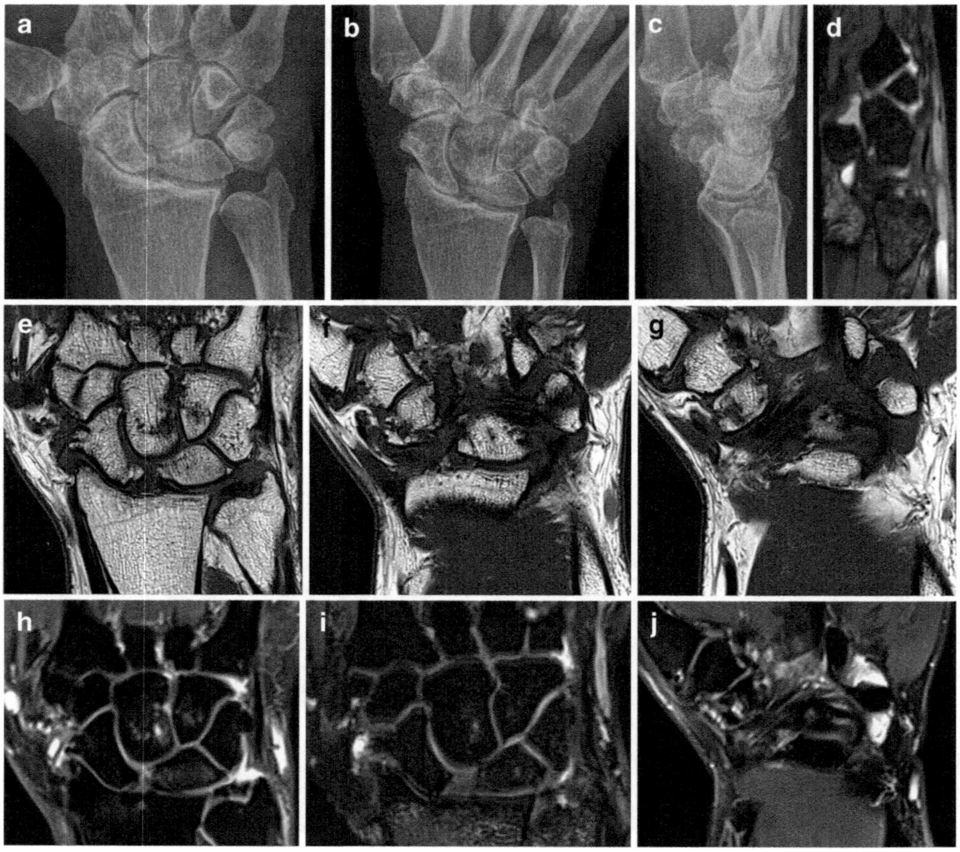

Fig. 33a Standard PA (**a**) with clenched fist (**b**), and Lateral (**c**) views; Sag 3D GRE (**d**); Cor T1-WI (**e**–**g**), T2-WI FS (**h**, **j**), and 3D GRE (**i**)

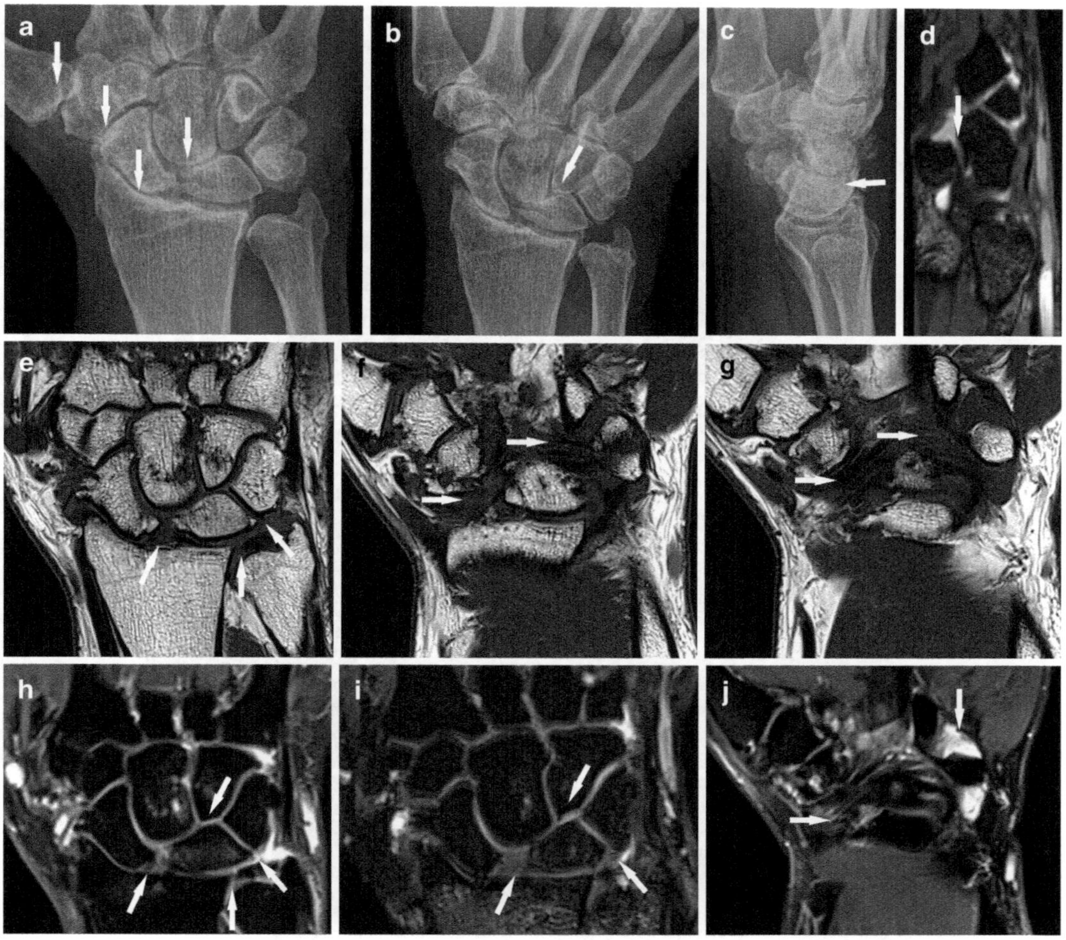

Fig. 33b OA CMC-I, STT, MC, and RC joint (**a**); static CID, SLAC grade 3 and DISI (**a**, **c**); HLA (**b**, **h**, **i**); hydrops, and OA Tri-P (**d**, **j**); SL, and LT tear (**e**, **h**, **i**); TFCC tear type I A (**e**, **h**); elongation palmar V (**f**, **g**, **j**)

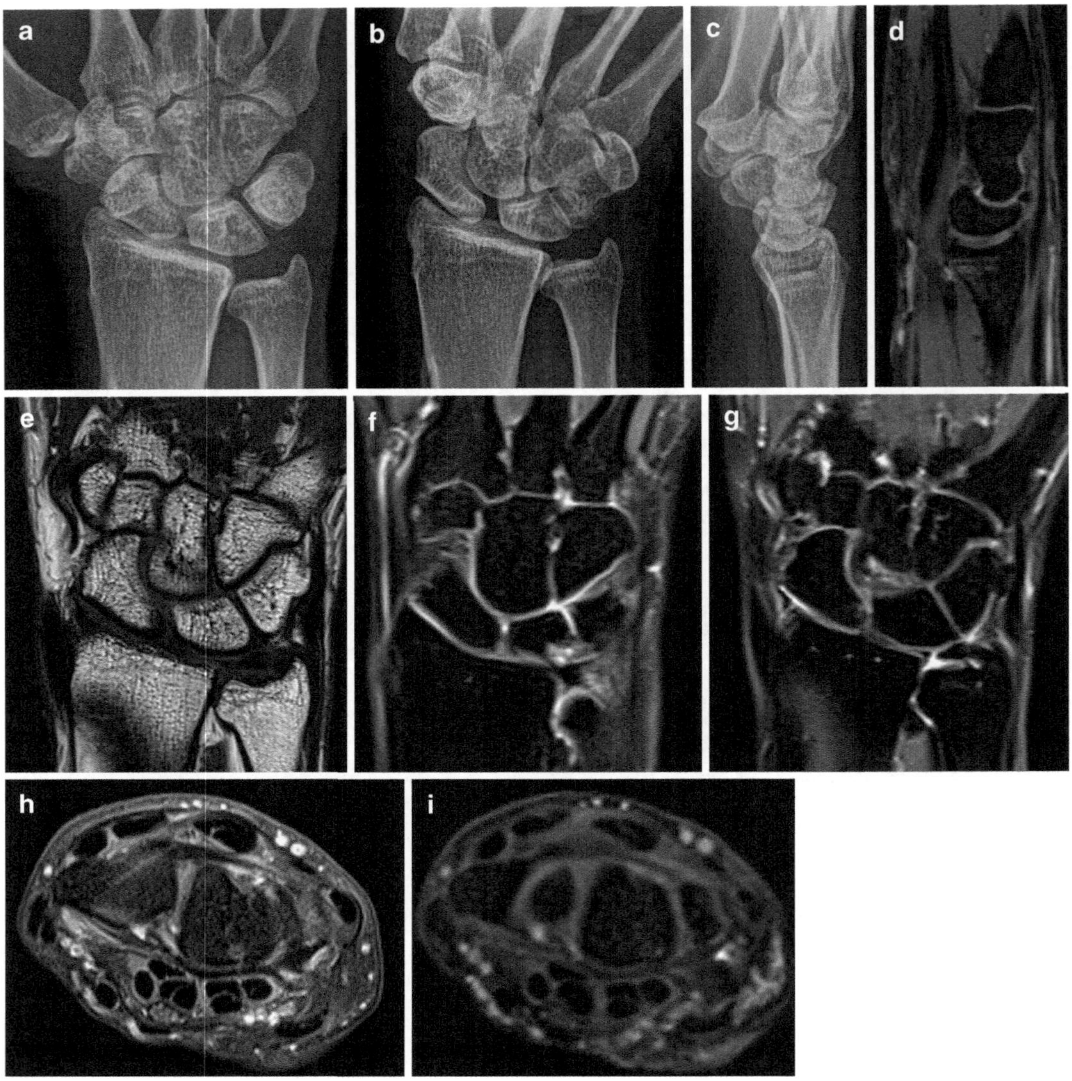

Fig. 34a Standard PA (**a**) with clenched fist (**b**) and lateral (**c**) views; Sag 3D GRE (**d**); Cor T1-WI (**e**), T2-WI FS (**f**), and 3D GRE (**g**); Ax T2-WI FS (**h**); and 3D GRE (**i**)

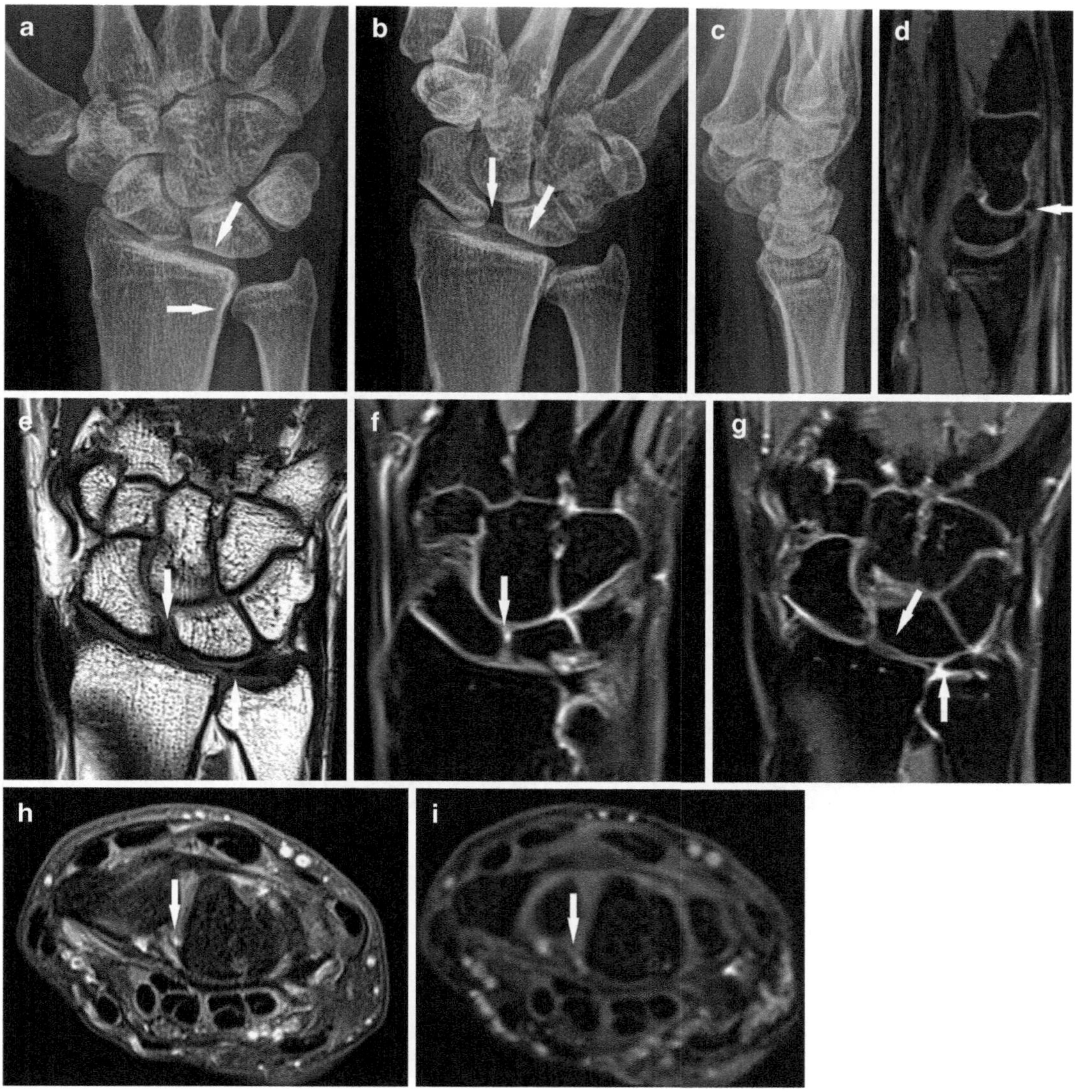

Fig. 34b Negative ulnar variance with starting impingement (**a**); sequel of AVN at the flattened radial side of the L (**a**, **b**, **g**); loose bone fragment at the dorsal pole of the L (**c**–**d**); TFCC tear type I A (**e**); SL tear (**e**, **f**, **h**, **i**) with dynamic CID (**a**, **b**)

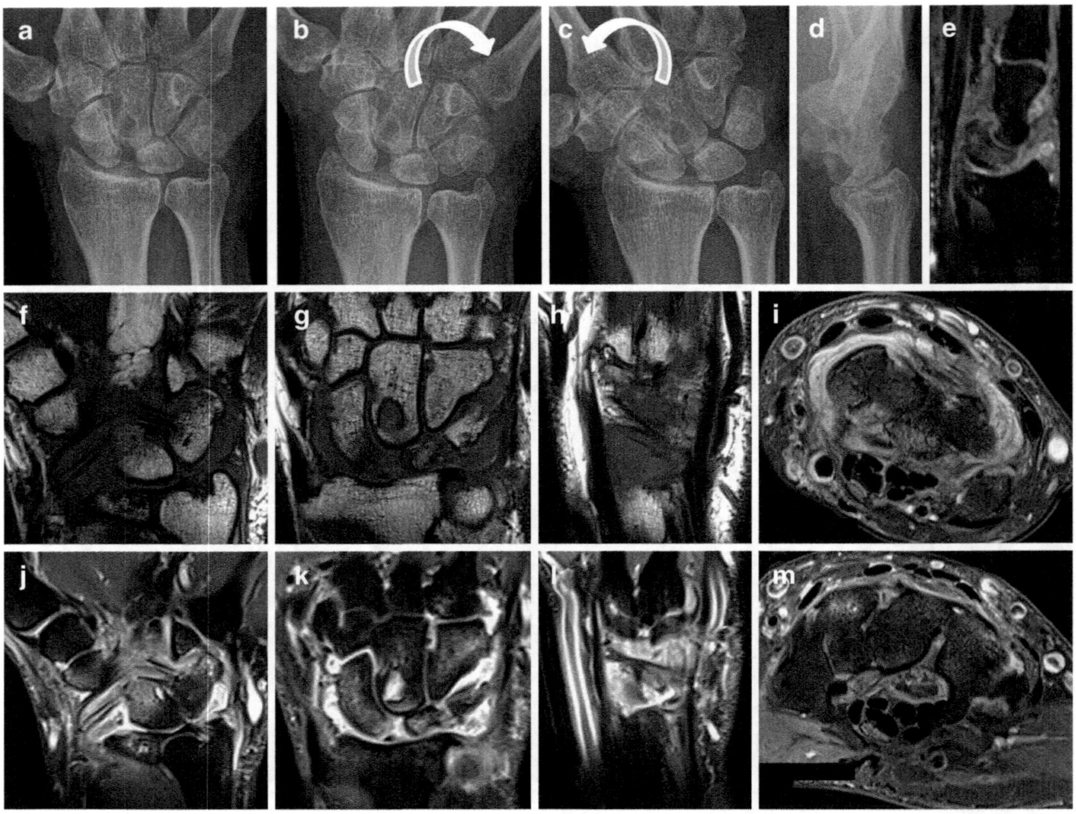

Fig. 35a Standard PA (**a**) in ulnar (**b**) and radial deviation (**c**), and lateral (**d**) views; Sag 3D GRE (**e**); Cor T1-WI (**f–h**); Ax (**i**) and Cor T2-WI FS (**j–l**); and 3D GRE (**m**)

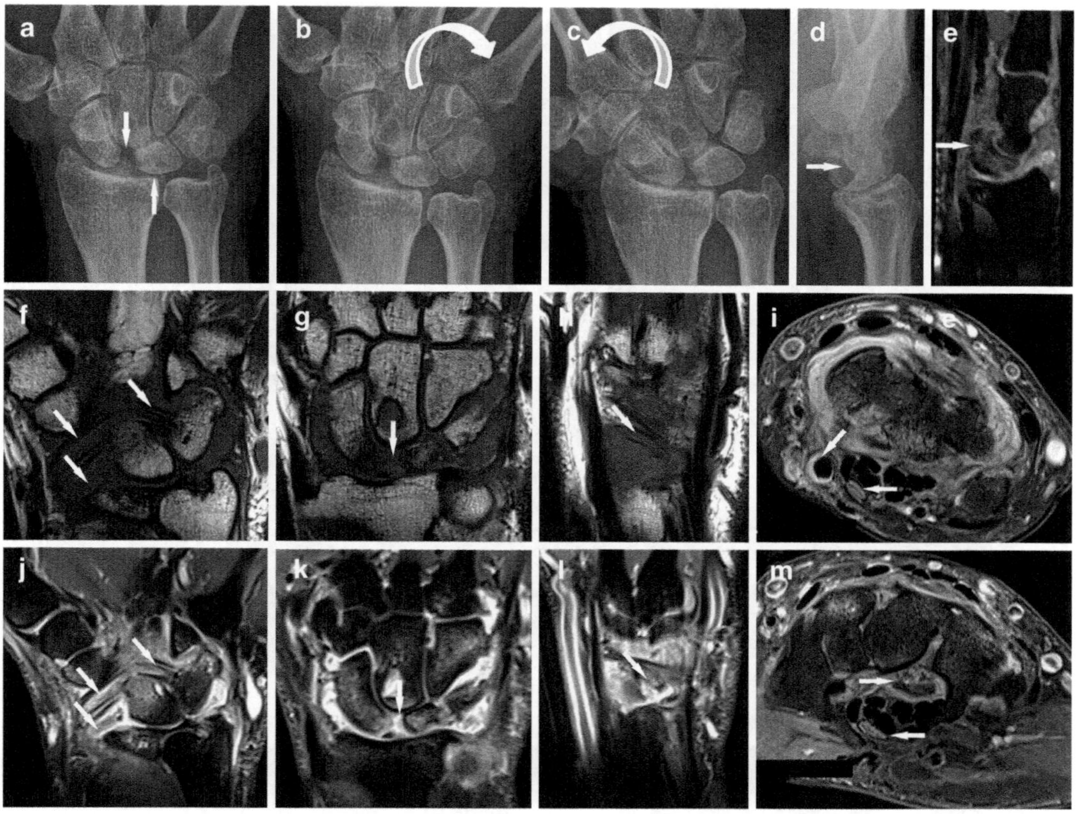

Fig. 35b Ulnar translocation type 2 (**a**); SL tear with static CID, DISI, and SLAC grade 3 (**a–e**, **g**, **k**); limited ulnar deviation (**b**); lunate tilted in the CT (**d**, **e**, **m**) with CTS (**m**); tenosynovitis fcr (**i**); oedematous infiltration of the palmar (**f**, **j**), and dorsal (**h**, **l**) extrinsic ligaments

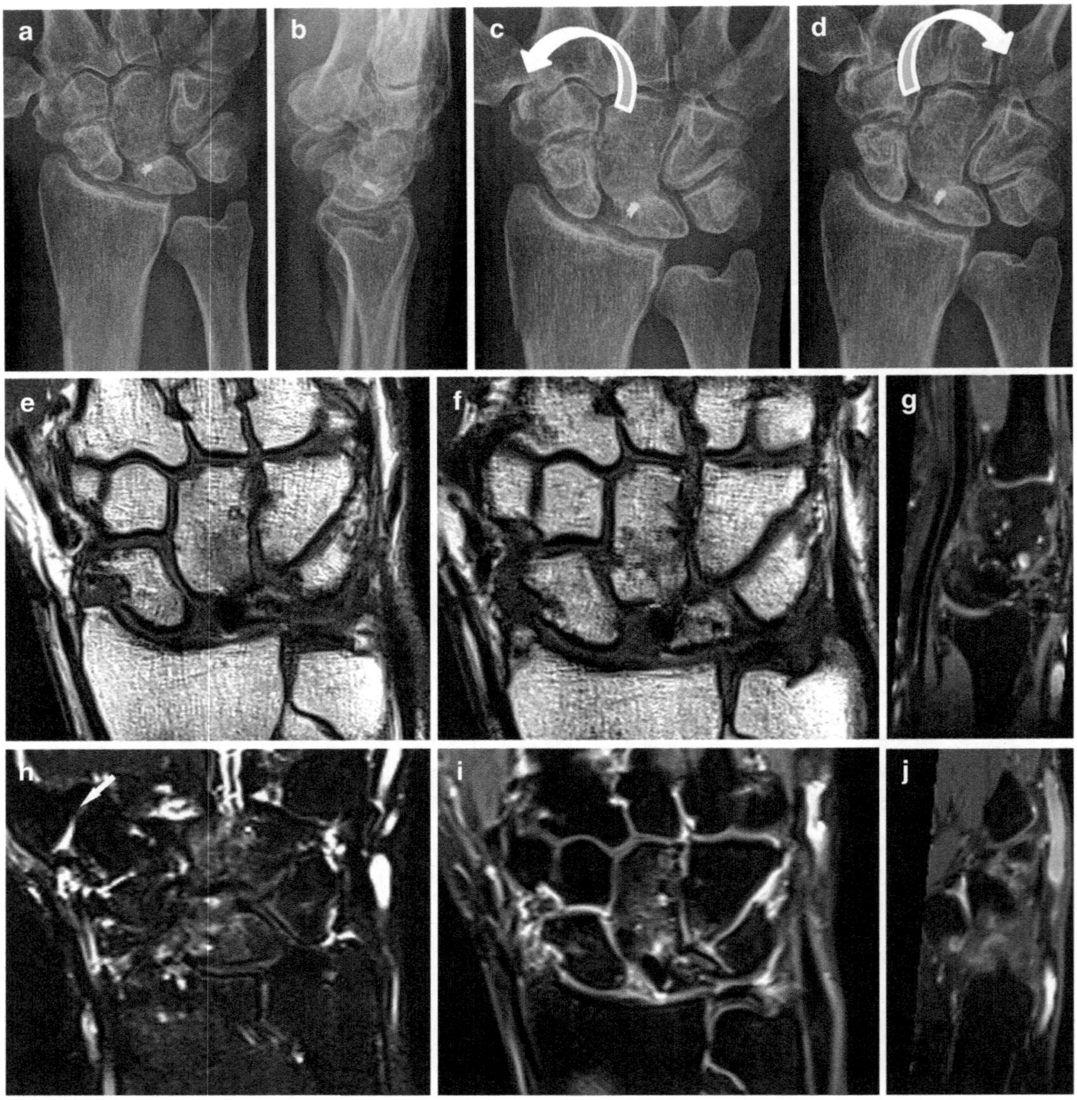

Fig. 36a Standard PA (**a**) and lateral (**b**) views; PA views in radial (**c**) and ulnar (**d**) deviation; Cor T1-WI (**e**, **f**), T2-WI FS (**h**, **i**); Sag 3D GRE (**g**, **j**)

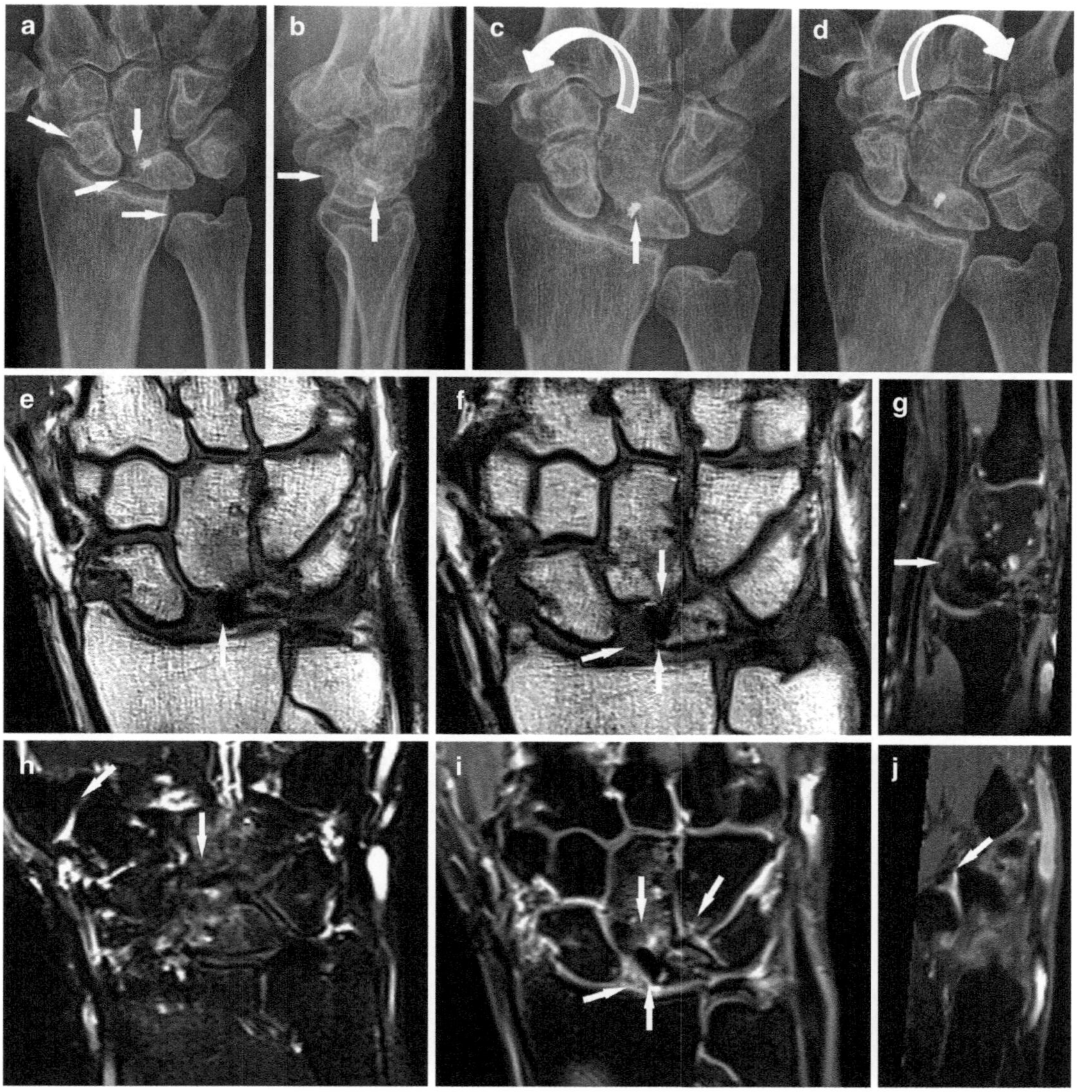

Fig. 36b Negative ulnar variance (**a**); failed SLL surgery (**b**, **c**, **e**, **f**, **i**) with rotatory subluxation of the S (**a**), static CID (**a**, **c**), DISI (**b**, **g**), SL diastasis (**a**, **f**, **i**), and SLAC grade 3 (**a**, **f**, **h**–**i**); limited radial (**c**), and ulnar (**d**) deviation at RC- and MC joint; BMO at C-L (**f**, **i**); HLA (**i**); OA, and hydrops at the Tri-P joint (**j**)

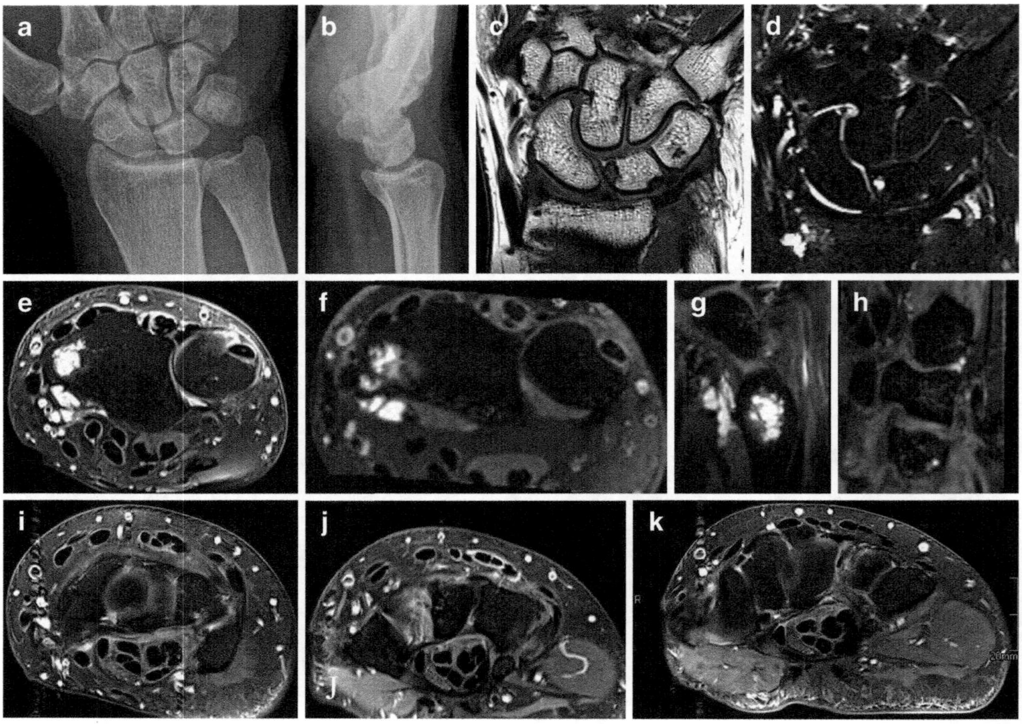

Fig. 37a Standard PA (**a**) and lateral (**b**) views; Cor T1-WI (**c**), T2-WI FS (**d**); Ax T2-WI FS (**e**, **i**–**k**), and 3D GRE (**f**); Sag 3D GRE (**g**, **h**)

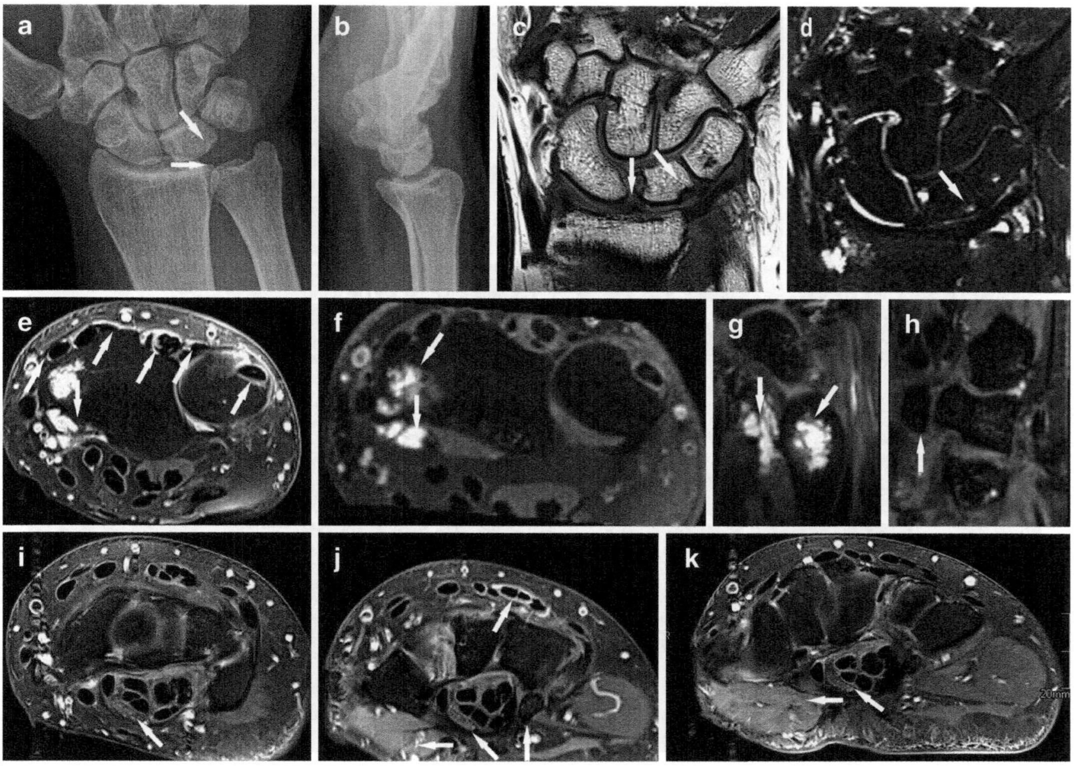

Fig. 37b Negative ulnar variance (**a**–**b**), and starting dynamic UA (**a**, **c**, **d**); SL tear (**c**) with palmar ASC (**f**, **g**); tenosynovitis extensor compartment 2–6 (**e**, **j**); intraosseous ganglion R (**f**, **g**); os hamuli proprium (**h**, **j**); CTS surgery sequel (**j**, **k**) with distal fibrous repair; compression, high signal, and fasciculation of the median nerve (**i**–**k**); starting denervation of the abductor pollicis brevis and opponens pollicis muscle (**j**, **k**)

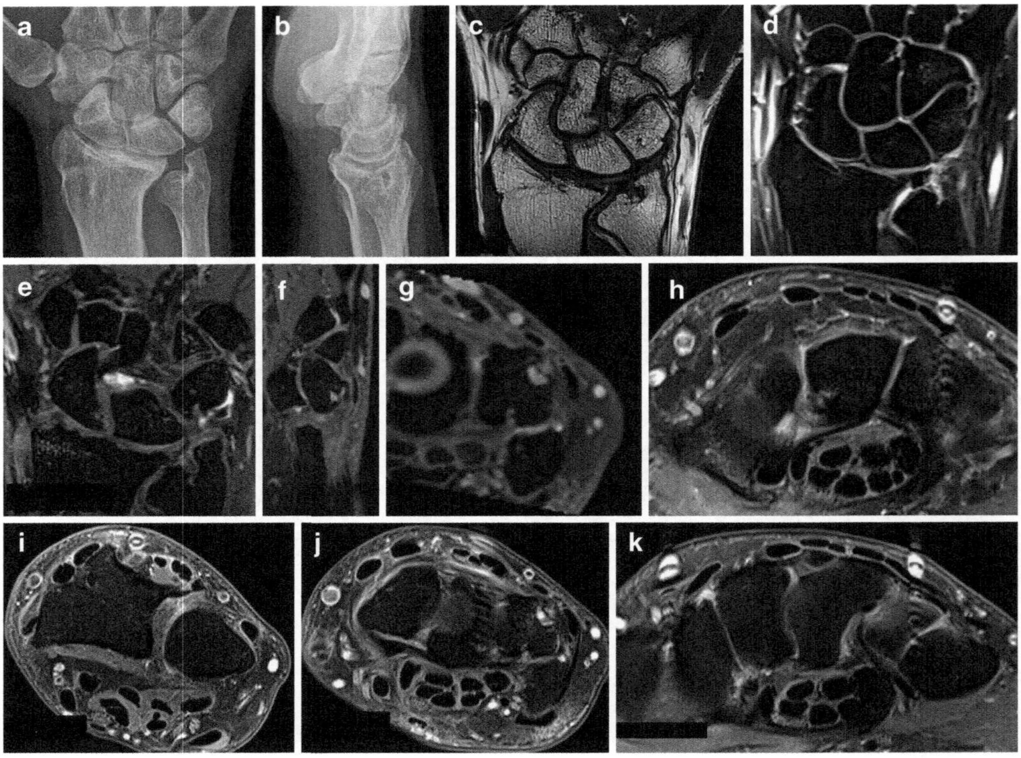

Fig. 38a Standard PA (**a**) and lateral (**b**) views; Cor T1-WI (**c**), T2-WI FS (**d**); Cor (**e**), Sag (**f**), and Ax (**g**) 3D GRE; Ax T2-WI FS (**h–k**)

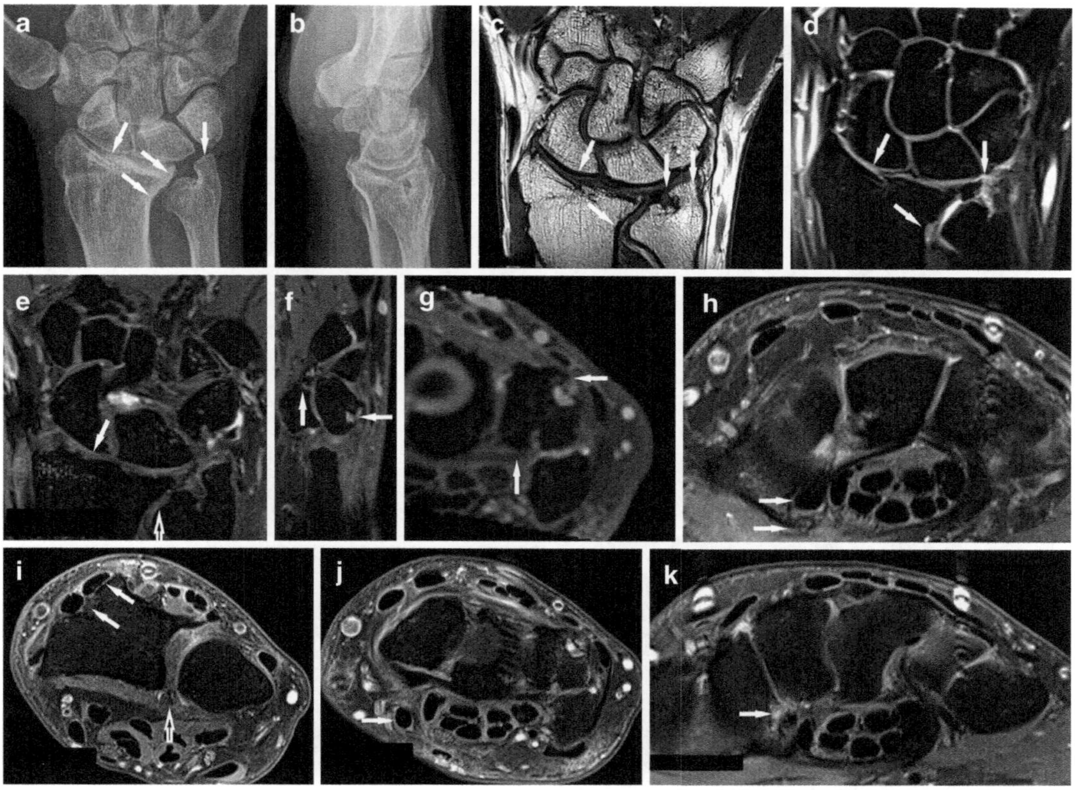

Fig. 38b Multiple post-traumatic consequences: deformed ulnar styloid (**a**–**d**); ulnar impingement (**a**, **c**, **d**); step off at the radial navicular fossa (**a**, **c**–**e**); deformed DRUJ (**a**, **c**, **d**); TFCC tear type I B (**c**, **d**); P # (**f**); dorsal Tri fracture (**f**, **g**); loose bone fragment tuberculum Tra (**h**) with tenosynovitis fcr (**h**, **j**, **k**); tenosynovitis extensor compartment 2 (**i**); tear of palmar DRU ligament (**i**)

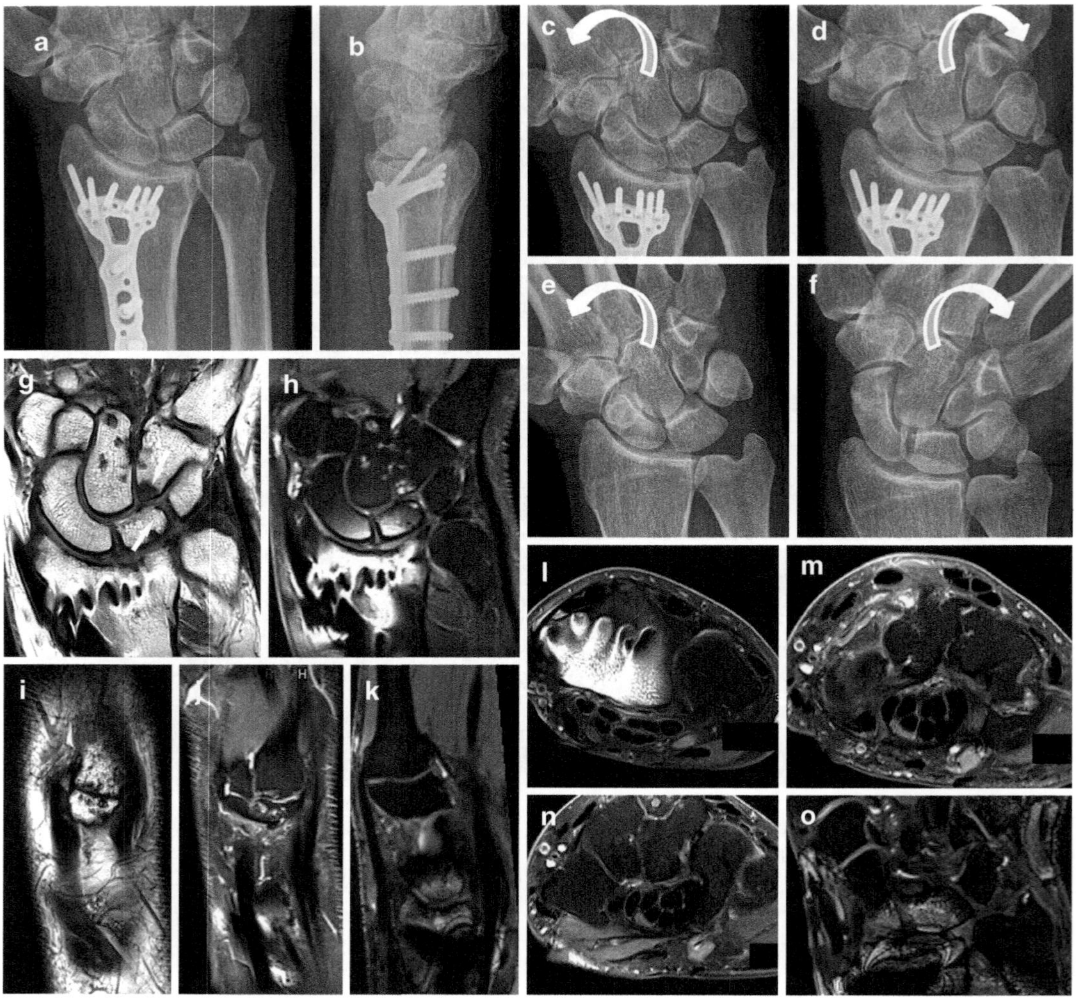

Fig. 39a Standard PA (**a**) and lateral (**b**) views; PA comparative views in radial (**c**, **e**) and ulnar (**d**, **f**) deviation; Cor T1-WI (**g**, **i**), T2-WI FS (**h**, **j**, **o**); Sag 3D GRE (**k**); Ax T2-WI FS (**l**–**n**)

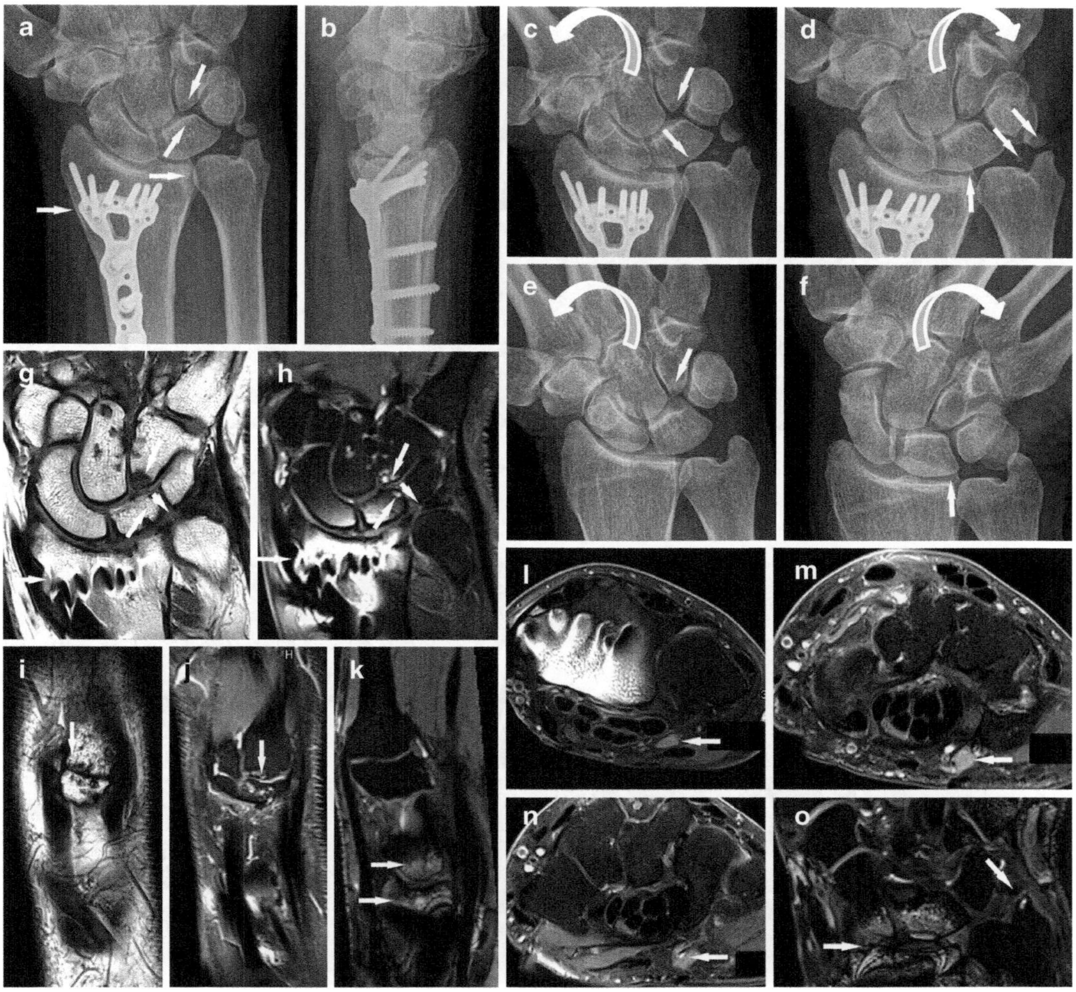

Fig. 39b Post-traumatic positive ulnar variance (**a**) with UA (**c**); (bilateral) HLA and Viegas type 2 L (**a**, **c**, **e**, **g**, **h**); metal (**a**, **b**) artefacts (**g**, **h**, **k**, **o**); carpal boss with degenerative changes (**i**, **j**); limited ulnar deviation at RCJ (**d**, **f**); large (neo-articulating) and small loose bone fragment at ulnar styloid (**d**, **o**); degenerative TFCC II D (**g**, **h**); ulnar neuritis (**l**–**n**)

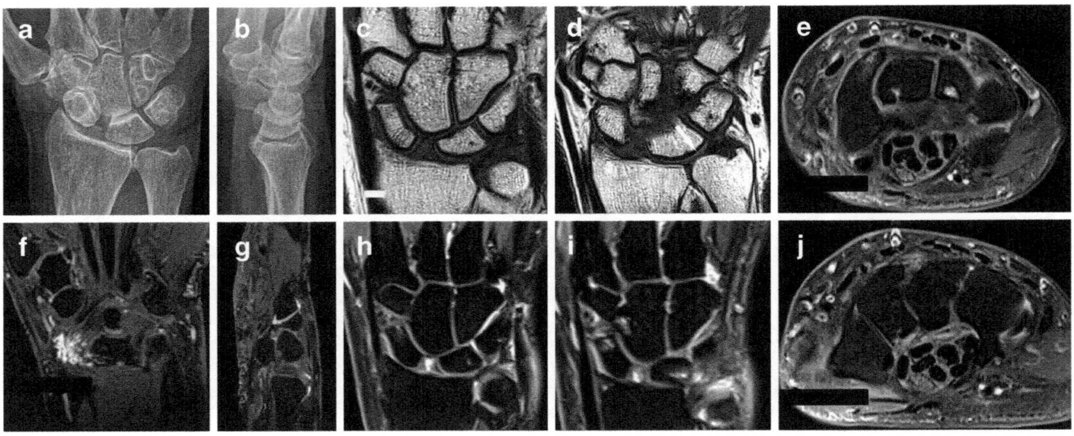

Fig. 40a Standard PA (**a**) and lateral (**b**) views; Cor T1-WI (**c–d**), Ax T2-WI FS (**e**, **j**); Cor (**f**), and Sag (**g**) 3D GRE; Cor T2-WI (**h**, **i**)

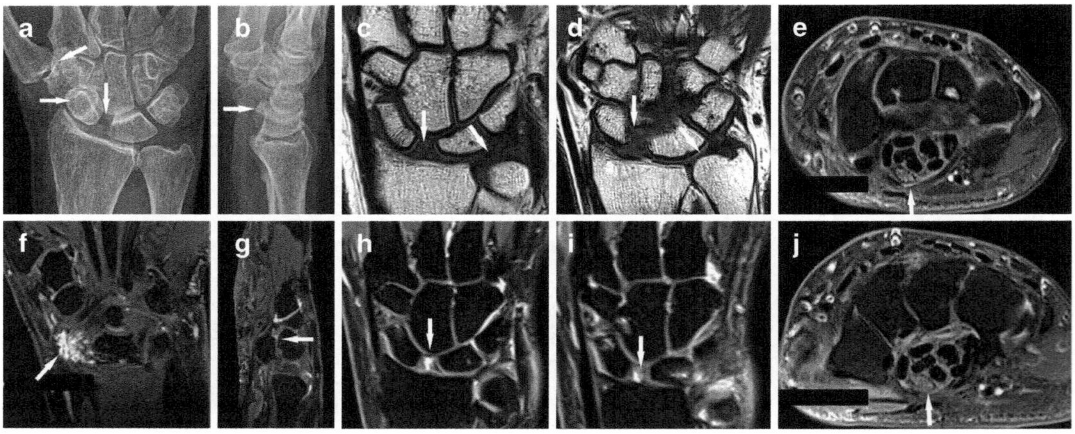

Fig. 40b OA CMC-I (**a**); S rotatory subluxation (**a**); SLL tear (**a**, **c**, **d**, **h**, **i**) with SLAC wrist grade 3 (**a**, **d**), DISI configuration (**b**), and radiopalmar ASC (**f**); degenerative TFCC II D (**c**, **d**); Tri-P subluxation (**g**); CTS after surgery (**e–j**)

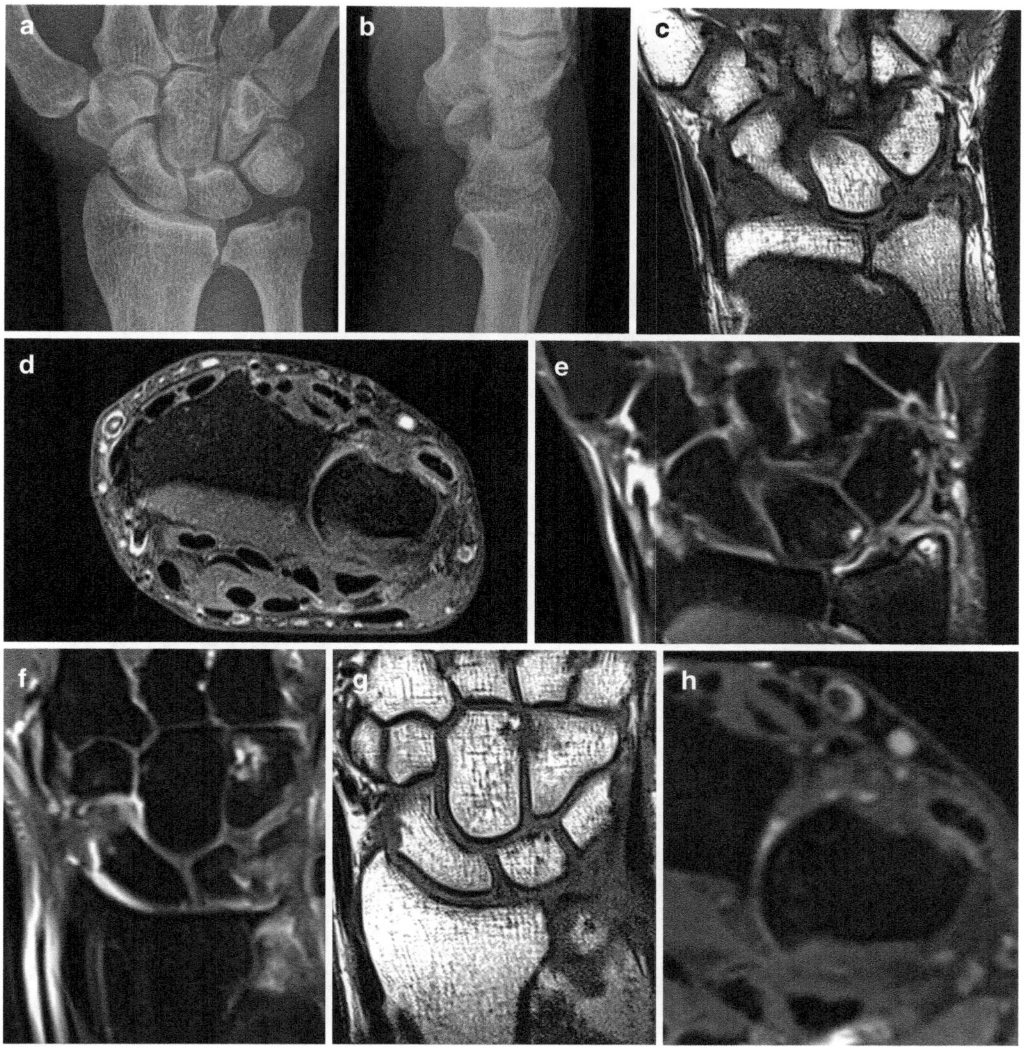

Fig. 41a Standard PA (**a**) and lateral (**b**) views; Cor T1-WI (**c**, **g**); Ax T2-WI FS (**d**); Cor T2-WI FS (**e**, **f**); Ax 3D GRE (**h**)

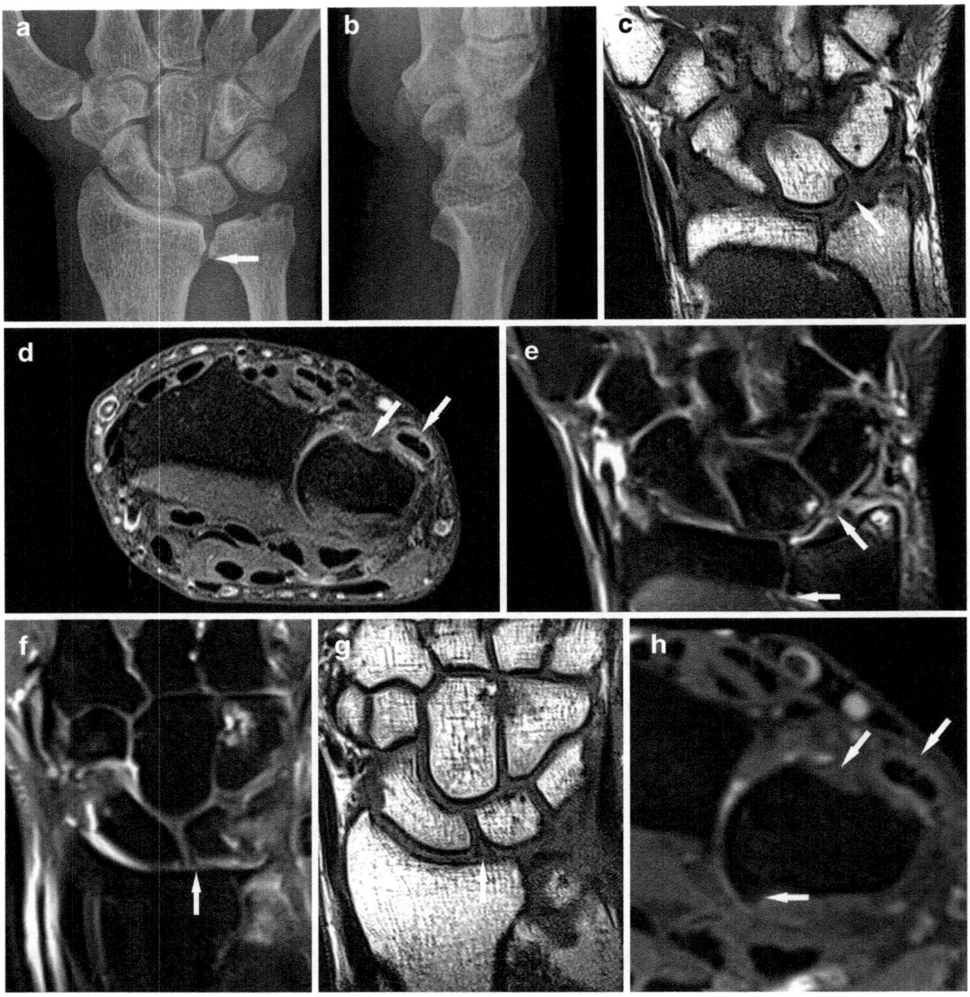

Fig. 41b OA DRUJ (**a**–**b**, **e**, **h**); degenerative TFCC II E (**c**, **e**); tenosynovitis, and subluxation ecu (**d**, **h**), SLL tear (**f**, **g**)

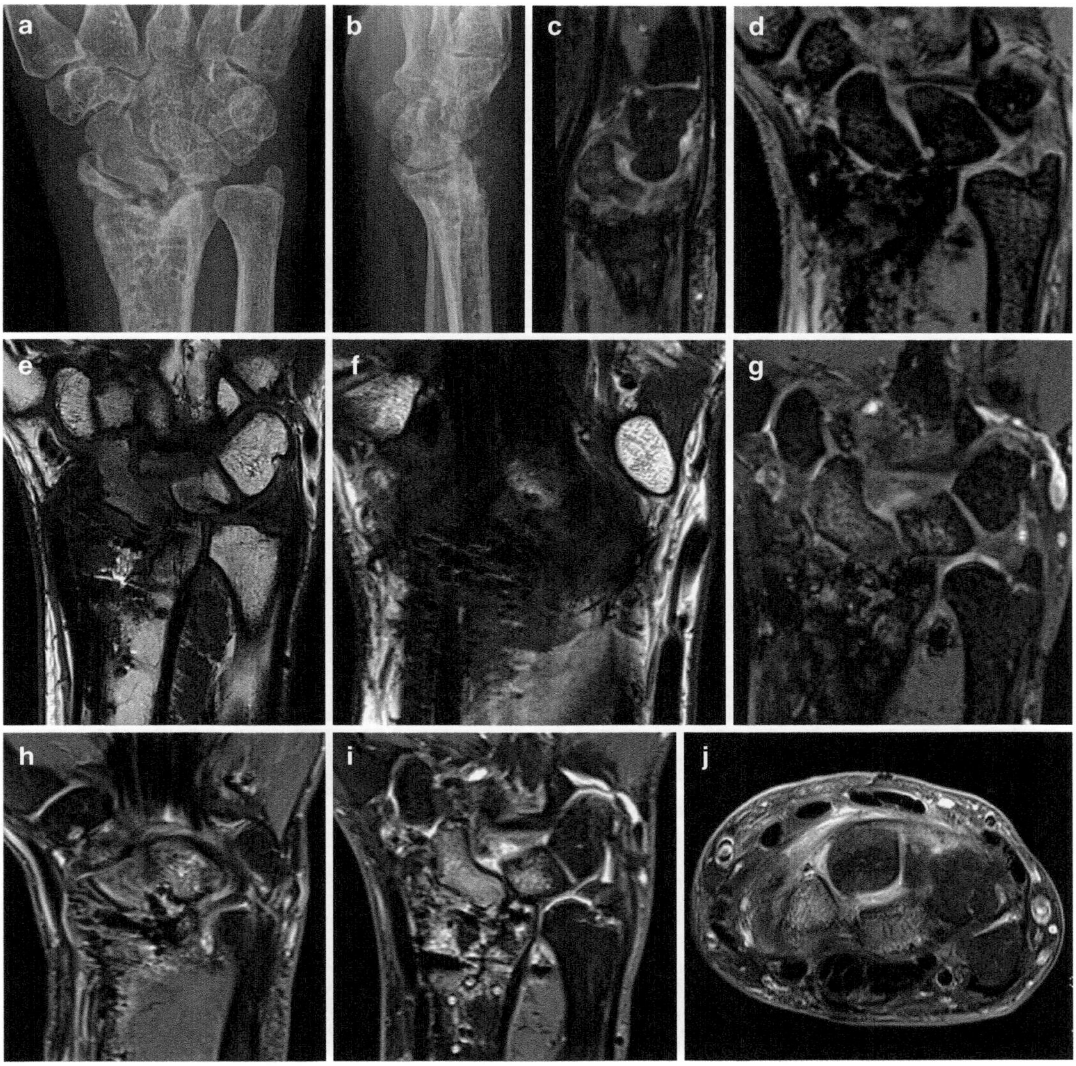

Fig. 42a Standard PA (**a**) and lateral (**b**) views; Sag (**c**), and Cor (**d**, **g**) 3D GRE; Cor T1-WI (**e**, **f**), and T2-WI FS (**h**, **i**)); Ax T2-WI FS (**j**)

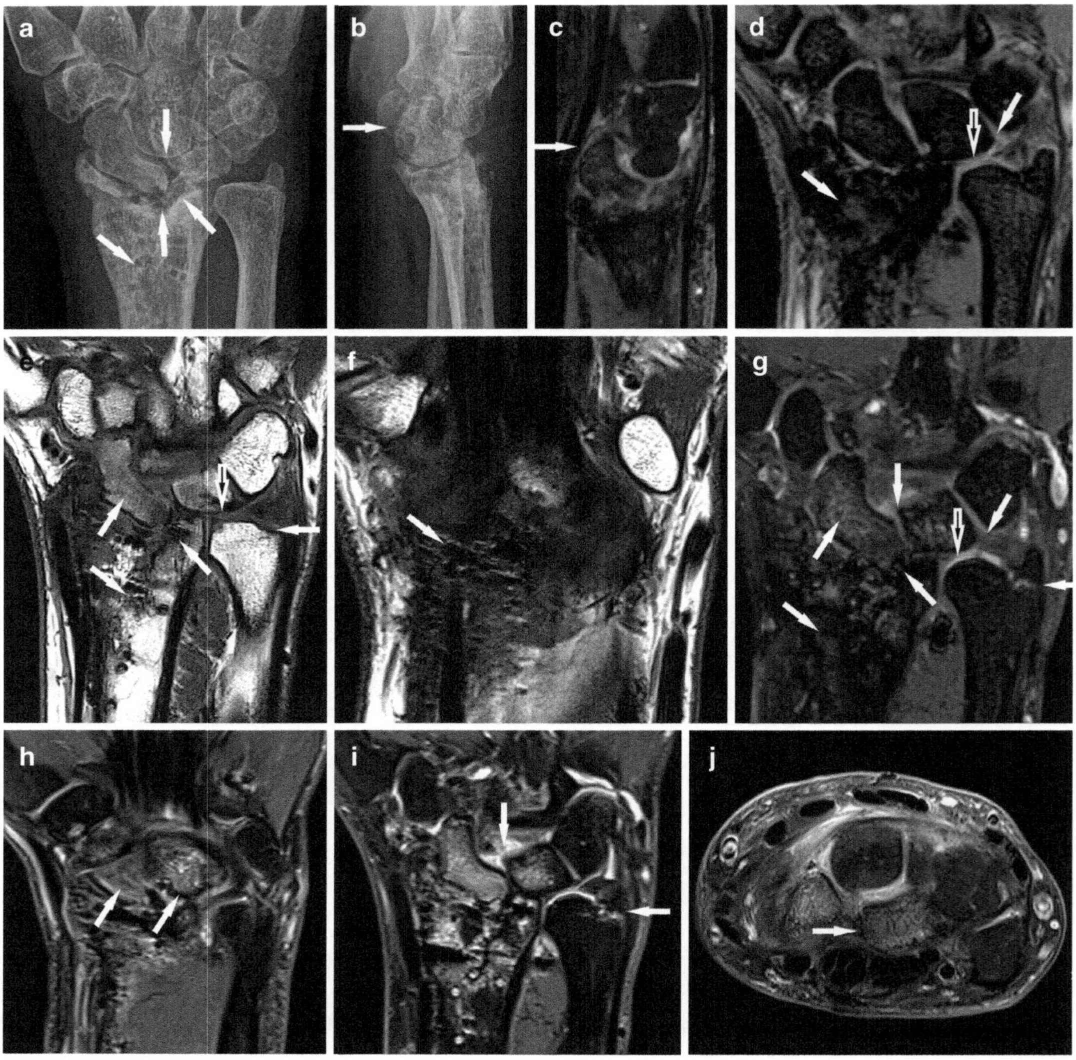

Fig. 42b Impaction # R (**a**); metal surgery artefacts (**a**, **d**, **e**–**g**); secondary abutment R-S (**a**, **e**, **g**); SL step off first, and second line of Gilula (**a**, **g**, **i**); DISI (**b**) with L tilted in the narrowed CT (**c**, **j**); TFCC II E lesion (**d**, **e**, **g**); LTL tear (**d**, **g**); diffuse BMO S, and L (**e**, **h**, **i**); pseudarthrosis at the base of the ulnar styloid (**e**, **g**, **i**)

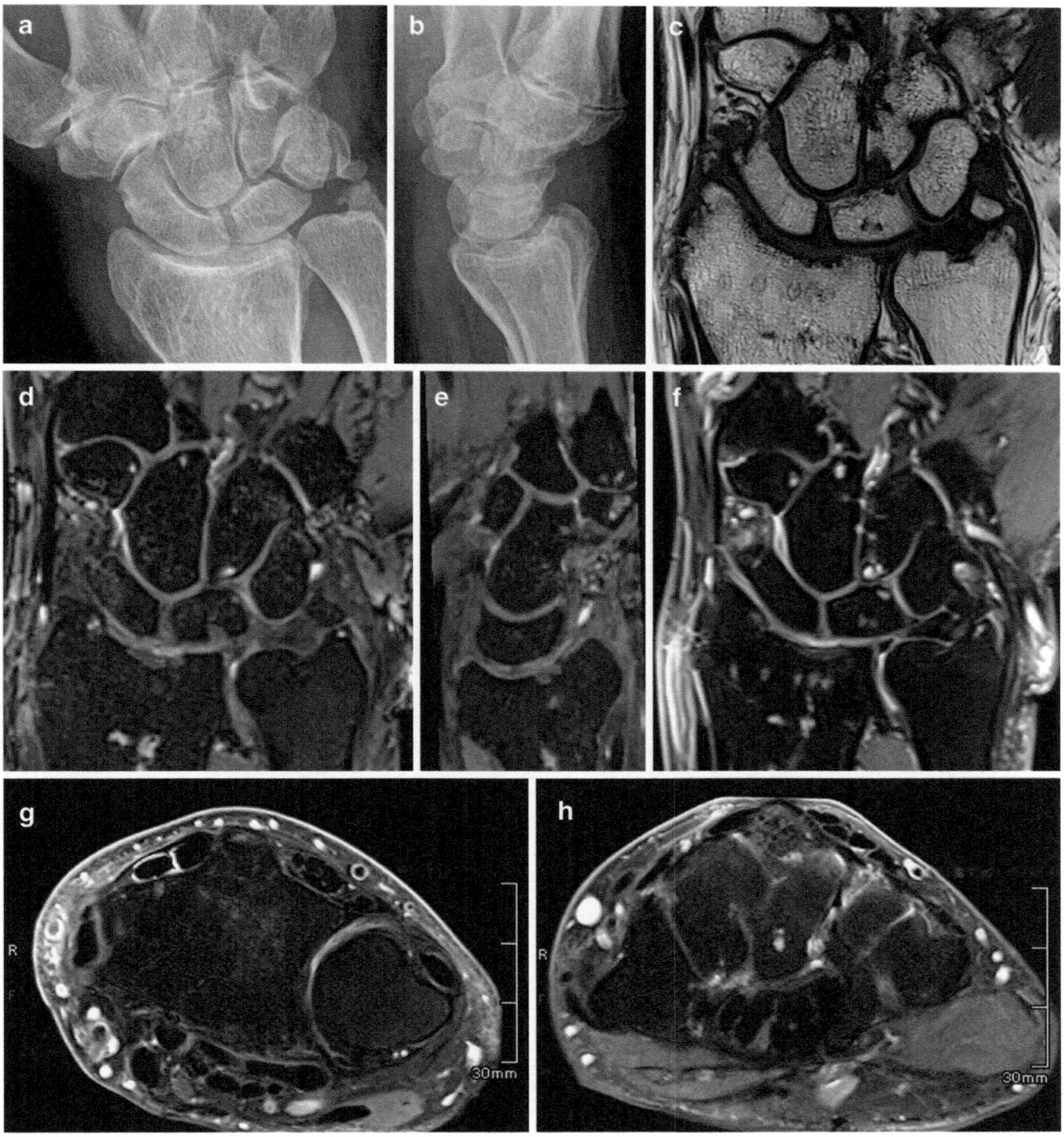

Fig. 43a Standard PA (**a**) and lateral (**b**) views; Cor T1-WI (**c**); Cor (**d**), and Sag (**e**) 3D GRE; Cor (**f**), and Ax (**g**, **h**) T2-WI FS

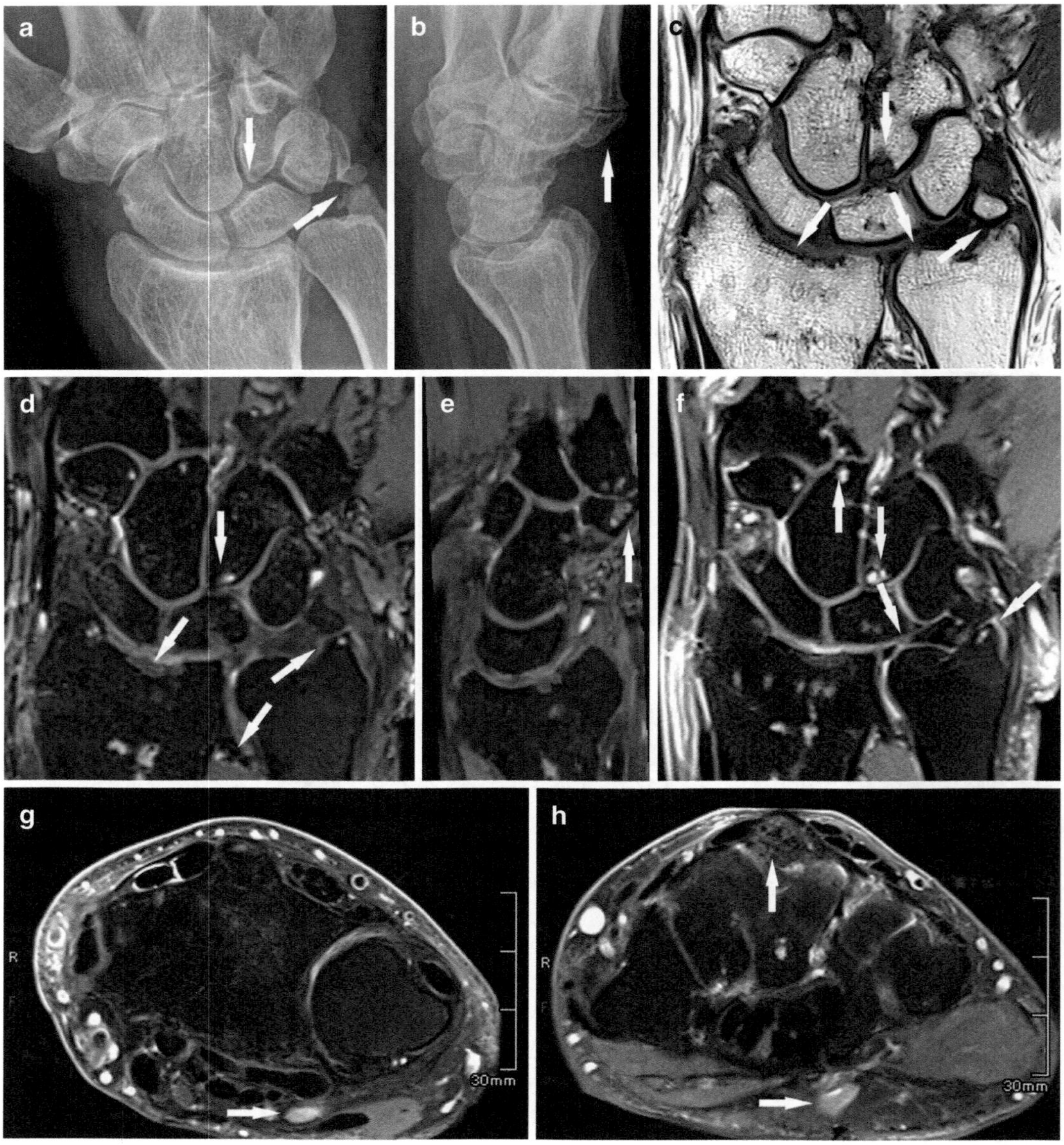

Fig. 43b HLA and L type 2 Viegas (**a**, **c**, **d**, **f**); sequel ulnar styloid # with pseudarthrosis (**a**, **c**, **d**); CB with os styloideum, and degeneration (**b**, **e**, **f**, **h**); oblique radial # into the deformed DRUJ (**c**, **d**); degenerative TFCC II C (**c**, **f**); peristyloidal neo bursa (**f**); ulnar nerve neuritis superficial branch (**g**, **h**)

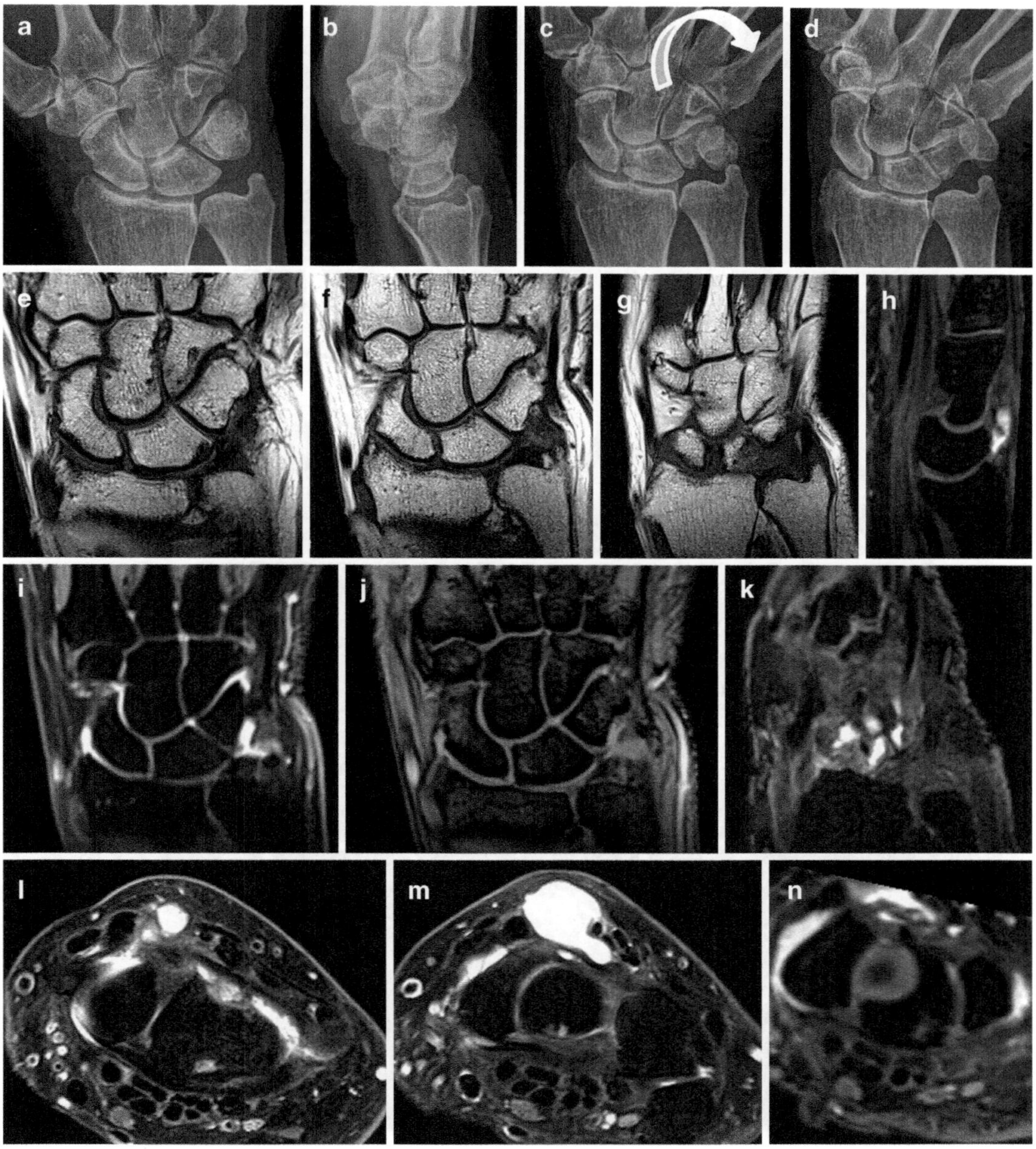

Fig. 44a Standard PA (**a**) and lateral (**b**) views; PA views in ulnar deviation (**c**) with clenched fist (**d**); Cor T1-WI (**e**, **g**); Sag 3D GRE (**h**); Cor T2-WI FS (**i**), 2D GRE (**j**), and 3D GRE (**k**); Ax T2-WI FS (**l**, **m**), and 3D GRE (**n**)

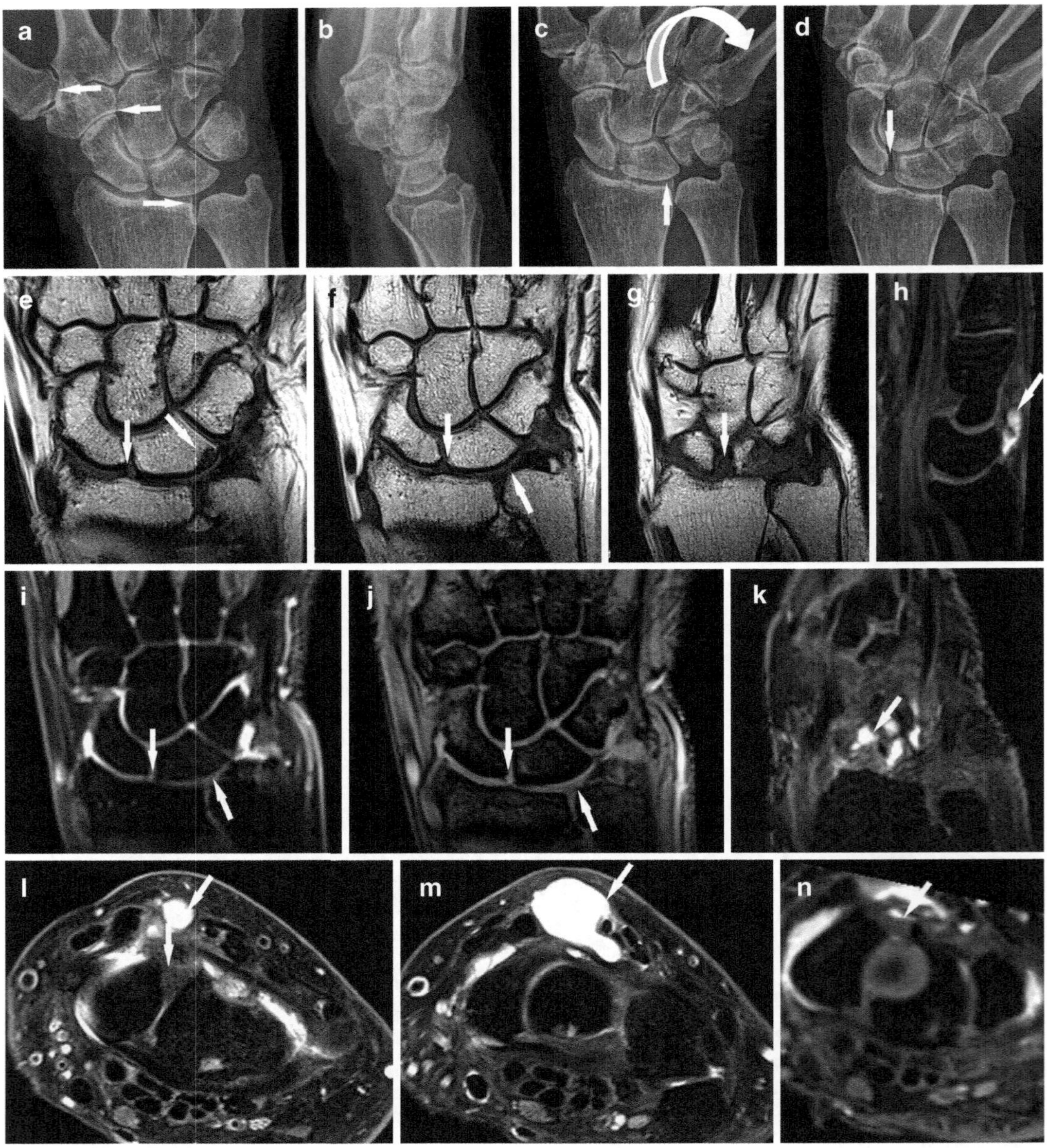

Fig. 44b OA CMC-I, and STT (**a**); positive ulnar variance (**a–b**); limited RC ulnar deviation (**c**); dynamic CID (**d**); UA (**e**); SL with scar tissue (**e–g**, **i**, **j**, **l**, **n**); degenerative TFCC II C (**f**, **i**, **j**); ASC starting from SLL (**h**, **k–m**)

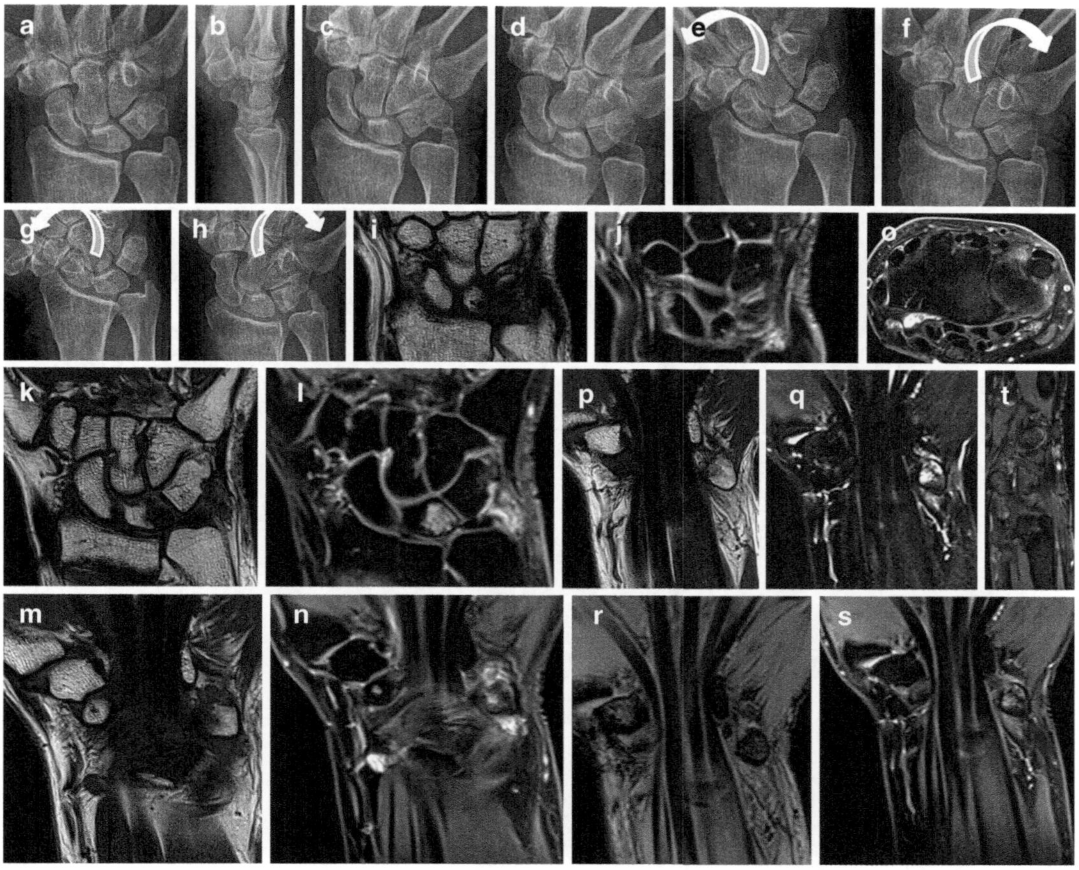

Fig. 45a Standard PA (**a**) and lateral (**b**) views; PA (**a**), and oblique views in ulnar deviation (**c**) with clenched fist (**d**); PA comparative views in radial (**e**, **g**) and ulnar (**f**, **h**) deviation; Cor T1-WI (**i**, **k**, **m**, **p**), T2-WI FS (**j**, **l**, **n**, **q**); Ax T2-WI FS (**o**); 2D GRE (**r**), and 3D GRE (**s**)

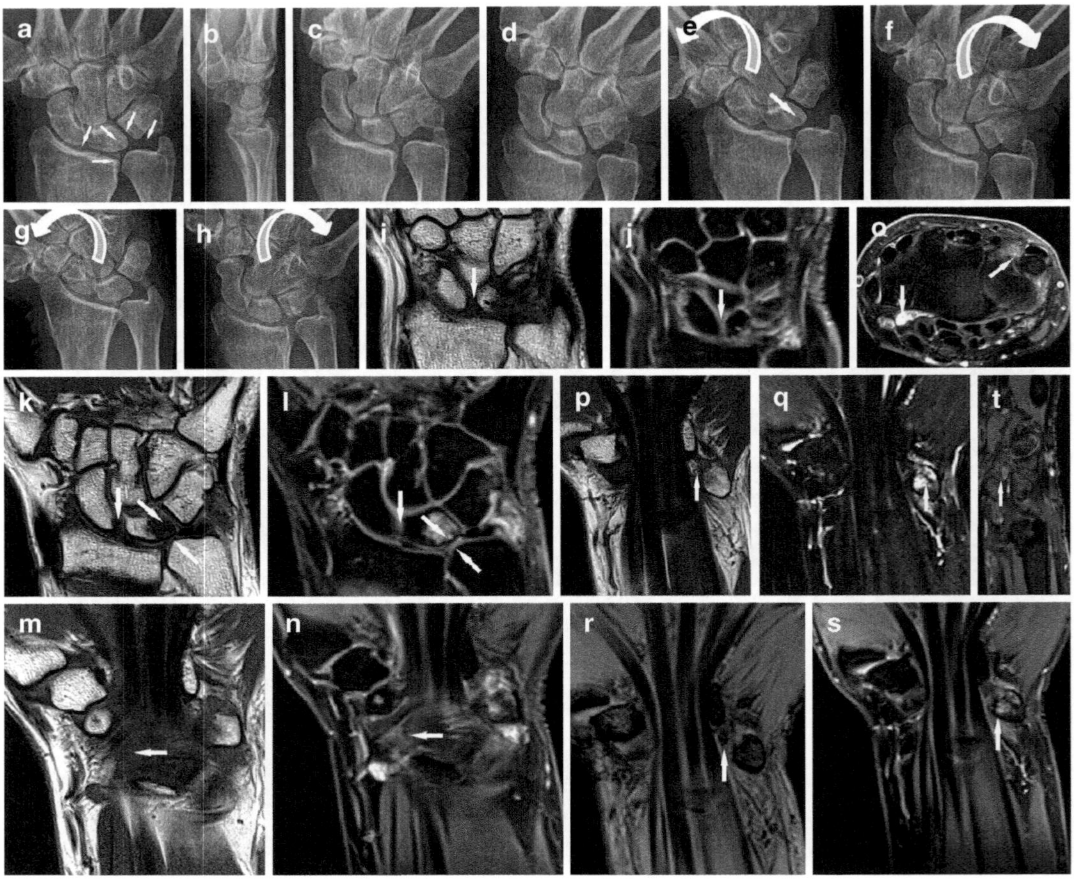

Fig. 45b CPPD RCJ, LT, and TFCC (**a**–**d**); UA (**a**, **e**, **k**, **l**); (bilateral) U+ (**a**, **g**); SLL lesion (**i**–**l**); degenerative TFCC II D (**k**, **l**); palmar V lesion (RLT) (**m**, **n**); ecu subluxation (**o**); radiopalmar ASC (**o**); distal P# with BMO (**p**–**t**). Despite multiple lesions no mobility restriction (**e**–**h**)

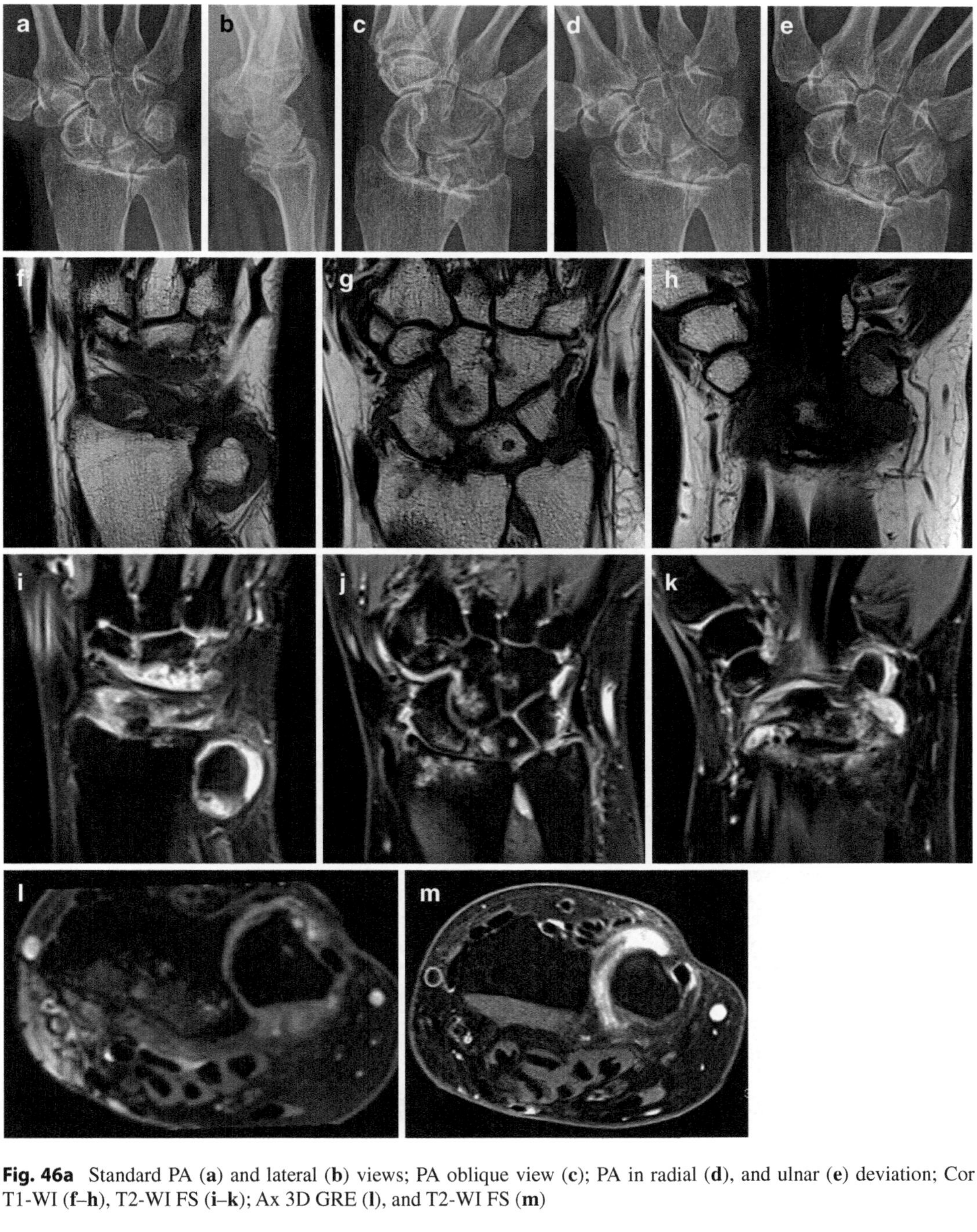

Fig. 46a Standard PA (**a**) and lateral (**b**) views; PA oblique view (**c**); PA in radial (**d**), and ulnar (**e**) deviation; Cor T1-WI (**f–h**), T2-WI FS (**i–k**); Ax 3D GRE (**l**), and T2-WI FS (**m**)

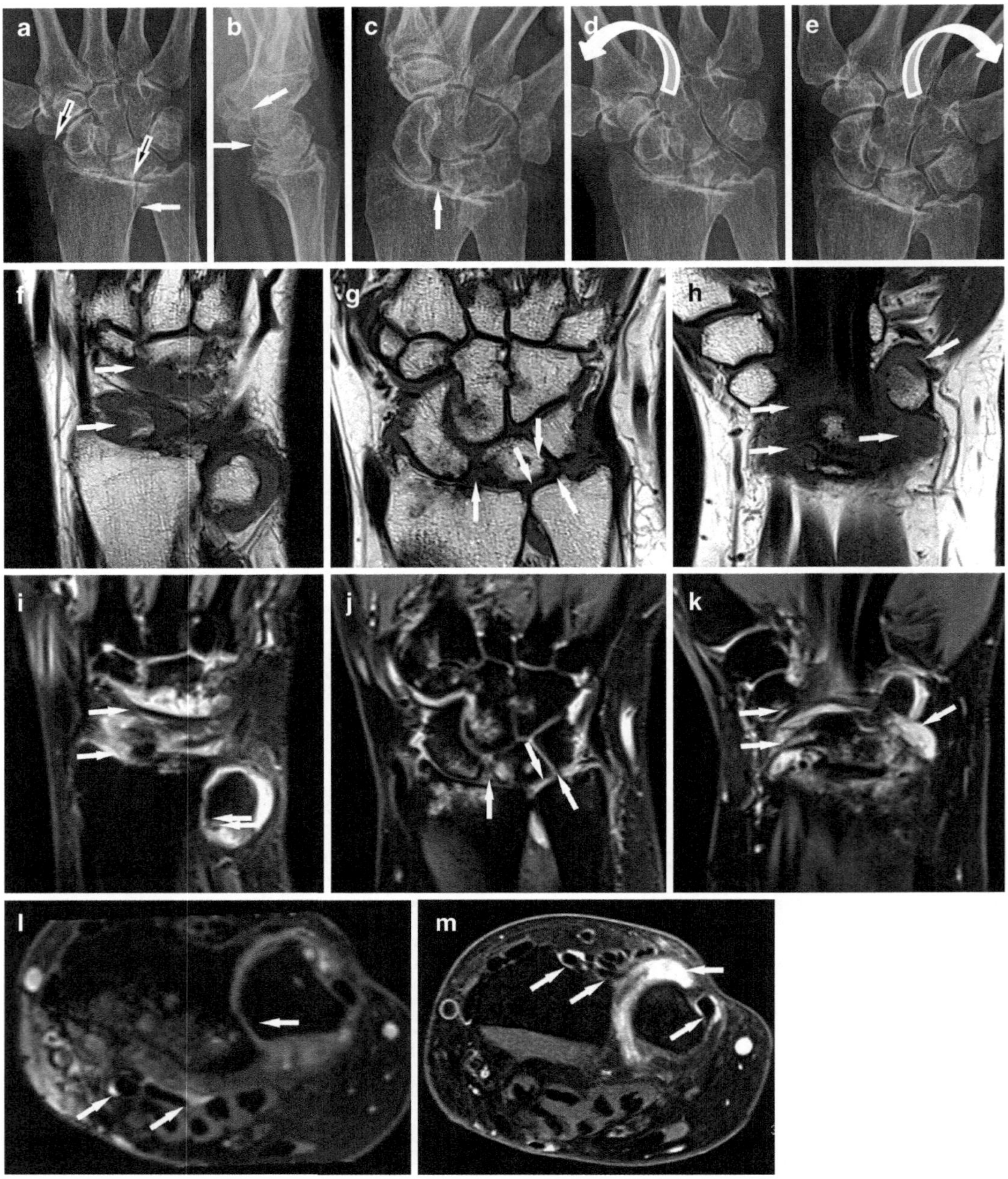

Fig. 46b Carpus translation type 1 (**a**); U+ (**a**); OA DRUJ with hydrops (**a**, **i**, **l**); DISI with SL diastasis (**b**–**c**); restricted mobility, mainly RC (**d**, **e**); Extrinsic dorsal (**f**, **i**) and ventral (**h**, **k**) ligament tears; LTL tear (**g**, **j**); UA (**g**, **j**); degenerative TFCC II E (**g**, **j**); OA Tri-P with hydrops (**h**, **k**); limited tenosynovitis extensor compartment 3–4, 6 (**m**). Underlying (old) RA?

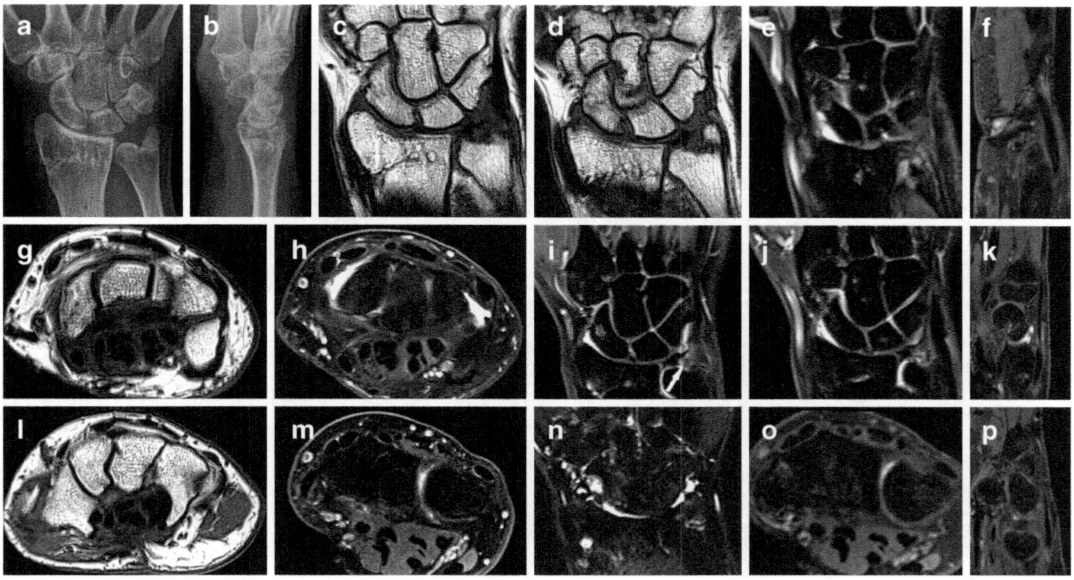

Fig. 47a Standard PA (**a**) and lateral (**b**) views; Cor T1-WI (**c**, **d**), and T2-WI FS (**e**, **i**, **j**, **n**); Sag 3D GRE (**f**, **k**, **p**); Ax T1-WI (**g**, **l**), T2-WI FS (**h**, **m**), and 3D GER (**o**)

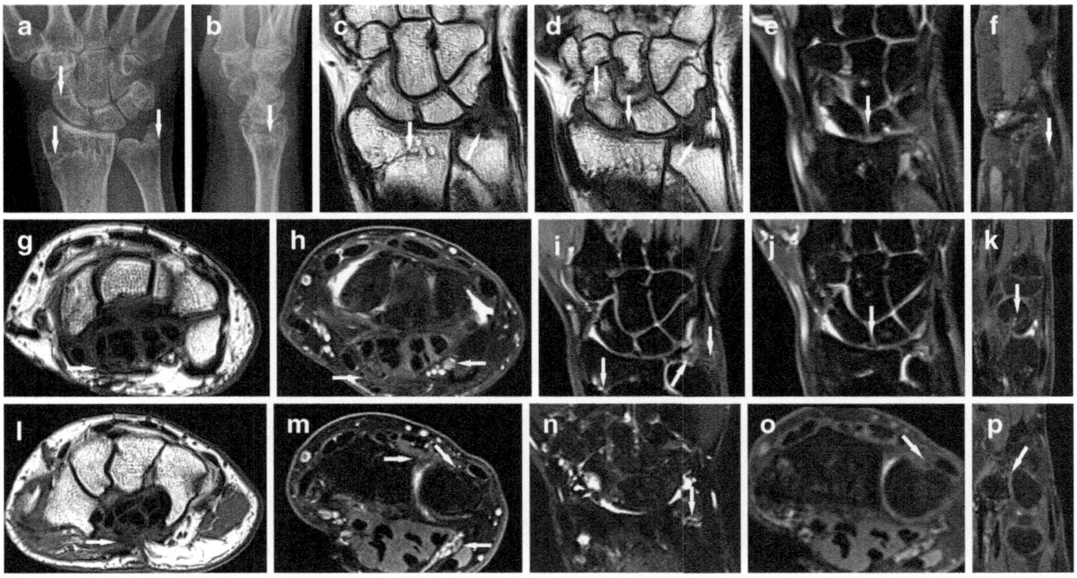

Fig. 47b Sequels of # at ulnar styloid with pseudarthrosis (**a**, **b**, **d**, **f**, **n**), R (**a**, **c**), and S (**a**, **d**, **k**); TFCC proximal insertion I B (**c**, **d**, **i**); SL (**d**, **e**, **j**); normal status after CTS surgery (**g**, **h**, **l**); neuritis n. ulnaris (**h**, **m**); dorsal R-U ligament (**m**), ecu subluxation (**m**, **o**); OA Tri-P (**p**)

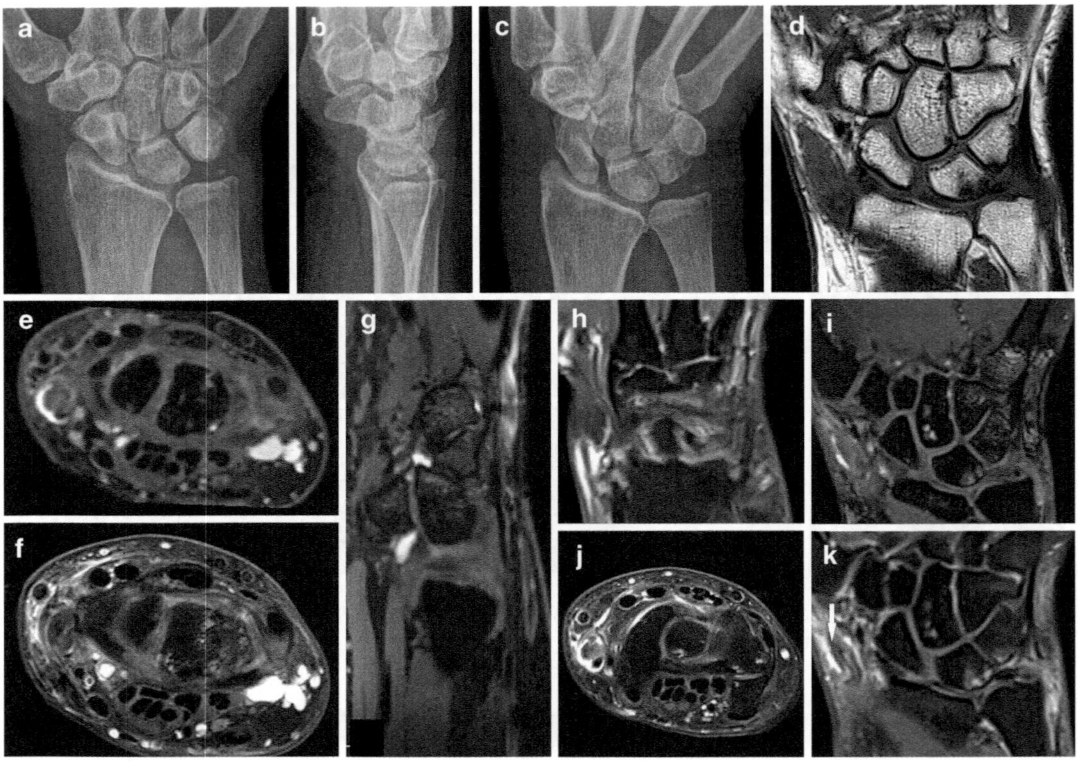

Fig. 48a Standard PA (**a**), lateral (**b**), and clenched fist (**c**) views; Cor T1-WI (**d**), Ax (**e**, **f**), and Sag (**g**) 3D GER; Cor (**h**), and Ax (**j**) T2-WI FS; Cor 3D GRE (**i**–**k**)

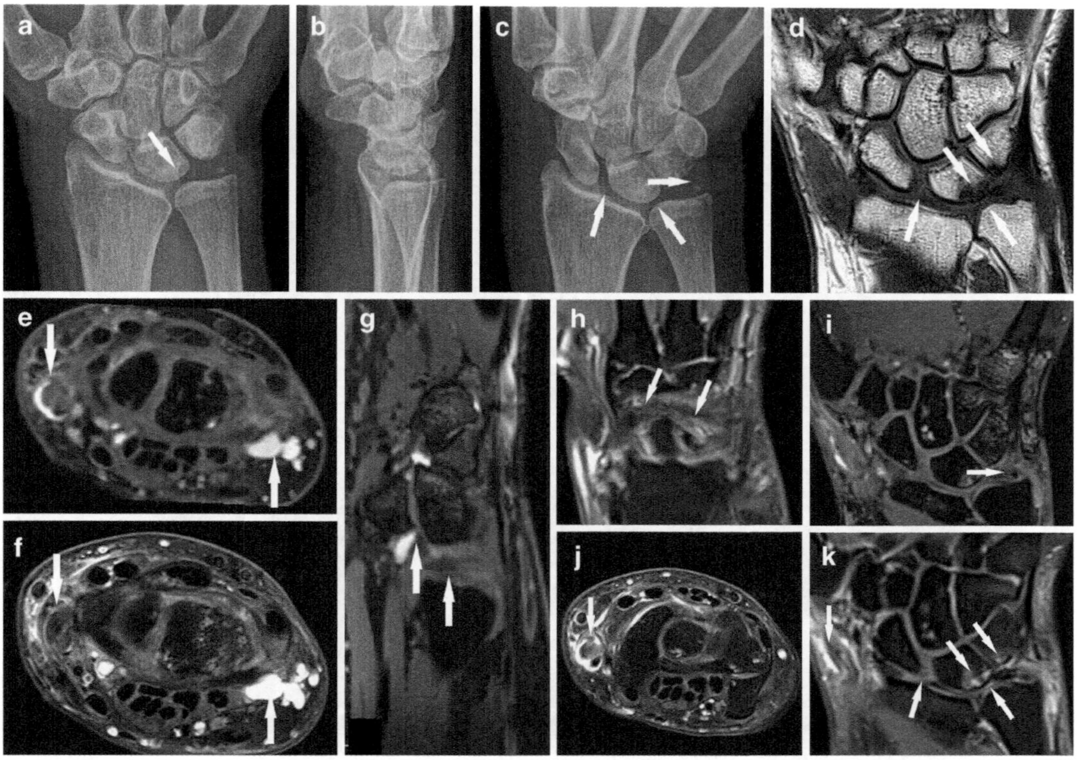

Fig. 48b U+ with UA on L and Tri (**a–d**, **k**); SLL tear (**c**, **d**, **k**) with dynamic CID (**c**); loose bone fragment of the ulnar styloid (**c**, **i**); degenerative TFCC II D (**d**, **e**); tenosynovitis extensor compartment 1 (**e**, **f**, **j**, **k**); OA Tri-P with hydrops (**e–g**); oedematous infiltration of palmar V (**h**)

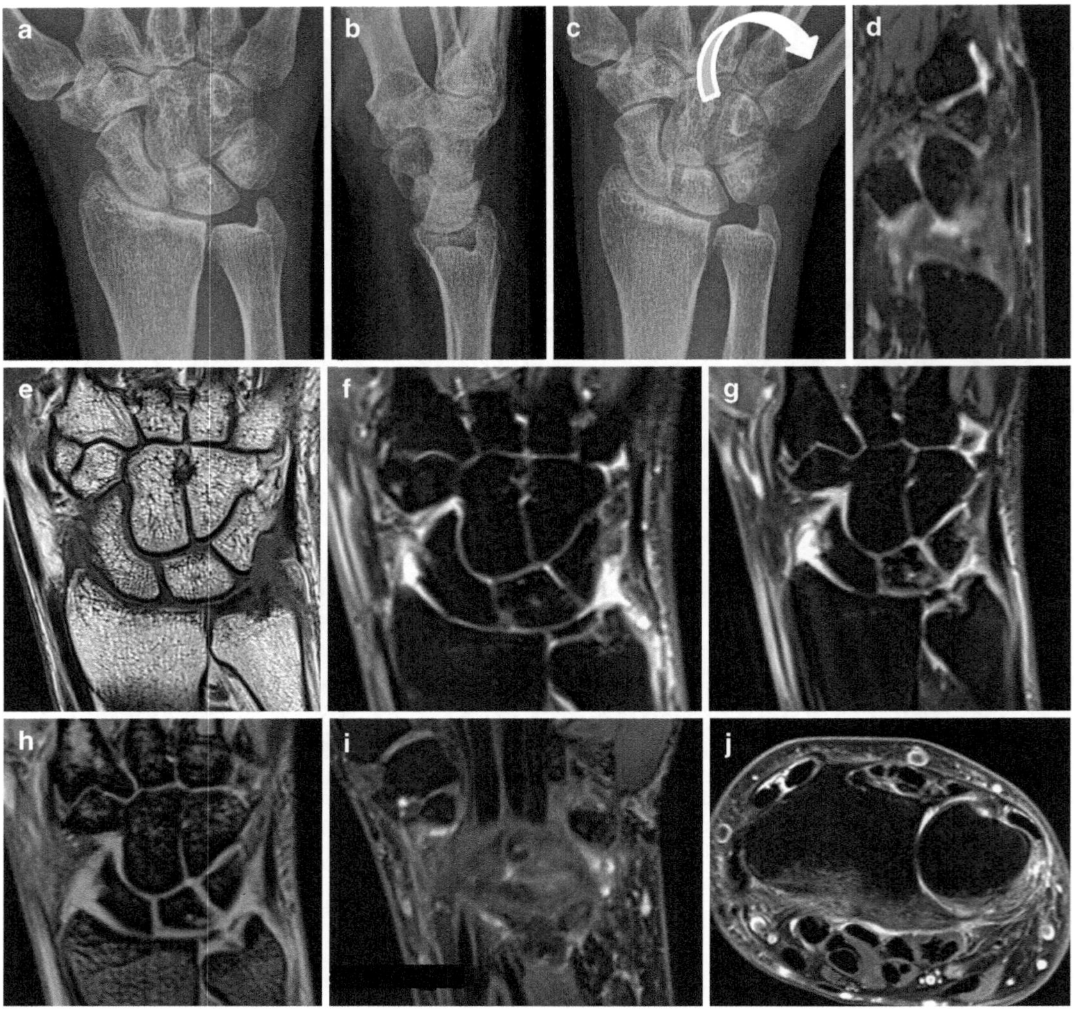

Fig. 49a Standard PA (**a**), lateral (**b**), and PA in ulnar deviation (**c**) views; Sag 3D GRE (**d**); Cor T1-WI (**e**), T2-WI FS (**f**–**g**), 2D (**h**), and 3D (**i**) GRE; Ax T2-WI FS (**j**)

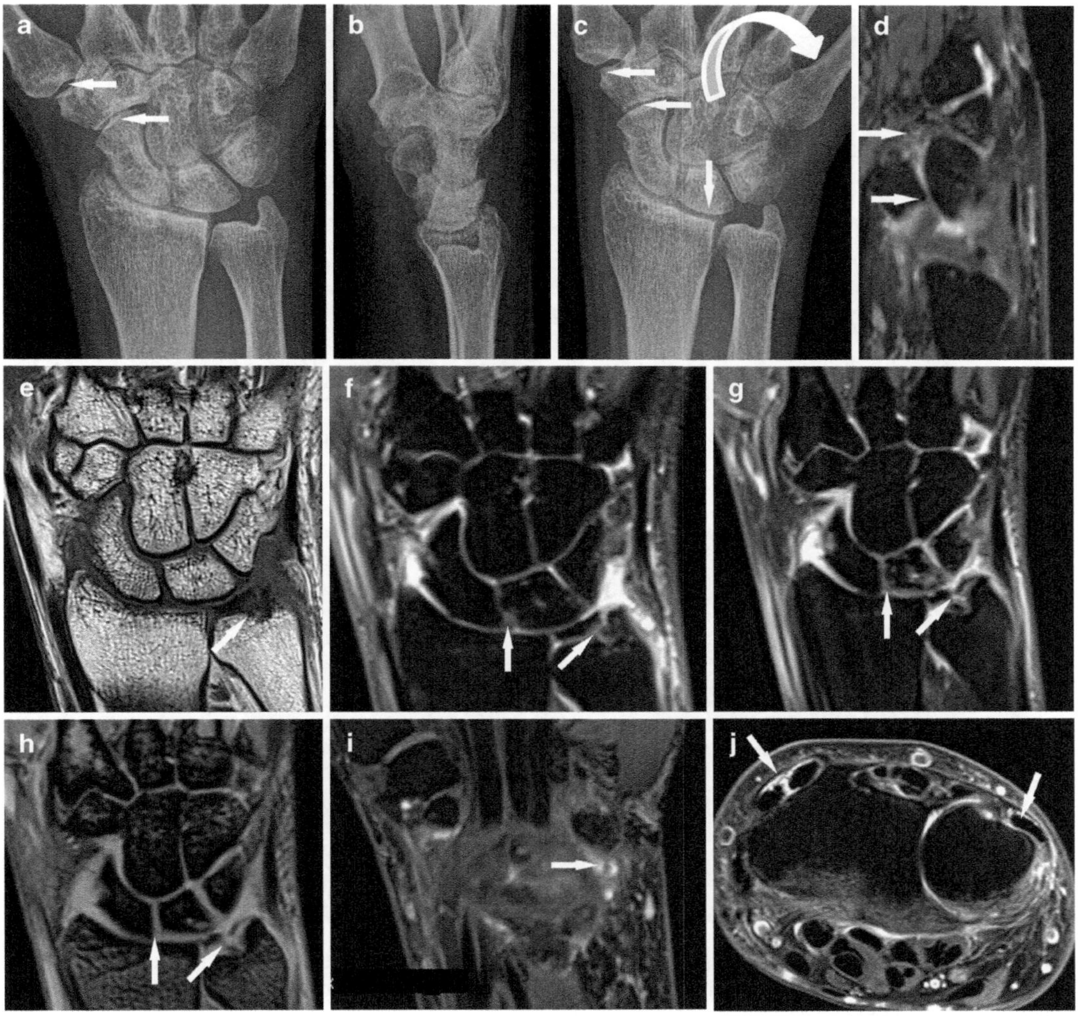

Fig. 49b OA CMC-I, and STT (**a**–**c**); ulnar deviation restriction (**c**); OA Tri-P with hydrops, and OCM (**d**, **i**), TFCC tear type I B (**e**–**h**); SLL tear (**f**–**h**); ecu subluxation (**j**); tenosynovitis extensor compartment 2 (**j**)

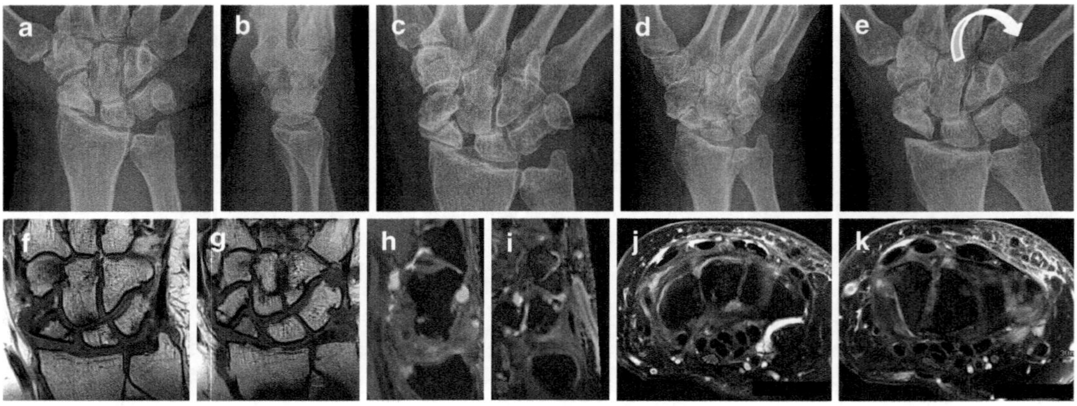

Fig. 50a Standard PA (**a**), lateral (**b**), PA with clenched fist (**c**), and oblique (**d**), PA in ulnar deviation (**e**) views; Cor T1-WI (**f**, **g**), Sag 3D GRE (**h**, **i**); Ax T2-WI FS (**j**, **k**)

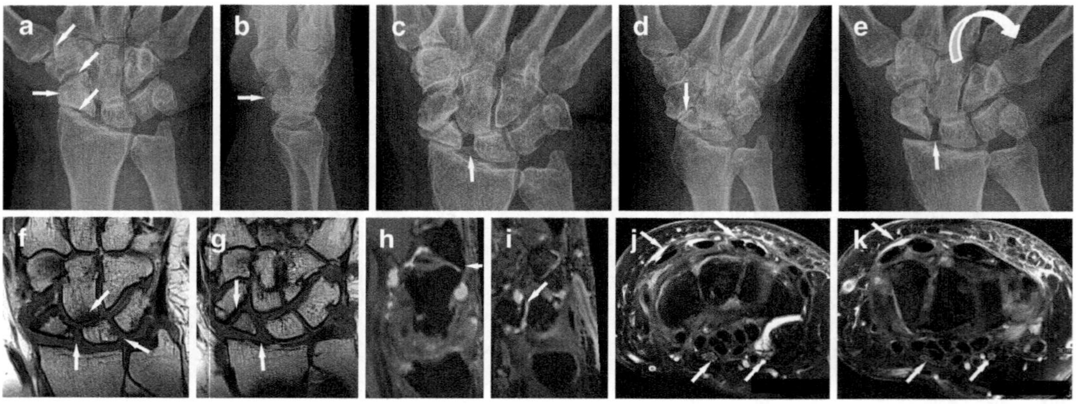

Fig. 50b OA CMC-I, STT, R-S (**a**); rotatory subluxation of S (**a**); SLAC grade 3 (**a**, **c**); tenosynovitis extensor compartment 2 and 4; DISI (**b**); SLL tear (**c**, **e–g**); pseudarthrosis S (**d**, **g**); LTL tear (**f**); CB (**f**); OA Tri-P with hydrops (**i**); neuritis median and ulnar nerve (**j**, **k**)

Further Reading

Beltran J (2004) MR imaging of the upper extremity. MRI clinics of North America. W.B. Saunders Company, Philadelphia, USA. ISSN 1064-9689

Berquist T (2003) MRI of the hand and the wrist. Wolters Kluwer/Lippincott Williams and Wilkins, Philadelphia. ISBN 0-7817-3796-6

Cooney WP III (2010) The wrist, diagnosis and treatment. Wolters Kluwer/Lippincott Williams and Wilkins, Philadelphia. ISBN 978-1-60831-390-7

Faletti C (2006) Sports traumatology imaging. UTET Scienze Mediche, Torino, Italy. https://books.google.be/books?id=P6bRtgAACAAJ

Gilula L, Ying Y (1996) Imaging of the wrist and hand. W.B. Saunders Company, Philadelphia. ISBN 0-7216-5125-9

Jans L, Chen M (2021) Arthritis imaging. Arthritis Imaging Publishing, Ghent. https://www.arthritisimaging.com

Jebson P, Kasdan M (2006) Hand secrets. Mosby Elsevier, Philadelphia. ISBN 1-56053-623-3

Kang H, Resnick D (2004) MRI of the extremities: an anatomic atlas. W.B. Saunders Company, Philadelphia. ISBN 0-7216-3071-5

Manaster B (2007) Diagnostic and surgical anatomy. Amirsys Inc, Salt Lake City, USA. ISBN 1-931884-31-5

Netter FH (2018) Atlas of human anatomy, 7th edn. Elsevier, Philadelphia

Resnick D (2022) Diagnosis of bone and joint disorders. W.B. Saunders Company, Philadelphia. ISBN 0-72168-921-3

Resnick D, Boutin R (1999) Musculoskeletal and soft tissue imaging (encyclopaedia of medical imaging volume III: 1). The Nicer Institute, Oslo, Norway. ISBN 82-91942-04-8

Saffar P (1987) Les traumatismes du carpe. Springer, Paris. ISBN 2-287-00010-0

Senwald G (1987) L'entité radius-carpe. Springer, Berlin. ISBN 3-540-16661-0

Shahabpour M, Isaac A, De Jonghe M (2021) MRI wrist and hand. Breitenseher Publisher, Horn, Austria. ISBN 978-3-02933-84-3

Vanhoenacker F, Maas M, Gielen J (2010) Imaging of orthopedic sports injuries. Springer, Berlin. ISBN 3-642-06532-5

General Conclusion

Keeping in mind that "the more you see, the more you learn and know", and that "you only see what you know" numerous MRI images from the daily practice were presented with the intention of training the visual memory of the radiologist. From obvious and basic to complex cases may have illustrated the challenging task of reporting a MRI of the wrist.

Systematic analysis of all images/sequences and comparison with standard views is essential, preferable also with abstraction of the clinical information in order to avoid diagnostic bias. Therefore, the technicians should follow as much as possible a standardised initial approach to each clinical problem, including any adjustments or sequences to be added. After reporting, a double check to correlate with the clinical information and the clinicians view in general (preferably complemented with a discussion) will provide optimal results for both radiologist and clinician.

M. Mespreuve, K. Waked, *MRI of the Wrist*, Medical Radiology,
https://doi.org/10.1007/978-3-031-63973-9

GPSR Compliance

The European Union's (EU) General Product Safety Regulation (GPSR) is a set of rules that requires consumer products to be safe and our obligations to ensure this.

If you have any concerns about our products, you can contact us on ProductSafety@springernature.com

In case Publisher is established outside the EU, the EU authorized representative is:

Springer Nature Customer Service Center GmbH
Europaplatz 3
69115 Heidelberg, Germany

Batch number: 10732799

Printed by Printforce, the Netherlands